B. E. GERBER   M. KNIGHT   W. E. SIEBERT (Eds.)

Lasers in the Musculoskeletal System

Springer-Verlag Berlin Heidelberg GmbH

B. E. GERBER
M. KNIGHT
W. E. SIEBERT

(Editors)

Lasers in the Musculoskeletal System

With 281 Figures, 86 in Colour
and 56 Tables

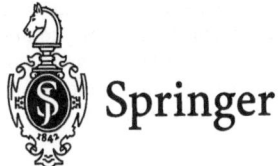 Springer

Bruno E. Gerber, MD
Clinique de Chirurgie Orthopédique
Hôpital Pourtalès
Rue de la Maladière 45
2000 Neuchâtel, Switzerland

Martin T. N. Knight, MD
Arbury Consulting Centre
Manchester Road
Rochdale, OL11 4LZ, UK

Prof. Dr. Werner E. Siebert
Orthopädische Klinik Kassel
Wilhelmshöher Allee 345
34131 Kassel, Germany

ISBN 978-3-642-62955-6   ISBN 978-3-642-56420-8 (eBook)
DOI 10.1007/978-3-642-56420-8

Library of Congress Cataloging in-Publication Data
Lasers in the musculoskeletal system / B.E. Gerber, M. Knight,
W.E. Siebert (eds.). p. ; cm. Includes bibliographical references
and index. ISBN 978-3-642-62955-6   1. Musculoskeletal
system-Diseases-Laser surgery. 2. Lasers in surgery. 3. Arthroscopy. I. Gerber, B.E. (Bruno Edoarda) II. Knight. M. (Martin)
III. Siebert, W. (Werner), 1953 [DNLM: 1. Musculoskeletal
Diseases-surgery. 2. Arthroscopy-methods. 3. Laser Surgery-
methods. WE 140 L343 001] RD732.L375 2001 617.4'7059-dc21

http://www.springer.de

© Springer-Verlag Berlin Heidelberg 2001
Originally published by Springer-Verlag Berlin Heidelberg New York in 2001
Softcover reprint of the hardcover 1st edition 2001

The use of general descriptive names, registered names,
trademarks, etc. in this publication does not imply, even in
the absence of a specific statement, that such names are
exempt from the relevant protective laws and regulations
and therefore free for general use.

Product liability: The publishers cannot guarantee the accuracy of any information about dosage and application contained in this book. In every individual case the user must
check such information by consulting other relevant literature.

Production: Pro Edit GmbH, 69126 Heidelberg, Germany
Cover Design: Erich Kirchner, Heidelberg, Germany
Typesetting: Hagedorn Kommunikation, 68519 Viernheim,
Germany

Printed on acid free paper
SPIN 10628711   24/3130 So   5 4 3 2 1 0

Disclaimer
The material presented in this book has been made available
by the international Musculoskeletal Laser Society for edu-
cational purposes only. This material is not intended to
represent the only, nor necessarily best, method or procedure appropriate for the medical situations discussed, but
rather is intended to present an approach, view, statement
or opinion of the faculty, which may be helpful to others
who face similar situations.
The International Musculoskeletal Laser society disclaims any
and all liability for injury or other damages resulting to any
individuals for all claims which may arise out of the use of
the techniques described in this book, whether these claims
shall be asserted by a physician or other party.

Preface

Laser procedures have been well established in several medical specialities such as ophthalmology, oto-rhino-laryngology, gynaecology, and dermatology for many years now. Their introduction into these fields was motivated by several factors:

▶ Surgical tissue interaction without subsequent scar formation, something which is a singular feature of lasers
▶ The stimulation of specific cellular functions
▶ Minimisation of surgical techniques
▶ Cutting without bleeding and without contact

The successful introduction of lasers into orthopaedics was delayed by the required development of very small diameter applicators and flexible fibres used to conduct the laser beam to the target in arthroscopy and mini-invasive spine surgery. Orthopaedic tissues such as cartilage and bone were sensitive to lasing at some wavelengths. Research results of the absorption profiles in these tissues and the results of empirical surgical treatments successively led to the elimination of harmful wavelengths. Subsequently experts in basic research and in clinical pilot trials have defined precisely the safe parameters for diverse surgical uses of laser energy. This information has been compiled in the table found on the next page (Table 1). Among these applications are a series of non-ablative laser applications to the locomotor tissues such as joint capsular shrinkage, synovitis coagulation or cartilage smoothing. These are specifically achieved by infrared lasers. Consequently these have become the preferential wavelengths in orthopaedic surgery. In this context some other biological tissue effects such as cellular stimulation or cellular inhibition in combination with dyes led to the development of orthopaedic photodynamic therapy.

Lasers can be used to achieve complex procedures such as spinal decompression by minimal means, but they can also simplify common and simple procedures such as the arthroscopic treatment of degenerative menisci, transsection of articular plicae, percutaneous reduction of disc herniation or open denervation in epicondylitis.

The present textbook has been written by experts with many years of experience with clinical orthopaedic laser surgery or with high standards and facilities for biological research. They are in a position to contribute to the actual state of the art in the field. Therefore this book should be used as an instructional publication to increase the general knowledge concerning the orthopaedic use of this technology. In so doing it also aims to prevent the inappropriate application of laser energy as has occurred in the past when lasers developed for completely different disciplines were used orthopaedically. At the same time this volume emphasises the proven advantages and favourable outcomes resulting from the use of laser energy in the musculoskeletal system and the reduced risks of these techniques when properly applied.

The spring of 2001

B. E. Gerber
M. T. N. Knight
W. E. Siebert

Table 1. Recommended surgical parameters for musculoskeletal laser applications. These values are based on the biophysical characteristics of the various laser systems and on results from different basic research and clinical study groups under the patronage of IMLAS.

Arthroscopy	Wavelength	Energy level per pulse	Power (W) and energy (kJ) supplied/joint	Repetition rates [pulse modes] [pulse duration]	Applicator(s) [beam: incidence, modality]
Knee					
Meniscus cutting (consistent flaps)	Ho, 2.1 µm	1.2–1.5 J	18–30 W	15–20 Hz	Front or side firing
			≤6 kJ	[Single/double] [short: ≤400 µs]	[Cutting plane for anatomical shaping focused]
Meniscus smoothing	Ho, 2.1 µm	0.8–1 J	10 W	10–12 Hz	Side > front firing, multifibre
			≤2 kJ	[Single/≤400 µs]	[Tangential shaping]
	(Excimer, 308 nm)	(45 mJ)	(1.8 W)	(40 Hz [60 ns])	(Vertically defocused)
Cartilage sealing	Ho, 2.1 µm	0.2–0.8 J	3–7.5 W	8–15 Hz	Side > front firing, multifibre
			≤1.5 kJ		[Tangential shaping]
	(Excimer, 308 nm)	(45 mJ)	(1.8 W)	(40 Hz [60 ns])	(Vertically defocused)
Capsular cutting (shelves, adhesions, lateral release)	Ho, 2.1 µm	≥1.5 J	~40 W	20–30 Hz	Front or side firing
			≤6 kJ		[Focused]
Shrinkage, haemostasis (Cyclops, capsuloraphy)	Ho, 2.1 µm	0.8–1 J	10 W	10–12 Hz	Side or front firing, multifibre
			≤3 kJ	[Single/≤400 µs]	[Defocused]
Synovectomy (accessory shrinkage)	Ho, 2.1 µm	≥1.5 J	40–60 W	20–40 Hz	Side or front firing, multifibre
			≤8 kJ		[Defocused]
Bone shaping	Ho, 2.1 µm	≥1.5 J	45–60 W	30–40 Hz	Side > front firing, multifibre [Tangential focused]
Shoulder					
Labrum smoothing	Ho, 2.1 µm	0.8–1 J	10 W	10–12 Hz [Single]	Side >front firing, multifibre [Tangential shaping, defocused]
	(Excimer, 308 nm)	(45 mJ)	(1.8 W)	(40 Hz [60 ns])	
Cartilage sealing	Ho, 2.1 µm	0.2–0.8 J	3–7.5 W	8–15 Hz	Side > front firing, multifibre
			≤1.5 kJ		[Tangential shaping]
	(Excimer, 308 nm)	(45 mJ)	(1.8 W)	(40 Hz [60 ns])	(Vertically defocused)
Capsular cutting (shelves, adhesions, frozen shoulder)	Ho, 2.1 µm	≥1.5 J	~40 W	20–30 Hz	Front or side firing
			≤6 kJ		[Focused]
Shrinkage, haemostasis (LACS, capsuloraphy)	Ho, 2.1 µm	0.8–1 J	10 W	10–12 Hz	Side or front firing, multifibre
			≤3 kJ	[Single/≤400 µs]	[Defocused]
Synovectomy (accessory shrinkage)	Ho, 2.1 µm	≥1.5 J	40–60 W	20–40 Hz	Side or front firing, multifibre
			≤8 kJ		[Defocused]
Bone shaping	Ho, 2.1 µm	≥1.5 J	45–60 W	30–40 Hz	Side > front firing, multifibre [Tangential focused]
Ankle, Elbow, Hip, Wrist	Analogous settings to those given above are used for analogous procedures				

Table 1. continued

Spine	Wavelength	Energy level per pulse	Power (W) and energy (kJ) supplied/joint	Repetition rates [pulse modes] [pulse duration]	Applicator(s) [beam: incidence, modality]
Percutaneous					
Intradiscal disc decompression	Ho, 2.1 µm Neodym, 1064 µm KTP	0.6–1 J	7–10 W	8–12 Hz	Bare fibre in guide tubespecial devices
			1.2–1.6 kJ	[Single/long]	[Defocused]
Foraminoscopic shaping, extradiscal disc treatment	Ho, 2.1 µm	0.8–1 J	10–24 W	12–20 Hz	Long side firing in combination with mechanical resection
			0.8–1.2 kJ	[Single/long]	
Foraminoscopic bony intraspinal decompression	Ho, 2.1 µm	1.2–1.5 J	12–30 W	10–20 Hz	Long side firing device
			1–1.5 kJ		
Open laser applications to the spine					
Open laser disc treatment with cooling lavage (OLDT)	Ho, 2.1 µm	0.8–1 J	7–10 W	8–12 Hz	Straight or side firing devices in combination with mechanical resection
			0.8–1.2 kJ	[Single/long]	
Laser haemostasis (peripheral venous plexus)	Ho, 2.1 µm	0.8–1 J	10–24 W	8–12 Hz	Straight or side firing devices in combination with mechanical tamponade
			0.8–1.2 kJ	[Single/long]	

Open laser applications to the locomotor system	Wavelength	Energy level per pulse	Power (W) and energy (kJ) supplied/joint	Repetition rates [pulse modes] [pulse duration]	Applicator(s) [beam: incidence, modality]
Elbow					
Wilhelm's denervation epicondylar circumcision	Ho, 2.1 µm	≥1.5 J	~40 W	20–30 Hz	Front firing surgical handpiece [Focused]
			≤3 kJ		
Synovectomy (elbow/larger joints)	Ho, 2.1 µm	≥1.5 J	~40 W	20–30 Hz	Front firing surgical handpiece [Focused]
			≤2 kJ/ ≤6 kJ		
Ligament debridement (radial anular/ulnar collateral)	Ho, 2.1 µm	0.8–1 J	10 W	10–12 Hz	Front firing surgical handpiece
			≤1.2 kJ	[Single/≤400 µs]	[Focused]
Jumper's knee/Achillodynia with cystic Achilles tendon					
Excision of cystic tissue	Ho, 2.1 µm	≥1.5 J	~40 W	20–30 Hz	Front firing surgical handpiece [Focused]
			≤3 kJ		
Sealing of tendon	Ho, 2.1 µm	0.8–1 J	10 W	10–12 Hz	Front firing surgical handpiece [Defocused]
			1.2 kJ	[Single/≤400 µs]	
Scarification of apex patellae	Ho, 2.1 µm	0.8–1.2 J	10–24 W	12–20 Hz	Front firing surgical handpiece in combination with mechanical resection
			0.8–1.2 kJ	[Single/long]	

By Bruno E. Gerber, as updated on 9 March 2001.

Contents

Part IV: Low Level Laser

Part V: Spine

List of Senior Authors

O. S. Atik
President, Turkish Joint Diseases
Foundation
Bilkent Camlik Sitesi
Arikusu Cikmazi D2-13
06530 Bilkent-Ankara, Turkey

M. E. Berend
Sports Medicine Section
Division of Orthopaedic Surgery
Dept. of Surgery
Duke University Medical Center
Durham, North Carolina 27704, USA

J. A. Botsford
Director, Dept. of Radiology,
The Deaconess Hospital
311 Straight St.
Cincinnati, Ohio 45219, USA

G. D. Casper
Medicare Population;
J. Oklahoma State Medical
Association Laser Spine
and Joint Center of Sw
1016 Sw 44th Street, Suite 500
Oklahoma City, Oklahoma 73109, USA

D. S. J. Choy
Laser Spine Center
& Columbia University
College of Physicians & Surgeons
170 E. 77 St.
New York, NY 10021, USA

I. Çilesiz
Biomedical Engineering Program
Dept. of Electronics and
Communication Engineering
Istanbul Technical University
80626 Maslak Istanbul, Turkey
e-mail: cilesiz@ehb.itu.edu.tr

K. Diehl
Chefarzt der Orthopädischen Klinik
der Bundesknappschaftsklinik
Krankenhaus Püttlingen
66346 Püttlingen, Germany

A. J. Freemont
Professor of Osteoarticular Pathology,
Dept. of Musculoskeltal Research
Stopford Building,
University of Manchester,
Oxford Road, Manchester M13 9PT, UK
e-mail: carol.a.denton@man.ac.uk

B. E. Gerber
Clinique d'Orthopédie et Traumatologie
Hôpital Pourtalès
Rue de la Maladière 45
2007 Neuchâtel, Switzerland
e-mail: bgerber@mail.vtx.ch

W. Glinkowski
Dept. of Orthopedics and Traumatology
of Locomotor System Medical University
of Warsaw ul. Lindleya 4
02-005 Warszawa, Poland

A. K. D. Goswami
Spinal Foundation
Manchester Road
Rochdale Lancs OL11 4LZ, UK

S. Götte
Albert-Schweitzer-Str. 9a
82008 Unterhaching

H. Graßhoff
Orthopädische Universitätsklinik
Otto-von-Guericke-Universität
Leipziger Str. 44
39120 Magdeburg, Germany

P. Guillen-Garcia
Dept. of Traumatology
FREMAP
Prevention and Rehabilitation Center
Carretera de Pozuelo a Majadahonda,
Km 3500
28220 Majadahonda (Madrid), Spain

K.-I. Ha
Dept. of Orthopaedic Sports Medicine
Samsung Medical Center
50 Iwon Dong, Kangnamku
135-230 Seoul, South Korea

K. Hayashi
Comparative Orthopaedic Research
Laboratory
Depts. of Medical and Surgical Sciences
School of Veterinary Medicine
University of Wisconsin-Madison
2015 Linden Drive West
Madison, Wisconsin 53706, USA

C. Hendrich
Abteilung Orthopädie
König-Ludwig-Haus
Universität Würzburg
Brettreichstr. 11
97074 Würzburg, Germany

D. W. L. Hukins
Dept. of Bio-Medical Physics
and Bio-Engineering
University of Aberdeen
Foresterhill, Aberdeen AB25 2ZD, UK
e-mail: d.hukins@biomed.abdn.ac.uk

A. B. Imhoff
Direktor der Abt. für Orthopädische
Sportmedizin
Technische Universität München
Connollystr. 32
80809 München, Germany

K. Inoue
Dept. of Orthopaedic Surgery
Tokyo Women's Medical University
School of Medicine, Daini Hospital
2-1-10 Nishiogu, Arakawa-ku
162 Tokyo, Japan

M. James
Head of Health Economics (R&D) Unit
and Senior Lecturer
Centre for Health Planning
and Management,
Keele University
Keele ST5 5BG, UK
e-mail: m.james@keele.ac.uk

M. T. N. Knight
Arbury Consulting Centre
Manchester Road
Rochdale Lancs OL11 4LZ, UK

R. Kosaka
Dept. of Orthopaedics,
Osaka Medical College
2-7 Daigaku-Machi, Takatsuki
Osaka 569, Japan

E. Kotilainen
Dept. of Neurosurgery and Surgery
Turku University Central Hospital
Kiinamyllynkatu 4-8
20520 Turku, Finland

J. Krott
Neurochirurgische Klinik
Klinikum Großhadern
Marchioninistraße 15
81377 München, Germany

M. Kunz
St. Elisabeth-Klinik Saarlouis
Kapuzinerstr. 4
66740 Saarlouis, Germany

S.-H. Lee
Wooridul Spine Hospital, Seoul, Korea
Spine Laser Clinic
16th F. Samboo Building
676 Yeoksam-Dong
Kangnam-Gu
Seoul, 135-080, Korea

J. R. Tatay Manzanares
C/Cardenal Jlundain N-3
Portal 41B,
41013 Sevilla, Spain

U. Mahlfeld
Orthopädische Universitätsklinik
Otto-Von-Guericke-Universität
Leipziger Str. 44
39120 Magdeburg, Germany

M. D. Markel
Comparative Orthopaedic Research
Laboratory
Depts. of Medical and Surgical Sciences
School of Veterinary Medicine
2015 Linden Drive West
University of Wisconsin-Madison
Madison, Wisconsin 53706, USA

Y. Nishijima
Dept. of Orthopedic Surgery
Kanazawa Medical University
Daigaku-Machi, Uchinada-Machi
Ishikawa-Ken 920-02 Japan
e-mail: nishi-yu@kanazawa-med.ac.jp.

T. G. Obenchain
Neurological Surgery Microsurgery
Diplomate American Board of
Neurological Surgery
355 East Grand Avenue
Escondido, California 92025-3336, USA

T. Okazaki
Dept. of Orthopaedics
Osaka Medical College
2-7 Daigaku-Machi, Takatsuki
Osaka 569, Japan

U. Pfeil
Orthopädische Klinik
Wilhelmshöher Allee 345
34131 Kassel, Germany

J. Raunest
Krankenhaus Neuwerk
Dünner Str. 214-216
41066 Mönchengladbach, Germany

J. A. Saunier
Sports Medicine Unit
Clinique Générale Beaulieu
1211 Genève, Switzerland

S. Schmolke
Medizinische Hochschule Hannover
Orthopädische Klinik
Heimchenstr. 1–7
30625 Hannover, Germany

C. L. Shields
Main Jobe Kerlan
Clinic Westchester
6801 Park Terrace
Los Angeles, LA
90045, USA

W. E. Siebert
Orthopädische Klinik
Wilhelmshöher Allee 345
34131 Kassel, Germany

M. Stanke
Orthopädische Klinik
Wilhelmshöher Allee 345
34131 Kassel, Germany

Ralf Stucker
Orthopädische Abteilung
Universitatsklinikum Freiburg
Hugstetterstr. 55
79106 Freiburg, Germany

I Introduction

History of Lasers in Orthopedic Medicine

W. E. Siebert

Introduction

When Albert Einstein first described the theory of stimulated emission in 1917 [10], he probably could not imagine that it would take less than 45 years for the establishment of the frist functional laser system, a ruby red laser constructed by Maiman in 1960 [31]. Already 1 year later this laser was being used clinically to treat dermatologic and ophthalmologic disorders [5, 15, 16].

However, many years would pass before orthopedic physicians discovered the interesting and intriguing possibilities of laser application in the musculoskeletal system. To name two milestones: in 1978 Whipple began his research on laser application in arthroscopic surgery using the CO_2 laser [54], and in 1986, more than 25 years after the laser was first used in medicine, Ascher and Choy conducted the first laser-assisted operation to remove herniated spinal disc tissue [8]. In the following, a short overview of the history of lasers in orthopedic medicine is given. In my opinion the future of lasers in orthopedic medicine will be just as interesting.

Lasers in Arthroscopy

The basic advantages of the laser compared to mechanical instruments, the compactness of the application instruments as well as the ablative and hemostatic effects, encouraged physicians to evaluate the performance of the laser in arthroscopic surgery.

As early as the 1960s, Jackson, known as the father of arthroscopy, became interested in lasers [37]. In 1978 Whipple conducted laser-assisted arthroscopies using the CO_2 laser and introduced his results in 1981 [54]. At around the same time Glick tested the 1.06 μm neodymium:YAG laser in a free beam mode for meniscectomy, the results of which were rather disappointing [14]. Inoue et al. found both the neodymium:YAG and the argon laser to be ineffective and recommended the CO_2 laser for arthroscopic surgery [23]. Both Siebert and Raunest found that the neodymium:YAG laser caused cartilage degeneration in experimental studies [39, 49]. In

1982, in the USA, Smith, who is also considered one of the fathers of arthroscopic laser surgery, used the 10.6 μm CO_2 laser for meniscectomy [52]. At the same time Philandrianos was conducting similar procedures in Europe [38]. In the USA, the pulsed 10.6 μm CO_2 laser was approved by the FDA for arthroscopic surgery in the mid 1980s and numerous hospitals in the USA possessed such a device at that time [7]. Brillhart was the first to use the 1.44 μm neodymium:YAG laser in arthroscopic surgery, in 1992. The tissue effects of the 1.44 μm neodymium:YAG laser are comparable to those of the holmium:YAG laser and should not to be confused with the 1.06 μm neodymium:YAG laser [6].

The 2.1 μm holmium:YAG laser, which was developed especially for arthroscopic surgery by Dillingham and Fanton in the late 1980s, has become the most accepted and prevalent laser for arthroscopic procedures [9].

Development of smaller application instruments and tips, using materials such as ceramic and sapphire, continued. Other lasers, such as the KTP laser, the excimer laser, the erbium:YAG laser and the thulium:YAG laser, have been tested for their feasibility in arthroscopic surgery [7, 21, 40, 41, 48]. However, holmium:YAG remains the most accepted system so far [30, 43, 51].

Laser-assisted arthroscopy was and is conducted not only in the knee, but also in smaller joints with good results [1, 4, 25, 55]. Based on experimental work by Markel and Hayashi [18, 32], the laser, usually the 2.1 μm holmium:YAG, was and still is used for capsular shrinkage of the shoulder [2, 17, 22, 53].

Brillhart estimated that by 1996 at least 6000 surgeons in the United States would have been trained in laser arthroscopy [7]. In the hands of well-trained surgeons, laser-assisted arthroscopy has become accepted all over the world.

Lasers in Spinal Surgery

Due to the fact that a major proportion of patients suffer from spinal disorders, often due to spinal disc hermia, many physicians and scientists have endeavored to find effective therapies. The first open operation to remove hemiated disc tissue was conducted by Mixter and Barr in 1934 [35].

To avoid the so-called postdiscectomy (failed back) syndrome, which may occur after open spinal disc surgery [26, 36], the search for less invasive procedures continued. Especially in the last 20 years a variety of minimal invasive techniques have been introduced including the lasser-assisted disc operation, first conducted by Ascher and Choy in 1986 [3, 8]. In the following years, non-endoscopic and endoscopic laser-assisted procedures have been developed alongside continuing improvement of laser systems and surgical application instruments. Several laser systems have been appraised for their effectiveness in spinal surgery, such as the CO_2 laser, erbium:YAG laser, neodymium:YAG laser, holmium:YAG laser and KTP laser [50].

Above all the KTP laser as well as the holmium:YAG and neodymium:YAG laser are now used for intradiscal, so-called blind intradiscal methods and/or endoscopics methods [50].

Basic Research

Alongside the research in clinical laser applications, basic research has been continuously conducted by a number of scientists and physicians. Especially the occurrence of tissue necrosis due to the laser's thermic effects has given incentive to develop less invasive and more effective laser systems [20, 42, 44].

In the middle of the 1980s the so-called excimer cold laser was developed, with a low occurrence of necrosis and carbonization [21, 27]. However, in the long run this laser has not been feasible for orthopedic applications due to its very low ablation rate [12]. Many other lasers, especially with wavelengths near infrared, were tested in numerous basic research studies as to their feasibility in orthopedic medicine [45, 48]. Based on these results, it has been revealed that the holmium:YAG laser is one of the most viable and is being used in spinal and arthroscopic surgery [13, 32, 56].

Parallel to the construction and development of high energy laser systems used in surgery, systems utilizing lower energies, such as the helium-neon laser and the gallium-arsenic laser, have been tested for their worth in medicine [11, 28, 29, 34, 47]. The Hungarian surgeon Mester can be considered the pioneer of low level laser medicine; he first tested the argon laser in 1964 [33].

The possibility to treat rheumatoid arthritis with photodynamic therapy utilizing laser energy has been researched in numerous experimental settings, but more research is necessary before clinical studies can be conducted [19, 46].

In more recent times Jackson has been testing tissue welding with lasers with some very intriguing results [24].

Future Outlook

Research on lasers in orthopedics is still quite necessary. There is still room for improvement of surgical methods and instrumentation and the laser systems. Furthermore many questions on the biochemical, photochemical and biomechanical tissue effects remain unanswered.

Orthopedic surgeons who wish to work with the laser must be familiar with laser biophysics and must understand the effects on human tissue. In-depth training and practice are mandatory. An untrained surgeon may apply the laser foolishly and not achieve the aspired results. Many skilled physicians routinely use the laser in a variety of clinical applications with large case numbers and little occurrence of side effects or complications. More basic research and many more prospective, randomized clinical studies are necessary in order to prove the long term merit of the laser for conservative and surgical therapy of the musculoskeletal system.

IMLAS, the International Musculoskeletal Laser Society, which was founded in 1993 in Paris, endeavors to develop and improve laser techniques in medicine, especially in the musculoskeletal system. IMLAS sponsors research programs, publications and regular meetings. It organizes training programs and courses for laser applications in orthopedic medicine. Annual congresses and meetings guarantee the exchange of current information and state-of-the-art techniques. Furthermore, IMLAS encourages and seeks to increase contact with other societies and organizations that utilize alternative energies, such as shock wave energies and radiofrequency, the physics of which are similar to laser energy.

For everyone interested in laser application in the musculoskeletal system, whether it is for surgical purposes or conservative treatment, membership in IMLAS is a must.

To join IMLAS contact:
IMLAS-Office, Orthopedic Hospital Kassel,
Wilhelmshoeher Allee 345, D-34131 Kassel, Germany,
Tel: +49/561-3084-246, Fax: +49/561-3084-204,
e-mail: imlas@okkassel.de,
web page: http://www.imlas.org

References

[1] Abelow S (1993) Use of lasers in orthopedic surgery: current concepts. Orthopedics 16:551–556
[2] Abelow S (1997) Laser capsulorrhaphy for multidirectional instability of the shoulder. Op Tech Sports Med 5:244–248
[3] Ascher P, Holzer, P, Sutter, B, Tritthart H (1991) Nukleuspulposus-Denaturierung bei Bandscheibenprotrusionen. In: Siebert WE, Wirth CJ (eds) Laser in der Orthopädie. Thieme, Stuttgart, pp 169–172
[4] Baker C, Graham J Jr (1993) Current concepts in ankle arthroscopy. Orthopedics 16:1027–1035
[5] Blancard P, Sorato M, Blanluet G, Iris L, Liotet S (1964) Therapeutic laser experiments. Bull Soc Ophthalmol Fr, Dec, 64:1009–1016
[6] Brillhart A (1993) Ablation efficiency determination using the 1.44 micron neodymium:YAG laser. SPIE Proc 1880: 29–30
[7] Brillhart A (ed) (1994) Arthroscopic laser surgery. Clinical applications. Springer-Verlag, Berlin, Heidelberg New York
[8] Choy D, Case R, Ascher P (1987) Percutaneous laser ablation of lumbar discs. A preliminary report of in vitro and in vivo experience in animal and four human patients. 33rd Annual Meeting, Orthopaedic Research Society 1987, 1:19
[9] Dillingham M, Fanton G (1990) The use of the holmium:YAG laser in operative knee arthroscopy – a double blind prospective study using a new arthroscopically guided laser system. Arthroscopy 6:152–153
[10] Einstein A (1917) Zur Quantentherorie der Strahlung. Physiol Z 18:121–128
[11] Gärtner C (1989) Analgesy by low power laser (LPL): a controlled double blind study in ankylosing spondarthritis (SPA). Lasers in Surgery and Medicine Suppl 1:30
[12] Gerber B, Siebert W, Morscher E (1996) Chirurgische Laseranwendung am Bewegungsapparat. Orthopäde 25:1–2
[13] Gerber B, Asshauer T, Delacrétaz G, Jansen T, Oberthür T (1996) Biophysikalische Grundlagenuntersuchungen zur Wirkung der Holmium-Laserstrahlung am Knorpelgewebe und deren Konsequenzen für die klinische Applikationstechnik. Orthopädie 25:21–29
[14] Glick J (1981) YAG laser meniscectomy. Presented at the Triannual Meeting of the International Arthroscopy Association. American Arthroscopy Association of North America. Rio de Janeiro, Brazil, 1981
[15] Goldman L, Siler V, Blaney D (1967) Laser therapy of melanomas. Surg Gynecol Obstet 124:49–56
[16] Goldman L, Rockwell R Jr (1968) Laser systems and their applications in medicine and biology. Adv Biomed Eng Med Phys 1:317–382
[17] Hardy P, Thabit G 3rd, Fanton G, Blin J, Jacob A, Benoit J (1996) Arthroskopische Behandlung der rezidivierenden vorderen Schulterluxationen durch Kombination der Labrumnaht mit einer anteroinferioren Kapselschrumpfung mit dem Holmium:YAG-Laser. Orthopäde 25(1):91–93
[18] Hayashi K, Thabit G 3rd, Vailas A, Bogdanke J, Cooley A, Markel M (1996) The effect of nonablative laser energy on joint capsular properties. An in vitro histologic and biochemical study using a rabbit model. Am J Sports Med 24(5):640–646
[19] Hendrich C, Hüttmann G. Diddens H, Seara J, Siebert W (1996) Experimentelle Grundlagen einer photodynamischen Lasertherapie für die chronische Polyarthritis. Orthopäde 25(1):30–36
[20] Hendrich C, Jakob P, Breitling T, Schäfer A, Berden A, Haase A, Siebert W (1996) Kernspintomographische Messung der Temperaturverteilung in Knorpelgewebe nach Lasertherapie. Orthopäde 25(1):17–20
[21] Hohlbach, G, Müller, K, Schramm U, Baretton G (1989) Experimentelle Ergebnisse der Knorpelabrasion mit dem Excimer-Laser. Histologische und elektronenmikroskopische Untersuchungen. Z Orthop 127:216–222

[22] Imhoff A, Ledermann T (1995) Arthroscopic subacromial decompression with and without the holmium:YAG-laser. A prospective comparative study. Arthroscopy 11(5):549–556
[23] Inoue K (1984) Arthroscopic laser surgery. IAA, London pp 29–39
[24] Jackson R, Judy M, Matthews J, Pollo F, Nosir H (1999): Light acctivated tissue bonding using 1,8 naphthalimide compounds. Presented at SICOT 99. Sydney, 18–23 April 1999, p 172
[25] Janis L, Kravitz R, Wagner S (1994) The pulsed holmium:yttrium-aluminum-garnet laser. Applications to ankle arthroscopy. Clin Podiatr Med Surg 11(3):483–498
[26] Krämer J (1987) Das Postdiskektomiesyndrom – PSD. Z Orthop 125:622–625
[27] Kroitzsch U, Laufer G, Egkher E, Wollene G, Horvath R (1989) Experimental photoablation of meniscus cartilage by Excimer laser energy. A new aspect in meniscus surgery. Arch Orthop Trauma Surg 108(1):44–48
[28] Kubota J, Ohshiro T (1989) The effects of fiode laser low reactive-level laser therapy (LOW LEVEL LASER) on flap survival in a rat model. Laser Therapie 1(3):127
[29] Lubart R, Wollman Y, Friedmann H, Rochkind S, Laulicht I (1992) Efffects of visible and nearinfrared lasers on call cultures. J Photochem Photobiol B 12:305–310
[30] Lübbers, C, Siebert W (1996) Die arthroskopische Holmium:YAG-Laseranwendung im Vergleich zu konventionellen Verfahren am Knie. Zweijahresergebnisse einer prospektiven Studie. Orthopäde 25(1):64–72
[31] Maiman T (1960) Stimulated optical radiation in ruby. Nature 6:493–494
[32] Markel M, Hayashi K, Thabit G 3rd, Thielke R (1996) Veränderungen am Gelenkkapselgewebe durch Holmium:YAG-Laserexposition in nichtablativen Energiedichten. Eine potentielle Anwendungsmöglichkeit zu Stabilisierungseingriffen. Orthopäde. 25(1):37–41
[33] Mester E et al (1968) Untersuchungen über die hemmende bzw. fördernde Wirkung der Laserstrahlen. Arch Klin Chir 322:1022
[34] Mester E et al (1988) Scientific background of laser biostimulation. LASER. J Eur Med Laser Ass 1(1):23
[35] Mixter W, Barr J (1924) Rupture of the intervertebral disc with involvement of the spinal canal. N Engl J Med 211:210–215
[36] Nachemson A (1996) Low back pain in the year 2000 – "back" to the future. Hosp Joint Diseases 55(3):119–121
[37] O'Brien S, Garrick J, Jackson R (1991) Symposium: lasers in orthopaedic surgery. Contemp Orthop 22:61–91
[38] Philandrianos G (1985) Le laser a gaz carbonique en chirurgie athroscopique du genou. Presse Med 14(41)2103–2104
[39] Raunest, J, Lohnert J (1989) Arthroskopische Synovektomie unter Anwendung des Neodym-YAG-Laser. Chirurg 60:782–787
[40] Raunest J, Löhnert J (1990) Arthroscopic cartilage debridement by excimer laser in chondromalacia of the knee joint. Arch Orthop Trauma Surg 109:155–159
[41] Raunest J, Sager M, Derra E (1994) Experimentelle Befunde zur Knorpelablation und Abrasionsarthroplastik mit thermisch und gepulsten UV-Lasern. Arthroskopie 7: 174–181
[42] Raunest J, Derra E (1996) Arthroseinduktion durch Lasereingriffe. Orthopäde 25(1):10–16
[43] Saunier J, Indermühle F, Compère J (1993) Use of the holmium 2.1 laser in surgical arthroscopy. Rev Med Suisse Romande 113(2):129–132
[44] Schlangmann B, Schmolke S, Berendsen B, Siebert W (1996) Temperatur-Ablationsmessungen bei der Laserbehandlung von Bandscheibengewebe. Orthopäde 25(1):3–9
[45] Schultz R, Krishnamurthy S, Thelmo W, Rodriguez J, Harvey G (1985) Effects of varying intensities of laser energy on articular cartilage. A preliminary study. Lasers Surg Med 5:577

[46] Seara J, Hüttmann G, Hendrich C, Housarek S, Lehnert C, Siebert W (1999) Experimentelle photodynamische Laser-therapie für die chronische Polyarthritis mit verschiedenen Photosensibilisatoren. Arthroskopie 12:50–54

[47] Siebert W, Seichert N, Siebert B, Wirth C (1987) What is the efficacy of "soft" and "mid" lasers in therapy of tendi-nopathies? Arch Orthop and Traum Surg 106:358–363

[48] Siebert, W, Kohn D, Klanke J, Wirth C, Scholz C, Müller G (1990) Rasterelektronenmikroskopische Untersuchungen zur Oberflächenbearbeitung von Knorpelschäden mit dem Neodym-YAG-Laser, dem CO_2-Laser, dem Excimer-Laser, dem Erbium-Laser, dem Holmium-YSSG-Laser und diversen motorgetriebenen Instrumenten. In: Glinz W, Kie-ser C, Munzinger U (eds): Arthroskopie bei Knorpelschä-den und bei Arthrose. Enke, Stuttgart

[49] Siebert W (1992) Laseranwendung in der Arthroskopie. Orthopäde 21:273–288

[50] Siebert W (1999) Perkutane Nukleotomieverfahren beim lumbalen Bandscheibenvorfall. Eine Bestandsaufnahme. Orthopäde, March/April 1999

[51] Siebert W (1999) Laser in der arthroskopischen Chirurgie. Medizinspiegel. Ärztejournal Schweiz 2:12–14

[52] Smith J, Nance T (1984) CO_2 laser energy for arthroscopic meniscus surgery. Presented to the American Academy of Sports Medicine, Anaheim CA, 25 July 1984

[53] Sommerfeld F, Pape H, Siebert W (1999) Minimalinvasive Schulterchirurgie: Welchen Stellenwert nimmt die laseras-sistierte Kapselschrumpfung (LACS) in der differentierten arthroskopischen posttraumatischer Schulterinstabilitäten ein? Orth Praxis 3

[54] Whipple T (1981) Applications of the CO_2 laser to arthro-scopic meniscectomy in a gas medium. Presented at the Triannual Meeting of the International Arthroscopy Asso-ciation. American Arthroscopy Association of North Amer-ica. Rio de Janeiro, Brazil, 1981

[55] Zangger P, Gerber B (1996) Laseranwendung in der Arthro-skopie des oberen Sprunggelenks. Indikationen, Technik, erste Ergebnisse. Orthopäde 25(1):73–78

[56] Zweifel K (1994) Laser tissue interactions: practical approach and real-time-MRI analysis of energy effects. 3rd Symposium on Laser-Assisted Endoscopic and Arthro-scopic Intervention in Orthopedics, Zürich, Switzerland, 26–27 May 1996

II Basics

Basic Laser Principles and Research: Introductory Remarks

B. E. GERBER

In this textbook the contributions to this first part, on the basics of laser and laser research, have been compiled with a view to allowing people who want to deal with surgical and other laser treatment of the musculoskeletal system access to the fundamental knowledge essential to an understanding of laser-tissue interactions without training as biophysical scientists.

Since the late 1980s much progress has been made in the primary basic science of laser interactions with dead tissues under laboratory conditions. These results, which led to an understanding that laser apparatus could be of special interest, are available elsewhere and served as the basis for a selection of significant utilizations in locomotor tissue which have been tested experimentally and are being developed or even introduced into the clinical setting.

This chapter therefore concentrates on the underlying physics and on the fundamentals of promising musculoskeletal laser applications for which basic research has already been able to focus on settings increasingly close to conditions of clinical use. Specific abilities of these technologies are explained together with their mechanisms of action in dependence on particular properties of the various laser wavelengths.

This should help to avoid inappropriate application of laser and inappropriate parameter settings, which can cause servere damage to patients, as has already occurred with the incorrect application of certain laser devices as soon as they were available on the medical market despite their having been developed for other fields.

In the first part of this part, well-known biophysicists teach us the basic physical principles of laser in relation to how laser apparatus and transmitting fibers work, and what tissue effects are produced, with an eye to present and future medical applications. Because a main advantage of laser technology is its good performance in minimally invasive surgery, the development of laser endoscopes for this purpose is then presented by specialized engineers. At the end of this first section of Part I, a clinician summarizes the basic knowledge required with an overview of the different types of laser, among which at present the holmium:YAG is the best performing, and about the specific possibilities of use in the locomotor system so far, in terms adapted to the clinician's needs including reference to the necessary laser safety precautions.

For the second section of this part, authors have been chosen who have carried out comprehensive studies of particular topics in the application of lasers to musculoskeletal tissues, from basic primary laboratory results to in vivo experiments in settings close to the conditions of clinical application. Aiming to be in some way representative of all the research done in the respective fields, these authors have based their contributions on their own successive studies as well as on complementary studies by other authors, giving an instructive presentation of the positive possibilities of laser technology, indicating both the optimized procedures that must be followed for success and the damage produced when such procedures are not respected. In this way, the range that is safe for therapeutic application is defined.

First the holmium-induced temperature profiles are measured using an MRI technique. Then a basic study describes the mechanisms that would allow tissue discrimination with a view to later clinical feedback ablation guided by optical selection. Effective clinical applications of laser which are already safely performable are joint capsular shrinkage and laser treatment of cartilage. The next two contributions outline the optimized procedures for these. By contrast, the photodynamic therapy of rheumatoid arthritis has been studied in an animal model using three substances that have yet to be approved for clinical use. Likewise, skeletal healing after osteotomy using an erbium laser not transmitted by classical fibers cannot yet be obtained clinically, because osteotomies made with available lasers show a much worse healing tendency.

At the end of the research part, cytological investigations evaluate the influence on cytokine production of rheumatoid synovial cells and the bactericidal effect of laser irradiation, and open up interesting supplementary treatment options.

The assembled information about the basics of lasers and laser research demonstrate that the present state of knowledge will allow well-targeted use of available laser technology and prevent foreseeable failures such as bad consolidation of an arthroscopic ankle arthrodesis after preparation of the bony surface with a currently available laser. In this way, oversimplified conclusions such as to reject all use of laser in this sort of surgery may be prevented- particularly since direct holmium laser treatment of the accompanying synovitis would in this case be very useful.

The different topics outlined here are of course constantly undergoing further investigation; the state of the art presented in this book will be updated in a later edition by further research results.

Basics, Laser Physics and Safety for the Clinician's Requirements

A. B. Imhoff

Introduction

The term LASER is an acronym standing for *light amplification by stimulated emission of radiation*. The atomic theories leading to the discovery of lasers were established by Einstein in 1917 [6]. The concept of using laser energy for medical applications dates from the early 1960s, when Theodore Maiman [27] built the first laser and found that a ruby crystal, when stimulated by a flash lamp, emitted red laser light at a specific wavelength of 0.69 µm. This laser was used in ophthalmology for photocoagulation and set the stage for the development of additional laser wavelengths for use in all types of medical applications.

Laser Physics

All lasers have at least these three essential components:

1. The *excitation source* pumps high electric energy into the lasing medium and stimulates electrons of the lasing medium to create photons. When atoms drop from a higher energy state to a lower energy level, they release energy in the form of photons. These photons are transmitted through a partially reflective mirror and emitted as a photon laser beam.
2. The *laser tube or resonator cavity* contains the laser medium and the two parallel mirrors.
3. The *lasing medium*, which is an excitable material and can be a gas, liquid, or solid, produces the photons and determines the precise wavelength of the resulting laser beam.

This resultant beam of light is *collimated* (all of the light waves are parallel), *coherent* (all of the light waves are in phase), and *monochromatic*. This monochromatic light wave can be in the visible or invisible portion of the electromagnetic spectrum. The original ruby laser beam was visible red light with a wavelength of 694 nm. Subsequent investigators have used various crystals and gases to develop lasers with many specific wavelengths in the electromagnetic spectrum, from the ultraviolet through the visible and out into the infrared portion of the spectrum.

The surgical efficacy (rate of tissue removal) of a laser is a function of the diameter of the laser beam in addition to the surface area or *"spot size"*. The laser beam is smallest at its focal point and diverges beyond this point. The power density is the power divided by the cross-sectional area of the beam at the place where it contacts the tissue. A small spot size will have a greater power density for any particular power rating. The power density is measured in watts per square centimetre. By changing the focal length, the spot size and the power density can be varied. Power density varies inversely with the square of the effective diameter of the laser beam. Therefore, if the laser beam is halved, the power density is increased fourfold. However, if the power is doubled and the beam diameter remains the same, the power density is only doubled.

Laser – Tissue Interaction

The optical properties of the material and the wavelength of the laser light determine the effectiveness of a given laser by controlling the interaction between the laser light and the tissue. The laser light may be *scattered* by particles in the liquid surrounding the tissue, *reflected* by the tissue, *transmitted* through and scattered within, or *absorbed* by the tissue.

Laser tissue ablations can be divided into three categories:

1. *Photothermal*, when laser light is absorbed by tissue with the tissue being heated and undergoing coagulation, necrosis, and vaporization. Photocoagulation is the process of heating tissues to induce necrosis on the surface and local scarring. Photovaporization requires enough heat to allow vaporization of intra- and extracellular fluids; it occurs during irradiation with long-pulse or continuous-wave lasers.
2. *Photochemical*, where absorption of photons, directly dissociates the molecular bonds. This photoablative process is only possible for ultraviolet laser wavelength [e. g. argon-fluoride laser with

a wavelength at 193 nm (excimer laser)]. Photodynamic therapy takes advantage of photochemical effects using a photosensitizer, which concentrates selectively in metabolically active tissue like tumours.

3. *Photomechanical*, where the deposited energy leads to increased stresses within the tissue. Ablation then occurs when stress exceeds the materials' strength. This process occurs during irradiation with short pulse laser and wavelength in the near-ultraviolet, visible, and near-infrared spectrum [33].

Laser tissue interactions can also be seen as *ionizing effects*, with photodisruption of tissue occurring in the targeted area through rapid ionization from a high-density laser beam that creates an acoustic shock wave [5, 49].

Orthopaedic Laser Systems

Lasers have been used in orthopaedics since the mid-1980s, primarily for arthroscopic procedures [17, 18, 37, 41]. Surgical lasers fall between the longest and shortest wavelengths, in the infrared, visible, and ultraviolet portions of the electromagnetic spectrum. Today, several surgical lasers are commercially available. The most frequently used medical lasers are the carbon dioxide (CO_2), argon ion, krypton ion, holmium:YAG (Ho:YAG), neodymium:YAG (Nd:YAG), doubled neodymium:YAG (KTP), helium neon (HeNe), visible dye, and excimer laser (XeF, XeCl, KrF, ArF).

CO_2 Laser

The CO_2 laser derives its energy from the electrical excitation of CO_2 gas with the resultant emission of photons with a wavelength of 1064 nm (10.6 μm). The CO_2 laser is highly absorbed by water with minimal scattering; therefore, gaseous insufflation of the joint is required. The CO_2 laser is a good cutting instrument that has some coagulation effects. The tissue is rapidly heated above boiling and is obliterated by the CO_2 laser with a small residue of ash. The thermal effect is to a depth of less than 200 μm and thermal necrosis less than 50 μm [44]. The CO_2 laser primarily creates a vertical incision with minimal lateral necrosis. The smoke must be evacuated from the joint during the procedure and the carbon ash residue should be removed with irrigation [43, 44]. The CO_2 laser cannot be transmitted through standard fibre-optic cables and requires an articulating arm with a channel of sensitive reflecting mirrors. Typically, the CO_2 laser uses a helium-neon laser beam because the CO_2 laser light is invisible. In 1984, Whipple et al. [56] performed one of the earliest

studies evaluating the CO_2 laser on New Zealand white rabbits. An arthrotomy and subtotal CO_2 laser meniscectomy were performed followed by staged histologic evaluations. The initial synovial response was characterized by hypertrophic changes with an increase in cell population and subsynovial interstitial fluid. Particulate organic material produced by the ablation of meniscal tissue was ingested by the synovium and caused a severe synovial reaction. After 8 weeks, no particulate matter could be localized. The authors concluded that the carbon ash residue was not especially noxious to the joint, but the synovial response was of sufficient severity to influence the authors not to use the CO_2 laser in humans.

In an experimental in vivo study Vangsness et al. [52] found no histologic evidence of healing or fibrous covering in superficial or deep laser lesions, and no adverse clinical effects (synovitis, infections) were seen in the laser group.

Sherk et al. [37] performed removal of polymethylmethacrylate by CO_2 laser in 117 patients undergoing revision operations. The CO_2 laser did not damage adjacent bone or soft tissue via lateral heat transfer. The maximum bone cortex temperature during CO_2 laser removal was 56 °C. This was lower than the 60 °C temperature encountered during initial cement insertion and curing. However, there was no statistical difference in surgical time, blood loss, or infection rate, and there were positively no cases of osteonecrosis caused by the laser.

The CO_2 laser requires gas insufflation of the joint; this can result in subcutaneous emphysema. Smith et al. [44] reported a 100 % incidence of subcutaneous emphysema which resolved rapidly. Retroperitoneal and mediastinal emphysema have been reported in patients in whom the knee joint had been distended with CO_2 [11, 37, 44].

For these reasons, the CO_2 laser has not gained significant acceptance in arthroscopic surgery [37, 41].

Excimer Laser

Excimer is the name given to a series of lasers that operate in essentially the same manner. These lasers use mixtures of a halogen and a rare gas to generate laser emission. The emitted wavelength depends on the elements used in the gas mixture: 193 nm for *argon-fluoride (ArF)*, 248 nm for *krypton-fluoride (KrF)*, 308 nm for *xenon-chloride (XeCl)*, and 351 nm for *xenon-fluoride (XeF)*. Excimer gases are triggered by a fast electrical discharge that raises the energy level of the rare gas atoms so that they react with the halogen molecules to form compounds such as ArF, KrF, or XeCl. These special compound molecules known as excimers *(excited dimers)* exist only briefly in the high-energy state. As they return to the ground energy level, they dissociate and fluoresce strongly in the ultraviolet spectrum. A high-energy pulse literally vaporizes a very thin tissue layer without heating the surrounding tissue. Layers on the order of several molecules can be removed per pulse. The effect is predominantly a surface effect with no measurable disruptions beyond 5–10 μm beneath the surface. The laser acts as a very high precision, non-heating, contact-free scalpel. This only occurs at energy levels above 200 mJ/cm^2.

This mechanism of ablation is quite different from the photothermal ablation of conventional laser beams. Material disintegration, which occurs by separating the molecules within the tissue, is generated without significant heat production. This process, known as *ablative photodecomposition* or *photo-ablation*, was initially described by Srinivasan et al. [46, 47]. Tissue is destroyed by *photodissociation* as the laser beam breaks the chemical bonds of the cell molecules. Excimer lasers therefore produce a "trench" in the tissue with extraordinarily sharp, cleanly defined boundaries. The non-thermal vaporization of tissue has been used for a variety of surgical treatments in ophthalmology since 1983 (to make fine incisions in the corneae to correct astigmatism and perform *radial keratotomy* with ArF laser), and in cardiovascular disease (*angioplasty*, to vaporize and remove plaque from clogged arteries with XeCl and KrF lasers), and in laryngeal surgery. Unlike the shorter wavelengths, only the 308-nm XeCl laser can be delivered fibre-optically and can be operated in a fluid environment.

The use of excimer lasers in arthroscopic procedures [2, 12, 13, 17, 18, 26, 31, 32, 34] and percutaneous nucleotomy [8, 24] has been investigated by several authors. Laboratory studies performed by Freedland [10] in 1988 showed that the excimer laser can ablate cartilage very precisely without infringing upon, or injuring the adjacent bone. Raunest et al. [31], in 1990, obtained excellent results in a prospective randomized clinical study of the arthroscopic treatment of chondromalacia patellae with the excimer laser. They compared the debridement of the defect with the laser and with the use of mechanical devices. The results were significantly better with regard to pain (p < 0.05) and postoperative irritative synovitis (p < 0.01). There were no differences between the groups in terms of disability or functional impairment. However, clinical and experimental studies by Imhoff and Leu [18] in 1989 determined that the ablation rate of the cold-cutting excimer laser was unsatisfactory.

The initial enthusiasm over the athermic excimer laser has diminished in the last few years due to its inadequate ablation rate. In experimental series, Imhoff and Leu [20] showed that an ablation rate of 4–5 μm per pulse was not adequate for ablation of meniscus cartilage. The results of Kroitsch et al. [22] are similar. A cut with a length of 5 mm and a depth of 3 mm needs 2.2 min of exposure at a pulse rate of 20 Hz.

There has been much concern over the potential mutagenic effects of the excimer laser. Laser wavelengths of 248 nm and 309 nm lie in the ultraviolet region. The wavelength of 248 nm is the most mutagenic wavelength. Many of the cells irradiated by the laser are ablated and effectively destroyed in comparison to a continous low dose of ultraviolet radiation.

Neodymium:YAG Laser

The beam of the neodymium:YAG laser is produced by means of excitation of the *neodymium-impregnated yttrium aluminium garnet (YAG) crystal*. The Nd:YAG laser emits light at a wavelength of 1.06 μm. This beam is invisible; therefore, a helium-neon laser beam is used. The Nd:YAG laser is highly absorbed by protein with a significant coagulation zone of 4–5 mm. In comparison with the CO_2 laser (0.1 mm), this is a very large coagulation zone. The typical tissue effect produced by the non-contact Nd:YAG laser is a broad and deep area of thermal necrosis. Unlike the CO_2 laser, the energy is not absorbed in the first 0.01 mm tissue. The depth of penetration varies with the amount of energy applied and the ability of the tissue to absorb the energy. Red, pigment-bearing tissue such as endometrium or synovium [14] absorbs the neodymium laser much more readily than white, uncoloured tissue such as tendon and fibrocartilage. Using an artificial sapphire or ceramic tip, the Nd:YAG laser works as a *contact laser*. The sapphire tips proved to be brittle and broke within the joint when the handpiece was used vigorously; the newer ceramic tips are much stronger without the risk of breakage. The fibre tip converts the laser beam into intense heat and functions as a heat probe to cut and vaporize tissue thermally [1]. The result is precise tissue cutting with reduced lateral tissue damage. The return of tactile sensation with this device is also advantageous.

O'Brien and Miller [29] demonstrated the regenerative ability of rabbit meniscal and articular cartilage tissue after being incised with the Nd:YAG contact laser. Characteristic remodelling and regeneration were seen in 75 % after scalpel meniscectomy, but a wide band of acellularity, which increased with time, was seen in all electrosurgical meniscectomies. After laser meniscectomy, some menisci showed regeneration similar to the scalpel lesions (fibrocartilaginous tissue). All of the articular cartilage defects created by the laser showed a vigorous healing response at 6 weeks, characterized by increased vascularity, chondrocyte proliferation, and fibrocartilaginous repair [35] (the subchondral bone interaction was not evaluated).

Recently, Sherk et al. [39] noted the effect of lasers on human meniscal tissue. With electrothermal coagulation, the depth and lateral extent of thermal necrosis was 250 µm (stained with heamatoxylin-eosin) and 478 µm (stained with trichrome). The Nd:YAG free-beam (continuous) laser had a thermal necrosis zone of 378 µm/870 µm compared to 60 µm/ 230 µm for the contact tip Nd:YAG (continuous) laser. The pulsed holmium:YAG laser produced an adjacent zone of tissue damage of 82 µm/552 µm while thermal necrosis from the excimer laser extended only 24 µm/0 µm.

Experimental studies have evaluated the use of lasers for tissue welding of skin (skin suturing), small arteries, and ureters (vessel reapproximation) [18, 53]. The possibility of a sutureless meniscal repair (tissue welding of meniscus) was reported by Sherk and Kollmer [38]. They carried out experiments in dogs to evaluate the healing of radial, full-thickness meniscal tears with lasers. By 6 weeks, they found no attempt at healing after a radial cut was made with a scalpel; however, cuts created by the laser cut had filled in with tissue which resembled immature fibrocartilage.

In contrast, Vangsness et al. [54] recently reported the results of an experimental study with 30 mature New Zealand white rabbits. The overall results showed no healing or fusion of a meniscal tear in the avascular zone in any of the 30 rabbits. The varying dose of the Nd:YAG laser demonstrated no gradient effect using only low-energy laser parameters (5 W/2 s = 10 J to 10 W/3 s = 20 J). Increased tissue response with greater inflammatory and synovial tissue reaction was noted in all lased areas. The greatest cellular inflammatory response was noted in the sutured and lased menisci.

The advantages of the Nd:YAG laser are its fibre-optic transmission and its ability to be used in aqueous media, unlike the CO_2 laser. The contact laser probe allows incision with extreme precision and minimal lateral tissue damage. A range of surgical handpieces is available that can be inserted into the joint like any other arthroscopic instrument. The clinical advantages of the laser "hot scalpel" over conventional instrumentation are the ability to cut, release, and coagulate tissue in an aqueous medium [14, 15, 45].

Argon Ion Laser

The argon laser emits light at a wavelength of 488 nm (blue range) or 514 nm (green range). This laser is excited by direct current electrical discharge and operates between a power range of 0 and 15 W. This laser beam can be delivered through a flexible fibre or through a slit lamp. The argon laser light is absorbed by tissue pigments such as haemoglobin and melanin. It can only coagulate small vessels and is used mainly in ophthalmology for photocoagulation; however, its absorption in pigmented tissue has made it useful in treating skin lesions such as port wine stains and haemangiomas.

KTP Laser

The frequency-doubled Nd:YAG laser emits light at a wavelength of 532 nm in the visible portion of the spectrum. This wavelength is exactly half the 1064-nm wavelength of the Nd:YAG laser. The beam produced by a Nd:YAG laser is passed through a potassium-titanyl-phosphate crystal. This doubles the frequency of the Nd:YAG beam and halves its wavelength. Output power typically reaches up to 20 W. The KTP laser has significant advantages over the argon laser. It requires no fibre cooling as the higher-powered argon does, and the energy can pass through a flexible fibre. The absorption characteristics are very similar to those of the argon laser.

Holmium:YAG Laser

The holmium:YAG laser emits light at a wavelength of 2.1 µm and can be transmitted through conventional optical fibres. The Ho:YAG laser has the ability to precisely and rapidly resect, cut, coagulate, vaporize, and ablate cartilaginous tissues. It causes a minimal amount of thermal necrosis while providing superior haemostatic control [40, 48]. This laser can function in a saline medium and may be used in direct contact with the tissue (surgeon feedback); however, a near-contact mode with a free beam is typically utilized [21, 23].

In clinical studies, excellent results were reported after meniscectomy using Ho:YAG laser. Fanton and Dillingham [7] noted less postoperative pain and swelling with a quicker return to full range of motion when comparing laser menisectomies to conventional meniscectomies. The results were not statistically significant. Lane et al. [23] also compared the clinical efficacy of the Ho:YAG and CO_2 lasers with that of mechanical techniques in arthroscopic debridement of the knee and reported similar results without statistical significance.

The in vitro analysis of laser meniscectomy by Vangsness [54, 55] showed that the excimer laser caused the least tissue changes; these changes were less extensive with the pulsed CO_2 laser than with the Ho:YAG, Nd:YAG, and KTP laser. The most surface disruption occurred with standard electrocautery. Histologic analysis of the necrosis at the laser-tissue interface showed that laser used in saline produced less tissue damage. A shortcoming of this study was that the total energy delivered and the time to cut was not addressed.

Experimental studies in our laboratory using the Ho:YAG laser (2100 nm) demonstrated that the highest efficiency in ablation of meniscal fibrocartilage can be achieved with a pulse rate of 10 Hz and 1.5 J or 15 Hz and 1.0 J. A higher pulse rate of 20 Hz cannot increase the ablation rate.

Lateral retinacular release performed using the Ho:YAG laser has shown reduced morbidity. When performing a lateral release, tightening of the medial retinaculum can give an added measure of success in cases with patellar subluxations. Shapiro et al. [36] reported in a comparative study that patients whose release was performed with a laser recovered more quickly than patients who had lateral release performed using an electrocautery device. The ability to photocoagulate as the laser cuts and ablates was the main reason given for the absence of postoperative bleeding in the laser-treated group, in contrast to the incidence of haemarthrosis in the electrocautery group. Recovery with respect to swelling, effusion, return of full active range of movement, pain, and completion of physical therapy was significantly better in the laser group.

After cartilage ablation, microscopic examination by Trauner et al. [50] revealed zones of thermal damage extending only 550 µm from ablation sites. Ablation rates were measured with a mass loss technique. The delayed biological response is not known. Above threshold, mass removal rates were proportional to laser radiant exposure. Threshold radiant exposure for ablation was 50 J/cm^2 for articular cartilage and 11 J/cm^2 for meniscal fibrocartilage. However, experimental work in our laboratory showed a proportional absorption in articular cartilage without threshold radiant exposure and for ablation it was only 30 J/cm^2 for articular cartilage.

In several studies, the use of the Ho:YAG laser was not superior to mechanical methods for remodelling and smoothing of fairly large chondral areas. In a comparative study in the rabbit arthrosis model, Moller et al. [28] found that after mechanical debridement, the articular surface was relatively smooth at 3 months, and tears and defects filled with fibrous repair tissue. However, after Ho:YAG laser debridement, the authors found chondral necrosis, occasionally with damage to the subchondral bone, and distinct inflammation in the marrow space. The surgical technique with regard to irradiation angle was not specified.

Recently, Collier et al. [3] reported on the effects of the Ho:YAG laser on equine articular cartilage and subchondral bone adjacent to traumatic lesions in terms of depth of damage and healing reponse over time. Cartilage adjacent to all lesions exposed to laser energy had better cellularity and proteoglycan content than did corresponding controls (p < 0.05). At higher energy levels (0.16 J and 0.2 J), there was loss of cellularity and necrosis in subchondral bone. However, they concluded that evidence of thermal injury to tissue adjacent to the laser-treated sites was minimal. The use of pulsed-laser energy significantly reduced the extent of thermal injury to adjacent tissues. The deleterious effect observed in subchondral bone at higher energy levels may have been partly due to damage from the photoacoustic effect. The peak power of each pulse can induce fissures in adjacent tissue (Moses effect) by vaporizing the thin intervening film of water.

In a recent study, Trauner et al. [51] evaluated the acute and chronic effects of the Ho:YAG laser on cartilaginous tissue. At 10 weeks, there was no healing of full- or partial-thickness defects in hyaline cartilage, and the filling fibrocartilaginous granulation tissue, seen at 2 and 4 weeks, was no longer evident. Chondrocyte necrosis extended to 900 µm distal to the edge of craters at 4 weeks. Increased damage may be attributed to the presence of a photoacoustic effect.

Synovectomies with Ho:YAG laser could be an alternative to existing therapeutic techniques in the treatment of rheumatoid arthritis and other synovial proliferative disorders such as synovial chondromatosis [19] or pigmented villonodular synovitis (PVNS) [17, 20, 42]. In an experimental study, Lind et al. [25] compared laser synovectomy using Ho:YAG laser to mechanical synovectomy in the knees of 48 rabbits after inducing chronic arthritis immunologically. In the laser group, edema, acute inflammation, and coagulation necrosis occurred immediately; however, after 1 week, the synovial layer showed slight fibrosis similar to that seen in the control group. One month later, the laser-synovectomized surface appeared to be smooth; in contrast, the mechanical abrasion group had pronounced haemorrhage, necrosis and fibrosis in all capsular layers. At 3 months, the synovial layer of knees in the mechanical abrasion group appeared coarse and villous. The results in the laser group were superior.

Erbium:YAG Laser

The erbium:YAG laser emits light at a wavelength of 2.940 µm (erbium:YSGG laser at a wavelength of 2.79 µm). This mid-infrared laser has a very high specificity for water and is used mainly for precise cutting and coagulation in ophthalmology, dermatology, and laryngeal surgery [16].

Tissue welding of a torn meniscus using an Er:YAG laser with a 1.3 μm wavelength was reported by Dew et al. in 1988 [5]. The laser was used to cause coagulation and sealing of tissue at the site of an experimentally created laceration on the meniscus with minimal associated tissue necrosis.

Histologic analysis of acute Er:YAG laser lesions reveals precise cutting effects with a minimal thermal damage zone of 40 μm. By comparison, the extent of thermal damage caused by the Er:YSGG and CO_2 laser is about twice as large. Tissue lesions induced with the argon and Ho:YAG lasers create a thermal damage zone of 200–300 μm.

Herdman et al. [16] recently compared the relative thermal damage caused by a surgical CO_2 laser and the Er:YAG laser when used to incise the human vocal fold in vitro. The depth of coagulative necrosis adjacent to an incision was reduced from 510 μm (± 75) using the CO_2 laser to 23 μm (± 12) using the Er:YAG laser and at the base was reduced from 125 μm (± 45) using the CO_2 laser to 12 μm (± 8) using the Er:YAG laser.

The Er:YAG laser can be used for osteotomies with minimal thermal necrosis. Bone healing subsequent to Er:YAG laser osteotomy takes the same course in time as secondary fracture healing. By contrast, bone healing after CO_2 laser application is delayed about two to three weeks.

Future Directions: Tissue Welding

Repair of torn tissue through tissue agglutination and tissue welding are interesting possible applications of the Ho:YAG laser. Using a *thulium-holmium-chromium:YAG laser* (THC:YAG laser) with a wavelength of 2.15 μm, Oz et al. [30] have shown that a laser-welded cholecystectomy in dogs, healed without evidence of leakage or infection by 2 weeks postoperatively and re-epithelialization was seen by 3 weeks after operation. By comparison, the suture-closed incisions made in the fundus of the gallbladder of the dogs were still without complete epithelialization 4 weeks after the procedure.

Laser-assisted fibrin clot soldering may allow the opposing edges of a meniscal tear to be held together. After irradiation with argon laser energy, the tensile strength of the laser-assisted fibrin clot-bonded menisci increased 40-fold over that of non-irradiated fibrin clot-bonded menisci [9].

Summary

Current orthopaedic lasers function in the ultraviolet (excimer) or in the infrared portion of the electromagnetic spectrum (CO_2, Nd:YAG, holmium). These lasers combine successfully the desired tissue effect and practical transmissibility for arthroscopic application. The laser energy is absorbed by cellular water and is converted to heat. This vaporizes the tissue with little or no thermal damage. Clinical applications for laser arthroscopy have expanded in the past 10 years. The holmium laser is the most widely used wavelength in arthroscopy. The holmium laser is clinically useful for meniscal cutting and ablation, lateral retinacular release, release of posttraumatic fibrosis, chondroplasty, synovectomy, debridement, ankle impingement decompression and debridement, and percutaneous nucleotomy. Current investigation with laser tissue photoagglutination and tissue welding may make it possible to repair torn meniscus by tissue welding with laser energy.

References

[1] Bickerstaff D, Wyman A, Laing, R, Smith T (1991) Partial meniscectomy using the neodymium:YAG laser. An in vitro study. Arthroscopy 7:63–67
[2] Buchelt, M, Papioannou T, Fishbein M, Peters W, Beeder C, Grundfest W (1991) Excimer laser ablation of fibrocartilage: an in vitro and in vivo study. Lasers Surg Med 11:271–279
[3] Collier M, Haugland L, Bellamy J, Johnson L, Rohrer M, Walls R, Bartels K (1993) Effects of holmium:YAG laser on equine articular cartilage and subchondral bone adjacent to traumatic lesions: a histopathological assessment. Arthroscopy 9/5:536–545
[4] Dew D (1995) Laser biophysics for orthopaedic surgeon. Clin Orthop 310:6–13
[5] Dew D, Supik L, Darrow C, Price G (1993) Tissue repair using lasers: a review. Orthopedics 16/5:581–587
[6] Einstein A (1917) Zur Quantentheorie der Strahlung. Phys Z 18:121
[7] Fanton G, Dillingham M (1992) The use of the holmium:YAG laser in arthroscopic surgery. Sem Orthop 7/2:102–116
[8] Fischer R, König K, Ruck A, Puhl W, Steiner R (1994) [Fluorescence spectroscopy in selective percutaneous nucleotomy using the excimer laser - experimental studies.] Einsatz der Fluoreszenzspectroskopie zur selektiven perkutanen Nukleotomie mit dem Excimer-Laser - Experimentelle Untersuchungen. Z. Orthop 132:9–15
[9] Forman S, Oz M, Lontz J, Treat M, Forman T, Kiernan H (1995) Laser-assisted fibrin clot soldering of human menisci. Clin Orthop 310:37–41
[10] Freedland Y (1999) Use of the excimer laser in fibrocartilaginous excision from adjacent bony stroma: a preliminary investigation. J Foot Surg 27/4:303
[11] Garrick J, Kadel N (1991) The CO_2 laser in arthroscopy: potential problems and solution. Arthroscopy 7:129–137
[12] Glossop N, Jackson R, Koort H, Reed S, Randle J (1995) The excimer laser in orthopaedics. Clin Orthop 310:72–81
[13] Grifka J (1993) Arthroskopische Therapie der Gonarthrose in Abhängigkeit vom Grad der Chondromalazie. Arthroskopie 6:201–211
[14] Grifka J, Schreiner C, Löhnert J (1994) Frühergebnisse der Nd:YAG-Laser-Synovektomie bei detritusindizierten Synovialitiden. Arthroskopie 7:154–157
[15] Grothues-Spork M, Bernard M, Cierpinski T, Hertel P, Noack W, Müller G (1994) Fünf Lasersysteme zur arthroskopischen Meniskuschirurgie im Tierversuch. Arthroskopie 7/2:68–75
[16] Herdman R, Charlton A, Hinton A, Freemont A (1993) An in vitro comparison of the erbium:YAG laser and the carbon dioxide laser in laryngeal surgery. Laryngol Otol 107:908–911

[17] Imhoff A (1991) [Knee arthroscopy: special diagnosis and surgical techniques.] Kniearthroskopie: Spezielle Diagnostik (Synovialis, Knorpelschäden) und Operationstechniken (Elektromesser, Lasersysteme). Akt Probl Orthop 40:44-63

[18] Imhoff A, Leu H (1991) Arthroscopic operations with the excimer laser. Initial experiences. In Siebert W, Wirth C (eds) [Lasers in orthopaedics.] Laser in der Orthopädie. Thieme, Stuttgart, pp 48-53

[19] Imhoff A, Schreiber A (1988) Synovial chondromatosis. Orthopäde 17:233-244

[20] Imhoff A, Schreiber A (1988) Etiology and pathogenesis of synovitis villonodosa pigmentosa. Orthopäde 17: 223-232

[21] Kautzky M, Susani M, Schenk P (1992) The holmium:YAG infrared laser and the UV excimer. Effects of lasers on the oral mucosa. Laryngorhinootologie 71:347-352

[22] Kroitsch U, Laufer G, Egkjer E, Wollenek G, Jprvath R (1989) Experimental photoablation of meniscus cartilage by excimer laser energy. Arch Orthop Trauma Surg 108:44-48

[23] Lane G, Sherk H, Mooar P, Lee S, Black J (1992) Holmium:YAG laser versus carbon dioxide laser versus mechanical arthroscopic debridement. Sem Orthop 7/2:95-101

[24] Leu H, Imhoff A, Schreiber A (1991) [Percutaneous nucleotomy with discoscopy: early results of photoablation with excimer laser.] Perkutane Nukleotomie mit Diskoskopie: erste Erfahrungen mit der Excimer Photoablation. In Siebert W, Wirth C (eds) [Lasers in orthopaedics] Laser in der Orthopädie. Thieme, Stuttgart, pp 163-167

[25] Lind B, Miller K, Schramm U, Baretton G, Trautmann C, Karcher K (1993) [Comparative experimental studies of mechanical and holmium laser synovectomy.] Vergleichende experimentelle Untersuchungen zur mechanischen und Holmium:YAG Laser-Synovectomie. Langenbecks Arch Chir 378:273-280

[26] Löhnert J, Raunest J (1994) Operationstechnik der arthroskopischen Knorpelablation mit dem 308 nm-Xenon-Chlorid-Excimer-Laser. Arthroskopie 7:170-173

[27] Maiman T (1960) Stimulated optical radiation in ruby. Nature 187:493

[28] Moller K, Lind B, Karcher K, Hohlbach G (1994) [Holmium laser versus mechanical cartilage resection. Comparative studies in the rabbit arthrosis model.] Holmiumlaser versus mechanische Knorpelabtragung. Vergleichende Untersuchungen am Arthrosemodell bei Kaninchen. Langenbecks Arch Chir 379:84-94

[29] O'Brien S, Miller D (1990) The contact neodymium-yttrium aluminium garnet laser (Nd:YAG laser) - a new approach to arthroscopic laser surgery. Clin Orthop 252:95-100

[30] Oz M, Popp H, Treat M, Bass L, Popilskis S (1991) In vivo comparison of THC:YAG laser welding to sutured closure of biliary tissue. Am Surg 57:275-279

[31] Raunest J, Sager M, Derra E (1994) Experimentelle Befunde zur Knorpelablation und Abrasionschondroplastik mit thermischen und gepulsten UV-Lasern. Arthroskopie 7:174-181

[32] Reed S, Jackson R, Glossop N, Randle J (1994) An in vivo study of the effect of excimer laser irradiation on degenerate rabbit articular cartilage. Arthroscopy 10:78-84

[33] Schaffer J, Dark M, Itzkan I, Albagli D, Perelman L, Von Rosenberg C (1995) Mechanisms of meniscal tissue ablation by short pulse laser irradiation. Clin Orthop 310:30-36

[34] Schreiner C (1994) Laser in der Arthroskopie. Arthroskopie 7:148-153

[35] Schultz R, Krishnamurthy S, Thelmo W, Rodriguez J, Harvey G (1985) Effects of varying intensities of laser energy on articular cartilage: a preliminary study. Lasers Surg Med 5:577-588

[36] Shapiro G, Fanton G, Dillingham M, Perkash R (1995) Lateral retinacular release - the holmium:YAG laser versus electrocautery. Clin Orthop 310:42-47

[37] Sherk H (1993) The use of lasers in orthopaedic procedures - current concept review. J Bone Joint Surg 75-A:768-776

[38] Sherk H, Kollmer C (1990) Meniscal repair with lasers. In Sherk H (ed) Lasers in orthopaedics. Lippincott, Philadelphia, pp 122-127

[39] Sherk H, Black J, Prodoehl J, Diven J (1995) The effects of lasers and electrosurgical devices on human meniscal tissue. Clin Orthop 310:14-20

[40] Shi W, Vari S, van der Veen M, Fishbeim M, Grundfest W (1993) Effect of varying laser parameters on pulsed Ho:YAG ablation of bovine knee joint tissues. Arthroscopy 9:96-102

[41] Siebert W (1992) The use of lasers in orthopaedics. Orthopäde 21: 273-288

[42] Siebert W, Saunier J, Gerber B, Lübbers C (1994) Holmium:YAG-Laser in der arthroskopischen Chirurgie des Kniegelenkes. Arthroskopie 7: 182-192

[43] Sisto D, Blazina M, Hirsh L (1993) The synovial response after CO2 laser arthroscopy of the knee. Arthroscopy 9/5:574-575

[44] Smith C, Johansen W, Vangsness C, Sutter L, Marshall G (1989) The carbon dioxide laser. A potential tool for orthopaedic surgery. Clin Orthop 242:43-50

[45] Spivak J, Grande D, Ben-Yishay A, Menche D, Pitman M (1992) The effect of low-level Nd:YAG laser energy on adult articular cartilage in vitro. Arthroscopy 8: 36-43

[46] Srinivasan R, Mayne-Banton V (1982) Self-developing photoetching of polyethylene therephtalate films by far-ultraviolet excimer laser radiation. Appl Phys Letts 41:576

[47] Srinivasan R, Wynne J, Blum S (1983) Controlled photoetching of organic material by far-ultraviolet (193 nm) laser radiation. Laser Focus 19:63

[48] Stein E, Sedlacek T, Fabian R, Nishioka N (1990) Acute and chronic effects of bone ablation with a pulsed holmium laser. Lasers Surg Med 10:384-388

[49] Thompson S (1989) Medical lasers: how they work and how they affect tissue. Cancer Bull 41:203-210

[50] Trauner K, Nishioka N, Patel D (1990) Pulsed holmium:YAG laser ablation of fibrocartilage and articular cartilage. Am J Sports Med 18/3:316-320

[51] Trauner K, Nishioka N, Flotte T, Patel D (1995) Acute and chronic response of articular cartilage to holmium:YAG laser irradiation. Clin Orthop 310:52-57

[52] Vangsness C, Smith C, Marshall G, Sweeney J, Johansen E (1995) The biological effects of carbon dioxide laser surgery on rabbit articular cartilage. Clin Orthop 310:48-51

[53] Vangsness C, Huang J, Smith C (1995) A spectrophotometer analysis of light absorption in the human meniscus. Clin Orthop 310:27-29

[54] Vangsness C, Akl Y, Marshall G, Subin W, Smith C (1994) The effects of the neodymium laser on meniscal repair in the vascular zone of the meniscus. Arthroscopy 10/2:201-205

[55] Vangsness C, Akl Y, Nelson S, Liaw L, Smith C, Marshall G (1995) In vitro analysis of laser meniscectomy. Clin Orthop 310:21-26

[56] Whipple T, Caspari R, Meyers J (1984) Synovial response to laser induced carbon ash residue. Laser Surg Med 3:291-295

Value of Infrared Radiometry to Medical Laser Applications with Reference to Temperature Feedback and Tissue Welding Options

I. ÇILESIZ

Thermometry in Medicine

The Medical Problem

As Barnes wrote in 1968 [1]:

> From the earliest days of medical practice, it has been known that thermal abnormalities or unusual localized areas of skin temperature, either elevated or depressed, usually denoted the presence of some underlying pathology or disease ... Until relatively recently, the physician who wished to examine his patient's skin temperature for diagnostic purposes had to rely strictly upon his own hand, usually the back of his hand, as his only thermal sensor ... Unsuccessful attempts were made to establish surface thermometry using a mercury thermometer whose bulb had been flattened to present a contact area of about 650 mm^2.

Modern devices such as thermocouples and thermistors have been used with considerably more success. Yet, they are difficult to use in non-aqueous non-homogeneous media, and like all contact methods these devices may alter the temperature of the tissue surface that they measure. Fortunately, "the human body continuously broadcasts thermal information, and to an IR *(infrared)* sensitive instrument, it behaves exactly as if it were truly incandescent, and it is these IR signatures that form the basis for medical thermography" [1].

Infrared Radiometry

Infrared (IR) radiation is a form of radiated electromagnetic (EM) energy "carrying heat". Thermal radiation is emitted by all objects at finite temperatures and it can be detected using transducers that convert IR radiation into electrical signals. IR radiation emitted by an exposed surface encompasses a large range of wavelengths and the amount of emitted radiation per unit wavelength varies with wavelength. Emitted radiation thus consists of a continuous non-uniform distribution of monochromatic (single wavelength) components [2, 3].

The spectral distribution of detected IR signals can be related to the temperature of the object of interest by the *Planck-Einstein Radiation Law* describing the monochromatic emissive power from an ideal radiator, called block body, as a function of body temperature

$$W_\lambda(T) = \frac{2\pi h c^2}{\lambda^5} \frac{1}{\exp(ch/\lambda kT) - 1} \quad [\mathrm{Wm^{-2}\mu m^{-1}}] \quad (1)$$

where $h = 6.625 \cdot 10^{-34}$ [Ws^2] is Planck's constant, $c = 3 \cdot 10^8$ [ms^{-1}] the speed of light, $k = 1.38 \cdot 10^{-23}$ [JK^{-1}] Boltzmann's constant, λ [m] or [μm] the emission wavelength, and T [K] the absolute temperature of the body. A convenient relationship derived from the Planck-Einstein Radiation Law is *Wien's Displacement Law* which relates the wavelength for maximum spectral emissive power to the absolute temperature of a body given as

$$\lambda_{max} T = 2897.8 \quad [\mu mK] \quad (2)$$

From Eq. 2 one can determine the most suitable wavelength band to look at targets of known temperature ranges, and, consequently, the type of detector one can use for the measurement of temperatures in that range.

The integral of the monochromatic emissive power over wavelength limits gives an expression for the radiant emittance known as the *Stefan-Boltzmann Law*

$$W(T) = \int_\lambda W_\lambda(T)d\lambda = \frac{2\pi^5 k^4}{15 c^2 h^3} T^4 = \sigma T^4 \quad [\mathrm{Wm^{-2}}]$$

$$(3)$$

where $\sigma = 5.67 \cdot 10^{-12}$ [Wm^{-2}K^{-4}] is the Stefan-Boltzmann constant. Note that Eqs. 1–3 are strictly valid for black bodies. A *black body* is defined as a perfect radiator that emits all the energy it absorbs. Most objects, however, do not radiate as effectively as black bodies. To describe the monochromatic emissive power of such objects, called *gray bodies*, emissivity, $\varepsilon_\lambda(T)$, is introduced as the ratio of the monochromatic emissive power of a gray body, $W_\lambda'(T)$, to the monochromatic emissive power of a black body at the same temperature:

$$\varepsilon_\lambda(T) = \frac{W_\lambda'(T)}{W_\lambda(T)} \qquad (4)$$

Emissivity is therefore a convenient measure of the degree to which an IR radiation source, i.e., gray body, approximates a black body. Emissivity is a function of the wavelength, type, and temperature of the material the gray body is made of, and its surface finish. For a black body, by definition $\varepsilon = 1$ for all T and λ of interest.

Like all other objects, human tissue is a gray body, and it emits IR radiation given by the *modified Stefan-Boltzmann Law*:

$$W'(T) = \int_\lambda \varepsilon_\lambda(T)W_\lambda(T)d\lambda \quad [Wm^{-2}]. \qquad (5)$$

Assuming $\varepsilon_\lambda(T) = \varepsilon(T) = $ constant for all λ, Eq. 5 reduces to

$$W'(T) = \varepsilon(T)\int_\lambda W_\lambda(T)d\lambda = \varepsilon(T)\sigma T^4 \quad [Wm^{-2}]. \quad (6)$$

However, due to atmospheric band-pass windows and spectral response limitations imposed by the available IR radiation detectors, the two presently used IR radiation wavelength bands are 3–5 μm and 8–12 μm, as shown in Fig. 1. As a result, the detected emissive power is less than the wide-band emissive power given in Eq. 6. The detected emissive power is obtained by integrating the monochromatic emissive power over the spectral response band ($\lambda_1 \rightarrow \lambda_2$) of the IR radiation detector as

$$W'(T,\lambda_1 \rightarrow \lambda_2) = \varepsilon(T)\int_{\lambda_1}^{\lambda_2} W_\lambda(T)d\lambda \quad [Wm^{-2}]. \quad (7)$$

Significance of IR Radiometry in Medicine

Non-contact thermometry by purely optical coupling between the object and the sensor, without physically contacting the object and/or perturbing the temperature field, provides convenience and feasibility when objects of interest are mechanically, electrically, physiologically or chemically fragile, or present a mechanical, electrical, chemical, biological or nuclear hazard [5].

Under standard environmental conditions thermal patterns that exist on exposed surfaces of objects are determined largely by the heat transferred to the surface from within the object or by EM radiation onto the object. Because IR thermometry, also referred to as IR radiometry, is entirely passive, making use *only* of the radiant energy spontaneously emitted by the object itself, it is entirely harmless to the object and may be used freely and as frequently as desired [1]. Therefore, it has been universally accepted as a powerful tool for non-destructive testing and diagnosis of problems in many fields, materials science, civil and aerospace engineering, zoology, and botany to name a few [6–8].

Although controversial, the emissivities of human tissues are in general considered to approach unity throughout the spectral region from about 2.5 to 15.0 μm, and the measured temperature is the actual surface temperature [3, 9]. A well-designed IR radiation instrument sensitive in one of the above-mentioned wavelength bands will thus be capable of measuring either the surface temperature or surface temperature differences of human tissue.

The diagnostic capability of IR radiation in medical applications is based on the following assumptions, most of which are proven facts [1, 10]: (1) all biological media above absolute zero emit diffuse IR radiation as an exponential function of their temperatures; (2) the emissive power of biological media may be optically collected, transduced into electrical signals, amplified, processed and displayed as

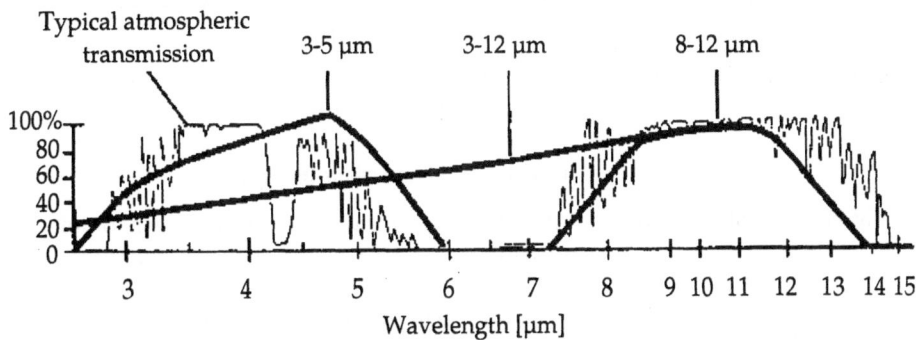

Fig. 1. Transmission of energy through typical atmosphere at sea level over a 0.3-km path a 26 °C and 5.7 mm precipitable water and the typical response of available IR detectors. Note that transmission varies primarily with optical path length and the concentrations of water and carbon dioxide in the atmosphere (modified from [4])

desired; (3) pigmentations such as are found in and on the tissues of different races, and in nipple areas, blemishes, sun tan, and the like do not alter the emissivity of the tissues; (4) the thermal patterns that occur on the surface of the tissue are generated largely by (4a) vascular patterns underneath, (4b) localized conditions of the tissue surface, such as necrosis and irritation, and (4c) thermal insult from outside the body, and temperature fields can be calculated using the heat conduction equation given as

$$\nabla^2 T(x,y,z,t) + \frac{Q_S(x,y,z,t)}{k^{\mathrm{app}}} = \frac{1}{\alpha} \frac{\partial T(x,y,z,t)}{\partial t} \quad [\mathrm{Km}^{-2}]$$

(8)

where T is the absolute temperature of tissue, $Q_s(x,y,z,t)$ [W/m^3] the heat source term in space-time domain incorporating metabolic heat and thermal insult from outside the body, and k^{app} [W/m-°C] and α [m^2/s] are the apparent thermal conductivity and the thermal diffusivity of tissue, respectively. k^{app} incorporates thermal conductivity, and heat losses due to blood perfusion within the tissue and convective heat transfer at the tissue/air interface.

IR Radiometers for Medical Applications

The first IR radiometer for skin temperature measurements was reported by Hardy in the 1930s [11]. Since then a number of radiometers and scanners have been developed to determine surface temperatures, with resolutions varying from 10 to 0.1 °C. Scanning IR radiometers have been developed to provide two-dimensional thermal maps of extended areas of a surface, called thermograms.

Definitions

A *radiometer* is a spot-measuring instrument to collect and measure EM radiation.

A *radiation thermometer* is a radiometer calibrated to indicate the temperature of a black body.

A *calibrated IR radiometer* senses the radiant flux from a target body of known emissivity and generates an output signal proportional to the surface temperature of that body.

Design Considerations

An IR radiometer generally consists of three basic parts:
- *Optics* for collection and focusing of the IR radiation on a detector,
- A *detector* to transduce the EM radiation into an electronic signal,
- An *electronic system* for signal processing.

In most IR systems the collecting and focusing part consists of optical components, such as optical fibers, lenses and mirrors. Greater accuracy can be achieved by alternately detecting the radiation from the source being measured and the radiation from a reference source. In this way errors due to detector responsivity drifts can be eliminated.

Common IR radiometer designs involve amplitude modulation (AM) of the IR radiation before it is collected by a detector. An AM modulated signal produced at detector output allows the use of limited bandwidth signal amplifiers to reduce electrical noise.

Signal processing is an essential part of an IR radiometer. Detection of very low level signals, such as the weak IR radiation of at most a few microwatts (10^{-6} W) emitted from objects at 0–100 °C, and suppression of broad band noise, such as the EM waves in free space and 50 or 60 Hz interference, requires synchronous heterodyne detection of the AM modulated IR signal. A lock-in amplifier (LIA) functions as a sharp band-pass filter by rejecting all other signals than the signals about the modulation frequency. Finally, a low pass filter (LPF) is employed for envelope detection of AM modulated temperature signals (see Fig. 2).

Significance of Temperature Feedback Control for Laser-Assisted Tissue Welding

Laser-Assisted Tissue Welding

Laser-assisted tissue welding (LTW) has been investigated as a surgical tool to improve the anastomosis of severed blood vessels, nerves and a variety of hollow organs. LTW can (1) provide immediate fluid-tight sealing, (2) reduce foreign-body reaction associated with healing around sutures, (3) preserve the mechanical integrity of the "weld" site, and (4) achieve successful anastomosis rates comparable to those of conventional suture techniques [12–14]. However, extensive training is required to form reproducibly successful bonds. The lack of satisfactory objective criteria for optimal laser exposure parameters required to produce an immediately durable weld has long been regarded as a major limitation of LTW [12, 15–19].

Photothermal Interactions During LTW

Absorption of laser light results in the generation of a distributive heat source in tissue. If sufficient laser energy is deposited, tissue components are thermally denatured. The thermal denaturation of proteins is believed to be the principal mechanism of heat-mediated welding and sealing of ruptured organs [16, 17, 20, 21]. Experience has shown that excessive irradiation may result in more thermal damage than needed for the "laser-induced" bond, while inadequate heat deposition results in tissue dehydration without effective fusion [12, 15, 17].

Temporal profiles of tissue temperature depend not only on irradiation parameters but also the optical and thermal properties of the tissue being irradiated. These properties are not constant and may quickly and dramatically change during laser irradiation [21–24]. Dehydration lowers thermal conductivity [25–28], which in turn tends to drastically increase local temperatures. In addition, light scattering is increased and often absorption is slightly decreased as a consequence of thermal damage [29–34]. As tissue dehydrates, laser-induced temperatures may exceed 100 °C before a surgeon can respond to visual changes in the tissue.

Rationale for Thermal Feedback Control

Surgeons typically look for subtle visual clues on the tissue surface, such as whitening, desiccation and shrinkage, as an endpoint for completion of a photothermal weld. Thus, success rates very much depend on surgical experience, subjective visual feedback and motor reflexes on the part of the surgeon. Ideally, automated dosimetry should be based upon indicators of thermal damage during laser irradiation. Yet, as the temperature and extent of coagulation along the severed edges *and* inside the tissue being irradiated are practically impossible to monitor, models were developed to determine dosimetry parameters prior to treatment, using simulations. Such models use optical and thermal properties of tissues to predict the photothermal response of tissues

[35]. Experience has shown that light penetrates less as tissue coagulates and dehydrates, leading to dramatic temperature increases [21, 24, 29, 30, 33, 34, 36]. In other words, both optical and thermal properties are functions of temperature and hydration levels inside the tissue during LTW. Therefore, computationally intensive real-time in vivo measurement of optical and thermal properties is required for simulation and open and/or closed loop control of photothermal coagulation.

On the other hand, denaturation has long been recognized as a rate process governed by the local temperature-time response hypothesized to be an indicator of tissue status during LTW [37, 38]. Since rate processes are exponential with temperature and linear with time, it is believed that regulation of tissue surface temperature at a quasi-constant level will result in a constant rate of denaturation. This narrow margin surface temperature feedback control (TFC), in return, will eliminate exponential increases in the rate of denaturation associated with excessive thermal insult, i.e., rapidly increasing temperatures.

Temperature Feedback Control Systems

Research Groups

Research on real-time dosimetry control for LTW in vivo has been carried out by several groups affiliated with (1) Tel Aviv University (TAU), (2) the University of Texas (UT), (3) ABIOMED R & D (ARD) and Harvard Medical School (HMS), and most recently, (4) Lawrence Livermore National Laboratory (LLNL) and the University of California (UC). In the current versions of their TFC systems, the TAU, UT, ARD and

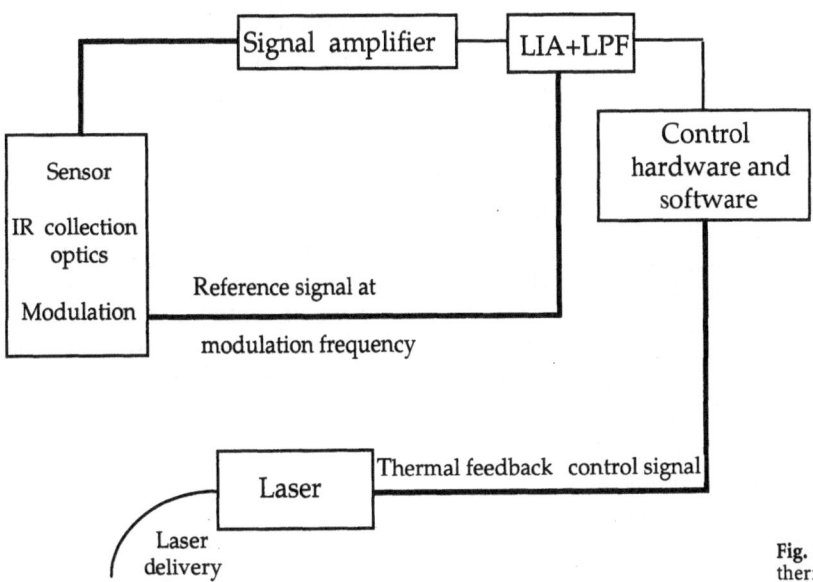

Fig. 2. Hardware block diagram for thermal feedback-controlled laser delivery. *LIA*, lock-in amplifier; *LPF*, low-pass filter

Table 1. Comparison of dosimetry control systems

System	Laser spot size (mm)	Detector range (µm)	Field of view (mm)	Response time (ms)	Accuracy (°C)	Laser irradiation control logic
Tel Aviv University (TAU) [39, 40]	= Field of view	2–20	= Spot size	> 100	0.2	On-off control of laser power
University of Texas (UT) [41]	1.5–2	2–5	0.75	50	1	On-off control with external laser beam shutter
ARD [42, 45]	0.7–1	8–13	0.4	~ 30	1	Laser output power adjustment
LLNL-UC [43]	3	2–6/2–12	1	~ 30	1	On-off control with external laser beam shutter; more recently, laser output power adjustment

ARD, ABIOMED R & D and Harvard Medical School; LLNL-UC, Lawrence Livermore National Laboratory and University of California.

LLNL-UC groups incorporated temperature sensing and laser delivery into the same "temperature sensor/laser delivery" housing for laboratory experiments [39–43]. The hardware block diagram of a sample thermal dosimetry control system is shown in Fig. 2 and a comparison of different sensing and delivery schemes in Fig. 3. Specifications of different TFC systems are compared and contrasted in Table 1.

While the UT group developed a co-aligned/confocal device, the TAU, ARD and LLNL-UC groups developed handpieces for experimental work in a hospital environment and for clinical trials. The TAU and LLNL-UC devices rely on all-fiberoptic temperature sensing and delivery [39, 40, 43]; in contrast, the ARD surgical handpiece delivers laser light with an optical fiber, but sensing is optical [42]; and the UT device is all-optical [41].

Description of TFC Systems

The TAU group developed an all-fiberoptic radiometric system for TFC of CO_2-laser-assisted LTW. A simplified diagram of their experimental setup is shown in Fig. 3 (a). A silver-halide fiber was used for laser delivery onto the tissue surface. IR radiation emitted by the irradiated tissue was collected by another silver-halide fiber, optically focused onto a photonic thermal detector and electronically processed by system hardware and software. Both delivery and collection fibers were held together using a holder to face the same spot and positioned 1 mm above the tissue surface to achieve maximal radiometric signal. The radiometric signal was processed by software and hardware to provide a feedback signal for on/off control of the laser and duty cycle adjustment of laser irradiation to achieve a stable tissue surface temperature [39, 40].

The UT group developed a stationary confocal laser delivery/temperature sensing device looking down on the specimen to be welded. Laser energy is delivered through an optical fiber and focused on the site of laser impact by optical components as shown in Fig. 3 (b). Temperature signals are collected from a field of view of 0.7 mm at the center of a 2- to 3-mm-diameter laser spot. The temperature signal is processed by control system hardware to provide a feedback signal for on/off control of a laser shutter placed on the laser beam path to adjust the duty cycle of laser irradiation and thus to achieve quasi-constant tissue surface temperature [41, 44].

ARD developed a microprocessor-based control system for temperature data acquisition and real-time laser power control. Fiberoptic laser delivery and optical IR radiometer were incorporated into a handheld surgical handpiece. A simplified diagram of their system is shown in Fig. 3 (c) [42, 45].

The LLNL-UC group developed an IR thermometer using a hollow glass optical fiber to collect IR radiation and a silica optical fiber for laser delivery. Like the design implemented by researchers at TAU, a handpiece containing the sensing and delivery fibers at a small angle is used by the operator to perform feedback-controlled LTW. The temperature signal is processed by the control system to provide a feedback signal for on/off control of a laser shutter placed on the laser beam path to achieve quasi-constant tissue surface temperature during LTW [43].

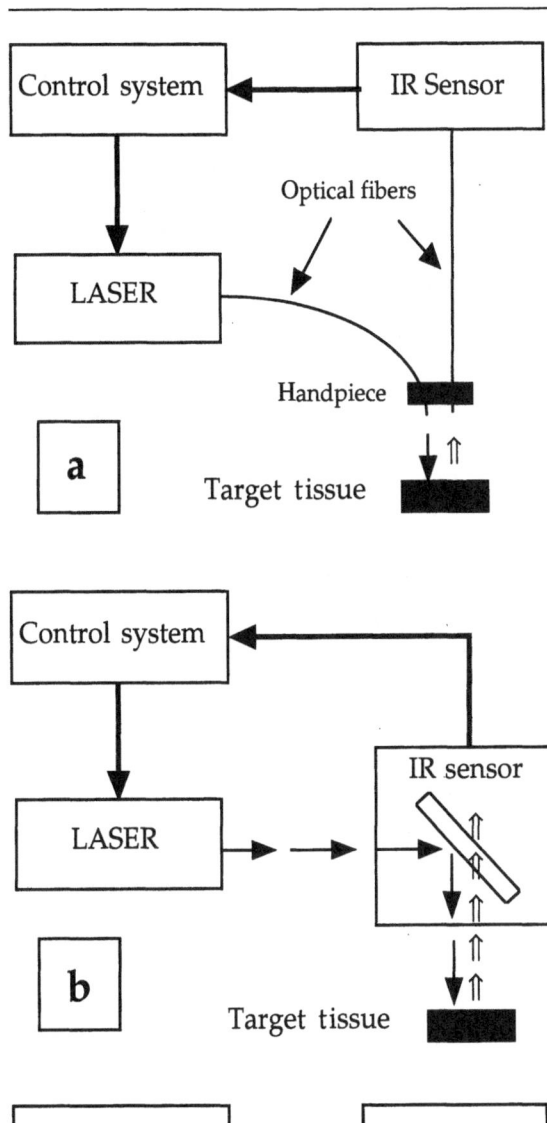

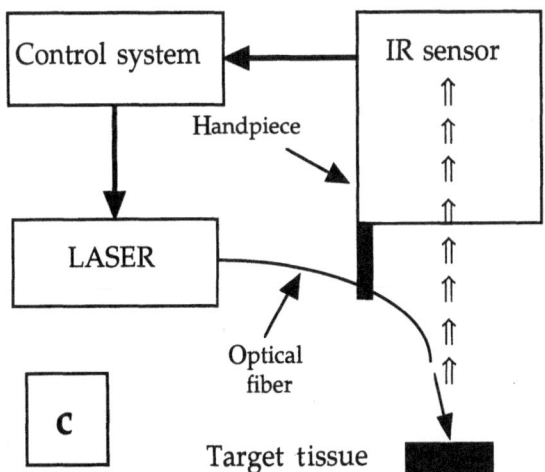

Fig. 3. Simplified diagrams of various dosimetry control systems: *a* Tel Aviv University and Lawrence Livermore National Laboratory – University of California systems, *b* University of Texas system, *c* ABIOMED R & D system

References

[1] Barnes, R (1968) Diagnostic thermotherapy. Appl Optics 7:1673–1685

[2] DeWitt D, Incropera F, Nutter GD (eds) (1988) Physics of thermal radiation. In: Theory and practice of radiation thermometry. New York, Wiley-Intescience, 21–88

[3] Incropera F, Witt D (1990) Fundamentals of heat and mass transfer. Wiley, New York

[4] Yates H, Taylor J (1960) Infrared transmission of atmosphere. ASTIA AD 240188. US Naval Research Laboratories, Washington, DC, (NRL report 5453)

[5] Yoder J (1968) Temperature measurement with an infrared microsope. Appl Optics 7:1791–1796

[6] Gates, D (1968) Sensing biological environments with a portable radiation thermometer. Appl Optics 7:1803–1809

[7] Hudson R Jr (1969) Infrared system engineering. Wiley Interscience, New York

[8] Sundstrom E (1968) Wide-angle infrared camera for industry and medicine. Appl Optics 7:1763–1768

[9] Shitzer, A, Eberhart R (eds) (1982) Heat transfer in medicine and biology, vol 2. Plenum, New York

[10] Shitzer A, Eberhart R (eds) (1982) Thermography in medical diagnosis. In: Heat transfer in medicine and biology, vol 2. Plenum, New York

[11] Hardy J, Soderstrom G (1937) An improved apparatus for measuring surface and body temperature. Rev Sci Instrum 8:419–422

[12] Neblett C, Morris J, Thomsen S (1986) Laser-assisted microsurgical anastomosis. Neurosurgery 19:914–934

[13] Costello A, Johnson D, Wishnow K (1990) Comparison of sutureless argon- and neodymium:YAG-welded ileo-ileal anastomosis using a biodegradable intraluminal stent. Proc SPIE 1200:33–37

[14] Dalsing M, Parker C, Kueppers P, Griffith S, Davis T (1992) Laser and suture anastomosis: passive compliance and active force production. Lasers Surg Med 12:190–198

[15] Quigley M, Bailes J, Kwaan H, Cerullo L, Brown J, Lastre C, Monma D (1985) Microvascular anastomosis using the milliwatt CO_2 laser. Lasers Surg Med 5:357–365

[16] Sorensen E, Thomsen S, Welch A, Badeau A (1987) Morphological and surface temperature changes in femoral arteries following laser irradiation. Lasers Surg Med 7:249–257

[17] Thomsen S, Morris J, Neblett C, Mueller J (1987) Tissue welding using a low microsurgical energy CO_2 laser. Med Instrum 21:231–237

[18] Flemming A, Colles M, Guillianotti R, Brough M, Brown S (1988) Laser assisted microvascular anastomosis of arteries and veins: laser tissue welding. Br J Plast Surg 41:378–388

[19] Costello A, Johnson D, Cromeens D, Wishnow K, von Eschenbach A, Ro J (1990) Sutureless end-to-end bowel anastomosis using Nd:YAG and water-soluble intaluminal stent. Lasers Surg Med 10: 179–184

[20] Murray L, Su L, Kopchok G, White R (1989) Crosslinking of extracellular matrix proteins: a preliminary report on a possible mechanism of argon laser welding. Lasers Surg Med 9: 490–496

[21] Thomsen S (1991) Pathologic analysis of photothermal and photomechanical effects of laser-tissue interactions. Photochem Photobiol 53: 825–835

[22] Thomsen S, Jacques S, Flock S (1990) Microscopic correlates of microscopic optical property changes during thermal coagulation of myocardium. Proc SPIE 1202:2–11

[23] Thomsen S, Vijverberg H, Hunag R, Schwartz J (1993) Changes in optical properties of rat skin during thermal coagulation. Proc SPIE 1882:230–236

[24] Jaywant S, Wilson B, Patterson M, Lilge L, Flotte T, Woolsey J, McCulloch C (1993) Temperature dependent changes in the optical absorption and scattering spectra of tissue: correlation with ultrastructure. Proc SPIE 1882:218–229

[25] Takata A, Zaneldi L, Richter W (1977) Laser induced thermal damage to skin. Final report. USAF School of Aerospace Medicine. (SAM-TR-77-38)

[26] Spells K (1960) The thermal conductivities of some biological media. Phys Med Biol 5:139–153

[27] Cooper T, Trezek G (1971) Correlation of thermal properties of some human tissue with water content. Aerospace Med 42:24–47

[28] Duck F (ed) (1990) Thermal properties of tissue. In: Physical properties of tissue, Academic Press, London, pp 9–42

[29] Derbyshire G, Bogen D, Unger M (1990) Thermally induced optical property changes in myocardium at 1064 nm. Lasers Surg Med 10:28–34

[30] Splinter R, Stevenson R, Littmann L, Tunfelder J, Chuang C, Tatsis G, Thompson M (1991) Optical properties of normal, diseased, and laser photocoagulated myocardium at the Nd:YAG wavelength. Lasers Surg Med 11:117–124

[31] Chambettaz F, Clivaz X, Marquis F, Salathé R (1991) Temperature variations of reflection, transmission, and fluorescence of the arterial wall. Proc SPIE 1427:134–140

[32] Chambettaz F, Marquis-Weible F, Salathé R (1992) Effect of dehydration on optical properties of tissue. Proc SPIE 1646:383–390

[33] Chambettaz F, Marquis-Weible F, Salathé R (1993) Temperature dependence of reflectance and transmittance of the artery exposed to air during laser irradiation. IEEE Trans Biomed Eng 40:105–107

[34] Çilesiz I, Welch A (1993) Light dosimetry: effects of dehydration and thermal damage on the optical properties of human aorta. Appl Optics 32:477–487

[35] Torres J, Motamedi M, Pearce J, Welch A (1993) Experimental evaluation of mathematical models for predicting the thermal response of tissue to laser irradiation. Appl Optics 32:597–606

[36] Agah R, Gandjbakhche A, Motamedi M, Nossal R, Bonner R (1996) Dynamics of temperature dependent optical properties of tissue:dependence on thermally induced alteration. IEEE Trans Biomed Eng 43:839–846

[37] Moritz A, Henriques F (1947) Studies in thermal injury II: the relative importance of time and surface temperature in the causation of cutaneous burns. Am J Path 23:695–720

[38] Pearce J, Thomsen S, Welch AJ, van Gemert MJC (eds) (1995) Rate process analysis of thermal damage. In: Optical thermal response of laser-irradiated tissue, Plenum Press, New York, pp 561–606

[39] Shenfeld O, Ophir E, Goldwasser B, Katzir A (1994) Silver halide fiber optic radiometric temperature measurement and control of CO_2 laser-irradiated tissues and application to tissue welding. Lasers Surg Med 14:323–328

[40] Eyal O, Zur A, Shenfeld O, Gilo M, Katzir A (1994) Infrared radiometry using silver halide fibers and a cooled photonic detector. Optic Eng 33: 502–509

[41] Çilesiz I, Thomsen S, Welch A (1997) Controlled temperature tissue fusion: argon laser welding of rat intestine in vivo, part I. Lasers Surg Med 21:269–277

[42] Stewart R, Benbrahim A, La Muraglia G, Rosenberg M, L'Italien G, Assott W, Kung R (1996) Laser assisted vascular welding with real time temperature control. Lasers Surg Med 19:9–16

[43] Small W, IV (4th) Celliers P, Silva L, Matthews D, Stolz B (1997) Two-color infrared thermometer for low temperature measurement using a hollow glass optical fiber. Proc SPIE 2977:115–120

[44] Çilesiz I, Thomsen S, Welch A, Chan E (1997) Controlled temperature tissue fusion: Ho:YAG laser welding of rat intestine in vivo, part II. Lasers Surg Med 21:278–286

[45] Poppas D, Stewart R, Massicotte M, Wolga A, Kung R, Retik A, Freeman M (1996) Temperature-controlled laser photocoagulation of soft tissue: in vivo evaluation using a tissue welding model. Lasers Surg Med 18:335–344

Tissue Discrimination and Selectivity in Laser Application

J. RAUNEST

Physical Aspects of Laser-Tissue Interaction

Laser irradiation of tissue samples leads to the phenomena of absorption, transmission, scattering and remittance. The light propagation in tissue determines the efficiency of laser exposure, creating more or less extended coagulation and tissue ablation effects. In addition to wavelength and specific output characteristics, laser-induced tissue alterations are critically dependent on the optical properties of the tissue. Chromophore and water content must be regarded as the most important correlates for optical tissue characterization. Distinction in the biochemical composition of different articular tissue classes, such as hyaline cartilage and fibrocartilage, as well as normal and degenerated tissue, such as healthy and malacic cartilage, may serve the purpose of selective or at least preferential tissue ablation in laser surgery [14].

The specific optical properties can be described in terms of optical density (OD), absorption (K) and back scattering (S). The optical density can be determined by analysis of transmission spectra. The values of I (transmission in the tissue area of interest), I_0 (transmission of the specimen assembly outside the tissue area) and the dark current of the system I_D have to be measured by photomultipliers. Optical density OD is calculated as

$$OD = \log\left[(I_0 - I_D) / (I - I_D)\right]. \qquad (1)$$

For determination of scattering and absorption coefficients, a model for light propagation in turbid and absorbing media was introduced by Kubelka and Munk [9, 10]. Figure 1 presents this model which separates light within the tissue into two diffuse fluxes propagating into (I) and outwards (J) from the sample. Remittance is defined as

$$R = J_0 / I_0. \qquad (2)$$

Depending on the thickness dx of the specimen, transmittance is calculated as

$$T = I_D / I_0 \qquad (3)$$

The model defines absorption (K) and scattering (S) coefficients and describes light propagation by the equations:

$$dI / dx = SI - KI + SJ \text{ and} \qquad (4)$$

$$dJ / dx = SJ + KJ - SI. \qquad (5)$$

With the values of remittance (R), transmittance (T), and thickness of the tissue sample (D), scattering and absorption coeffients S and K can be calculated as:

$$S = 1 / D \left[(1 + R^2 - T^2 / 2R)^2 - 1\right]^{-} \\ \times \cot^{-1}\{(1 - R^2 + T^2) / \\ \left[(1 + R^2 - T^2 / 2R)^2 - 1\right]^{-1/2}\} \qquad (6)$$

and

$$K = S\{[(1 + R^2 - T^2) / 2R] - 1\}. \qquad (7)$$

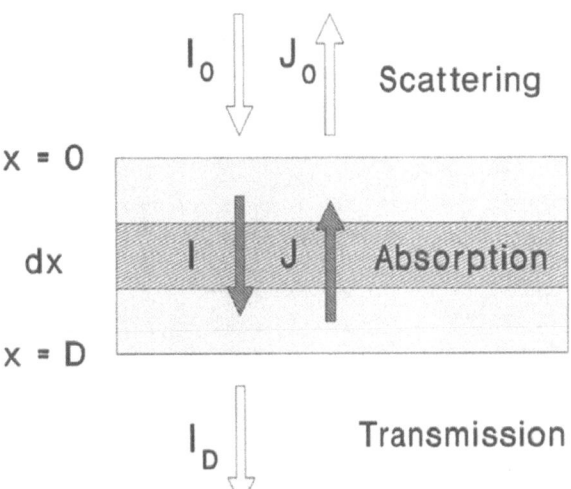

Fig. 1. Model of light propagation in tissue according to Kubelka and Munk [9, 10]. I_0 is the incident light, J_0 is the remitted light, I_D is the transmitted light, and D is the thickness of the specimen. Under the assumption that light is propagated diffusely through the tissue, changes in I und J can be described with differential equations. Concerning boundary conditions these equations can be solved for incident radiation (I_0), transmittance (I_D/I_0), and remittance (J_0/I_0) to give absorption and scattering coefficients in terms of measurable quantities.

For a very small value of T, such as in regions of high absorption or in a thick tissue sample, Eq. 7 can be approximated to

$$K = S\,[(1 - R)^2 \,/\, 2R]. \tag{8}$$

One of the most obvious shortcomings in the model presented above is that it ignores remittance and refraction phenomena occurring at the tissue boundaries. Furthermore, the model assumes that inhomogeneities within the sample are small, that scattering is symmetric, and that the incident light is diffuse. However, these errors from inadaquate modeling are likely to be small because absorption is much greater than scattering in cartilage and synovial tissues. This assumption is corroborated by calculations based upon experiments performed in vascular tissue presenting a close agreement between the S and K coefficients and calculations according to Beer's law, which completely ignores scattering phenomena [15].

Optical Properties of Articular Tissue

Figure 2 shows the experimental setup for the determination of optical density [16, 17]. For transmission spectroscopy, an ultraviolet transmission microscope is employed in combination with a xenon high-pressure light source and a prism monochromator. The monochromatic light is projected on the object stage of the microscope. After being collected by a glycerol immersion objective the transmitted light is projected onto a photomultiplier tube with the area of the tissue analyzed restricted by a luminous field stop. The amplified signal of the photomultiplier is digitized and recorded on a computer also controlling the wavelength and slit width of the monochromator by stepping motors.

For the measurement of total transmission and diffuse reflection an integrating sphere setup is necessary (Fig. 3). The light from a xenon lamp passes through a prism monochromator and then monochromatic light is projected onto the tissue

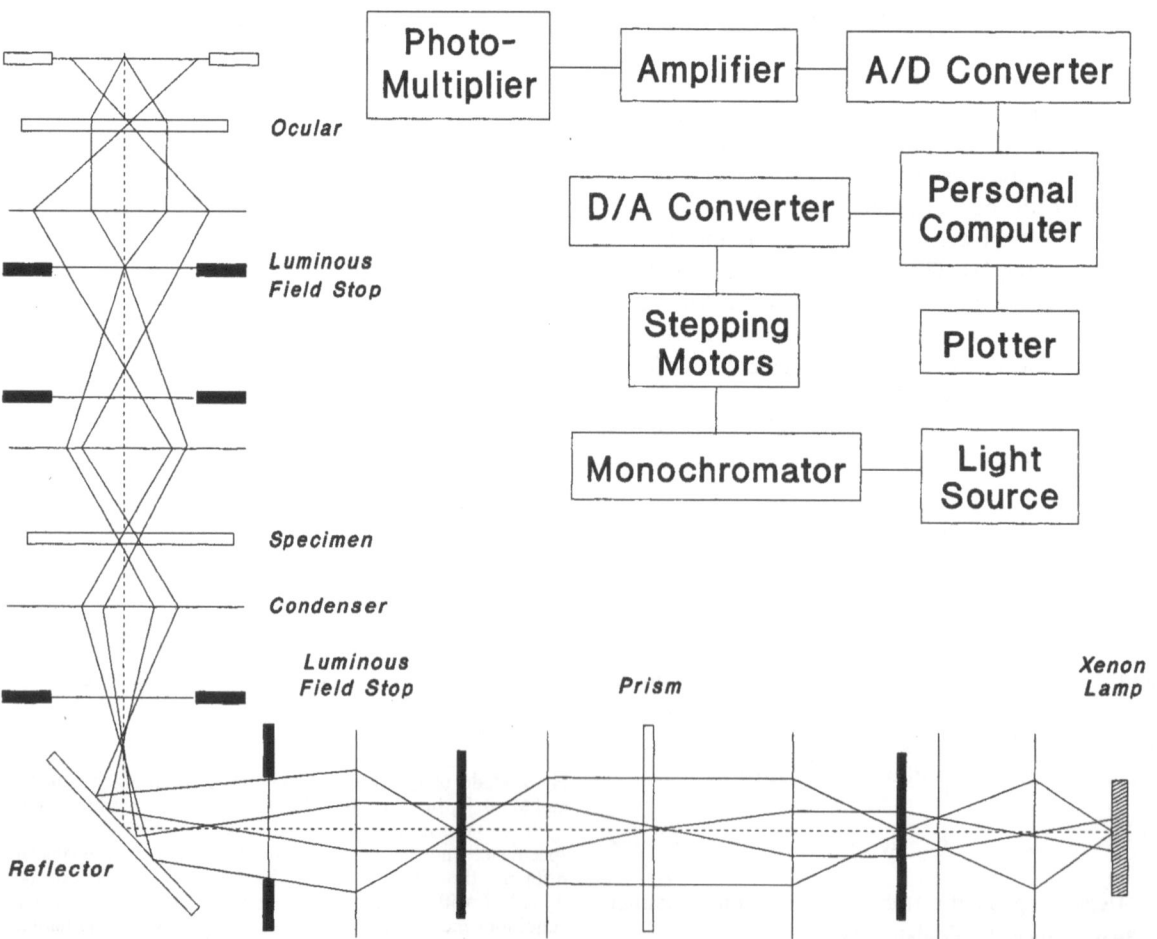

Fig. 2. Experimental setup for measurement of optical tissue density related to spectral range. Modified according to Schwarzmaier et al. [17, 18]

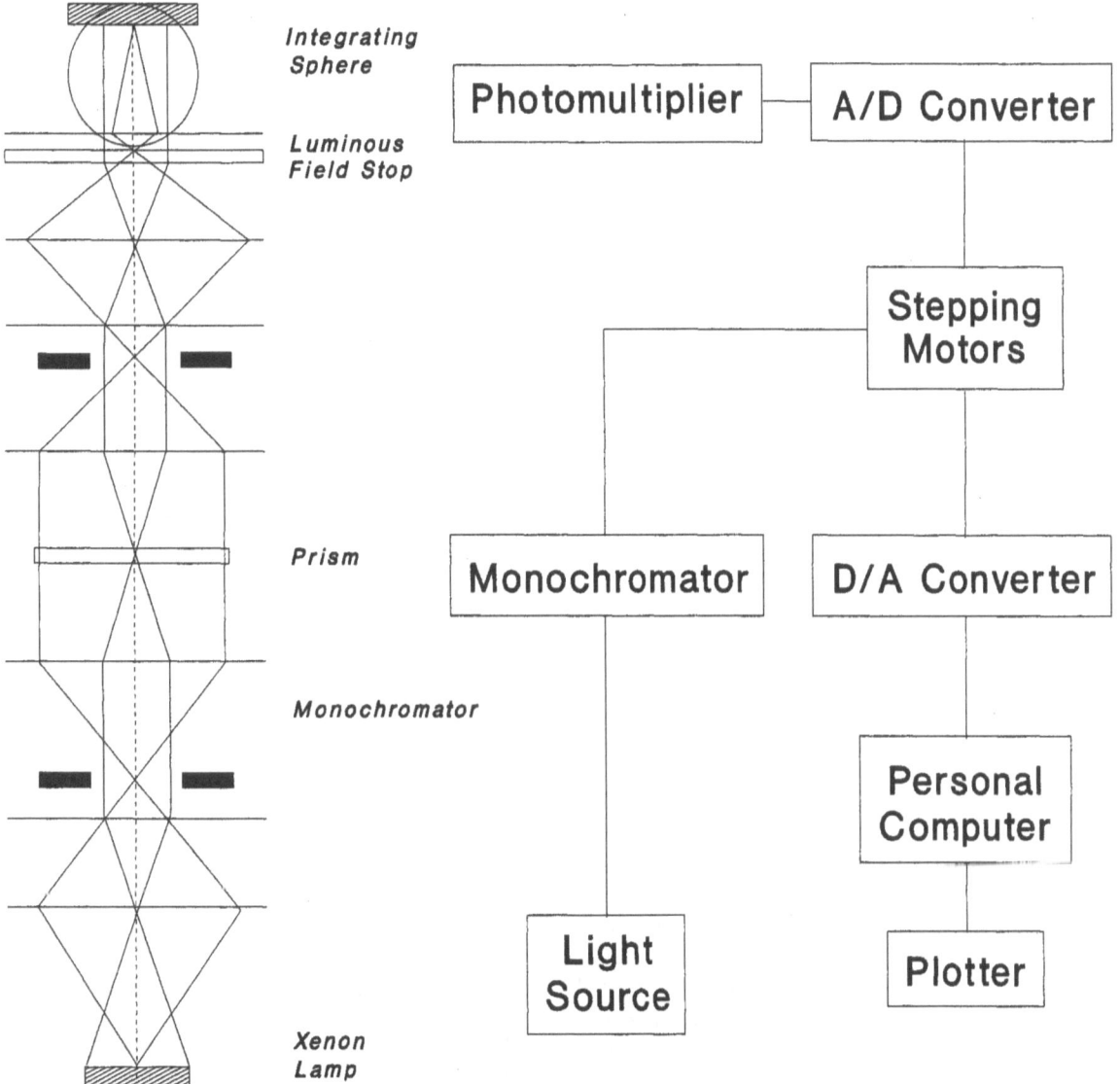

Fig. 3. Experimental setup for the measurement of diffuse tissue reflection. Technique according to Prince and Schwarzmaier [15, 18]

sample. The transmitted light is measured within an integrating sphere by a photomultiplier. For the determination of diffuse reflection, the tissue sample covers the hole where light leaves the integrating sphere. Measurements are performed by a photomultiplier tube positioned in the path of the sample beam within the integrating sphere [15, 20].

The results of the digitized and averaged spectra for articular tissue structures are presented in Fig. 4. In normal hyaline cartilage, transmission spectra exhibit increased absorption at 280 nm. After a trough at 260 nm, the optical densities increase again with shorter wavelengths towards the ultraviolet end of the spectrum analyzed. Over the whole visible spectral range, the optical density curves steadily decrease, with no other relevant chromophores being present between 320 and 770 nm. Compared to hyaline cartilage, mensical tissue exhibits a 30 % increased optical density. It also exhibits maxima in the ultraviolet spectrum. However, there is no second absorption maximum at 280 nm common to spectra obtained from hyaline cartilage. Towards the infrared end of the spectrum analyzed, synovium exhibits a 1.2-fold higher optical density over meniscal tissue and a 1.6-fold higher density over hyaline cartilage [16].

The optical densities of normal and degenerated hyaline cartilage are shown in Fig. 5. With increasing degeneration an augmentation in optical density can be observed over the entire spectral range examined. The relative optical density, defined as the relation in optical densities of degenerated cartilage to normal

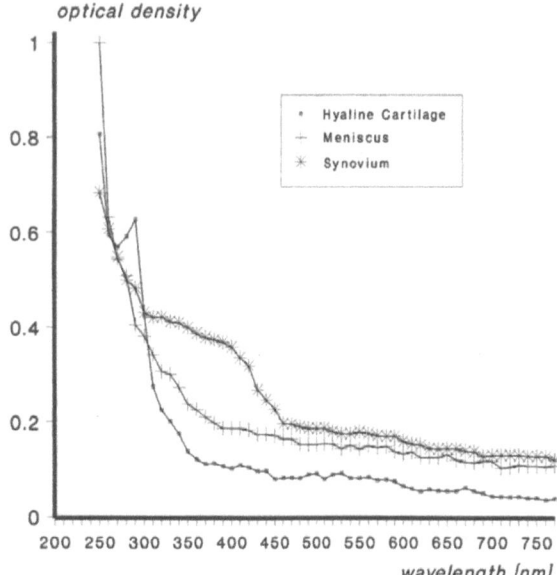

Fig. 4. Optical densities of normal hyaline cartilage, meniscus, and synovium measured by microspectrophotometry

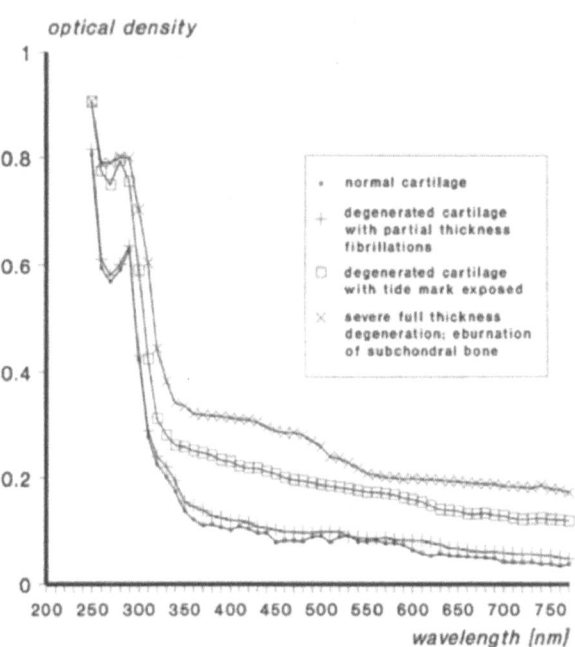

Fig. 5. Discrimination of optical tissue properties in hyaline cartilage. Correlation between the degree of degeneration and optical density

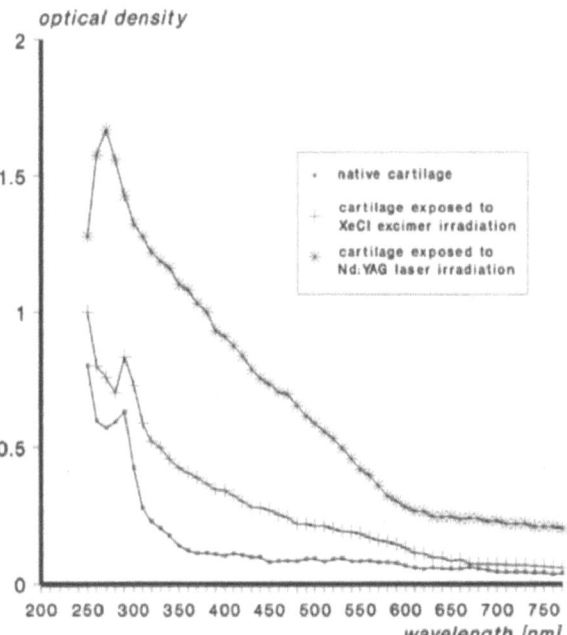

Fig. 6. Modification of optical tissue properties by exposure with ablative and thermal lasers

tissue at the respective wavelength, shows a significant increase towards the infrared end of the spectrum analyzed.

Spectroscopic analysis of optical properties in biological tissue is one of the key issues in determining mechanisms of laser-tissue interaction. These models were intended to predict thermal energy deposition in tissue, suggesting subsequent tissue removal. Furthermore, tissue-specific absorption characteristics related to the spectral range of the transmitted light may contribute to the problem of selective tissue ablation [22]. In respect of articular tissue, Vangsness et al. [21] have analyzed absorption characteristics of meniscal tissue in a spectral range from 300 to 2500 nm resulting in a uniform spectrum for both normal and degenerated tissue. Based on equivalent results measured from water, the authors concluded that light absorption is mainly affected by the water content of the tissue in the infrared portion of the spectrum. At the ultraviolet range of the spectrum, however, articular tissue structures reveal significantly differing absorption maxima for the respective tissue structures due to optical interaction by amino acids, nucleic acids, and amide groups, which allow a differentiation of hyaline cartilage, meniscal tissue, and synovial membrane including the respective histopathologic subtypes.

However, ablation and coagulation effects induced by pulsed ultraviolet and continuous wave lasers relate to optical properties provided not by native tissue but by irradiated tissue structures [18]. Figure 6 presents the modification of optical tissue characteristics in a hyaline cartilage specimen exposed to XeCl

excimer and Nd:YAG laser irradiation. Nd:YAG laser coagulation leads to substantial changes in optical tissue properties with a wavelength-dependent 2- to 9.5-fold increase in optical density in a spectral range extending from 250 to 770 nm by coagulation and carbonization activity. Hyaline cartilage exposed to XeCl excimer laser irradiation exhibits an increased optical density over native tissue preferentially in the ultraviolet and parts of the visible spectral range. The transmission properties in excimer-irradiated areas differ substantially from data obtained following Nd:YAG laser exposure. In spite of significant modifications in optical tissue properties by laser irradiation, some tissue features remain unchanged, especially with the use of ablative laser systems, and corroborate the hypothesis that optical tissue characteristics may form a basis for preferential laser application. Furthermore, data obtained from spectral analysis may contribute to the selection of appropriate laser systems in articular surgery [7, 19].

Feedback Systems for Selective Laser Ablation

In addition to optical tissue properties characterized in terms of absorption, remittance, and scattering, laser-induced fluorescence seems to be another important feature of laser-tissue interaction. The observation of fluorescence emission spectra is based upon the existence of fluorophores, which are defined as an idividual molecular group or bond that has a nonzero fluorescence quantum yield. The preequisite for recording fluorescence emission

scans is the excitation of tissue at a distinct wavelength by laser irradiation (Fig. 7). For fluorescence analysis, tissue samples must present fluorophores in sufficient concentrations, which appreciably absorb the excitation beam and have a reasonable quantum for fluorescence. Although articular tissues contain a number of potentially observable chromophores, only a few contribute to the fluorescence spectrum obtained at a single wavelength [11]. So the fluorescence bands observed differ widely depending on the spectral range of tissue excitation. Concerning hyaline cartilage and meniscal tissue, a suitable excitation wavelength seems to be the ultraviolet and near-ultraviolet range [13].

With the help of fluorescence emission spectroscopy, quantitative analysis of the tissue scans allows fibrocartilage to be distinguished from hyaline cartilage (Fig. 8). The few studies concerned with the monitoring of fluorescence emission scans in human articular tissue present widely differing and in some respects contradictory results. The divergence in fluorescence profiles may be explained by the variable experimental designs, especially concerning the spectral range of laser excitation and the laser tissue interface [12].

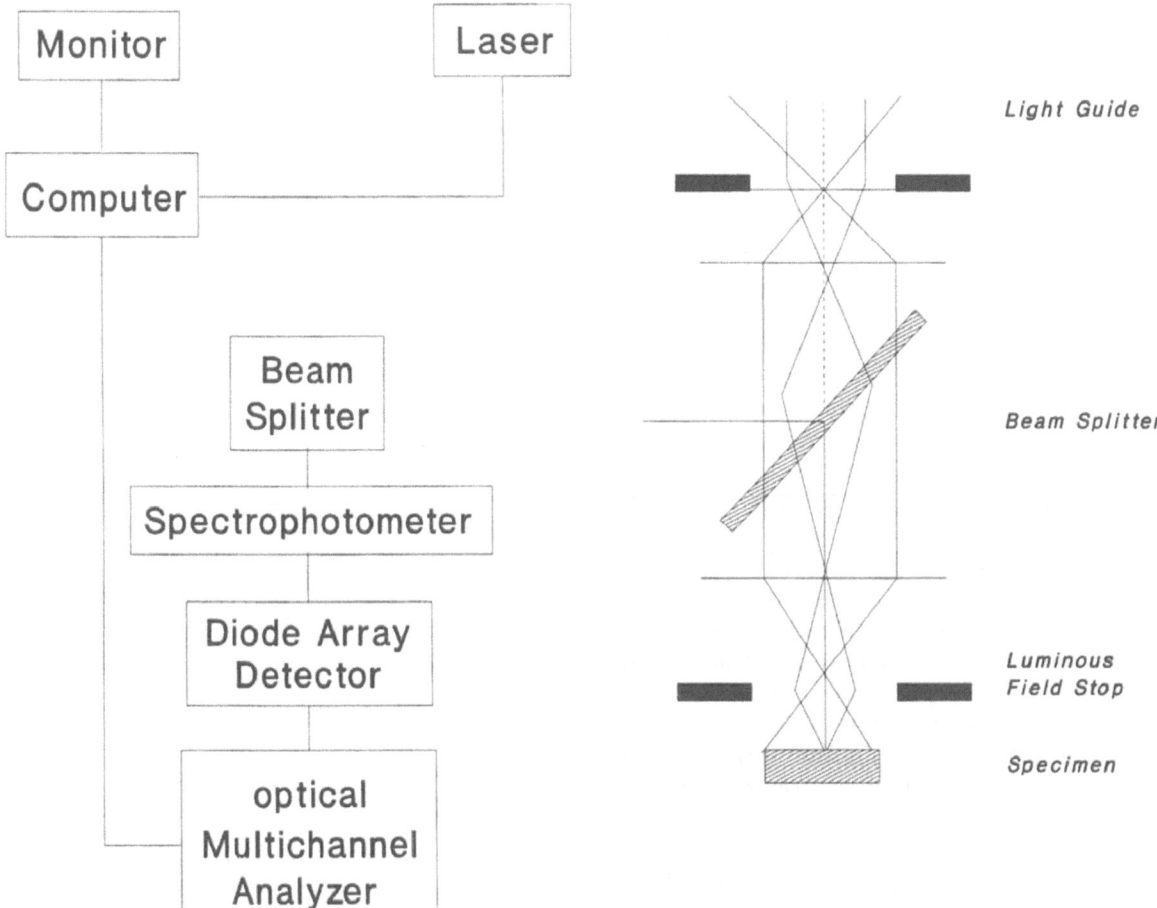

Fig. 7. Diagram of a laser-induced fluorescence spectroscopy system

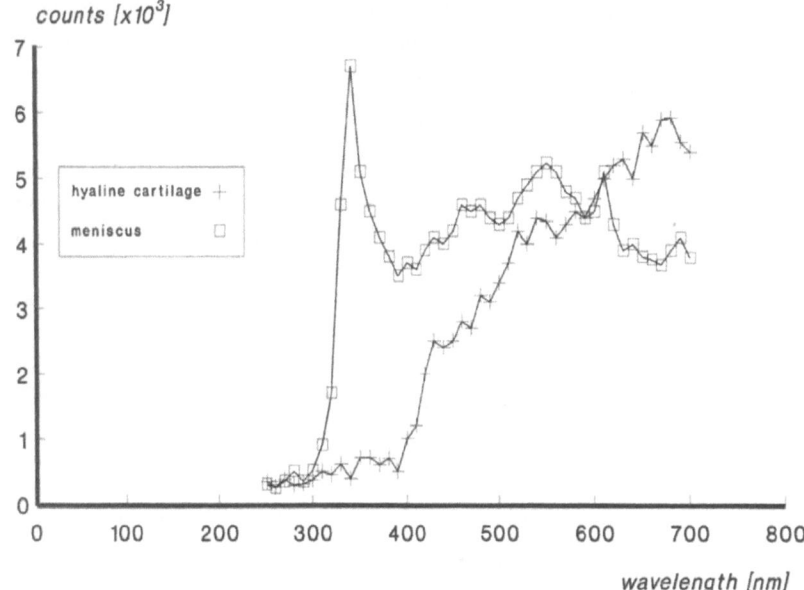

Fig. 8. Typical fluorescence spectra obtained from a hyaline cartilage and meniscus specimen

The laser-induced fluorescence pattern reflects the content and distribution of biochemical compounds in a tissue structure, so the fluorescence scan yields quantitative biochemical and morphological in vivo information about the tissue composition [1, 2]. The characteristic distribution of chromophores allowing articular tissues to be distinguished and even discrimination between normal and degenerated or inflamed structures can serve for in vivo monitoring of the laser ablation process, thus minimizing the removal of healthy tissue [6]. The approach of a fluorescence-guided laser system has been used in connection with a XeCl excimer laser under clinical conditions. As shown in Fig. 7 the laser system is equipped with an optical shutter that is controlled by a computer system. The typical fluorescence pattern is continuously recorded during the ablation process. After digitizing, the fluorescence scans are compared to scans of the target tissue. A divergence between the on-line registration and the typical scan profile of the tissue, indicating a failure in tissue ablation, interrupts the laser beam [4, 5]. Although the feedback system has the advantage of in vivo application, clinical experience is not encouraging so far. Due to the variety in fluorescence patterns even within the same tissue, the specificity of the system is insufficient for effective performance. However, fluorescence spectroscopy-guided lasers may contribute to selective laser application and avoid iatrogenic lesions in articular laser surgery provided further improvements to the system, especially with regard to the spectral resolution, are successful.

Fig. 9. Modification of the optical tissue properties by in vitro incubation with diclofenac in a hyaline cartilage specimen

Pharmacological Modification of Optical Tissue Properties

The paucity of chromophores in cartilaginous structures has led to experiments aiming at a modification of tissue optical properties by dye incorporation into hyaline cartilage, both to increase ablation efficiency and to create a basis for selective tissue ablation. In vitro experiments demonstrated a significant increase in ablation rate at 308 nm in hyaline cartilage samples incubated with diclofenac or vitamin B complex [8]. Figure 9 represents the optical densities

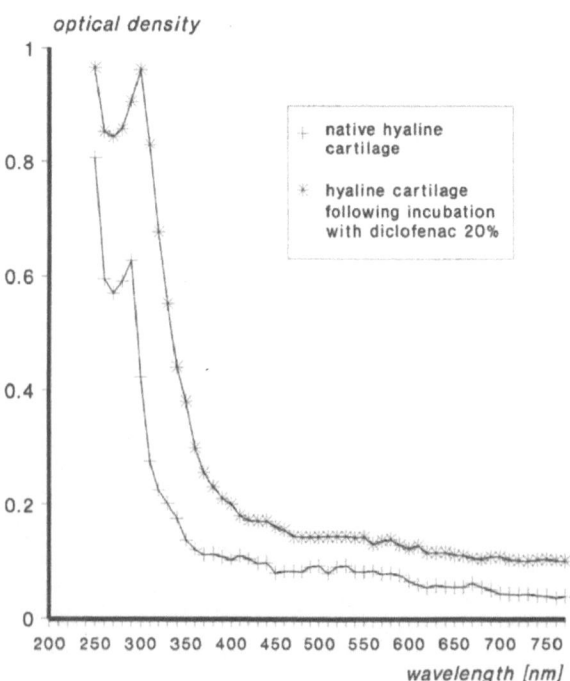

at 250–770 nm of native cartilage and a tissue sample incubated in diclofenac 24 h before microspectrophotometry. Over the whole spectral range examined, a significant rise in optical density is achieved by incorporation of diclofenac. These results are in close agreement with reports about improved ablation with pharmacological treatment of hyaline cartilage [8]. Although these data seem promising with regard to selective tissue labeling and ablation, widespread application in clinical practice has not yet been established. As to the pharmacokinetics, in vivo tissue impregnation leads to a poor increase in the ablation rate, far below the values expected from experimental results, while on the other hand, a general uptake of the dye substance into cartilage tissues following intraarticular application prevents selectivity in laser ablation [3].

Clinical Implications

At present, the approach of selective tissue ablation by feedback systems based upon laser-induced tissue fluorescence, pharmacological labeling of articular tissue, or selecting specific laser output characteristics according to optical properties has not been developed up to the state of a clinical routine procedure. As the differences between normal and degenerated tissue structures obtained via microspectophotometry are relatively small, the range for tissue discrimination remains restricted. Therefore laser surgery has the potential for preferential tissue ablation without offering the chance of selective tissue treatment. However, experimental results presented so far may justify further research especially with regard to the development of more sophisticated algorithms in fluorescence-guided laser systems.

References

[1] Banga, I, Bihari-Varga M (1974) Investigations of free and elastic bound fluorescent substances present in the atherosclerotic lipid and calcium plaques. Connect Tissue Res 2:237–243

[2] Baraga J, Rava R, Taroni P, Kittrell C, Fitzmaurice M, Feld M (1990) Laser induced fluorescence spectroscopy of normal and atheroscelrotic human aorta using 306–310 nm excitation. Lasers Surg Med 10:245–261

[3] Brooks S, Ashlex S, Fisher J, Davies G, Griffiths J, Kester R, Rees M (1992) Exogenous chromophores for the argon and Nd:YAG lasers: a potential application to laser tissue interactions. Lasers Surg Med 12:294–302

[4] Buchelt M, Katterschafka T, Horvat R, Kutschera H, Kickinger W, Laufer G (1991) Fluorescence guided excimer laser ablation of intervertebral discs in vitro. Lasers Surg Med 11:280–286

[5] Deckelbaum L, Lam J, Cabin H, Clubb K, Long M (1989) Discrimination of normal and atherosclerotic aorta by laser induced fluorescence. Lasers Surg Med 7:330–335

[6] Deckelbaum L, Desai S, Kim C, Scott J (1995) Evaluation of a fluorescence feedback system for guidance of laser angioplasty. Lasers Surg Med 16:226–234

[7] Derbyshire G, Bogen D, Unger M (1990) Thermally induced optical property changes in myocardium at 1.06 μm. Lasers Surg Med 10:28–34

[8] Grothues-Spork M, Bernard M, Kirgis A, Hertel P, Noack W (1993) Die Modifikation der Absorption gelenkbildender Strukturen und dessen Einfluss auf die arthroskopische Laserchirurgie. Lasers Med Surg 9:48–56

[9] Kubelka P (1954) New contributions to the optics of intensely light-scattering materials. J Opt Soc Am 44:330–335

[10] Kubelka P, Munk F (1931) Ein Beitrag zur Optik der Farbanstriche. Z Tech Phys IIA:593–601

[11] Mahadevan A, Mitchell M, Silva E, Thomsen S, Richards-Kortum R (1993) Study of the fluorescence properties of normal and neoplastic human cervical tissue. Lasers Surg Med 13:647–655

[12] Pelinka H, Janousek A (1991) Differenzierung verschiedener Kniegelenkstrukturen durch die fluoreszenzspektroskopische Analyse des Laserlichtes. In: Siebert W, Wirth C (eds) Laser in der Orthopädie. Thieme, Stuttgart, pp 70–71

[13] Perk M, Flynn G, Smith C, Bathgate B, Tuklip J, Yue W, Lucas A (1991) Laser induced fluorescence emission: the spectroscopic identification of fibrotic endocardium and myocardium. Lasers Surg Med 11:523–534

[14] Perkampus H (1986) UV-VIS-Spektroskopie und ihre Anwendungen. Springer, Berlin, Heidelberg, New York

[15] Prince M, Deutsch T, Mathews-Roth M, Margolis R, Parrish J, Oseroff A (1986) Preferential light absorption in atheromas in vitro: implications for laser angioplasty. J Clin Invest 78:295–302

[16] Raunest J, Schwarzmaier H (1995) Optical properties of human articular tissue as implication for a selective laser application in arthroscopic surgery. Lasers Surg Med 16:253–261

[17] Schwarzmaier H, Hennig T, Betz P, Kaufmann R, Wolbarsht M (1990) Optical density of human arterial vessel wall and atheromatous plaque as a basis for pulsed laser angioplasty. SPIE 1201:10–14

[18] Schwarzmaier H, Heintzen M, Müller W, Kaufmann R, Wolbarsht M (1992) Optical density of vascular tissue before and after 308-nm excimer laser irradiation. Opt Eng 31:1436–1440

[19] Thomsen S, Jacques S, Flock S (1990) Microscopic correlates of macroscopic optical property changes during thermal coagulation of myocardium. SPIE 1202:2–7

[20] van Gemert M, Schets G, Stassen E, Gijbers G, Bonnier J (1985) Optical properties of human blood vessel wall and plaque. Lasers Surg Med 5:235–237

[21] Vangsness C, Huang J, Smith C (1991) Light absorption characteristics of the human meniscus: application for laser ablation. SPIE 1424:16–20

[22] Walsh J, Cummings J (1994) Effect of the dynamic optical properties of water on midinfrared laser ablation. Lasers Surg Med 15:295–305

Measurement of Holmium:YAG Laser-Induced Temperature in Musculoskeletal Tissues Using an Experimental MRI Technique[1]

C. Hendrich · T. Breitling · P. M. Jakob · A. Berden · A. Schäfer · C. Hillenbrand · V. Krenn · A. Haase · W. E. Siebert

Introduction

In the field of orthopedics, laser systems coupled in by fibers have been in use for the past 10 years. Today, together with the excimer and the neodymium:YAG laser, the holmium:YAG laser is the most common in clinical use [21, 23]. Because it is possible to miniaturize the instruments, the main indications for use of the Ho:YAG laser are percutaneous surgery of the intervertebral disc [25] and arthroscopy [16]. Using the laser has proved to be the method of choice for percutaneous treatment of protrusions of the intervertebral disc. In the field of arthroscopy, especially in treating damaged cartilage, lasers allow a surface treatment of much higher quality than mechanical instruments [6]. However, histologic analysis has shown that using the Ho:YAG laser is accompanied by a small thermically damaged zone (200–800 µm, depending on the power) [2, 22]. In the recent past some publications have warned that a deeper-seated damaged zone exists which is not assessable by light microscopy [4, 5], and which in some cases is supposed to be responsible for the development of osteochondronecrosis after arthroscopy [3, 19]. Reports also exist describing MRI signal enhancements in the cartilage adjacent to the subchondral bone after laser decompression which might be mistaken for spondylodiscitis [20]. Therefore it has become important to establish what temperatures actually do occur during the operation, in order to be able to assess the possibility of damage realistically and to be able to fix suitable laser parameters.

All trials carried out so far to measure the temperature directly have suffered from the same weaknesses: they neither had the necessary resolution, nor did they allow measurement under clinical conditions. Recently MRI procedures have been suggested for this purpose [13, 15, 27]. One of these methods [13] is based upon the shift in the resonance frequency of water protons, which is dependent on the change in temperature. This method allows a high spatial and temporal resolution. In this paper we report the possibility of monitoring the temperature by means of MRI after using laser in vitro on cartilaginous and intervertebral disc tissue.

Materials and Methods

Laser System and Choice of Parameters

The experiments were performed with a Dornier MediLas H Ho:YAG laser (Daimler-Benz Aerospace, Dornier Medizintechnik GmbH, Germering, Germany) with an impulse width of 250 µm. The laser energy was led to the samples via 600-µm quartz fibers for the cartilage specimens and 400-µm fibers for the intervertebral disc samples. The degree of transmission of the fiber was evaluated with the integrated powermeter and according to this the power of the laser was adjusted automatically.

Cartilage Samples

Fresh preparations of cartilage with grade II or III damage according to the Outerbridge classification [17] were taken from donated corpses. For the irradiation experiments the preparations were fixed in a special sample cell with constant irrigation with Ringer's lactate. The angle of laser irradiation was either 30° or 90° in relation to the surface of the cartilage. Four preparations were prepared for each combination of parameters. For irradiation experiments pulse energies of 1.0 and 1.3 J were used. The frequency remained at 10 Hz. Except where otherwise indicated, the distance between fiber tip and preparation was 1 mm.

Samples of the Intervertebral Discs

Fresh intervertebral discs were taken from donated corpses as complete vertebral motor segments. The adjacent osseous tissue was removed up to the cartilaginous tissue near the subchondral bone by means of a diamond-coated running belt saw (Exakt Apparatebau, Norderstedt, Germany). Then the isolated

---

[1] This work was performed with generous support from Dornier Medizintechnik GmbH, Germering, Germany.

intervertebral discs were punctured from posterolateral by an 18-gauge plastic cannula, so that the end of the cannula came to lie in the center of the disc, while the whole preparation was embedded in agargel. For the irradiation experiments a 400-µm fiber was placed in the plastic cannula in such a way that the tip of the fiber was 5 mm longer than the cannula. The laser parameters were 1 J and 10 Hz and 100 pulses were applied continuously over 10 s. Four samples each were treated with these parameters.

Basics of Measuring Temperature by MRI

In recent years a number of studies have demonstrated the possibilities of MRI for spatially resolved quantitative measurement of temperature [15, 27]. Using these thermometric MRI methods for dynamic temperature measurement does not seem sensible because of the real-time resolution required. In contrast to this, the recently suggested proton-shift method [13] combines high temporal with high spatial resolution. It is known that the resonance frequency of water protons varies linearly with temperature with a sensitivity S of 0.01 ppm/°C [12]. Therefore the change in temperature ΔT can be seen as a phase shift in a spoiled gradient echo MRI image which allows the calculation of two-dimensional temperature maps [13]. Apart from the change in temperature, this phase shift $\Delta\phi$ is dependent on echo time and the available strength of the magnetic field B_0:

$$\Delta\phi\,(\Delta T) = \gamma\, TE\, S\, \Delta T\, B_0$$

with γ = gyromagnetic ratio.

Temperature dependence of the susceptibility can be neglected. To calculate the changes in temperature, the phase difference between a reference image (before application of the laser) and a current measurement (e. g., during or after laser application) is used. The forming of the phase difference allows suppression of artifacts evoked by inhomogeneities of the magnetic field. A detailed description of this MRI method ist presented elsewhere [14].

The gradient-echo procedure was implemented by means of an ultrafast snapshot FLASH sequence [8] in a 7-T experimental system (Bruker BIOSPEC, Bruker, Karlsruhe, Germany). The hardware components in use allowed image measuring time of up to 512 ms for a 128 × 128 imaging matrix with a local resolution of up to 200 µm. This extremely short examination time is suitable for monitoring the development of temperature during laser application.

Definition of the Calibration Curve

In order to verify the relation [1], samples of cartilage or intervertebral discs were placed in the sample cell within the magnet, heated up by temperable irri-

gation, and afterwards cooled down. The temperature of the irrigation was controlled by a thermocouple. After adjusting thermal equilibrium between the tissue and water the MRI phase measurements were performed for various temperatures between 20 °C and 55 °C.

Measuring Cartilage Temperature During Laser Irradiation

The tissue specimen was placed in the magnet with the positioned laser fiber. Before, during, and after laser application a series of 10–40 MRI phase images with a temporal resolution of 512 ms - 1 s for each image were taken. Afterwards (offline) the phase images were evaluated in relation to each other by means of an IBM 6000 workstation with IDL imaging software and converted into temperature images.

Results

The result of a representative calibrating measurement is shown in Fig. 1. The calibration curve shows a shift of the resonance frequency with the temperature at a rate of $S = 0.0078 \pm 0.0005$ ppm/°C. A sensitivity higher than $S = 0.01$ ppm/°C was seen in none of the experiments. Therefore this value was employed for all the further evaluations so that the following temperatures have to be regarded as maximum temperatures.

In cartilage samples laser irradiation at 1.0 J, 10 Hz for 1 s showed an immediate rise in temperature of 5° at the border of an elliptical area with an aver-

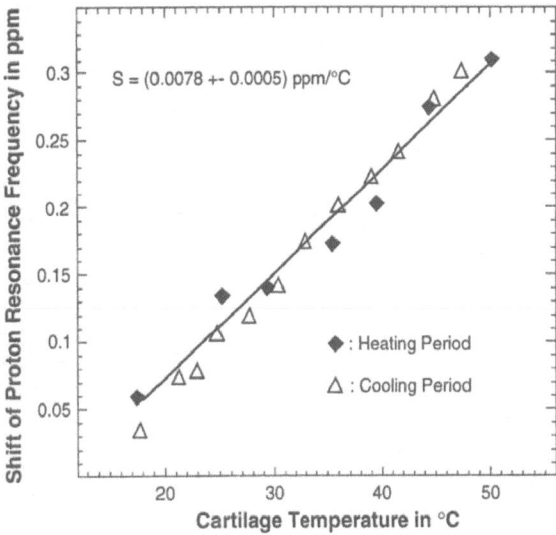

Fig. 1. Experimentally obtained calibration curve for the shift in proton resonance frequency according to the change in temperature in the cartilage. In the observed range of temperature between 20 °C and 55 °C there is a linear relation between resonance frequency and temperature. The slope of the straight line is $S = 0.0078 \pm 0.0005$ ppm/°C. Measurements were performed with a snapshot FLASH sequence (image measuring time 512 ms, TR = 4.0 ms, TE = 2.2 ms)

Fig. 3. Data from MRI images of a representative cartilage sample for an irradiation at 1.3 J, 10 Hz for 1 s. Sixteen consecutive MRI temperature images from before irradiation until 13 s after irradiation are depicted. The time of laser exposure is indicated. ▶ In this series of experiments the laser fiber was in direct contact with the cartilage surface

age width of 4 mm and a depth of 2 mm. In four independent experiments we found a maximum rise in temperature of 27 °C in the center (Fig. 2). This change in temperature was measured once; in the other experiments it was 25°. The spreading of these temperature peaks was limited to an area of 400 × 200 µm. After 1 s the temperature had fallen by 10°, after 2 s by another 4°. Changing the angle of irradiation to 30° to the surface of the cartilage did not have a relevant effect on the temperature (not more than 27°).

After laser irradiation at 1.0 J, 10 Hz for 5 s, the zone in which the rise in temperature was 5° also had an elliptical shape, with an average width of 6 mm and a depth of 3 mm. In four independent experiments the maximum change in temperature at the center was 34-35 °C in an average area of 400 × 800 µm. The temperature decreased by 6 °C in the first second and by another 4.5° in the next. At no time at all was an increase in temperature of more than 10 °C observed near the subchondral bone.

Irradiating the cartilage samples at 1.0 J and 10 Hz for 1 s at no distance led to a maximum rise in temperature of 30°. Using a pulse energy of 1.3 J and a frequency of 10 Hz the maximum rise in temperature was 27° in four different experiments (Fig. 3).

In intervertebral discs after laser application of 100 J, an elliptical zone of enhanced temperature showed in the center directly in the plane of the fiber which measured 8 by 4 mm. In the center of this zone we found a maximum rise in temperature of 54 °C in an area of 600 × 1200 µm. In the plane of the cartilage adjacent to the subchondral bone we saw in four independent experiments, with the fiber positioned in the center, a maximum rise in temperature of 12 °C in an area of 4 × 2 mm. After another 50 s no further rise in temperature was measurable surrounding the end plate (Fig. 4).

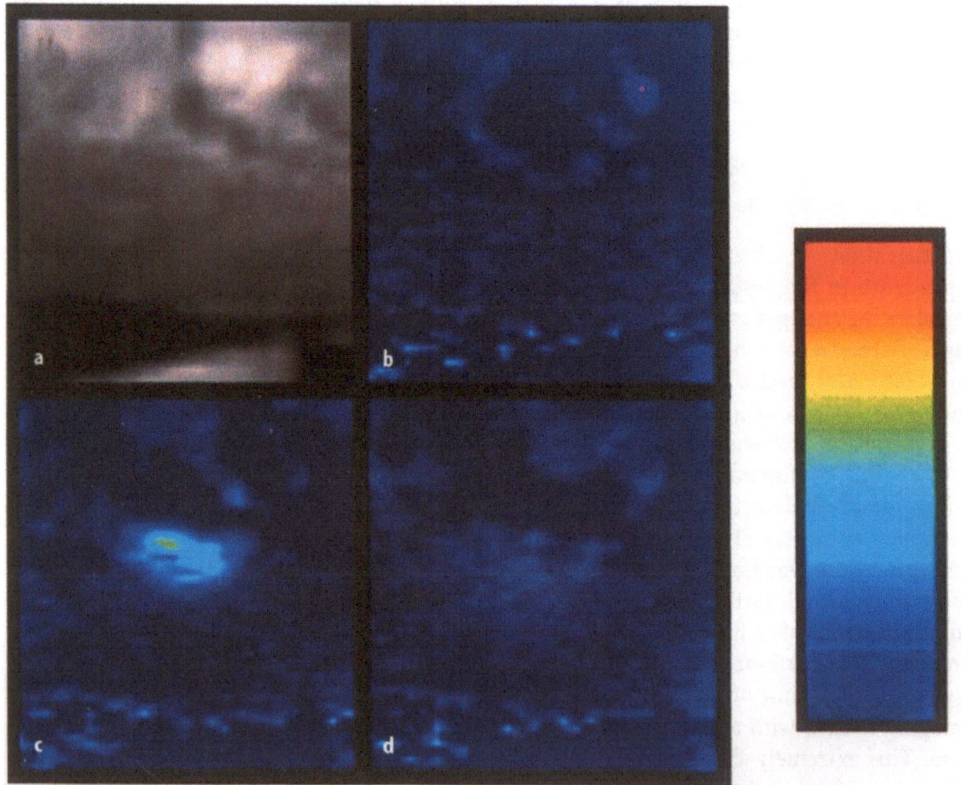

Fig. 2. Data from the MRI images of a representative cartilage sample for irradiation at 1.0 J, 10 Hz for 1 s. **a** Magnified proton cut. **b** MRI temperature image at the end of irradiation. **c** MRI temperature image, 2 s after irradiation. **d** MRI temperature image, 4 s after irradiation

Fig. 4. Data from MRI images of a representative intervertebral disc for an irradiation at 1.0 J, 10 Hz for 5 s. The *first row* indicates the proton images in four different horizontal planes of the disc (slice 1: proximal end plate; slice 2: between end plate and center of the disc; slices 3 and 4: near the center of ▶ the disc), the *second row* shows the temperature images after 14 s, the *third row* those after 60 s

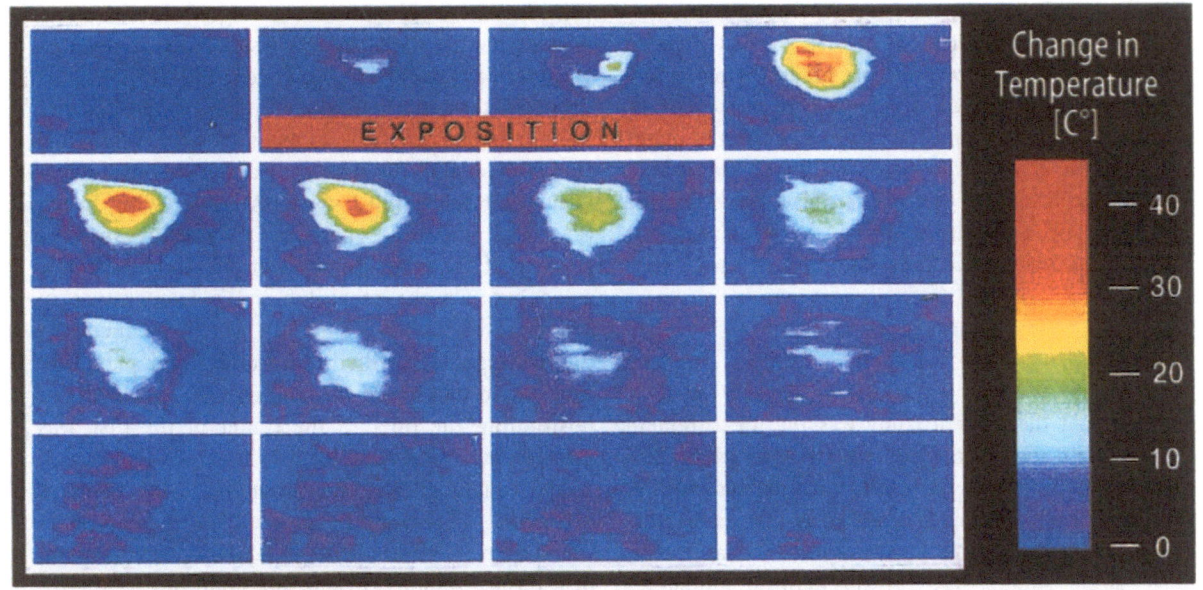

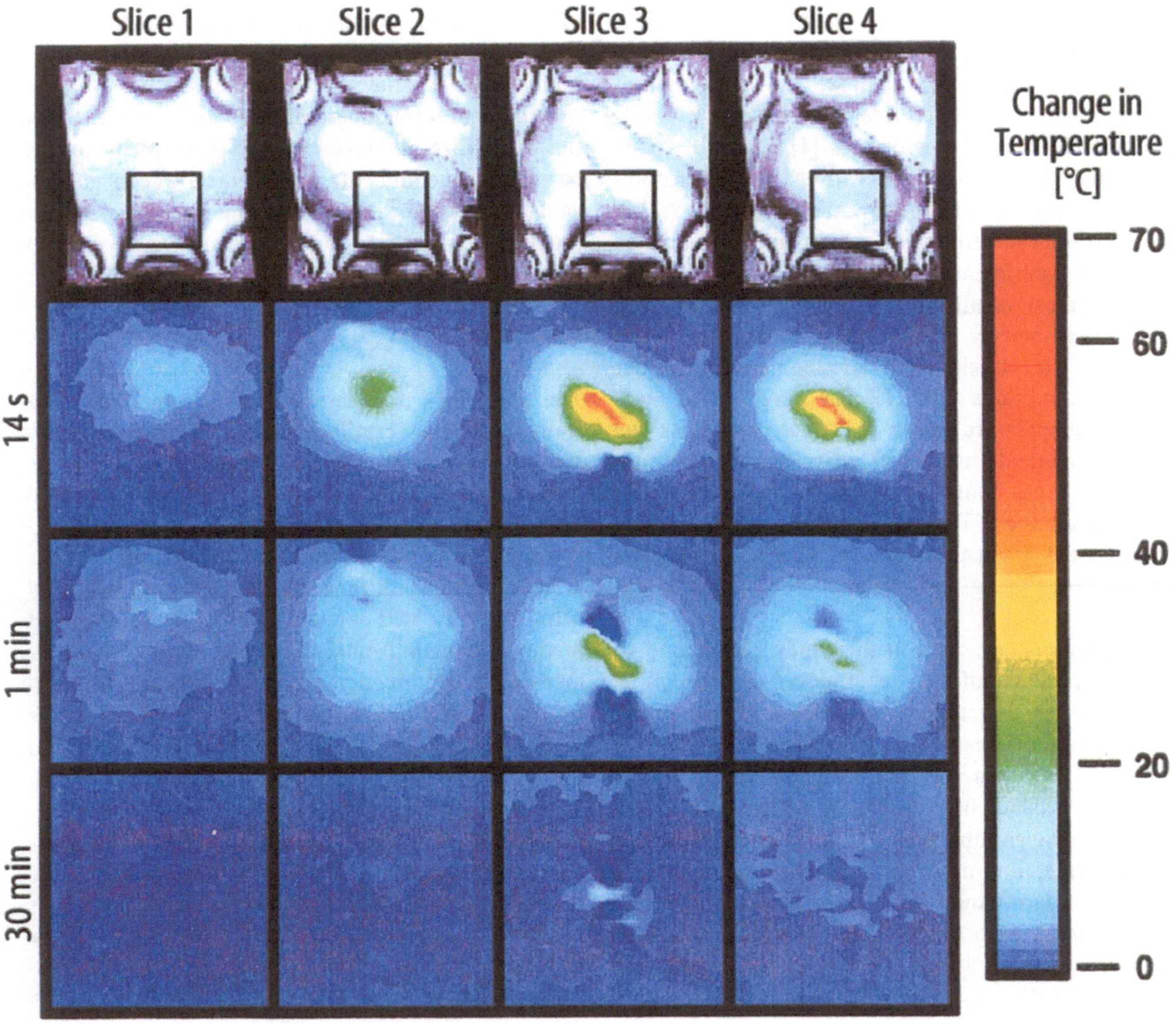

The usable measuring range in the case of cartilaginous and intervertebral disc tissue lies between 20 and 55 °C. In temperature ranges above 55 °C this method is limited by changes in susceptibility because of the denaturation of tissue. Errors in determining the temperature were estimated to ± 5 °C, mainly explicable by the phase noise. Mistakes due to magnetic field drift during the measurements were ruled out by the short duration of the experiments.

Discussion

The aim of the present study was the measurement of temperature in cartilage and intervertebral disc tissue by means of MRI after irradiation with a Ho:YAG laser. Although the Ho:YAG laser already has a place in arthroscopy and in minimally invasive spine surgery [7, 24] no definite guidelines exist which laser parameters are most appropriate for which kind of tissue. In the end the parameters must be adjusted individually by each surgeon on the basis of his or her experience or of visual monitoring of the effect on each tissue. Particularly in regard to the temperature during treatment, data are insufficient at present. In the case, chiefly, of treatment of hyaline cartilage, the temperatures brought about by laser treatment have a key role in possible damaging processes [1].

Studies to date have concentrated on the histologic consequences of laser irradiation [4, 18, 2, 26]. So far, direct measurement of temperature has failed because experimental conditions differ so greatly from clinical conditions [1, 4]. For the moment, MRI thermometry seems to be the only way to observe the development of temperature under clinical conditions [10, 11]. For purposes of measuring temperature under real-time conditions the T1-map methods used so far have measuring times which are too long. By contrast, the proton-shift method on the 7-T experimental system has much shorter measuring times and a higher spatial resolution [14], allowing us to simulate the clinical situation.

The parameters used in this study correspond to the favorable conditions of unmoved laser application. The rise in temperature which occurred in the cartilaginous tissue of the joint after irradiation of one spot for 5 s at 1 J and 10 Hz was no more than 35 °C. The depth of penetration at the time of the highest temperature was 4 mm. Considering the body temperature of 37 °C , the worst assumed peak in temperature would be 72 °C, which drops below 60 °C after 1 s and below 55 °C after 2 s, whereas long-term damage of the tissue can only be assumed if temperatures of 55 °C persist for more than 10 s

[9]. In these circumstances significant thermal damage to the cartilaginous tissue can be avoided with the parameters mentioned here [10]. In the case of intervertebral discs, a rise in temperature of no more than 12 °C was shown surrounding the cartilage adjacent to the subchondral bone after application of a total of 100 J via a laser fiber lying in the center of the disc. Therefore thermically induced damage of the cartilaginous end plates can be safely ruled out. On the other hand, the temperature in the plane of the fiber came up to 54°, so incorrect positioning of the fiber near to the end plate will lead to certain thermal damage. The necessity of positioning the fiber in the center of the disc was mentioned several times.

To conclude: the thermometric MRI method described allows specification of "safe" parameters for the treatment of cartilaginous and intervertebral disc tissue. Under experimental conditions the proton-shift method is already suitable for gaining a lead on the temperatures occurring when lasers are used in the musculoskeletal system. More exact knowledge about the coherence between temperature and phase shift is needed for further development of this method of measurement [11]. As a long-term goal, the development of this method up to the point where it allows real-time observation of the development of temperature seems possible. With the possibility of measuring temperature by means of an MRI method, the orthopedic surgeon gains a valuable indicator for optimizing laser therapy in the field of arthroscopy and minimally invasive spinal surgery.

Summary

The possibility of measuring temperature resulting from irradiating cartilage with a Ho:YAG laser by means of dynamic magnetic resonance imaging is demonstrated. Human cartilage and intervertebral disc specimens were irradiated using a Ho:YAG laser via 600-μm or 400-μm quartz glass fibers under clinical conditions. Temperature was measured using a 7-T MRI system with the proton-shift method. In chondromalacia grade II and III specimens a maximum increase in temperature of 35 °C was found after irradiation at 1.0 J and 10 Hz for 5 s at a distance of 1 mm between the laser fiber and the cartilage surface. In no case was an increase in temperature of more than 10 °C observed in the cartilage adjacent to the subchondral bone. In intervertebral disc specimens after 100 J total energy in the central plane, a maximum temperature of 54 °C was observed. However, in the plane of the end plates a temperature elevation of 12 °C was measured. Measuring time for a single MR image was 512 ms at a resolution of 200 µm. These results demonstrate the possibility of MRI thermometry at high resolutuion for tissue specimens (cartilage) and organoid structures (intervertebral disc). In principle, MRI methods may therefore be used to monitor the evolution of temperature induced by lasers in the musculoskeletal system. For the surgeon, the results may give a valuable indication by which to estimate thermal damage during the operative procedure.

References

[1] Bressem M, Meyer D, Bickelmann K, Foth H.-J. (1995) Die thermische Belastung von Knorpel durch Holmium-Laser-Strahlung. Lasermedizin 11:85

[2] Collier M, Haugland L, Bellamy J, Johnson L, Rohrer M, Walls R, Bartels K (1993) Effects of Holmium:YAG laser on equine articular cartilage and subchondral bone adjacent to traumatic lesions: a histopathological assessment. Arthroscopy 9:536–545

[3] Fink B, Schneider T, Braunstein S, Schmielau G, Rüther W (1996) Holmium:YAG laser-induced aseptic bone necroses of the femoral condyle. Arthroscopy 12:217–223

[4] Fischer R, Krebs R, Scharf H (1993) Cell vitality in cartilage tissue culture following excimer laser radiation: an in vitro examination. Lasers Surg Med 13:629–637

[5] Fischer R, Hibst R, Schröder D, Puhl W, Steiner R (1994) Thermal side effects of fiber-guided XeCl excimer laser drilling of cartilage. Lasers Surg Med 14:278–286

[6] Gerber B, Guggenheim R, Mathys D, Düggelin M, Litzistorf Y, Gudat F (1991) Ultrastrukturelles Bild des Excimer-Laser-Effektes der Knorpelvaporisation – eine in-vitro Pilotuntersuchung. In: Siebert W, Wirth CD (eds) Laser in der Orthopädie. Thieme, Stuttgart, pp 62–69

[7] Grifka J (1993) Arthroskopische Therapie der Gonarthrose in Abhängigkeit vom Grad der Chondromalazie. Arthroskopie 6:201–211

[8] Haase A (1990) Snapshot FLASH MRI. Applications to T1, T2 and chemical-shift imaging. Magn Reson Med 13:77–89

[9] Helfmann J, Brodzinski T (1989) Thermische Wirkungen. In: Berlien H-P, Müller G (eds) Angewandte Lasermedizin. Landsberg: Ecomed II-3.3:1–8

[10] Hendrich C, Jakob P, Breitling T, Schäfer A, Berden A, Haase A, Siebert W (1996) Kernspintomographische Messung der Temperaturverteilung in Knorpelgewebe nach Lasertherapie. Orthopäde 25:17–20

[11] Hendrich C, Jakob P, Breitling T, Schäfer A, Berden A, Krenn V, Haase A, Siebert W (1996) Thermometrische Kernspintomographie bei Holmium:YAG Lasereinsatz an Knorpelgewebe. Lasermedizin 1:3–8

[12] Hindman J (1966) Proton resonance shift of water in gas in liquid states. J Chem Phys 44:4582–4592

[13] Ishihara Y, Calderon A, Watanabe H, Mori K, Okamoto K, Suzuki Y, Sato K, Kuroda K, Nakagawa N, Tsutsumi S (1992) A precise and fast temperature mapping method using the water proton chemical shift. Proceedings of the 11th Annual Meeting of the Society of Magnetic Resonance in Medicine, Berlin, 1992, p 4803

[14] Jakob P, Hendrich, C, Breitling T, Schäfer A, Berden A, Haase A (1998) Real time monitoring of laser induced thermal changes in cartilage in vitro using snapshot FLASH. Magn Reson Med 37:805–808

[15] LeBihan D, Dellannoy J, Lvin R (1989) Temperature mapping with MR imaging of molecular diffusion. Radiology 171:853–857

[16] Lübbers C, Siebert W (1996) Die arthroskopische Holmium:YAG-Laseranwendung im Vergleich zu konventionellen Verfahren am Knie: Zwei-Jahres-Ergebnisse einer prospektiven randomisierten Studie. Orthopäde 25:64–72

[17] Outerbridge R (1961) The etiology of chondromalacia patellae. J Bone Joint Surg [Br] 43:752–757

[18] Reed S, Jackson R, Glossop N, Randle J (1994) An in vivo study of the effect of excimer laser irradiation on degenerate rabbit articular cartilage. Arthroscopy 10:78–84

[19] Rozbruch S, Wickiewicz T, DiCarlo E, Potter H (1996) Osteonecrosis of the knee following arthroscopic laser meniscectomy. Arthroscopy 12:245–250

[20] Schlangmann B, Schmolke S, Siebert W (1986) Temperatur- und Ablationsmessungen bei der Laserbehandlung von Bandscheibengewebe. Orthopäde 25:3–9

[21] Sherk H (1993) The use of lasers in orthopaedic procedures. J Bone Joint Surg [Am] 75:768–776

[22] Shi W, Vari S, van der Veen M, Fishbein M, Grundfest W (1993) Effect of varying laser parameters on pulsed Ho:YAG ablation of bovine knee joint tissues. Arthroscopy 9:96–102

[23] Siebert W (1992) Laseranwendung in der Arthroskopie. Orthopäde 21:273–288

[24] Siebert W (1993) Percutaneous laser disc decompression: the European experience. Spine: State of the Art Reviews 7:103–133

[25] Siebert W, Berendsen B, Tollgaard J (1996) Die perkutane Laserdiskusdekompression (PLDD) – Erfahrungen seit 1989. Orthopäde 25:42–48

[26] Trauner K, Nishioka N, Flotte T, Patel D (1995) Acute and chronic response of articular cartilage to Holmium:YAG laser irradiation. Clin Orthop 310:52–57

[27] Young I, Hand J, Oatrige A, Prior M, Forse G (1994) Further observations on the measurement of tissue T1 to monitor temperature in vivo by MRI. Magn Reson Med 31:342–347

Fundamental Studies of Laser Energy for Joint Capsular Shrinkage

K. Hayashi · M. D. Markel

Background

A recent pilot clinical study has demonstrated that the application of nonablative laser energy to the glenohumeral joint capsule in patients with glenohumeral instability stabilized the shoulder joint in the majority of the patients treated [17]. In this multi-institutional clinical trial, a nonablative level of holmium:yttrium-aluminum-garnet (Ho:YAG) laser energy was applied to patients with glenohumeral instability in order to shrink the redundant capsuloligamentous tissues of glenohumeral joint under arthroscopic guidance. At a mean follow-up time after surgery of 6 months (range 2-12 months), for all patients, regardless of arm dominance, age, sex, or direction of instability, postsurgical subjective scores were significantly higher than presurgical scores [presurgical subjective score 17 ± 1.9 (mean $\pm$ SEM); mean postsurgical subjective score 68 ± 2.2] ($p < 0.0001$). Although this pilot study did not have a comparable nonoperated control population or an operated open surgical repair group, the results indicated that nonablative reduction of redundant glenohumeral joint capsule using the Ho:YAG laser is potentially an effective treatment for joint instability in certain subgroups.

The interactions between laser energy and tissue are based on photothermal, photochemical, photomechanical, and/or photoacoustic effects, which are mainly determined by the wavelength of the laser light and the absorption characteristics of the tissue [3, 13, 15, 16]. Laser applications in surgery have mainly focused on its tissue ablative action, which is primarily caused by the photothermal effect of laser energy [13, 15, 16]. When a laser beam is directed at biological material, light can be reflected from, transmitted through, scattered within, or absorbed by the tissue. Light energy absorbed by the tissue is transformed into effective thermal energy. Thermal shrinkage of collagen is a well-described phenomenon that has been studied in a number of experimental models [1, 2, 4, 5, 12, 18].

Recent scientific studies evaluating laser energy for tissue welding and thermokeratoplasty have indicated that long-lasting alterations of collagenous tissue architecture can be achieved without a concomitant inflammatory response [6, 14]. Based on the collective findings of these studies, we hypothesized that thermal modification of dense collagenous tissues such as joint capsule, ligament, and tendon may allow precise alteration of these tissues mechanical and/or structural properties to enhance joint function, and that thermal modification of these tissues can be achieved by applying nonablative laser energy. To test these hypotheses, we have performed a series of in vitro and in vivo animal studies.

In Vitro Studies

The effect of laser energy at nonablative energy densities on joint capsular mechanical, biochemical, histological and ultrastructural properties was evaluated in an in vitro rabbit model [8, 10, 11]. Joint capsular specimens (5 mm x 20 mm) were collected from the medial and lateral portion of the femoropatellar joint; thus, four specimens were collected from each rabbit (right medial, right lateral, left medial, left lateral). Specimens were divided into four groups using a randomized block design: a control group and three at different laser power settings (5 watts, 10 watts, 15 watts; the groups being designated 5W, 10W, and 15W, respectively). Laser energy was applied using the Ho:YAG laser in four transverse passes across the tissue at a velocity of 2 mm/s and distance from the tip of the handpiece to the synovial surface of the specimen set at 1.5 mm in a 37 °C tissue bath of lactated Ringer's solution.

The application of laser energy resulted in 9 %, 26 %, and 36 % reduction respectively in capsular tissue length in the 5W, 10W, and 15W groups. Tissue shrinkage was significantly and strongly correlated with energy density ($p < 0.0001$; $R^2 = 0.80$) (Fig. 1). Laser energy caused a significant decrease in tensile stiffness in the 10W and 15W groups ($p < 0.05$). There was a significant but weak correlation between energy density and post-laser stiffness values ($p < 0.0001$; $R^2 = 0.34$). Laser energy did not change the relaxation properties of capsular tissue at any

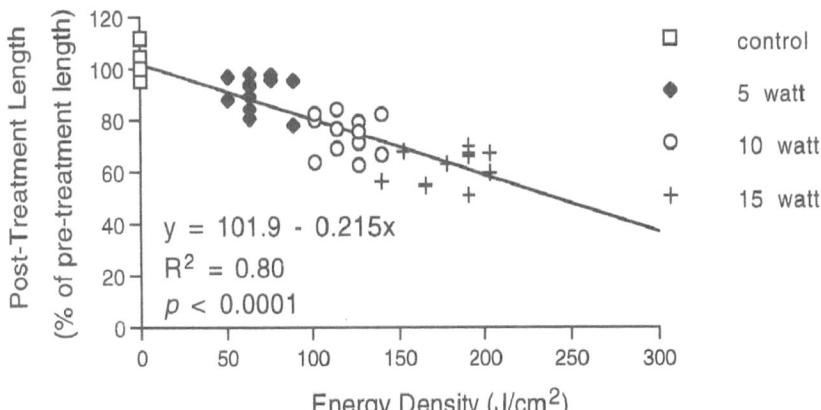

Fig. 1. Correlation between laser energy density and joint capsular shrinkage

energy density when compared to prelaser values ($p > 0.05$; $\Delta = 29\%$ at power $= 0.8$). There was no significant correlation between energy density and relaxation properties of the tissue ($p > 0.05$). The loads required to return specimens to their original length were significantly lower for the 5W group (3.6 ± 5.1 N) than for the 10W (15.0 ± 6.2 N) and 15W (14.0 ± 5.2 N) groups (Fig. 2). There was a significant correlation between energy density and the load required to return the specimen to its original length ($p < 0.0001$; $R^2 = 0.58$) (Fig. 2).

Biochemical analysis indicated that application of laser energy did not cause significant alteration of collagen content [hydroxyproline (Hyp) concentration] and nonreducible crosslinks [hydroxylysylpyridinoline (HP) concentration] at any energy density.

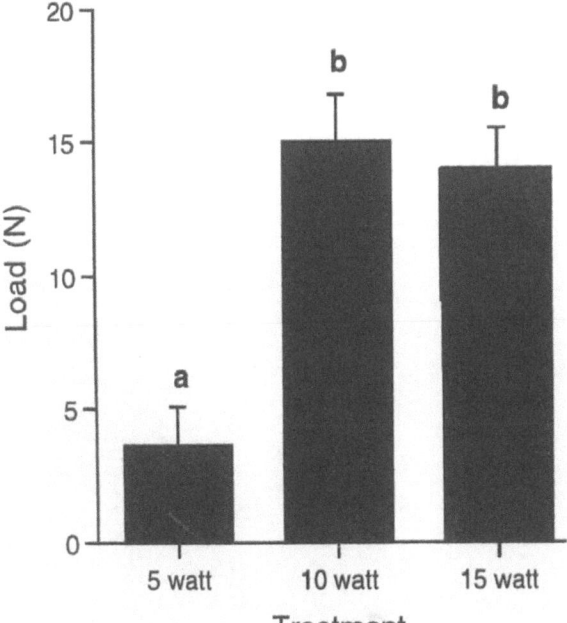

Fig. 2. Loads required to return specimens to their original length (mean $\pm$ SE), comparing the three laser treatment groups. *Bars* with differing letters were significantly different from each other ($p < 0.05$)

There were no significant differences in collagen content among groups: 47.6 ± 10.8, 46.1 ± 5.3, 46.8 ± 9.8, and 45.9 ± 10.0 (mg Hyp/mg dry weight; mean $\pm$ SD) in the control, 5W, 10W, and 15W groups, respectively ($p > 0.05$; $\Delta = 20\%$ at power $= 0.8$). In addition, there were no significant differences in nonreducible collagen crosslinks among groups: 0.75 ± 0.17, 0.85 ± 0.17, 0.87 ± 0.17, and 0.87 ± 0.16 (mole HP/mole collagen; mean $\pm$ SD) in the control, 5W, 10W, and 15W groups, respectively ($p > 0.05$; $\Delta = 23\%$ at power $= 0.8$).

Histological examination of the tissue revealed evidence of thermal damage of the tissue at all laser energy densities, which was characterized by hyalinization of collagen and pyknotic nuclear changes in fibroblasts; each subsequently higher laser energy caused significantly greater morphologic changes over a larger area (Fig. 3).

Transmission electron microscopy revealed alteration of the collagen architecture, with significantly increased fibril cross-section for each of the treated groups compared to controls. The fibrils began to lose their distinct edges and their periodical cross-striations at subsequently higher energy densities. The results of ultrastructural morphometry of fibril diameter distributions revealed that each subsequently higher laser energy caused a significant increase in collagen fibril diameter ($p < 0.05$). Mean fibril diameter was significantly correlated with energy density ($p < 0.0001$; $R^2 = 0.51$).

This study demonstrated that significant capsular shrinkage can be achieved with the application of nonablative Ho:YAG laser energy without detrimental effects on the viscoelastic properties of the tissue, although at higher energy densities, laser energy did lessen capsular stiffness properties. Application of laser energy did not cause significant alteration of biochemical parameters evaluated in this study; however, histological/ultrastructural analysis revealed thermal changes in the tissue and significant alteration of collagen ultrastructure.

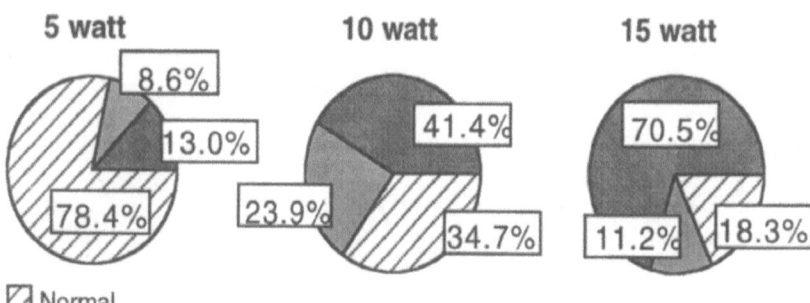

5 watt **10 watt** **15 watt**

8.6%
13.0%
78.4%

41.4%
23.9%
34.7%

70.5%
11.2% 18.3%

☑ Normal

▨ Total Affected Area - Area of Hyalinization

■ Area of Hyalinization

Fig. 3. The effect of laser energy on percent area with histological alterations caused by laser energy. The percent area with collagen hyalinization and the percent area with any change observed were significantly different among laser-treated groups ($p < 0.05$)

In Vivo Studies

The effect of nonablative laser energy on the short term histological properties of joint capsular tissue was evaluated in an in vivo rabbit model [9]. Rabbits were randomly assigned to one of three groups (0, 7, and 30 days post surgery). Both stifles of each rabbit were prepared for surgery and the femoropatellar joint was exposed via a patellar tenotomy. One randomly selected stifle was treated with laser energy, and the contralateral stifle was sham operated. Laser energy (0.5 J/10 pulses per second) was applied to the femoropatellar joint capsule in lactated Ringer's solution using the Ho:YAG laser. The laser hand piece was held approximately 1.5 mm away from the synovial surface and moved over the tissue in a paint brush motion. Animals were euthanized immediately after surgery (day 0), or at 7 days after surgery, and 30 days after surgery, and the femoropatellar joint capsule was harvested immediately after euthanasia. Control tissues obtained from animals euthanized immediately after sham operations showed no significant histological lesions. Laser-treated samples at day 0 showed diffuse hyalinization of collagen with nuclear karyorrhexis and nuclear streaming of fibroblasts in treated regions (Fig. 4). Laser-treated tissue at 7 days after surgery revealed similar histological changes to control tissue along with fibroblast proliferation around and into acellular hyalinized collagen regions. Laser-treated tissues at 30 days after surgery showed fibrosis with cellular and disorganized connective tissue. Hyalinized collagen regions were greatly reduced by 30 days after laser treatment as large reactive fibroblasts migrated to the site and secreted new matrix to replace the hyalinized tissue (Fig. 5).

The effect of nonablative laser energy on the long-term mechanical, histological, and ultrastructural properties of joint capsular tissue has also been evaluated in an in vivo sheep model [7]. Femoropatellar

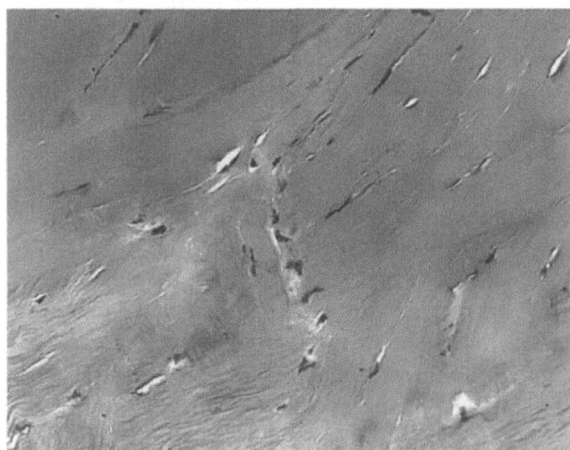

Fig. 4. Light micrograph of laser-treated day 0 capsular tissue demonstrating hyalinization of collagen and karyorrhexis of fibroblasts (hematoxylin-eosin stain, original ×50).

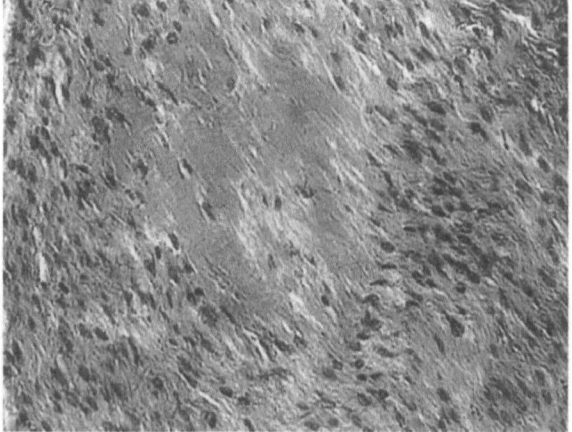

Fig. 5. Light micrograph of laser-treated capsular tissue at 30 days after surgery demonstrating greatly reduced hyalinized acellular regions with surrounding fibroblasts (hematoxylin-eosin stain, original ×50).

joint capsule was treated with the Ho:YAG laser via arthroscope, and tissues were harvested immediately after surgery (day 0), or at 3, 7, 14, 30, 60, 90, or 180 days after surgery. Laser treatment caused significant decrease in tissue stiffness from 0 to 7 days after surgery, then stiffness improved after 14 days. Tissue strength was lowest at 3 days after laser treatment. Histology demonstrated immediate collagen hyalinization and cell necrosis, followed by active cellular reparative response characterized by extensive fibroblast migration and capillary sprouting, and tissue maturation. Transmission electron microscopy revealed that the treated region was infiltrated with fibroblasts and replaced with fine collagen fibrils by 90 days after surgery. This study illustrates an active and prompt tissue response to the tissue modification, with concomitant improvement of mechanical properties by 30 days after surgery.

Discussion

The thermal modification of musculoskeletal collagenous tissues by nonablative laser energy may have the potential for a number of applications to address joint disorders and other abnormalities. In vitro studies have demonstrated that the effect of laser energy on joint capsular tissue is energy-dependent, and that at relatively low Ho:YAG laser power settings, significant capsular reduction could be achieved without significant alteration of the tissue's mechanical properties. In vivo studies demonstrated that initially decreased tissue stiffness regained its pre-treatment value as fibroblasts migrating from the adjacent regions actively secreted and deposited new collagen. The thermal treatment induced an active cellular response including angiogenesis and fibrogenesis without causing a severe inflammatory response.

Experimental studies have suggested that laser treatment has many advantages over the conventional treatments for joint instability in terms of diminishing redundancy of the tissue and joint volume, minimally invasive surgery, no foreign body reaction, no bleeding, and an active reparative response without a severe inflammatory reaction. These advantages may result in a less painful postoperative course and faster healing than conventional treatments. We propose that thermal modification of joint capsular tissue has the potential to become a minimally invasive and simply performed surgical procedure that addresses capsular redundancy and helps stabilize the joint, allowing patients to return to their previous level of activity without limiting function. However, the tissue's mechanical properties were inferior immediately after laser application, and therefore the joint must be protected during this period. A carefully controlled clinical trial with long term follow-up should be performed to further clarify the advantages and disadvantages of this technique.

References

[1] Allain J, Le Lous M, Cohen-Solal L, Bazin S, Maroteaux P (1980) Isometric tension developed during the thermal swelling of rat skin. Conn Tiss Res 7:127-133
[2] Danielsen C (1982) Precision method to determine temperature of collagen using ultraviolet difference spectroscopy. Collagen Rel Res 2: 143-150
[3] Duffy S, Davis M, Sharp F (1992) Preliminary observation of Holmium:YAG laser tissue interaction using human uterus. Lasers Surg Med 12:147-152
[4] Flory P, Garrett R (1958) Phase transition in collagen and gelatin systems. J Am Chem Soc 80:4836-4845
[5] Flory P, Weaver E (1959) Helix coil transition in dilute aqueous collagen solutions. J Am Chem Soc 82:4518-4525
[6] Guthrie C, Murray L, Kopchok G (1991) Biochemical mechanisms of laser vascular tissue fusion. J Invest Surg 4:3-12
[7] Hayashi K, Hecht P, Vanderby R, Peters D, Cooley A, Xiang Z, Thabit G III, Fanton G, Markel M (1998) The long term effect of laser energy on joint capsular tissue. Orthop Res Soc 23:1026
[8] Hayashi K, Markel M, Thabit G III, Bogdanske J, Thielke R (1995) The effect of non-ablative laser energy on joint capsular properties: an in vitro mechanical study using a rabbit model. Am J Sports Med 23: 482-487
[9] Hayashi K, Nieckaez J, Thabit G III, Bogdanske J, Cooley A, Markel M (1997) Effect of nonablative laser energy on the joint capsule: an in vivo rabbit study using holmium:YAG laser. Lasers Surg Med 20:164-171
[10] Hayashi K, Thabit G III, Bogdanske J, Mascio L, Markel M (1996) The effect of nonablative laser energy on the ultrastructure of joint capsular collagen. Arthroscopy 12:474-481
[11] Hayashi K, Thabit G III, Vailas A, Bogdanske J, Cooley A, Markel M (1996) The effect of non-ablative laser energy on joint capsular properties: an in vitro histological and biochemical study using a rabbit model. Am J Sports Med 24:640-646
[12] Kronick P, Maleeff B, Carroll R (1988) The locations of collagen with different thermal stabilities in fibrils of bovine reticular dermis. Conn Tiss Res 18: 123-134
[13] LeCarpentier G, Motamedi M, Mcmath L (1993) Continuous wave laser ablation of tissue: Analysis of thermal and mechanical events. IEEE Trans Biomed Eng 40:188-200
[14] Moreira H, Campos M, Sawusch M (1993) Holmium laser thermokeratoplasty. Ophthalmology 100:752-761
[15] O'Brien S, Miller D (1990) The contact neodymium-yttrium aluminum garnet laser. Clin Orthop 252:95-100
[16] Sherk H (1993) The use of lasers in orthopaedic procedures. J Bone Joint Surg 75-A:768-776
[17] Thabit G III (1994) Treatment of unidirectional and multidirectional glenohumeral instability by an arthroscopic holmium:YAG laser-assisted capsular shift procedure: a pilot study. Laser application in arthroscopy. 1st Congress of International Musculoskeletal Laser Society
[18] Verzar F, Zs.-Nagy I (1970) Electronmicroscopic analysis of thermal collagen denaturation in rat tail tendons. Gerontologia 16:77-82

In Vitro and Experimental Animal Research on Arthroscopic Laser Treatment of Cartilage – Setup Near to Clinical Application Conditions

B. E. Gerber · M. Zimmer · T. Asshauer · S. Preiss · M. Norberg · G. Delacretaz · H. Pratisto · M. Frenz

Introduction

Since laser systems became available for arthroscopic surgery a certain number of clinical uses have been reported. One of the special applications is the smoothing of the fibrillated hyaline cartilage, which is not possible by the customary mechanical or motorized instruments without leaving in place a toothbrush-like surface with bad mechanical properties and the risk of an enlarged degeneration area. The actual advantage of a cartilage debridement had only been the elimination of locking flaps, with the danger of tearing down more of the cartilage by the shaving procedure. In any case a wider surface treatment was abandoned because of the subsequent impairment of the cartilage often observed [29, 57].

For a new consideration of that sort of surgery the 308 nm excimer-laser, available for intraarticular application since the late 1980s, seemed to offer particular possibilities due to its low penetration rate and its "cold-laser" characteristics [16, 21, 50, 51, 62, 64]. On this account it was chosen for a preliminary experimental study even if the known, low general tissue ablation rate was unsatisfactory for meniscectomies or other resection procedures, for which different infrared laser sources actually are preferred [8, 58, 60, 61, 63]. Its immediate effects on the intact hyaline cartilage (energy related volumetric ablation rate, in vitro histology of the resection borders) have been investigated in several laboratories in especially well-measurable experimental settings [22, 32, 34, 62, 64]. Nevertheless ablation of broad healthy cartilage areas or drilling holes into an intact hyaline surface [22, 62. 64] will bring certain essential information, but it does not correspond to a useful clinical indication.

Preliminary In Vitro Pilot Study

For that reason we set up an in vitro pilot study, published in 1990 [16], to investigate a situation with real clinical applicability.

On fresh condyles of pig knees from slaughterhouse material a mechanical standard lesion was pro-

duced by scratching off the cartilage surface, wiping it with mid-granulated sand-paper in several directions. Thus about one third of the cartilage thickness was ablated, obtaining a fibrillated dim surface aspect similar to the one known from stage II-III osteoarthritis in human arthroscopy. One third of these areas was then treated by oblique irradiation with an excimer laser at a 50 Hz pulse repetition rate at a distance of 2–3-mm from the glass-fiber tip in one passage per surface unit. The laser source was a MAX 10 ultraviolet xenonchloride excimer laser, produced by Technolas/Germany, emitting at a wavelength of 308 nm. Corresponding areas were exposed to three passages or left further untreated. Intact condyle areas were used as controls, part of them after taking off the patina as a minimal surface layer.

Full thickness specimens were then fixed in 2.5 % Na-cacodylate buffered glutaraldehyde and used for scanning electron microscopy (SEM) investigation. Toluidine blue stains in EPON in light microscopy gave the gross orientation for osmium transmission electron microscopy (TEM) and indirectly for SEM. After critical-point drying (CPD) SEM specimens were mounted on Al-plates, gold-sputtered at 20 nm and imaged at 10 kV in different angles.

The superficial roughening by sand paper of the hyaline cartilage, compared to intact areas with regular parallel collagen fibers under the patina (Fig. 1a), created a surface lesion (Fig. 1b) very similar to SEM and TEM aspects of early human osteoarthritis [23, 24] in spite of the evident absence of any biological reaction [16]. By the wide superficial photoablation with the 308 nm excimer laser a smoothing was obtained immediately similar to the one we knew from the arthroscopic images of clinical laser treatments [21, 35, 50]. The investigations by TEM and special light microscopy stains showed variable features under the obtained surface. SEM areas were found with a close-meshed short-fragment fiber network very different from the scratched collagen fiber pattern after roughening (Fig. 1c) and other areas with a melted, absolutely smooth closing layer (Fig. 1d). A clear distinction of the melted layers from the slightly wrinkled patina of intact cartilage was

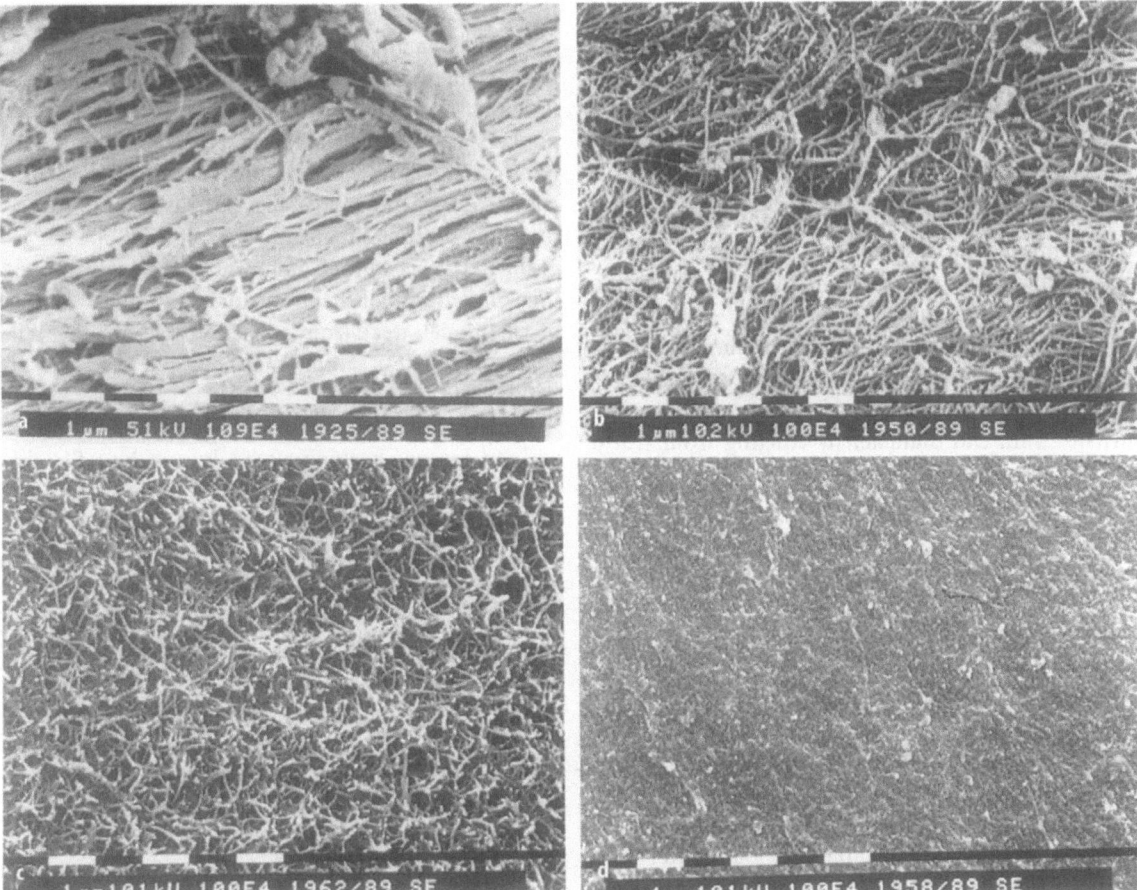

Fig. 1. a Normal parallel collagen fiber arrangement under the surface of intact cartilage after opening of the cover patina (SEM, high magnification). **b** Irregular collagen fiber mesh at a deeper level after scratching off the superficial one third of the cartilage by sand paper (in vitro OA model; SEM, high magnification). **c** Close-meshed short-fragmented fiber network forms as a new surface immediately after superficial smoothing of the scratched, OA model cartilage by photoablation with a 308 nm excimer laser (one passage; SEM, high magnification). **d** Melted, absolutely smooth closing layer after treatment of the scratched, OA model cartilage by photoablation with a 308 nm excimer laser (three passages; SEM, high magnification)

not always possible. Although the surgical procedure itself was specially designed to be realizable in clinical practice, an experimental setting for an in vivo study without previous induction of an osteoarthritis (OA) model [22, 51] could not allow any conclusions about the follow-ups after laser application transferable to human conditions.

First Experimental Animal Series

We therefore developed the experimental, in vivo OA model with induction of an installed OA reaction previous to the evaluation of the tested surgical procedure.

The other purpose of that study was to appreciate the impact of sealing of osteoarthritic fibrillated cartilage, by excimer laser smoothing onto the natural history of an induced early OA. The comparison of the corresponding results obtained by observation of the mentioned protocol with the ones without a laser application permits an evaluation of the particular therapeutic contribution of this procedure, all

the more so since the starting point is quite exactly comparable to the state created by a traditional motorized shaver abrasion [29, 57, 62].

Experimental Animal Series

On a series of 24 individuals of open breed pigs the model OA standard lesion was applied in a first open surgical procedure to roughen the cartilage within reach of the right knee only (OA inducing session). All animals recovered their gait ability within 10 days. About 4 weeks after the first operation a second open surgical intervention was performed to treat half of the cartilage surface previously roughened with the model lesion by excimer laser smoothing (treatment session).

This series was split up into three groups. The first eight animals were killed 3 days after the second surgical session to catch the early effects of the laser sealing and the reactive inflammatory response to the second operation. The second eight animals were killed at an average of 6 weeks after the treatment session for a short follow-up. The third group was killed at an average of 20 weeks after the treatment session for longer lasting observation of the therapy effects.

Surgical Procedures

To produce the standard lesion an antero-lateral arthrotomy of the right knee was performed under inhalation general anesthesia in a supine position, under Terramycin single shot cover and usual sterile conditions. The complete exposable femoral cartilage and the whole retropatellar surface was roughened as homogeneously as possible with a motorized dentist's burr of 2 mm end diameter by ablating from 1/3 to 1/2 of the overall thickness. After intensive joint lavage the incision was closed layer by layer and a spray cover was applied instead of a surgical dressing.

After an OA induction period of 4 weeks, on average under identical surgical conditions, a rearthrotomy of the right knee was done by the same approach. Before the laser energy was applied to the half of the exposable surface, chisel marks were created by ablating the cartilage with the subchondral bone in a transverse furrow in the middle of the femoral condyles in flexion and in the middle of the patella, to define a precise cartographical distinction of the laser treated areas. We thus obtained a uniform load pattern for the treated areas allowing a comparison to corresponding areas with the standard lesion only. Then the smoothing laser therapy was applied onto the areas provided for by irradiation with constant laser parameters until a macroscopic smoothing was achieved. The laser source was again a MAX 10 ultraviolet xenonchloride excimer laser emitting at a wavelength of 308 nm. The pulse duration was of 60 ns and the repetition rate of 40 Hz. The chosen pulse energy of 45 mJ was situated above the threshold of photoablation.

Evaluation Protocol

The harvesting of specimens from the right knees excised in toto was performed by the following defined procedure (2 controlateral knees for intact cartilage control were prepared in the same manner): The femur was dissected to apply a standardized impaction by a special "Bioimpactor" (RUSSEN-BERGER, Schaffhausen, CH) on an area with standard lesion only and on an area which subsequently was smoothed by superficial excimer laser photoablation.

For scanning electron microscopy (SEM) osteochondral pieces were taken by a circular chisel with a diameter of 1 cm, from impacted and nonimpacted surfaces, and fixed in Na-cacodylate buffered glutaraldehyde [44]. These specimens were processed by critical-point-drying and sputter coating with 20 nm gold and photographed at 10 kV with magnifications

from 25× for full surface up to 1000× and 10,000× for detail imaging. By knowledge of the pathoanatomical structure of hyaline cartilage we developed criteria that allowed a documented statistical evaluation of every specimen: roughness, clefts/edges, different fiber mesh features, filling substance density, imaged chondrocytes and deposite layers. Based on these criteria two persons independent from the SEM imager evaluated the codified pictures. Then we examined the concordance of the evaluators and the distinction of OA model areas from treated areas with the Wilcoxon test, U test (Mann-Whitney) and the Kruskal-Wallis test.

For light microscopy (LM), squares of 0.25 mm^2 with an osseous backing were taken off by a flat chisel and fixed in formaldehyde 4 % with saframin-O adjunction [56]. For these specimens different stainings were applied such as alcyan blue/PAS, H & E, and soluphenyl red, and compared to the features of human osteoarthritis specimens. A qualitative random sample examination occurred in magnifications from 10× to 15× by standard light microscopy or under polarization. From the ultra-thin search cuts of the 197 light microscopy samples, black and white overview paper prints were used for quantitative morphometric measurements: surface-layer thickness, cellular density per mm^2 and cell dispositions in the deeper layers as well as vascular ingrowth were recorded in conformity with the six different follow-up groups and the three depth layers. The counted fields were squares of 500 μm of sidelength taking into account the different magnifications ranging from 80× to 640×.

For transmission electron microscopy (TEM) we excised wedges of 2 mm of thickness with an osseous corner opposite to the examined cartilage surface and fixed them in glutaraldehyde [47]. Then these specimens were pretreated by osmic acid and tannin and, after localizing typical features by the means of search-cuts, paper prints were taken in magnifications ranging from 1200× to 12,000×. The imaged cartilage layers (superficial/intermediate/deep) of each follow-up group were evaluated separately with regard to the ratios of vital and dead chondrocytes. In the vital cells degenerative signs typical for osteoarthritis such as glycogen agglomerations, widening of the rough endoplasmic reticulum, lipoid inclusions, peripheral membrane indentations, and pericellular halo formations were scored by attribution of each cell to a scale of "none or few" (1 point), "middle" (2 points), or "important" (3 points). This scoring allows calculation of a mean chondrocyte factor (ϕ) of viability and cell activity for a specific time – and treatment-related follow-up group with regard to every one of the above-mentioned cytological TEM criteria by means of the following equation:

$$\phi = \frac{v^2}{\Sigma \cdot t}$$

where v is the number of vital cells in a group, Σ is the sum of degenerative TEM score points, t is the total number of investigated cells (vital and dead cells); $\phi = 0$ indicates a cell population without any viability composed exclusively of dead cells and cell debris, and $\phi = 1$ describes a cell population with full vitality, in which all degenerative criteria have been graded "none or few".

The fragments for immunoassays (IA) were purely cartilaginous and stored in 0.9 % saline at −90 °C [59]. These samples for proteoglycan analysis underwent determination of glycosaminoglycan contents and of keratan-sulfate epitopes with antibody "12-1" in relation to the water content and the dry weight and were evaluated according to the six follow-up groups.

From all investigated parameters human values concerning normal cartilage and OA were determined by the same procedures. For harvesting of the human comparison material the same four kinds of samples as from the animals were taken from the resection sites in the knees to be provided with an endoprosthesis, partly from the severely fibrillated worn compartments, partly from healthy border areas with intact cartilage.

For evaluation we took into account the fact that the animals were very closely related due to the open breeding and that the specimens for OA model only and for the excimer laser sealing were harvested from the same knees and the normal controls from controlateral knees. Therefore all pictures of the different imaging methods and all samples for IA taken from an identical group were put together for common evaluation. The human samples were placed in one separate group.

Regarding the different histomorphological parameters, both for the morphometrically investigated light microscopy (LM) overviews as well as for cytological signs on the TEM images, all groups were evaluated according to three layers: a superficial layer of ongrown fibrous tissue or of horizontal longitudinal chondrocytes, an intermediate layer of cartilage and a deep cartilage layer adjacent to the subchondral bone.

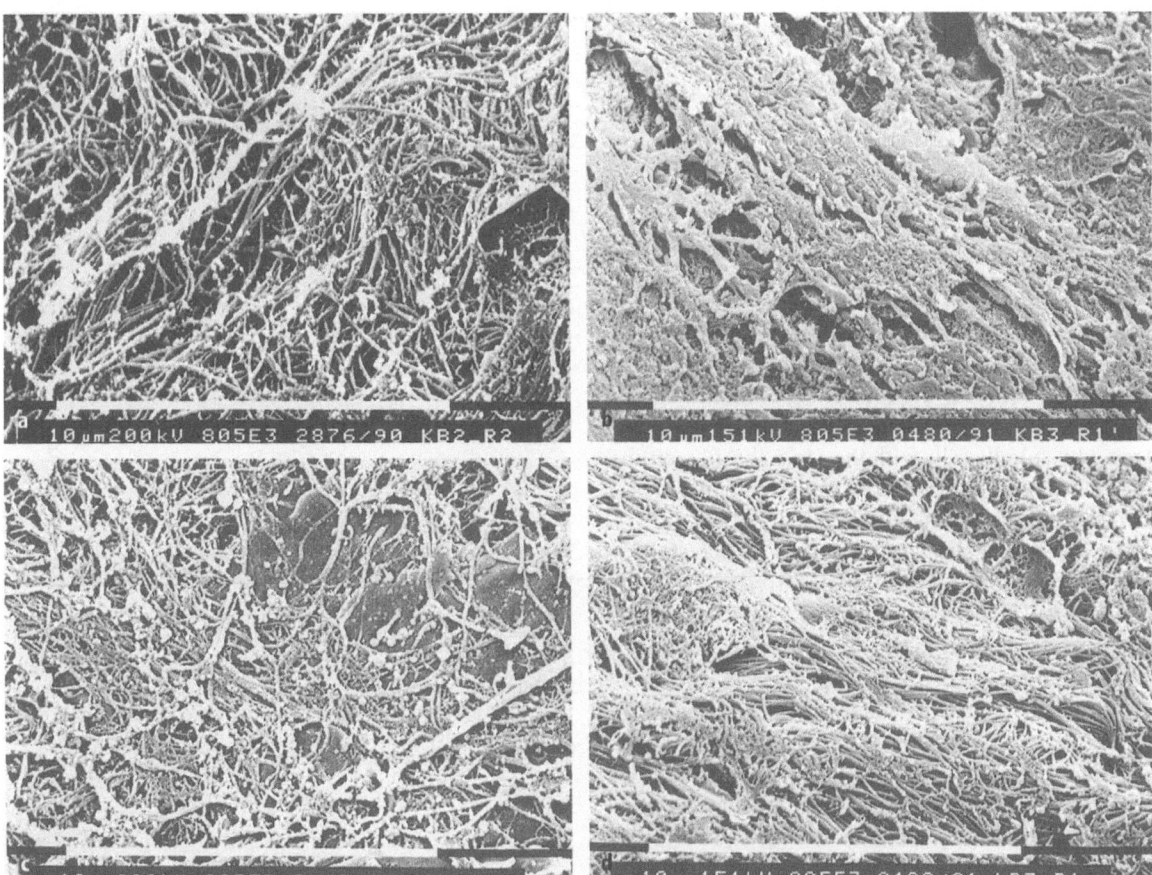

Fig. 2. Irregular fibrous surface cover **a** 9 weeks after lesion; note the low density of the fiber mesh (SEM, high magnification). **b** A more dense fiber mesh forms 24 weeks after lesion (SEM, high magnification). **c** Six weeks after lasering, note the low density of the fiber mesh (SEM high magnification). **d** A more dense fiber mesh forms 20 weeks after lasering (SEM, high magnification)

Results of In Vivo Evaluation
After Excimer Laser Exposure

Ultrastructural Results

Scanning Electron Microscopy

The comparative SEM investigation of normal untreated cartilage samples with induced OA and samples after excimer laser sealing (122 samples by 4–10 images each) proved that onto all the surfaces on which the standard lesion had been applied with less than about 5 mm of interspace an irregular fibrous tissue cover grows without discontinuity within approximately 6–10 weeks, independent of the applied surface treatment. Before that a fibrin layer remains fixed during the first postoperative phase. With increasing follow-up time a significant density repair of the collagen fiber tissue up to the 20th–24th week occurs (Fig. 2). The areas smoothed by laser application are not significantly distinguishable from the roughened ones. By the same distribution the mechanical resistance to a standardized impaction is diminished in the superficial cartilage of all areas. We found comparable deep clefts as a sign of diminished mechanical resistance (Fig. 3a,b). Both the roughened and laser-treated surfaces appear different from the healthy cartilage of the contralateral knee, on which no fibrous cover is formed and the mechanical resistance to the standardized impaction is not diminished. It only shows a slight impaction halo that can hardly be distinguished in SEM images (Fig. 3c).

Light Microscopy

The investigation of the section plane by LM according to 197 photographs evaluated by morphometry (from 61 samples by 3–7 images each, i. e. 28 pictures per group) confirms the constant presence in all treated groups of a superficial fibrous tissue layer infiltrated by spindle cells with the same sharply outlined difference in staining from an underlying hyaline cartilage as found in human OA.

In the superficial layer 3–4 weeks after standard lesion chondrocytes are found disposed in cluster formations (Fig. 4) according to 1.5 cluster/mm^2 versus 1.2 cluster/mm^2 immediately after lasering. A constant increase of clusters is seen in OA model areas and a successive stabilization in laser-treated areas. Vascular ingrowth (Fig. 4) was found with a maximum at 6–10 weeks for both groups, but about half as intensive after lasering. In the healthy cartilage neither clusters nor vascular ingrowth were observed in this layer.

In the deeper layers in all samples a well definable stratum of vital residual cartilage was found between the fibrous infiltrated surface layer and the subchondral bone. No spindle cells were found at this tissue

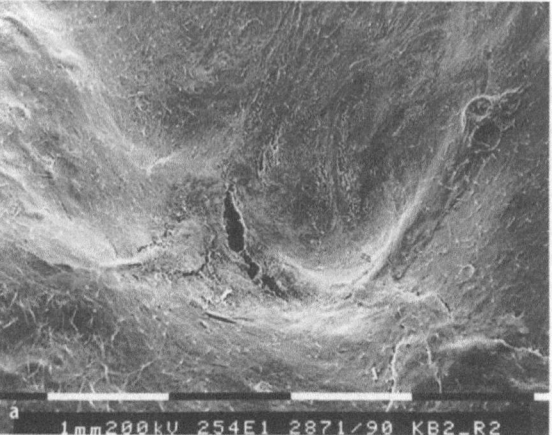
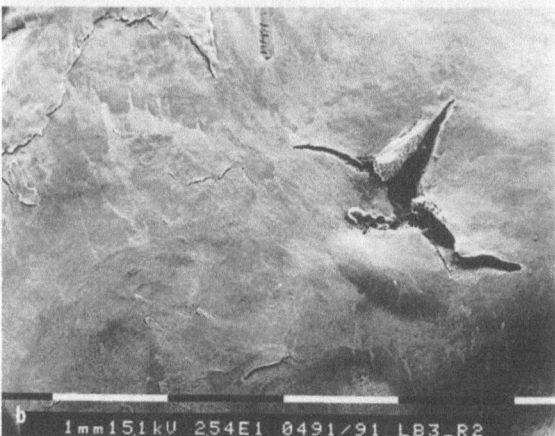
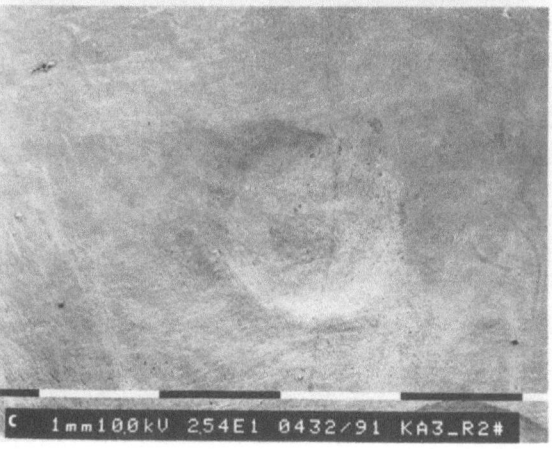

Fig. 3a–c. Mechanical resistance as observed by SEM. **a** Ruptured surface by standardized impaction 10 weeks after OA lesion, demonstrating the impaired mechanical resistance. **b** Ruptured surface by standardized impaction 6 weeks after lasering, also demonstrating an impaired mechanical resistance. **c** Impaction halo on a healthy cartilage surface by the same standardized impaction; (low magnification)

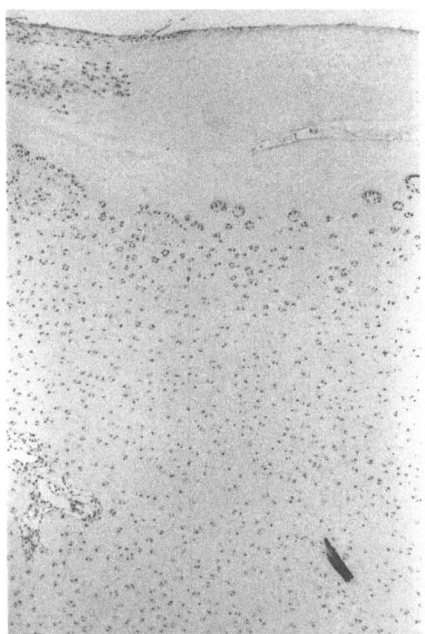

Fig. 4. Fibrous cover shown by light microscopy: vascular ingrowth and intensive cluster formations 10 weeks after model standard lesion; hematoxy lin/eosin, low magnification

level. The combined thickness of deeper layers with preserved hyaline cartilage was 964 µm on average. Rare clusters at the beginning in standard lesion areas are followed by significant multiplication, but after laser exposition the cluster incidence is much less intense.

Transmission Electron Microscopy

The investigation of qualitative cytological signs by TEM was conducted based on 906 images, with an average of 37.8 pictures per animal (151/follow-up group and 50.3/layer group), the different layers being represented by 266 pictures of the superficial, by 314 pictures of the middle layer and 326 pictures of the deep one. The calculation of the viability factor ϕ (see equation above) was done on the basis of 1789 chondrocytes by 74.5 cells per animal, the layers being represented by 470 chondrocytes in the superficial layer, 630 in the middle and 689 in the deep one. After separate counting of the dead cells and definable cell debris, the cytological TEM scoring for the single ultrastructural criteria of glycogen accumulation, lipoid inclusions, enlarged endoplasmic reticulum, membrane indentations and pericellular halo formations (Fig. 5, Fig. 6) was run on 1249 viable chondrocytes by 52 cells/animal, the layers being represented by 123 viable chondrocytes in the superficial layer, 513 in the middle layer and 613 in the deep one.

The overall evaluation of the different degenerative signs corresponding to the findings in human OA

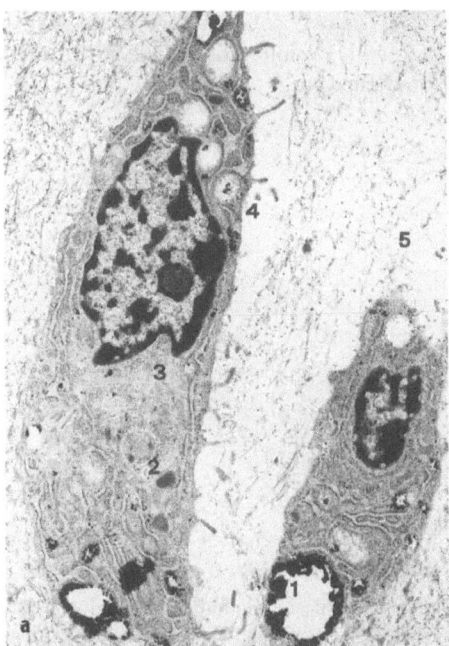
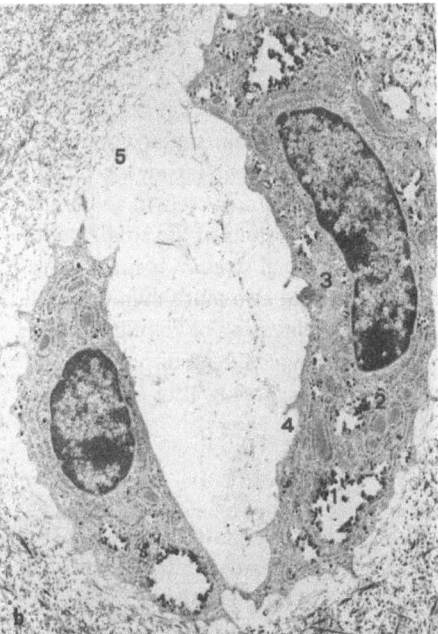

Fig. 5a,b. Pairs of chondrocyte in the middle layer after 6–10 weeks with degenerative TEM signs. *1* increased glycogen accumulation; *2* lipoid inclusions; *3* enlarged endoplasmic reticulum; *4* membrane indentations; *5* pericellular halo formations (TEM, higher magnification). **a** Experimental OA model; **b** laser

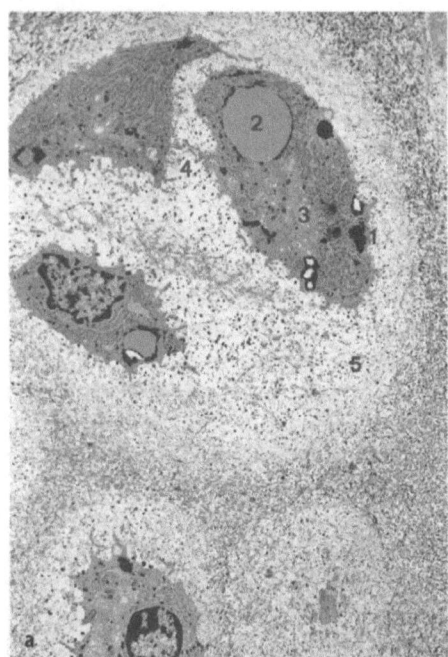
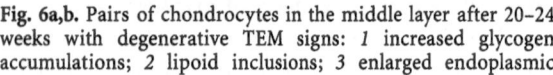
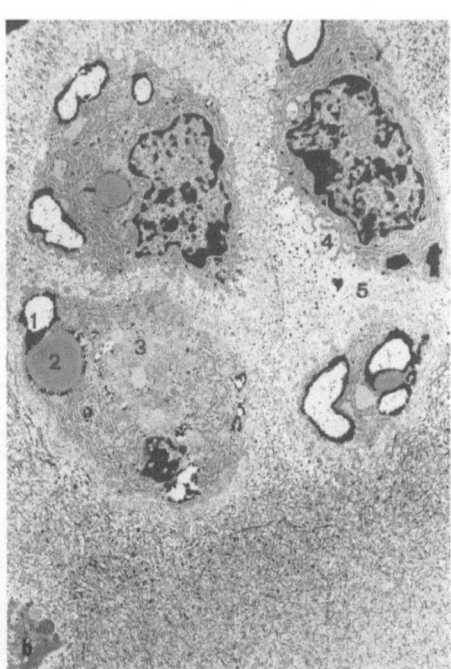

Fig. 6a,b. Pairs of chondrocytes in the middle layer after 20–24 weeks with degenerative TEM signs: *1* increased glycogen accumulations; *2* lipoid inclusions; *3* enlarged endoplasmic reticulum; *4* membrane indentations; *5* pericellular halo formations (TEM, higher magnification; 180x). **a** Experimental OA model; **b** laser

gave the following time-related distribution of the general cell viability for the two main groups (OA model and laser-treated areas) and the three depth layers taken together: 4 weeks after induction of OA by the standard lesion the chondrocytes in the model areas show a viability of 28 %. Three days after laser smoothing the chondrocytes of the three depth layers in these areas have an overall viability of 20 %; 10 weeks after lesion the viability of the OA model chondrocytes is 35 % and 6 weeks after lasering the cells have recovered a viability of 32 %. Some 24 weeks after roughening in the OA model surfaces the viability of the chondrocytes attains 44 %, the cells of laser exposed areas regain a viability of 43 %. The separate observations of the single depth layers show that the superficial stratum is much more involved than the deeper and also more than the middle one, where the early depression of viability, a little more evident after lasering, is less important and returns to a stability of 50 % already after 6–10 weeks.

Biochemical Results

Immunoassays

For this evaluation 58 full-thickness cartilage specimens without adjacent bone were available from the different follow-up groups. The evolution curves for the content of glycosaminoglycans (GAG) and keratansulfate (KS) in % of dry weight (Fig. 7) start with normal values for both parameters and both

treatment groups. Thereafter the model group with standard lesion shows a decrease after 6 more weeks, to a level comparable with human OA values which remains until the end of the study. In the laser group the mean contents fall after 6 weeks to levels lower than human OA values and recover nearly to the starting level at the end of follow-up. Human normal values confirmed by our own specimens were nearly double those of the corresponding values for human OA.

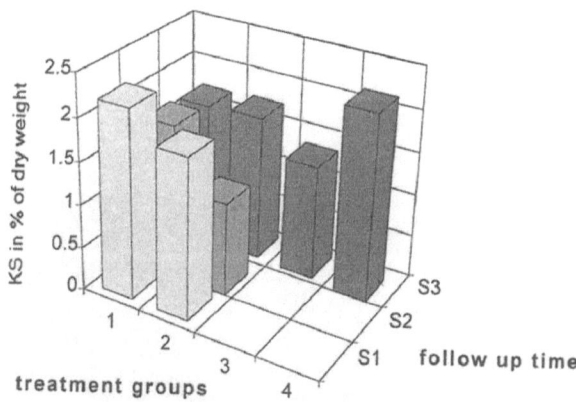

Fig. 7. Biochemical evolution curves of glycosaminoglycan und keratan sulfate contents during follow-up after standard lesion and laser exposition (human values for comparison). *1* OA model; *2* laser; *3* human osteoarthritis; *4* human normal values; *S1* early; *S2* 6–10; *S3* late

Conclusions from In Vivo Data After Excimer Laser Smoothing

Laser sealing has been proposed as the only technique for smoothing of the fibrillated osteoarthritic cartilage and has been used clinically mainly in arthroscopic procedures [8, 58, 60, 63]. The biological effects to the underlying cartilage already damaged by OA were still uninvestigated even though there are many in vitro studies [12, 34, 61, 62, 64]. Some newer research has been done in vivo on the effect of surface application of lasers to the healthy cartilage [22, 51] which does not correspond to any clinical situation. In the early times of clinical application the 308 nm excimer laser was considered as a safe tool because of its "cold" ablation without production of a carbonization zone. For this reason it has been chosen for the testing on early osteoarthritic surfaces on which installation of degenerative disease has been performed by an in vivo OA model before the laser sealing has been applied. This allows observation of its influence on the natural history of OA and the possibilities of salvage of the underlying cartilage as well as of local biomechanical debridement effects. The resulting experimental findings create a basis to be put in relation to the immediate surgical advantages in clinical use described by several authors [8, 21, 35, 50, 55] and are superimposable on our own clinical experience [63]. In this way an explanation may be found for the improved clinical outcomes after laser sealing, with better symptom relief as well as less and later recurrence compared to mechanical debridement by a shaver abrasion. The clinical results of the latter are the same as after a simple arthroscopic joint lavage [21, 50]. The only additional effect of a mechanical abrasion treatment seems to consist in a elimination of impinging tissue flaps but it maintains and even supports an OA-like cartilage state.

The first aim of this research project was: (1) to develop an in vivo model for producing early OA in a simple procedure especially appropriate for testing surgical, mainly arthroscopic, surface treatments under test conditions similar to the ones encountered when the indication to application in humans may be discussed [16] and (2) to prove the relevance of this model for induction of chondromalacia, comparable to early osteoarthritic lesions in humans. It had to fulfill the following critieria:

- At the time of experimental treatment a OA-like surface lesion of the cartilage must be visible macroscopically. It has to develop in a reasonable interval.
- Typical OA signs in histological, biochemical and biomechanical parameters must be obtained reproducibly within a suitable period.
- A sufficient follow-up without spontaneous healing on one hand and without development of relevant joint deformation on the other hand is essential.
- A persistence of the OA producing factor has to be avoided during the whole observation period.
- A transfer of the observations to human conditions must be possible.
- The standard OA lesion should be easily achieved on a suffcient amount of weight bearing surface area.

The testing without induction of an OA-like lesion [22, 50] is misleading because the available surgical techniques do not allow an absolutely homogeneous processing of the cartilage [16] and therefore intermediate areas of normal aspect may not reflect a good result of treatment but only inhomogeneous application of the model lesion.

Examining the important range of known OA models we distinguished two essential types: chemical and mechanical [1, 2, 15, 25, 37, 42, 48, 49, 53, 65]: Chemical lesions, induced by injections of corticoids, enzymes or other irritative agents, may lead to the biochemical changes of early OA in a sufficient portion of cartilage but the absence of a real surface lesion does not allow a surgical smoothing. Mechanical models without arthrotomy (patellofemoral contusions [15, 65], permanent compression by external fixator [53]) may not produce a sufficient OA area and the pathological process will occur more under the joint surface and thus not be visible enough. Mechanical models with meniscectomy [42] or ligament transsections [1, 37, 49] keep the OA producing factor permanent and the surgically treated area undergoes the same effects, which would have been eliminated in humans by ligament reconstructions or osteotomies. Moreover these sorts of lesions rapidly induce an advanced and deforming stage of OA.

None of the known in vivo models could fulfill the criteria mentioned above. Therefore the development of a new OA in vivo model was necessary. The model is independent from the tested treatment. The standard lesion can be applied either in an open or an arthroscopic procedure. A large cartilage surface can be exposed, e. g., in a pig knee, and is thus available for examination of different parameters. Comparable control and treatment areas can be marked and cartilage samples of control and treatment areas can be investigated in comparison.

The SEM investigations show an increasing repair of the cartilage surface with time. But, as the macroscopic, LM and TEM view prove, a fibrous layer grows rapidly onto the surface and the morphological type of the real cartilage surface is not detectable by SEM. First adhesion of a blood clot appears and then an increasingly fibrous layer develops over the injured cartilage with increasing density of collagen fibers. The variation in thickness of this fibrous layer may be explained by unequal mechanical wear and/or by preparation artifacts. In LM this layer has the same sharply outlined difference of staining as found in human OA. This is in agreement with results from immediate rearthroscopy in humans [29]. As expected this effect is not found on untouched cartilage surfaces of the intact contralateral knee.

The morphometric evaluations of the LM specimens and special stains show the induction of degenerative signs and hyperrepair features (cluster formations, vascular ingrowth, atopic collagen) comparable to the findings in human OA [23, 24, 43, 54, 68]. In TEM the viability factor calculation based on the evaluated degenerative criteria demonstrates a diminution of the viability, stabilized at about 50 % of healthy chondrocytes both for specimens after induction of our OA models by the standard lesion and for our human samples.

The IAs for obtaining dry weight contents of proteoglycans also give values comparable to early human OA [59, own measurements], where the exaggerated repair induced production of proteoglycans by the cluster cells seems to balance the proteoglycan loss in this early stage of the disease.

All the induced alterations can still be found after 6 months, comparable to the natural history of real OA. Open breed pigs prove to be essentially similar to humans in cartilage response patterns.

By the fact that a typical biological reaction is released and an implication of the whole cartilage surface within reach is observed, investigations about the homogeneity of surgical and especially of arthroscopic procedures like shaving or laser sealing are possible. The presented in vivo model for early OA fulfills all citeria mentioned above. Thus it is a good model for examining various methods of treatment which may be applied to an osteoarthritic cartilage.

The second part of this study deals with the comparative results of excimer laser smoothing tested by this model protocol and with the specific question of its influence on the spontaneous outcome of the experimentally induced OA.

Since a fibrous cover grows onto all treated surfaces the biological information obtained by SEM is limited to the following facts: The laser smoothing does not impede the superficial repair reaction nor modify it in quality. The successive density increases occur in the same manner as for the model lesion alone. But, apart from the elimination of impinging irregularities of the surface, the mechanical properties of the ongrown cover are not further improved.

In LM the morphometric investigations show that the excimer laser sealing preserves a constant layer of vital hyaline cartilage. The same sort of degenerative signs, with proteoglycan loss, diminution of chondrocyte density and thinning of the hyaline cartilage layer, is found at a lesser intensity than in the fully stimulated osteoarthritic response in the experimental OA model as well as the hyperrepair reaction of cluster formation.

In TEM a defined factor of mean vitality of the chondrocyte populations after lasering shows a more or less strong early depression of vitality according to the different layers and a recovery of the mean vitality up to values in the range of OA model areas.

The IAs show even a better recovery of proteoglycan contents from a considerable depression immediately after laser smoothing.

Based on the overall results of the biological follow-up parameters investigated in this study, no arguments were found that would constrain to renounce the mechanical benefit of arthroscopic surface smoothing on installed early human OA. In clinical mid-term follow-up studies this method leads to significant improvements compared to mechanical debridment [8, 21, 50].

This favorable situation for clinical laser applications to treat osteoarthritic cartilage surfaces arthroscopically still included two weak points: In a longer lasting observation of excimer lasers in clinical application, specifically the ablation rates on menisci and cartilage flaps as well as the absence of any hemostatic effect in synovial resections, led to the gradual abandonment of this wavelength, produced moreover in quite bulky machines. Also, knowledge of biophysical active mechanisms of pulsed lasers was only very rudimentary; neodymium:YAG lasers, which were available clinically in continuous wave form, were increasingly taken as a substitute for treating joint tissues albeit in undue indications, causing relevant damage. In the meantime, important developments were achieved particularly on pulsed near infrared lasers as holmium, and later on erbium. These wavelengths allowed significantly more rapid and effective tissue ablation than excimer lasers. The relatively easy development of application devices for holmium leading to a quick expansion in its clinical use called for basic research investigations clearing up the biophysical mechanisms in order to avoid detrimental applications and to point out optimal exploitation conditions for its favorable effects.

In Vitro Basic Research on Holmium Laser Effects to the Cartilage

At that stage of the investigations the fact was known that infrared laser pulses delivered in a fluid environment like in arthroscopy or angioplasty create transient vapor bubbles [6]. Subsequently dissections of vascular tissue by laser induced cavitation during angioplasty had been reported [11]. Cell damage and vitality decreases on cartilage tissue and in cultures were attributed to these photoacoustic effects [9,11] independent of the levels of applied energy or other parameters that may influence their modulability.

After the generation of pressure transients during holmium laser ablation and the dynamics and collapse of the induced bubbles had been investigated systematically in free water and on polyacrylamide gel tissue models [3, 4, 6, 7], the dependence of the bubble formation and collapse-induced pressure on pulse energy, fiber diameter and puls duration was taken into account in the setup of the in vitro study on cartilage tissue. Respecting the significant decrease of peak pressures by reduction of fiber diameter and pulse energy, the effects of cavitation bubbles on cartilages specimens in saline were studied as a function of the laser irradiance and the angle of incidence of the delivering fiber. The used laser parameters covered the range of clinical application [18].

Materials and Methods of the In Vitro Holmium Experiment

The positioning of the different devices in the experimental setup is shown in Fig. 8. A Cr:Tm:holmium:YAG laser working at a wavelength of 2.12 μm was used. Laser pulse energies of 0.5, 1.0 and 1.5 J were investigated. The pulse duration was kept at 250 μs (340 μs required for 1.5 J pulses). The laser light was coupled into a 600 μm core diameter quartz fiber. The processes taking place on the cartilage samples were imaged by standard time-resolved flash videography [5] using a white light xenon flash lamp (Hamamatsu L4633) synchronized with the laser source by a delay generator (Stanford Research Systems DGD 535), allowing imaging at variable delay times ranging from 0 to 1000 μs after the laser pulse. The acoustic measurements [6, 7] were performed with a piezoelectric needle hydrophone (Imotec). Measuring the exact distance of the hydrophone from the bubble collapse center for each experiment, for comparison purposes, all pressure data were normalized to a standard distance of 1 mm. Freshly harvested, cylindrical, porcine femur, patellar groove cartilage samples 6–8 mm in diameter and 2–3 mm thickness stored under saline at 4 °C were used as target. The videography and pressure results were obtained from single pulses on virgin sample sites at least 2 mm away from each other to avoid accidental interactions between subsequent irradiations.

The presented histomorphometric data are taken from these same cartilage sample sites after single pulse irradiation and from analogous sample sites after irradiation by five consecutive pulses without any changes in setup or laser parameters. Immediately after laser exposure the cartilage samples were placed in a buffered 4 % formalin solution for 5 days, then decalcified and imbedded in parafin and cut to slices of 5 μm thickness. The samples were stained with azan and safranin-O light green [33, 56]. We analyzed alterations in the intercellular substance and structure modifications in cell morphology according to a defined geometrical relation to the center of laser impaction with the following criteria: (1) variations of staining of the nuclei, cyto-

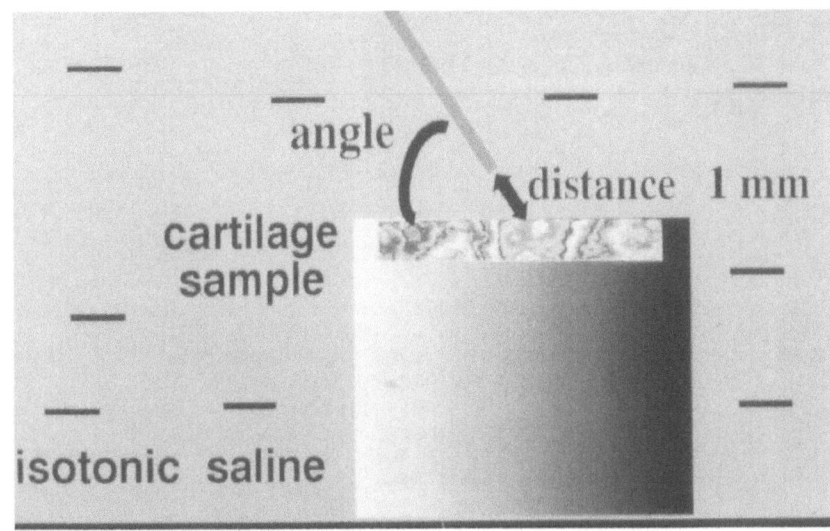

Fig. 8. Experimental setup of the in vitro holmium experiment

plasm and intercellular substance, (2) shape and size of the nuclei compared to the chondrocyte cavity, and (3) position of the nuclei inside the chondrocyte cavity.

Results of In Vitro Experimentation with Holmium Laser

Biophysical Results

Effects of Perpendicular Irradiation

In the typical bubble dynamics after perpendicular delivery of a 0.5 J energy pulse, shown in Fig. 9a, during the initial expansion phase the bubble develops as it would in free water (100 µs). Then it reaches the cartilage surface and starts to be influenced by the latter (200 µs). After having passed its maximum extension the bubble collapses modified by this interaction, becomes almost hemispherical (400 µs) and moves its center towards the cartilage surface exposing it to shock waves (600 µs). The recorded collapse pressure peaks do not increase with rising pulse energy (Fig. 10). The process which leads to this leveling is at best illustrated by the bubble dynamics induced by the highest investigated pulse energy (Fig. 9b): the initially purely vapor-filled bubble (100 µs) in the further course is increasingly per-

turbed in its symmetry once the water layer between fiber tip and tissue is removed and ejection of ablation products from the cartilage surface starts (200 µs). Most of these are propelled through the vapor before being decelerated in the surrounding water layers at 400 µs. After the bubble collapses some solid ablation particles remain visible in the fluid around the fiber tip (630 µs).

Fig. 9. a Typical bubble dynamics after perpendicular delivery of a 0.5 J energy pulse (standard time-resolved flash videography). **b** Bubble dynamics induced by the highest investigated pulse energy (1.5 J energy pulse, 90°, 1 mm distance to fiber tip): initially there is a purely vapor-filled bubble (100 µs), increasingly perturbed in its symmetry by ejected ablation products from the cartilage surface (200 µs) (standard time-resolved flash videography). **c** At an irradiation angle of 30° (1.0 J energy pulse, 1 mm distance to fiber tip), the bubble first develops undisturbed until the vapor channel from the fiber tip to the cartilage surface is opened (100 µs–200 µs). Then the strong absorption of laser energy in the upper cartilage layers leads to an ejection of ablation particles perpendicular to the surface (300 µs) resulting in an impressive distortion of the bubble (400 µs; standard time-resolved flash videography).

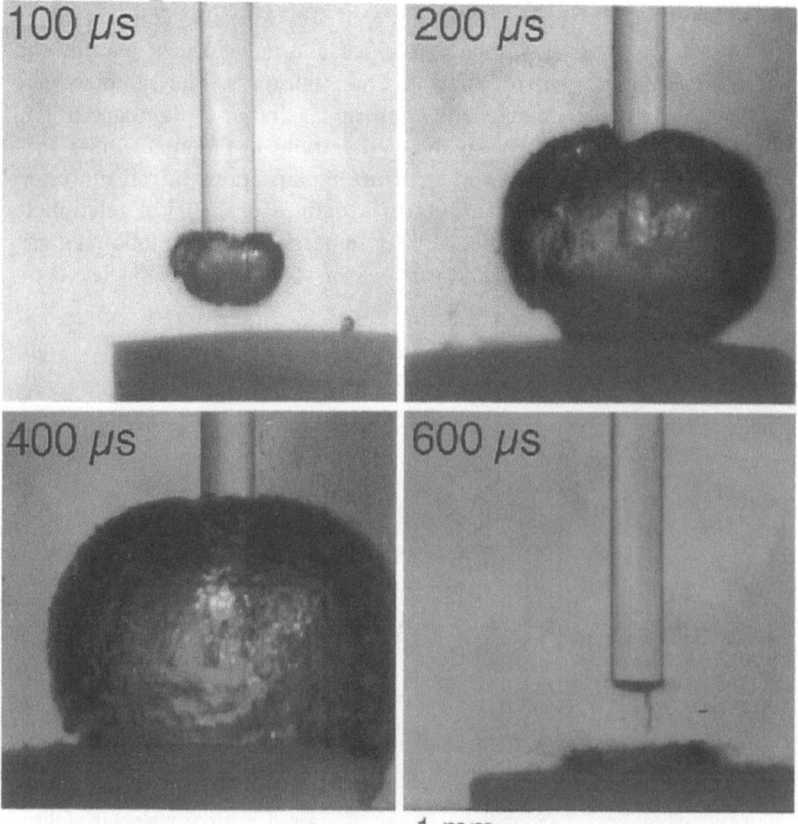

a   ⊢————⊣ 1 mm   Fig. 9a

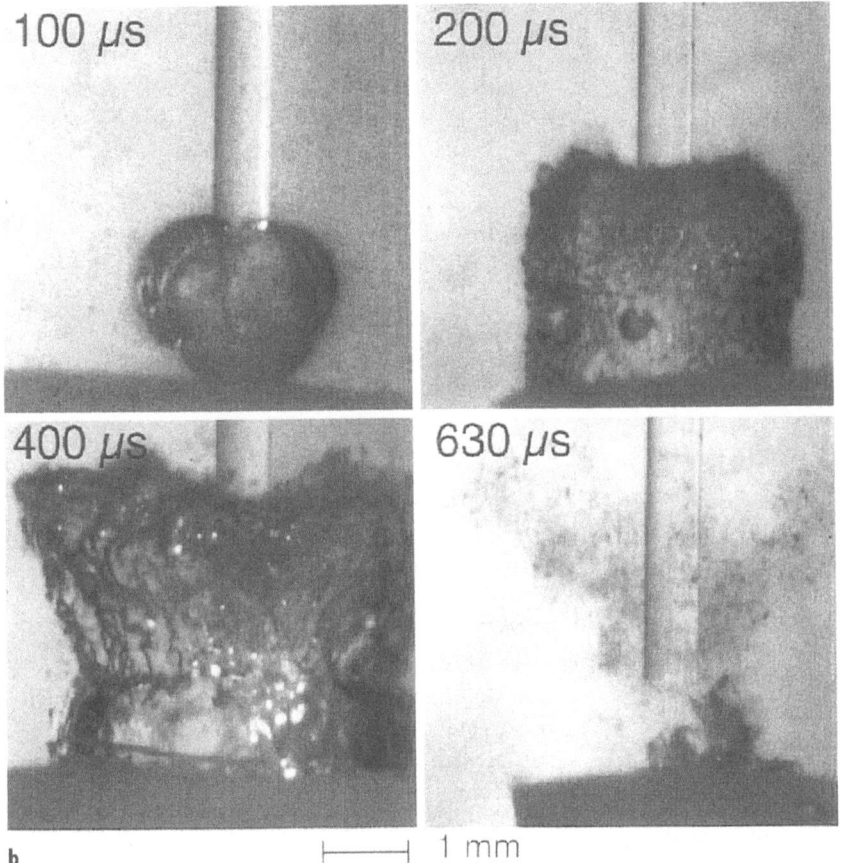

100 µs   200 µs

400 µs   630 µs

b   ⊢———⊣ 1 mm   *Fig. 9b*

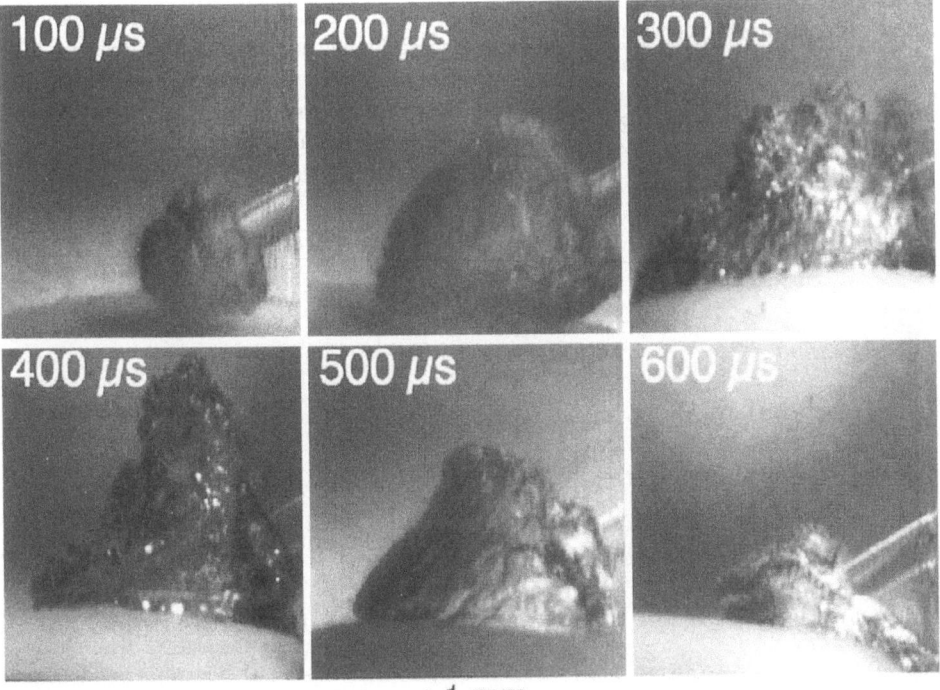

100 µs   200 µs   300 µs

400 µs   500 µs   600 µs

c   ⊢———⊣ 1 mm   *Fig. 9c*

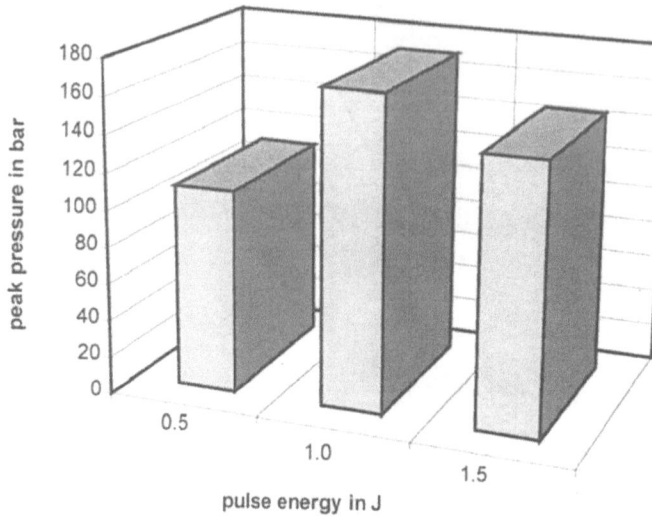

Fig. 10. Maximum bubble collapse pressure peaks with 90° fiber angle as a function of pulse energy

Effects of Variable Angles of Irradiation

The perturbation of the bubble symmetry increases significantly when the delivery fibers are tilted to increasingly oblique angles of incidence (Fig. 9c). At an irradiation angle of 30° the bubble first develops undisturbed until the vapor channel from the fiber tip to the cartilage surface is opened (100 µs–200 µs). Then the strong absorption of laser energy in the upper cartilage layers leads to an ejection of ablation particles perpendicular to the surface (300 µs) resulting in an impressive distortion of the bubble (400 µs) even though the ablated volume is less significant than at 90° with identical pulse energy. A significant reduction of the collapse pressure peaks for small angles of irradiation (Fig. 11) is the result. At 0° of incidence no particle ejection from the tissue surface is observed, but the bubble symmetry is particularly perturbed by the competing attractions of the cartilage surface and the fiber tip. Therefore the peak pressures measured at 80 bar are the smallest [5].

Histological Results

Perpendicular Single Pulse Irradiation

Single Holmium laser pulses applied at 90° of incidence create a circumscript lesion on intact porcine cartilage with characteristic tissue modifications in azan staining situated around a central ablation crater. The depth of the tissue removal and the surrounding alterations depends on the laser pulse energy. For pulses of 1.5 J energy the ablation crater has a mean depth of 300 µm and a width of 450 µm. It shows an irregularly disrupted bottom line. Just underneath the remainders of the intercellular substance are slightly condensed with some vacuolae. In the adjacent area the chondrocyte cavities are empty. Then follows a zone where the intercellular substance is brightened up as are the nuclei of the chondrocytes. This corresponds quite precisely to results of in vitro experiments on laser induced cartilage welding using confocal microscopy and differentiating living from dead cells after exposure of

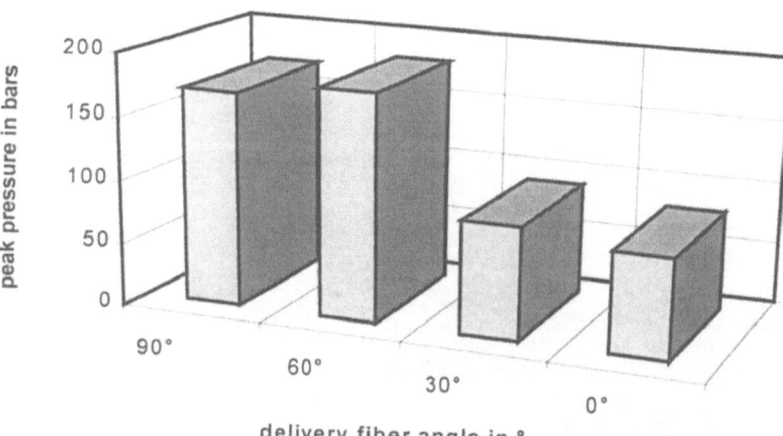

Fig. 11. Maximum bubble collapse pressure peaks with constant pulse energy (1 J) as a function of fiber angle

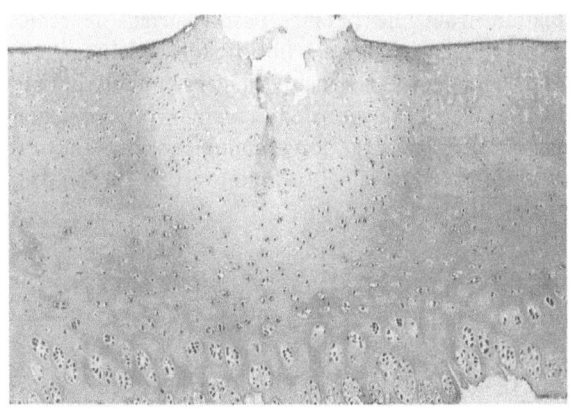

Fig. 12. Single holmium laser pulse (1.5 J/200 µs) applied at 90° of incidence on intact porcine cartilage; safranin-O, × 15

bone-cartilage specimens held alive in PBS solution [40]. The threat to cell vitality reaches down twice as far as the cell destruction seen in usual histological stainings. In the next tissue band normal nuclei are displaced eccentrically in the cell cavities with regard to the crater center at the level of the surface line in a sucessively densifying pattern of intercellular staining. The border of the area of tissue modifications is again marked by a slightly condensed intercellular substance and reaches down to 950 µm from the surface line with a diameter of 900 µm in a parabolic disposition (Fig. 12). The cartilage beyond this border line is normal in all histological parameters.

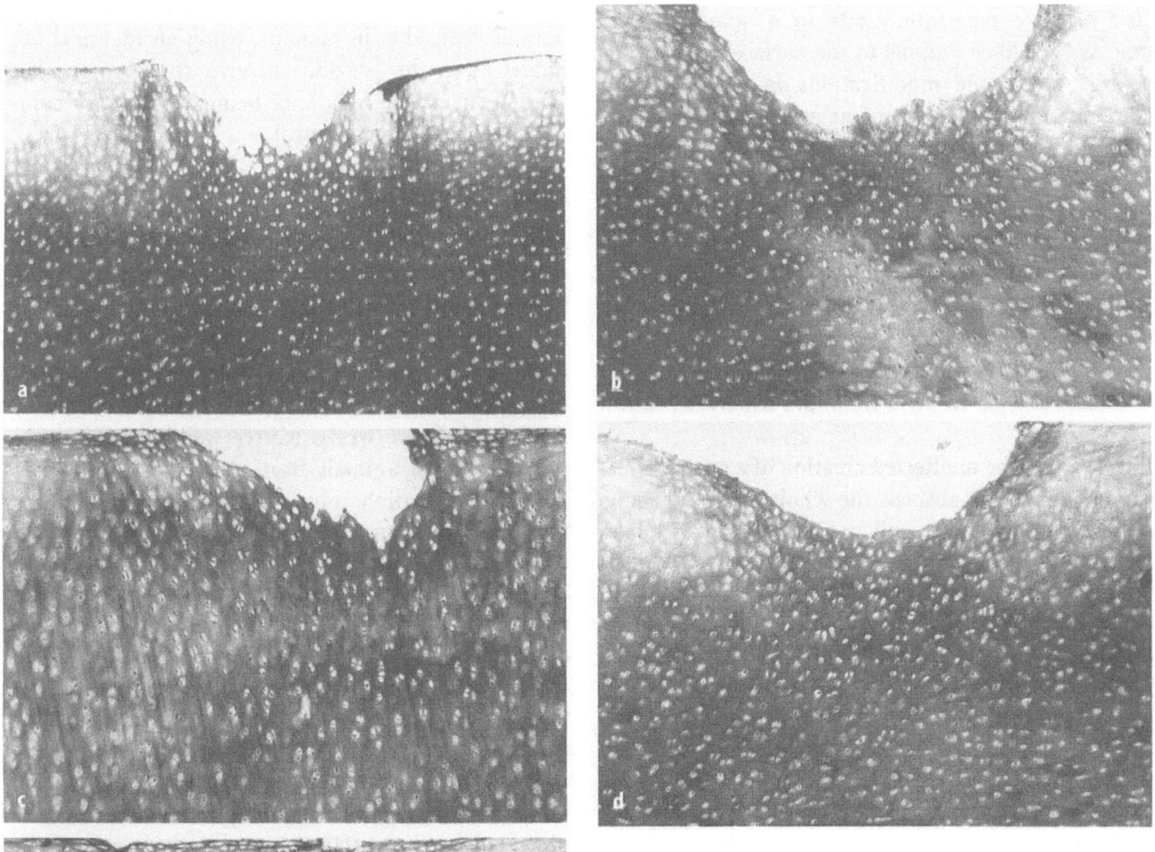

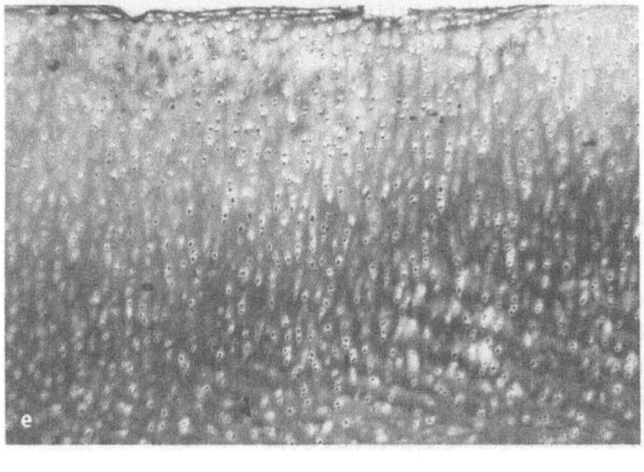

Fig. 13. a Symmetrically parabolic ablation crater in an intact porcine cartilage at 90° (1 pulse, 1.0 J). **b** Nearly unchanged crater after exposure to five pulses (90°, 1.0 J). **c** Diminished crater depth and increased width at 30° with deepest point at the bottom shifted opposite to the fiber tip and the surface disruption only present on that side (1 pulse, 1.0 J). **d** Smooth crater line after five pulses at 30°. **e** With a fiber parallel to the surface no crater is visible (1 pulse, 1.0 J). The tissue modifications in the successive adjacent zones are the same as at 90°, but their geometrical distribution remains strictly epicentric with regard to the bubble collapse point facing the deepest modification area about 300 µm from the surface line (toluidine blue, × 40)

Histological Consequences of Irradiation Angles and Pulse Repetition

The most influential factor to the shape of the histological appearance of the ablation by the laser irradiation is the impact angle of the beam. At 90° the ablation crater of one pulse is symmetrically parabolic (Fig. 13a), shows the smallest width and reaches furthest down into the tissue (450 µm). After five pulses the crater shape remains nearly unchanged but shows a smoother inner surface (Fig. 13b). With diminishing fiber angle the crater depth diminishes and its width increases at 60° to 215 µm and 690 µm, at 30° to 130 µm and 950 µm, respectively. The deepest point at the bottom of the crater does not remain in its center but shifts opposite to the fiber tip and the surface disruption well seen on both sides at 90° is only present on that side at 30°. A pulse repetition leads to a smooth crater line. With a fiber parallel to the surface no crater is visible. The tissue modifications in the successive adjacent zones are the same as at 90°, but their geometrical distribution remains strictly epicentric with regard to the bubble collapse point facing the deepest modification area. The dimensions of these zones diminish more slowly than the ones of the ablation crater. So at 0° these zones of tissue modification without destruction are still found reaching down overall to about 300 µm.

Conclusions from In Vitro Holmium Experimentation

In free water the unaffected creation of a symmetrical vapor bubble that absorbs the whole pulse energy is followed by a bubble collapse generating 350 bars of maximum pressure for a 1 J pulse [4]. To open up a 1 mm thick saline layer to a vapor bubble, in which the holmium wavelength is not absorbed any more, a 0.5 J pulse needs almost 200 µs. Its whole pulse duration is generally 250 µs. Thus only 20 % of its laser energy is available for tissue ablation, whereas from a 1.5 J pulse about 70 % of the energy is absorbed by the tissue. Subsequent analogous experimentation with an erbium laser conducted by a conjoint group of researchers, apart from a basically different shape of the bubbles, gave similar results. Irradiating perpendicularly to a tissue surface, the leveling of the pressure peaks at less than one half by ejected ablation particles is due to a loss of symmetry of the bubble as was demonstrated in free water by the biophysicist members of our group; the pressure amplitude per pulse energy decreased strongly when the bubble shape was deviated from spherical symmetry [4, 18]. With decreasing irradiation angles, the loss of symmetry is even more important, leading to a peak pressure reduction to less than one fourth at 0°, where no

ablation from the parallel tissue surface is seen. Inversely, osteoarthrotic fibrillations sticking out from the cartilage cover are hit perpendicularly and ablated. Yet all the recorded maximum pressures are below a critical range for a biological sensibility of skeletal hard tissues as we found in our subsequent in vivo study.

Holmium and Erbium Laser Effects to the Cartilage Surface In Vivo

Thus the easiest mode for clinical arthroscopic application, i. e. an utmost tangential irradiation, appeared in vitro to be the least damaging in the deeper layers and the most efficient in ablating surface irregularities. We were therefore able to design an in vivo protocol adopting exactly the same arthroscopic procedure as realizable in humans, using an identical OA model as in the previous in vivo study on the left knee of sheep, the right knee being available for comparison as an intact control.

Materials and Methods

Under general anesthesia in lateral decubitus ten sheep were operated on the left knee in a first session by a parapatellar arthrotomy to create experimental osteoarthritis by scratching with a gross rasp in random directions all the cartilage surfaces at reach on the patella, the groove and both femoral and tibial condyles. After 6 weeks of free walking, which was possible for all animals from the second day on, in the same operation room setting a surgical arthroscopy was performed using a 30° Storz arthroscope connected to a Hopkins camera through an anterolateral portal. The 70° side-firing Coherent hand-pieces were either used unmodified for holmium application or adapted by gluing a zirkonium fluoride fiber in contact with a sapphire at their tip for erbium lasering. The handling and the beam exit were strictly identical.

In a predetermined turnover mode the osteoarthritic cartilage was tangentially irradiated by scanning each of the surfaces on patella, groove and the femoral condyles. The osteoarthritic tibial surfaces were left for observation of the natural history of the osteoarthritis model.

All laser applications were conducted at 12 Hz with a pulse duratiuon of 500 µs, up to a monitored total energy of 400 J/area of ~ 1 cm². Two areas were treated with a holmium laser (Versapuls/Coherent) at 0.6 J/pulse and 0.8 J/pulse, respectively, two other areas with an erbium laser (experimental prototype) at 0.12 J/pulse and at 0.18 J/pulse, respectively. From the same day on, full weight bearing in free walking was again allowed.

Five animals were killed 6 months after surgery and the other five after 1 year. The patellae and the distal femurs and tibial condyles of the operated knees and from eight controlateral intact knees were decalcified and the transverse microtome cut slices were stained with safranin-O and examined at 15× and 40× of magnification. We assessed the surface quality, the chondrocytes, cluster formations, the intensity of intercellular staining and the thickness of the persisting cartilage.

Results of Arthroscopic Holmium and Erbium Irradiation of Osteoarthritic Cartilage

The clinical recordings of the free walking ability showed that all of the sheep studied moved without limping or swelling of the operated knee within 2 weeks.

In the histomorphometric evaluation we found the following results: Compared to the intact healthy sheep cartilage, which has a histological appearance

Fig. 14. a Intact cartilage from opposite knee of a sheep from the in vivo experimental series on arthroscopic infrared laser treatment of osteoarthritic cartilage. **b** Scratching osteoarthritis model area after 1 year follow-up (safranin-O, × 15)

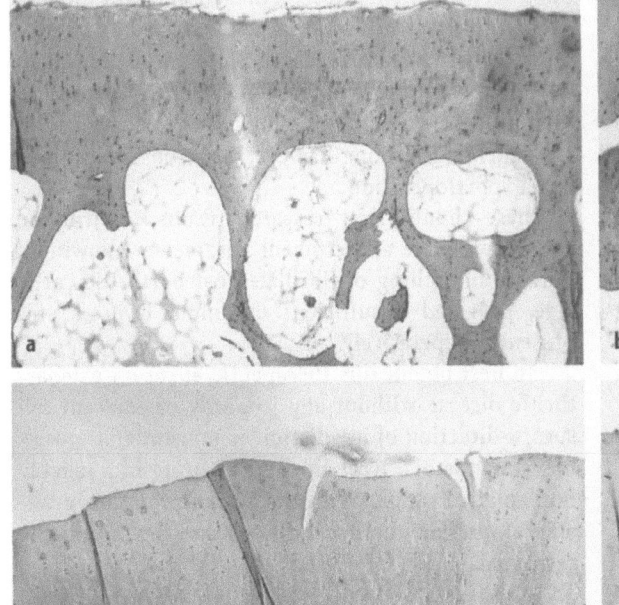

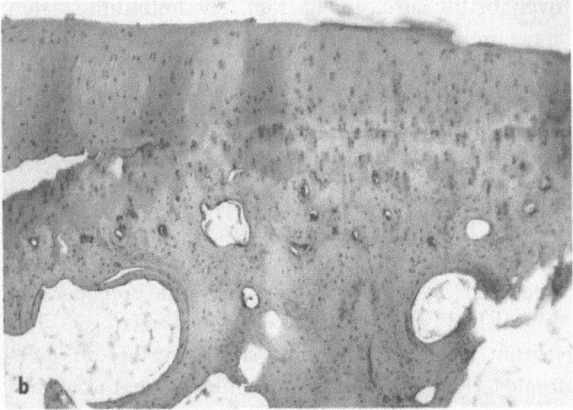

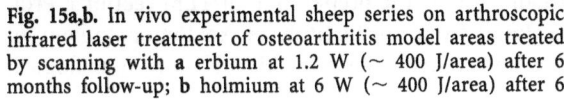

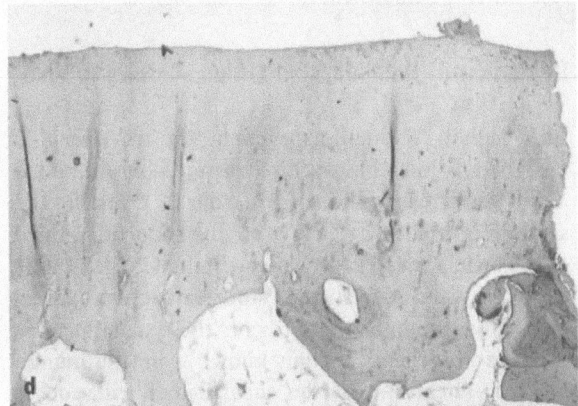

Fig. 15a,b. In vivo experimental sheep series on arthroscopic infrared laser treatment of osteoarthritis model areas treated by scanning with **a** erbium at 1.2 W (∼ 400 J/area) after 6 months follow-up; **b** holmium at 6 W (∼ 400 J/area) after 6 months follow-up; **c** erbium at 1.2 W (∼ 400 J/area) after 1 year follow-up; **d** holmium at 8 W (∼ 400 J/area) after 1 year follow-up (safranin-O, × 15)

almost identical to that of human (Fig. 14a), the scratching OA model areas from 6 months follow-up on (Fig. 14b) show a means residual cartilage layer of two thirds the original thickness and an incidence of cartilage defects down to bone on each seventh, nonoverlapping examined area. The superficial part of this residual cartilage contains a constantly persisting agglomeration of clusters still unchanged after 1 year. Variable vascular ingrowth is seen.

Six months after laser exposure specific features are observed according to the infrared wavelength used: erbium, at the beginning, produces a slightly undulatory surface (Fig. 15a). Significant cluster formations remain present even after 1 year of follow-up. In contrast the more condensed surface after holmium treatment no longer shows clusters after 6 months (Fig. 15b). In both cases the preserved vital cartilage is of a means thickness of about half the original intact one. The incidence of cartilage defects down to bone is the same as on OA model areas in the specified observation time and further on up to 1 year. The subchondral bone is inconspicuous. One year after infrared laser smoothing the cartilage layer thickness increases again up to two thirds that of intact cartilage. Erbium treated areas still contain a significant amount of clusters and present a relatively brittle surface (Fig. 15c). The holmium treated areas only show very rare clusters and the dense superficial line persists in continuity with a zone of less cellular density underneath (Fig. 15d). None of the subchondral bone beneath the holmium and erbium treated areas shows any signs of bony necrosis at 1 year.

The biochemical evaluation by immunoassays gave the following results: The proteoglycan content measured by immunoassays is still considerably diminished compared to healthy cartilage, but erbium treated areas show similar values to non-treated OA areas whereas holmium treated areas are less different from healthy cartilage zones.

Discussion of Holmium and Erbium Results In Vivo

This in vivo animal experiment on ten sheep is designed to resemble as closely as possible the routinely performed clinical procedure. Overall, the scratching model, by taking off the superficial third of the articular cartilage, which eliminates the closing cover, in sheep as well as pigs or goats, creates a real OA within 2 months that presents the typical histological and biochemical signs known from the human disease. The fact that the superficial fibrillation is less pronounced is taken into account by a standardization of the arthroscopic procedure otherwise exactly performed as in clinical conditions, as well

as of the instrumentation material and the surgical technical details. The energy applied to each surface unit has been kept constant and a precise cartographic delimitation has allowed histomorphometric and biochemical analysis of the areas in every knee treated by the predetermined respective wavelengths and parameters used on the various locations. To our knowledge the observed follow-up duration of 1 year is among the longest experimental follow-ups found in the literature.

None of the sheep showed prolonged limping, which indicates a favorable functional impact of the examined treatment. The histological features found after analysis of the different arthroscopic treatment settings, chosen within a non-ablative laser intensity, confirm that this sort of surgical therapy does not create supplementary lesions. The irregularities and defects in the remaining cartilage layer are at the same incidence in pure model areas as in laser treated areas, where vital cartilage, as a rule, is preserved at a thickness of 1 mm at least. With a more condensed surface line the typical cluster formations induced by the model OA almost disappear after holmium treatment, whereas erbium primarily creates a less modified, new surface under which chondrocyte clustering persists. Due to the less significant penetration depth erbium less fully treats the osteoarthritic middle cartilage layer, and the disease at 1 year is not as notably influenced as by holmium, where only sporadic clusters are observed. At our energy settings, up to somewhat higher values than we recommend for clinical use, no effect of the subchondral bone has ever been observed up to 1 year post-operation.

These chonroplasty research results confirm the existence of safe and efficient parameters allowing a durable smoothing of fibrillated osteoarthritic cartilage, provided a sufficient minimum layer is still present preoperatively.

To best obtain this therapeutic effect on osteoarthritic disease without any jeopardy of adjacent tissues, a direction of irradiation as tangential as possible is mandatory, with an energy setting in a reliably non-ablative range. With the instrumentation available at present these conditions can be thoroughly respected.

■ Acknowledgments. The authors would like to thank the Hoffmann La Roche Company for placing at our disposal the infrastructure of animal experimentation, Prof. R. Guggenheim from the Scanning Electron Microscopy Laboratory of the University of Basle for the SEM-imaging support, Mrs. C. Champion for the preparation of TEM sections, Prof. G. Jundt from the Institute of Anatomopathology of the University of Basle for his advice in pathological interpretations and M. Seibel MD for the immuno-assays. The excimer laser in vivo project has been supported by the Swiss National Foundation (N° 32–28 586.90). Special thanks also to Prof. W. E. Siebert who has placed at our disposal his junior collaborators T. Jansen and T. Oberthür for the histomorphometric evaluation of the holmium in vitro specimens with the help of the teams of Division I of the Institute of Anatomopathology (Prof. A. Georgii) and of Division III of the anatomy, cell biology and electron microscopy (Prof. E. Reale/Prof. L. Luciano) departments of the Hannover Medical College. The combined holmium and erbium laser project was supported by the University Council of the Swiss Fed. Inst. of Technology in the priority project "Optics" (Project N° 421).

References

[1] Adams M, Pelletier J (1988) Canine anterior cruciate ligament transsection model of osteoarthritis. Handbook of animal models for the rheumatic desease. Greenwald R, Diamon H (eds) CRC, Boca Raton, Fl, II:57

[2] Annefeld M, Erne B, Rasser Y (1990) Ultrastructural analysis of rat articular cartilage following treatment with dexamethasone and glycosaminoglycan-peptide complex. Clin Exp Rheum 8:151

[3] Asshauer T, Jansen E, Frenz M, Delacrétaz G, Welch A (1994) Acoustic transients in pulsed holmium laser ablation: Effects of pulse duration. In: Jacques S, Katzir A (eds) Laser interaction with hard and soft tissue, Proc SPIE 2323:117

[4] Asshauer T, Jansen T, Oberthür T, Delacrétaz G (1995) Holmium laser ablation of cartilage: Effect of cavitation bubbles. In: Jacques S, Katzir A (eds) Laser tissue interaction IV, Proc SPIE 2391 A, 379, SPIE, Bellingham

[5] Asshauer T, Oberthür T, Jansen T, Gerber B, Delacrétaz G (1996) Holmium laser ablation of cartilage: Effects of delivery fiber angle of incidence. In: Jacques S, Katzir A (eds) Laser tissue interaction and tissue optics, Proc SPIE 2624:49

[6] Asshauer T, Rink K, Delacrétaz G (1994) Acoustic transient generation by pulsed holmium-laser-induced cavitation bubbles. J Appl Phys 76:5007

[7] Asshauer T, Rink K, Delacétaz G, Salathé R, Gerber B, Frenz M, Pratisto H, Ith M, Romano V, Weber H (1994) Acoustic transient generation in pulsed Holmium laser ablation underwater. Proc SPIE 2134 A, 423, SPIE, Bellingham

[8] Brillhart A (1991) Arthroscopic laser surgery. Am J Arthroscopy 1:5

[9] Buchelt M, Kutschera H, Katterschafka T, Kiss H, Schneider B, Ulrich R (1992) Erb:YAG and Hol:YAG laser ablation of meniscus and intervertebral discs. Lasers Surg Med 12:375

[10] Burmann M, Finkelstein H, Mayer L (1934) Arthroscopy of the knee. J Bone Joint Surg 16:255

[11] Doukas A, McAucliffe D, Flotte T (1993) Biological effects of laser-induced shock waves: structural and functional cell damage in vitro. Ultrasound Med Biol 19:137

[12] Draenert Y (1978) Die Gefriertrocknung des Gelenkknorpels. Diss, Bern University

[13] Fischer R, Krebs R, Scharf H (1993) Cell vitality in cartilage tissue culture following Excimer laser radiation: An in vitro examination. Laser Surg Med 13:629

[14] Garino J, Lotke P, Sapega A, Reilly P, Esterhai J (1995) Osteonecrosis of the knee following laser-assisted arthroscopic surgery: A report of six cases. Arthroscopy 11/4:467

[15] Gédéon P, Mazières B, Ficat P (1978) Un nouveau modèle d'arthrose expérimentale: la contusion du cartilage. Rev Rhum 45:40

[16] Gerber B, Guggenheim R, Mathys D, Düggelin M, Litzistorf Y, Gudat F (1991) Ultrastrukturelles Bild des Excimer-Laser-Effektes der Knorpelversiegelung – eine In vitro-Pilot-Untersuchung. In: Sieber W, Wirth C (eds) Laser in der Orthopädie. Thieme, Stuttgart:62

[17] Gerber B, Zimmer M, Guggenheim R (1991) Excimer-Laser-Effekte bei der Knorpelversiegelung In vivo im Tierexperiment. Orthop Mitt 21:155

[18] Gerber B, Asshauer T, Delacrétaz G, Jansen T, Oberthür T (1996) Basic investigations on holmium laser effects on articular cartilage and their impact on the clinical application technique (Biophysikalische Grundlagenuntersuchungen zur Wirkung der Holmium-Laserstrahlung am Knorpelgewebe und deren Konsequenzen für die klinische Applikationstechnik) Orthopäde 25/1:21

[19] Ghosh P (1989) Therapeutic modulation of cartilage catabolism by nonsteroidal antiinflammatory drugs in arthritis. Semin Arthritis Rheum 18/3, Suppl 1:2

[20] Grifka J, Moraldo M, Krämer J (1990) Apparative und technische Voraussetzungen für die arthroskopische Chirurgie am Kniegelenk. Orthopäde 19:60.

[21] Grifka J (1993) Arthroskopische Therapie der Gonarthrose in Abhängigkeit vom Grad der Chondromalazie. Arthroskopie 6:20

[22] Grothues-Spork M, Bernard M, Cierpinski, T. Hertel P, Noack W, Müller G (1994) Fünf Lasersysteme zur arthroskopischen Meniskuschirurgie im Tierversuch. Arthroskopie 7:68

[23] Hesse I, Mohr W, Hesse W (1990) Morphologische Veränderungen in frühen Stadien der Arthrose. Orthopäde 19/1:16

[24] Hesse W, Reichelt A, Hesse I (1981) Funktionsabhängige, präarthrotische und arthrotische Veränderungen der Ultrastruktur des Gelenkknorpels. Akt Rheimatol 6:21

[25] Ishimaru J, Goss A (1992) A model for osteoarthritis of the temporomandibular joint. J Oral Maxillofac Surg 50:1191

[26] Jackson R, Silver R, Marans H (1986) Arthroscopic treatment of degenerative joint disease. Arthroscopy 2:114

[27] Jansen D, van Leeuwen T, Mtamedi M, Borst C, Welch A (1994) Temperature dependence of the absorption coefficient of water for midinfrared laser radiation. Lasers Surg Med 15:258

[28] John T, Scheller E, Rahmanzadeh R (1995) Is cartilage regeneration with low-level laser therapy possible? An in vitro cell culture assay. Abstract N° 464, End Congress of EFORT, Munich, 4–7 July 1995

[29] Johnson L (1986) Arthroscopic abrasion chondroplasty historical and pathological perspective: present status. Arthroscopy 2:54

[30] Johnson L (1991) Characteristics of the immediate post arthroscopic blood clot formation in the knee joint. Arthroscopy 7:14

[31] Jungmichel D, Weber H, Gratzsche L (1988) Gelenkwaschung – eine Behandlungsmöglichkeit bei aktivierter Arthrose. Beitr Orthop Traumatol 35:51

[32] Kar H, Excimer laser. In: Berlien H, Müller A (eds) Angewandte Laser-Medizin, Lehr- und Handbuch für Praxis und Klinik. Laser Medizin Zentrum Berlin, ecomed, Landsberg, II-2.4.6

[33] Kiviranta I, Jurvelin J, Tammi M, Säämänen A, Helminen H (1985) Microspectrophotometric quantitation of glycosaminoglycans in articular cartilage sections stained with Safranin O. Histochemistry 82:249

[34] Kroitzsch U, Laufer G, Egkher E, Wollenek G, Horvath R (1989) Experimental photoablation of meniscus cartilage by excimer laser energy. A new aspect of meniscus surgery. Arch Orthop Trauma Surg 108/1:44

[35] Löhnert J, Raunest J (1994) Operationstechnik der arthroskopischen Knorpelablation mit dem 308nm-Xenon-Chlorid-Excimer-Laser. Arthroskopie 7:170

[36] Lübbers C, Siebert W (1996) Die arthroskopische Holmium:YAG-Laser-Anwendung im Vergleich zu konventionellen Verfahren am Kniegelenk: Zwei-Jahres-Ergebnisse einer prospektiven randomisierten Studie. Orthopäde 25/1:64

[37] Lukoschek M, Boyd R, Schaffler M, Burr D, Radin E (1986) Comparison of joint degeneration models. Surgical instability and repetitive impulsive loading. Acta Orthop Scand 57:349

[38] MacConail M (1951) The movements of bones and joints. 4. The mechanical structure of articulating cartilage. J Bone Joint Surg 33B:251

[39] Magnuson P (1941) Joint debridement and surgical treatment of degenerative arthritis. Surg Gynecol Obstet 73:1

[40] Mainil-Varlet P et al. (1998) personal communication

[41] Mankin H (1962) Localization of tritiated thymidine in articular cartilage of rabbits. J Bone Joint Surg 44A:682

[42] Moskowitz R (1973) Experimentally induced degenerative joint lesions following partial meniscectomy in the rabbit. Arthritis Rheum 16:397

[43] Nakata K, Bullough P (1986) The injury and repair of human articular cartilage: a morphological study of 192 classes of coxarthrosis. J Jpn Orthop Ass 60:763

[44] O'Connor P, Brereton J, Gardner D (1984) Hyaline articular cartilage dissected by papain: light and scanning electron microscopy and mecromechanical studies. Ann Rheum Dis 43:320

[45] Otte P (1958) Die Regenerationsfähigkeit des Gelenkknorpels. Z Orthop 90:299

[46] Outerbridge R (1962) The etiology of chondromalacia patellae. J Bone Joint Surg [Br] 43:752

[47] Paukkonen K, Helminen H (1987) Chondrocyte ultrastructure in exercise and experimental osteoarthritis. A stereologic morphometric study of articular cartilage of young rabbits using transmission electron microscopy. Clin Orthop Relat Res 224:284

[48] Phillips T, Gurr K (1989) Preconditioned arthritic hip model. J Arthoplasty 4:193

[49] Pond M, Nuki G (1973) Experimentally induced osteoarthritis in the dog. Ann Rheum Dis 32:387

[50] Raunest J, Löhnert J (1990) Arthroscopic cartilage debridement by excimer laser in chondromalacia of the knee joint. A prospective randomized clinical study. Arch Orthop Trauma Surg 109:155

[51] Raunest J, Sager M, Derra E (1994) Experimentelle Befunde zur Knorpelablation und Abrasionschondroplastik mit thermischen und gepulsten UV-Lasern. Arthroskopie 7:174

[52] Raunest J, Derra E (1996) Lasermeniskektomie: Analyse des inhärenten Potentials zur Arthrose-Entwicklung. Orthopäde 25/1:10

[53] Refior H (1978) Das Verhalten des hyalinen Gelenkknorpels nach Immobilisation und Remobilisation im Tierexperiment – Mikro-strukturelle Untersuchungen zur Definition des Präarthroseprozesses. Z Orthop 116:436

[54] Rehak H-C, Hermann G, Schain F (1991) Pathophysiologie des Gelenkknorpels. Dtsch Z Sportmed 42/7:316

[55] Rogri-Hansen B, Elltisgaard N, Funch M, Jensen M, Prieske J (1991) Low level laser treatment of chondromalacia patellae. Int Orthop 15:359

[56] Rosenberg L (1991) Use of safranin-O in the study of articular cartilage. J Bone Joint Surg 53A:69

[57] Schmid A, Schmid F, Tiling T (1985) Electron microscopy findings after cartilage shaving. In: Müller W, Hackenbroch W (eds) Surgery and arthroscopy of the knee. Springer, Berlin Heidelberg New York Tokyo, p 426

[58] Schreiner C (1994) Laser in der Arthroskopie. Arthroskopie 7:148

[59] Seibel M (1989) Komponenten der extrazellulären Gewebematrix als potentielle "Marker" des Bindegewebe-, Knorpel- und Knochenmetabolismus bei Erkrankungen des Bewegungsapparates. Z Rheumatol 48/1:6

[60] Sherk H (1993) The use of lasers in orthopedic procedures. J Bone Joint Surg 75/A:768

[61] Shi W, Vari S, van der Veen M, Fishbein M, Grundfest W (1993) Effect of varying laser parameters on pulsed Ho:YAG ablation of bovine knee joint tissues. Arthroscopy 9:96

[62] Siebert W, Kohn D, Klanke J, Wirth C, Scholz C, Müller G (1990) Rasterelektronenmikroskopische Untersuchungen zur Oberflächebearbeitung von Knorpelschäden mit dem Nd:YAG-Laser, dem CO_2-Laser, dem Excimer-Laser, dem Er-YAG-Laser, dem Ho-YSSG-Laser und diversen motorgetriebenen Instrumenten. Fortschr Arthrosk 6:82

[63] Siebert W, Saunier J, Gerber B, Lübbers C, IMLAS Study Group (1994) Lasers in Arthroscopic Surgery: Ho:YAG-Laser in der arthroskopischen Chirurgie des Kniegelenks. Arthroskopie 7:182

[64] Srinivasan R (1986) Ablation of polymers and biological tissue by ultraviolet lasers. Science 234:559

[65] Thompson R Jr, Oegema T Jr, Lewis J, Wallace L (1991) Osteo-arthrotic changes after acute transarticular load. An animal model. J Bone Joint Surg 73A:990

[66] Trauner K, Nishioka N, Flotte T, Patel D (1995) Acute and chronic response of articular cartilage to holmium:YAG laser irradiation. Clin Orthop 310:52

[67] Vangsness C, Watson T, Saadatmanesh V, Moran K (1995) Pulsed Ho:YAG laser meniscectomy: Effect of pulsewidth on tissue penetration rate and lateral thermal damage. Lasers Surg Med 16:61

[68] Von der Mark K, Glückert K (1990) Biochemische und molekular-biologische Aspekte zur Früherfassung humaner Arthrosen. Orthopädie 19/1:2

[69] Wittenberg H, Müller K (1988) Untersuchungen über das Schneideverhalten von Knorpelfräsen bei Gonarthrose. Arthroskopie 1:138

Effects of Laser Irradiation on Cytokine Production of Rheumatoid Synovial Cells

K. Inoue · T. Nishimura

Introduction

There have been various reports of positive clinical results of laser therapy for rheumatoid arthritis [2], but the mechanisms of these effects are unknown. Although there have been some reports of investigations of proliferation rates and cytokine production after low-power laser irradiation [3, 5, 8], the results concerning its effects on cell cultures are inconsistent. It is generally assumed that the resulting cellular changes depend mainly on the irradiation intensity and the irradiation time of the laser. To determine the mechanism of the effects of laser irradiation, we have investigated the effects of low-powered Nd:YAG laser irradiation on cytokine production of rheumatoid synovial cells.

Materials and Methods

Synovial cells were obtained from seven rheumatoid arthritic patients during total knee arthroplasty. Cells were seeded at a concentration of 1×10^6 cells/ml into 24-well plates, 1 ml in each, and divided into four groups. Cells in group A were nonirradiated and used as controls, cells in group B were irradiated with 1 W for 1 min (30 J/cm^2), cells in group C were irradiated with 1 W for 5 min (150 J/cm^2), and cells in group D were irradiated with 3 W for 5 min (450 J/cm^2).

The laser beam was conducted through a quartz fiber, and its intensity was measured with an optical power meter. The trypan-blue exclusion method was used to assess viability of the cells before and after laser treatment.

Supernatant for measurement of cytokine concentrations was harvested at 0, 1, 2, and 3 days after irradiation. The concentrations of interleukin-1β (IL-1β), interleukin-6 (IL-6), interleukin-8 (IL-8), and tumor necrosis factor-α (TNF-α) in supernatants of the cells were determined in a quantitative enzyme-linked immunosorbent assay (ELISA).

The results are expressed as mean ± standard deviation (SD). Student's t-test was applied to compare two group means for significance of difference. p was considered significant below the 0.05 level.

Results

All the cases showed almost the same pattern of cytokine production over time, but the cytokine levels in each case were quite different, so for easy comparison we calculated the changes in the form of percentage differences compared with the nonirradiated control group showing the maximum cytokine concentration.

Figure 1 shows the cytokine production after laser irradiation. For IL-1β, the difference between group A and group B was not significant; however, the production of IL-1β was inhibited in group C and group D. For IL-6 and IL-8, no significant differences were detected between any of the groups. The production of TNF-α was slightly inhibited in group C, but no significant differences were detected in group B and group D.

Figure 2 shows the cytokine production of a typical case for each group. As group A shows, IL-1β increased up to day 2 and decreased thereafter. IL-6 and IL-8 showed a continual and gradual rise up to day 3. TNF-α peaked on day 1 and then gradually decreased. The production of IL-1β was inhibited in group B, group C and group D, compared to group A, the control group. However, the production of IL-6, IL-8, and TNF-α was not inhibited.

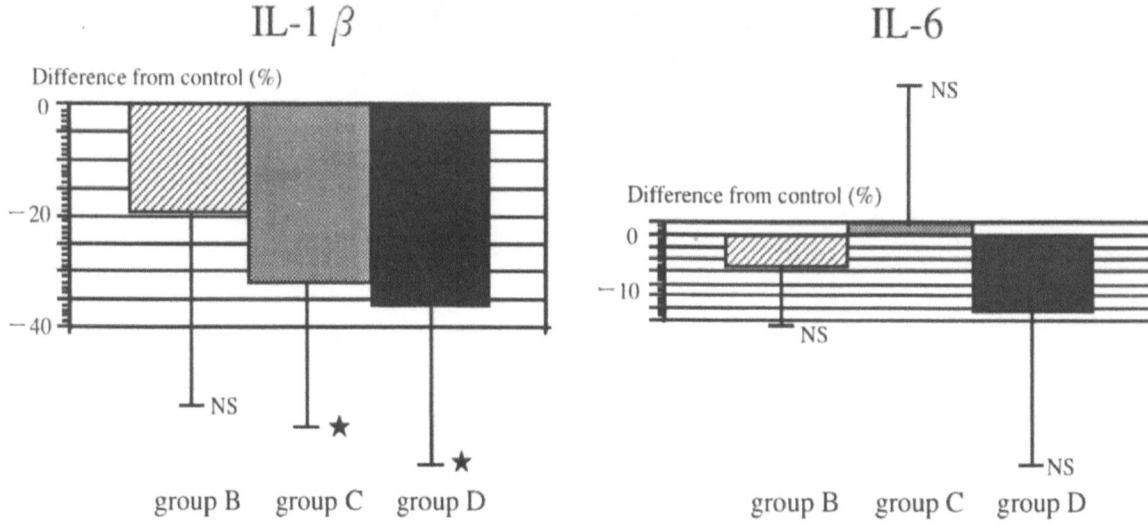

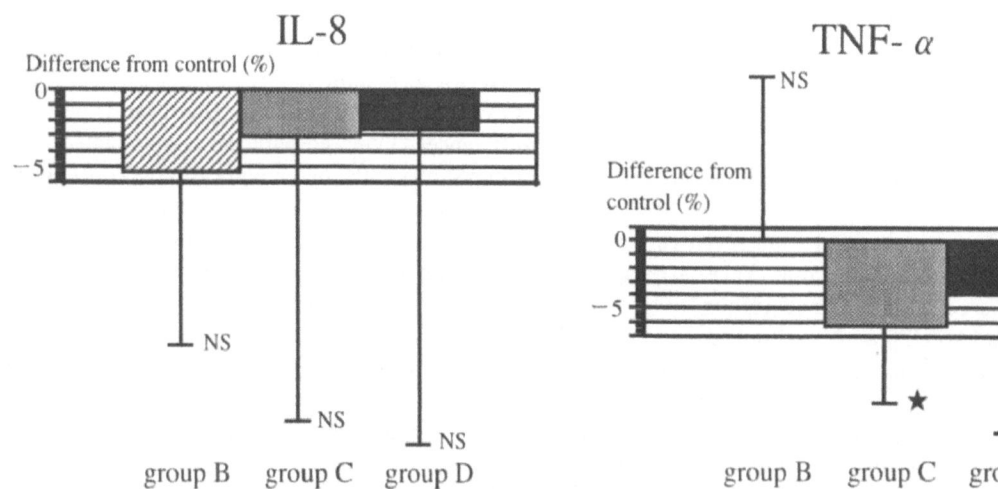

Fig. 1. Cytokine production after laser irradiation. Data presented as percentage differences of cytokine concentrations in irradiated cultures compared to nonirradiated controls. Values are given as mean ± SD. *Asterisks* indicate significance ($p < 0.05$). For IL-1β, the difference between group A (control group) and group B was not significant; however, the production of IL-1β was inhibited in group C and group D. For IL-6 and IL-8, no significant differences were detected between any of the groups. The production of TNF-α was slightly inhibited in group C, but no significant differences were detected in group B and group D

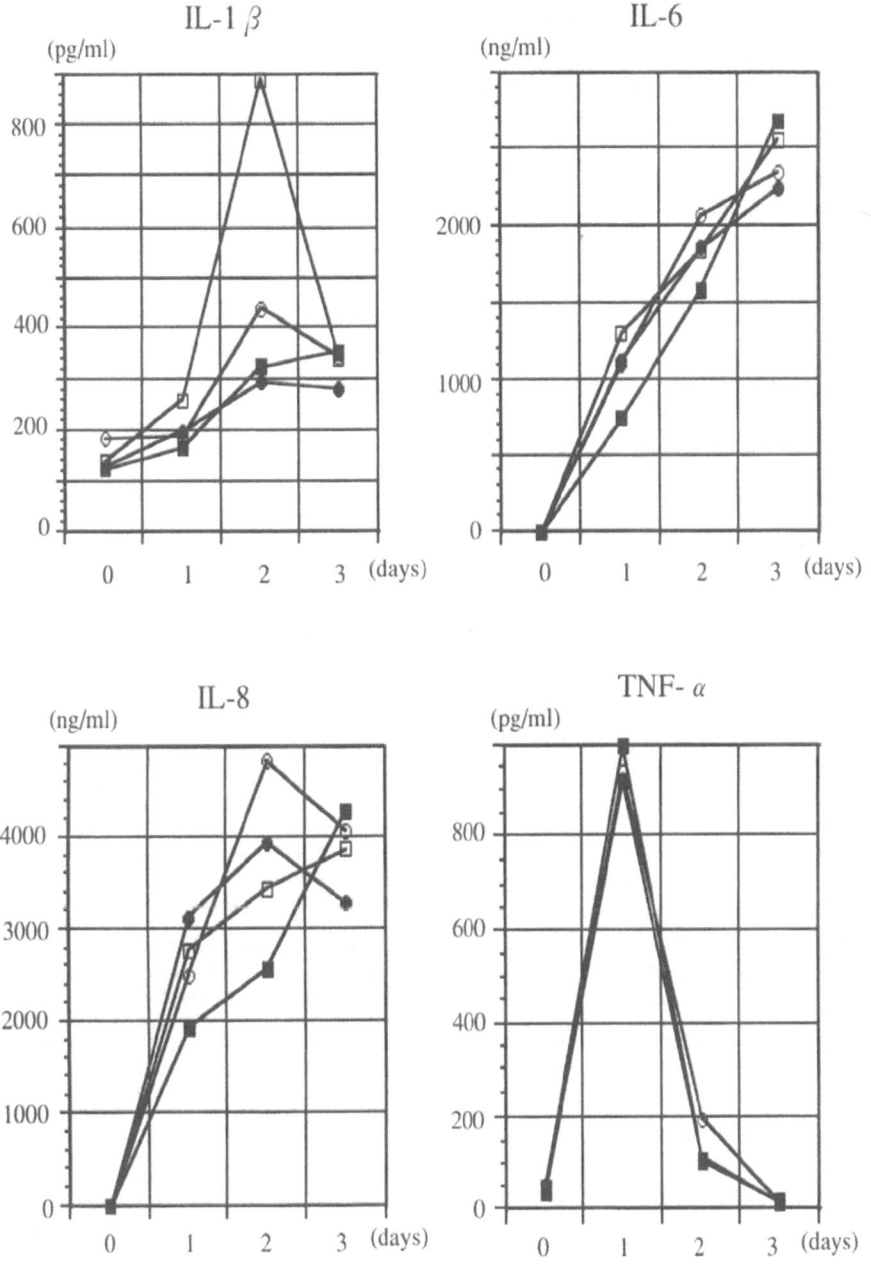

Fig. 2. Cytokine production, in a typical case for each group. The production of IL-1β was inhibited in group B, group C, and group D compared to group A, the control group. However, the production of IL-6, IL-8, and TNF-α was not inhibited. □: Group A, ○: Group B, ■: Group C, ●: Group D

Discussion

Low-power laser irradiation, that is, laser without thermal effects, is considered very effective and has been demonstrated to be safe in inflammatory diseases such as rheumatoid arthritis. A pain-killing effect by modulating nerve conduction, enhanced wound healing by normalizing blood flow and stimulating cell proliferation, and interference with immunological functions have been thought to be the mechanisms of these effects; however, these are only inferences because there have been very few detailed descriptions of such effects on the cellular level.

There have been many studies of photobiological effects in vitro and in vivo following low-power laser irradiation of unsensitized cells or tissues. The results concerning the effects of low-power lasers are inconsistent: either stimulatory or inhibitory effects have been reported [1, 5, 6, 9], and in some studies no effect at all was observed [4, 8, 10, 11]. Bosatra et al. [3] found ultrastructural changes in the mitochondria and Golgi apparatus. Funk et al. [5] reported that He-Ne laser light induces enhanced cytokine production at lower energy densities (18.9 J/cm^2) and decreased cytokine production at higher energy densities (37.8 J/cm^2). Kupin et al. [8] failed to demonstrate altered IFN-α or IFN-γ concentrations in cultures of isolated human lymphocytes which were irradiated with a He-Ne laser at very low intensity (0.3 mW/cm^2). Meyers et al. [10] failed to show any increase in DNA production in irradiated lymphocytes or any potentiation of mitogenic effect of phytohemagglutinin.

The present study demonstrated that the Nd:YAG laser decreased production of IL-1β by rheumatoid synovial cells. The result indicates that laser irradiation controls rheumatoid synovitis by decreasing production of IL-1β both directly and indirectly through the cytokine network. It is suggested that laser irradiation controls rheumatoid synovitis by decreasing cytokine production of rheumatoid synovial cell.

In this study, no effect was seen in group B, but effects were seen in group C and group D. This indicates that more than 5 min irradiation or more than 150 J/cm^2 energy is neccessary for efficacy. This contradicts claims that lasers with a power of less than 1 W are effective clinically. There are two possible explanations for this. One is that the laser irradiation was applied only once in this experiment in contrast to repeated irradiation in the clinical cases. Kubasova et al. [7] reported that single irradiation of primary human embryo fibroblasts with He-Ne laser of 1 J/cm^2 did not affect the cell surfaces, however, laser treatment repeated four times caused functional alterations. If we irradiated repeatedly, less than 1 W would be enough to achieve efficacy. The other possible explanation is that only a pain-killing effect can be expected in clinical tests, and thus, a power of more than 1 W may be necessary to control cytokine production.

Clinically, we use Nd:YAG laser for nonsurgical treatments, because the Nd:YAG laser penetrates tissue more deeply than other kinds of laser, which are more feasible as surgical tools.

Conclusion

This study demonstrated that the Nd:YAG laser decreased production of IL-1β by rheumatoid synovial cells. It is suggested that laser irradiation controls rheumatoid synovitis by decreasing cytokine production by rheumatoid synovial cells.

References

[1] Abergel, R, Lyons R, Castel J, Dwyer R, Uitto J (1987) Biostimulation of wound healing by laser: experimental approaches in animal models and in fibroblast cultures. J Dermatol Surg Oncol 13:127–133
[2] Asada K, Yutani Y, Sakawa A, Shimazi A (1991) Clinical application of GaAIAs 830 nm diode laser in treatment of rheumatoid arthritis. Laser Ther 3:77–82
[3] Bosatra M, Jucci A, Olliaro P, Quacci D, Sacchi S (1984) In vitro fibroblast and dermis fibroblast activation by laser irradiation at low energy. An electron microscopic study. Dermatologica 168:157–162
[4] Colver G, Priestlex G (1989) Failure of a helium-neon laser to affect components of wound healing in vitro. Br J Dermatol 21:179–186
[5] Funk J, Kruse A, Kirchner H (1992) Cytokine production after helium-neon laser irradiation in cultures of human peripheral blood mononuclear cells. J Photochem Photobiol B 16:347–355
[6] Haas F, Isserroff R, Wheeland R, Rood P, Graves P (1990) Low-energy helium-neon laser irradiation increases the motility of cultured human keratinocytes. J Invest Dermatol 94:822–826
[7] Kubasova T, Kovacs L, Somosy Z, Unk P, Kokai A (1984) Biological effect of He-Ne laser: investigations on functional and micromophological alterations of cell membranes, in vitro. Lasers Surg Med 4:381–388
[8] Kupin V, Sorokin A, Ivanov A, Lapteva R, Polevaya E (1987) The effect of nondamaging intensity laser irradiation on the immune system. Neoplasma 34:325–331
[9] Lam T, Abergel R, Meeker C, Castel J, Dwyer R, Uitto J (1986) Laser stimulation of collagen synthesis in human skin fibrolblast cultures. Lasers Life Sci 1:61–77
[10] Meyers A, Joyce J, Cohen J (1987) Effects of low-watt helium-neon laser irradiation on human lymphocyte cultures. Lasers Surg Med 6: 540–542
[11] Rood P, Haas A, Graves P, Wheeland R, Isserroff R (1992) Low-energy helium-neon laser irradiation does not alter human keratinocyte differentition. J. Invest Dermatol 99:445–448

Bactericidal Effect of Argon Laser Irradiation with Dyes

T. Okazaki · T. Yonezawa · T. Onomura · M. Abe · T. Goto · K. Sano · M. Nakai

Introduction

In orthopedic surgery, we often encounter infectious conditions such as osteomyelitis and decubitus. As one of the causative agent of these infections, MRSA (methicillin-resistant *Staphylococcus aureus*) has been a major problem. The infections are sometimes life-threatening for patients with severe underlying conditions, because the bacteria are highly resistant against many antibiotics. In this study, we examined a new method of killing bacteria by laser irradiation with food coloring agents.

Materials and Methods

Bacteria and Culture

MRSA was maintained in heart infusion slant agar (HIA, Difco) and bacteria were precultured overnight at 37 °C in heart infusion broth (HIB, Difco). Five microliters of precultured bacterial suspensions were plated on 6 ml medium and cultured for 14 h. After culturing, bacterial suspensions were centrifuged for 15 min at 3000 rpm. Pelleted bacteria were resuspended in phosphate buffer saline (PBS) and bacterial suspensions were recentrifuged and washed twice with PBS. Again, the pelleted bacteria were resuspended in PBS.

Laser Systems and Laser Irradiation

Argon laser (wavelength 514 nm, Coherent Co. Ltd) was employed. Irradiation was continuous-wave (CW) transmitted via a quartz fiber and was noncontact. A handpiece was attached at the tip of the fiber. The laser was directed perpendicularly to the white supporting table. The distance from the tip of the handpiece to the surface of the agar plate was 20 mm. Irradiation power was set at 0.2, 0.4, 0.6, 0.8, or 1.0 W, and irradiation time was 5, 10, 15, 20, or 25 s.

Dye Solutions and Measurement of Absorbency

The dyes added to the bacteria were red food colors no. 2, no. 3, and no. 102 (supplied by Kiriya Chem. Co. Ltd). The absorbency of each dye solution (1.0 mg/ml) diluted by PBS was measured using a double beam spectrophotometer (Hitachi).

Differences in Bactericidal Effect of Laser Irradiation with Various Dyes

Two hundred microliters of bacterial solutuon and 5 ml 1.0 mg/ml dye solution was mixed. After incubating for 30 min at 37 °C, the bacteria in dye solution were centrifuged and the sediment was suspended in PBS. Two hundred microliters of solution were dropped on the HIA plates, and were applied to the entire culture surface with a Conradirod. The laser irradiation was performed using the same method as described above. After the irradiated HIA plates were cultured at 37 °C for 24 h, a growth inhibition circle was seen.

The Optimum Condition Presenting the Most Effective Bactericidal Action in Case of Addition of Food Color Red No. 3 to Bacteria

Bacterial cells were mixed with food color no. 3 at a concentration of 1.0 mg/ml. Bacterial cells with dye were reacted for 10 min or 30 min and spread evenly as described above. After culturing at 37 °C for 24 h, a growth inhibition circle was seen.

In the same way, bacterial cells reacted at three different concentrations (0.1, 1.0, 10 mg/ml) for 30 min were spread on HIA plates, and growth inhibition circles were observed.

In order to examine the retention of dye, the growth inhibition circles of bacterial solutions with dye washed with PBS twice were compared with those without washing.

Results and Discussion

The first report of laser irradiation of bacteria was published by Klein et al. [2], who used a ruby laser to irradiate *Serratia*, *S. aureus*, and *P. acruginosa*. However, the output power of the laser oscillator was low and the reported bactericidal effect using laser irradiation alone was low. More recently it was reported that the bactericidal effect was enhanced by adding dyes such as methylene blue [6], trypan blue [5], and hematoporphyrin [4] to the bacterial cell at the time of laser irradiation. However, these pigments have some toxic effects on the living body. On the other hand, the safety for the living body of the food colors used in this study has been sufficiently discussed [1], and they are more easily applied to clinical medicine than other dyes that have been reported.

Concerning the bactericidal effect of argon laser, we have reported that argon laser irradiation had a bactericidal effect without the addition of dye [4]. However, very high energy with more than 30 s exposure time at 0.6 W was needed to obtain the growth inhibition circle, and the diameter of the growth inhibition circle was as small as about 1 mm. To obtain a bactericidal effect with a low laser irradiation output and to widen the area of bacterial inhibition, the addition of food color to the bacteria was needed before irradiation. In this study, the dye solutions

used did not reveal any bactericidal effect at the concentrations employed (data not shown).

We selected three food colors (Red nos. 2, 3, and 102) that showed higher absorption at 514 nm, the emission wave length of the argon laser used in this experiment. Of three food colors, Red no. 3 indicated the highest absorption in 514 nm, followed by Red no. 2 and Red no. 102 (Fig. 1). We also examined the differences in bactericidal action among the food colors. With the addition of Red no. 3 to bacterial cells, a growth inhibition circle started at an irradiation output of 0.2 W and an exposure time of 5 S (Table 1). Next was Red no. 2 at an irradiation output of 0.4 W and an exposure time of 15 s followed by Red no. 102 at an irradiation output of 0.4 W and an exposure time of 25 s. Thus, the absorption of food colors at the 514 nm emitted by argon laser correlated to the bactericidal effect. It was speculated that laser light was absorbed efficiently in molecules of Red no. 3 adherent to the bacterial wall or incorporated into the bacterial cytoplasm.

In order to clarify the optimum conditions for the most effective bactericidal action in the case of Red no. 3, we investigated the reaction time (10 min or 30 min) of food color to bacteria, the concentration of the dye solutions (0.1, 1.0 or 10 mg/ml), and the presence or absence of washing with PBS after incubation. Concerning the reaction time to bacteria and retention of dye, there was not obvious difference in

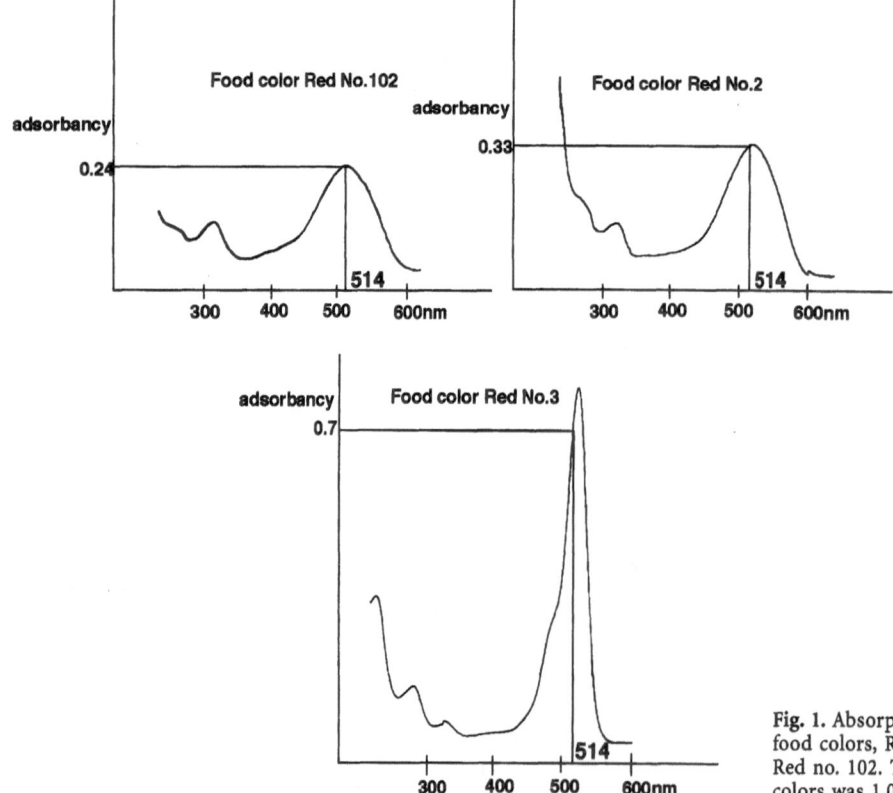

Fig. 1. Absorption spectra of three different food colors, Red no. 2, Red no. 3, and Red no. 102. The concentration of all food colors was 1.0 mg/ml

Table 1. Emergence of the growth inhibition circle in relation to irradiation power and duration for the three different added food colors

Duration (s)	Irradiation power (W)				
	0.2	0.4	0.6	0.8	1.0
Red no. 102					
5	−	−	−	+	+
10	−	−	−	+	+
15	−	−	+	+	+
20	−	−	+	+	+
25	−	+	+	+	+
Red no. 2					
5	−	−	−	+	+
10	−	−	+	+	+
15	−	+	+	+	+
20	−	+	+	+	+
25	−	+	+	+	+
Red no. 3					
5	+	+	+	+	+
10	+	+	+	+	+
15	+	+	+	+	+
20	+	+	+	+	+
25	+	+	+	+	+

+ Growth inhibition circle appeared.
− Growth inhibition circle did not appear.

Table 2. Comparison of diameter (mm) of growth inhibition circles for Red nor. 3 in bacterial solutions washed twice with PBS versus unwashed bacterial solutions

Duration (s)	Irradiation power (W)				
	0.2	0.4	0.6	0.8	1.0
Unwashed solutions					
5	3	4	5	5	6
10	4	5	6	6	7
15	5	6	6	7	8
20	6	7	7	8	9
25	6	7	8	8	9
Washed solutions					
5	1	1	1	1	1
10	1	1	1	1	1
15	1	1	1	1	1
20	1	1	1	1	1
25	1	1	1	1	1

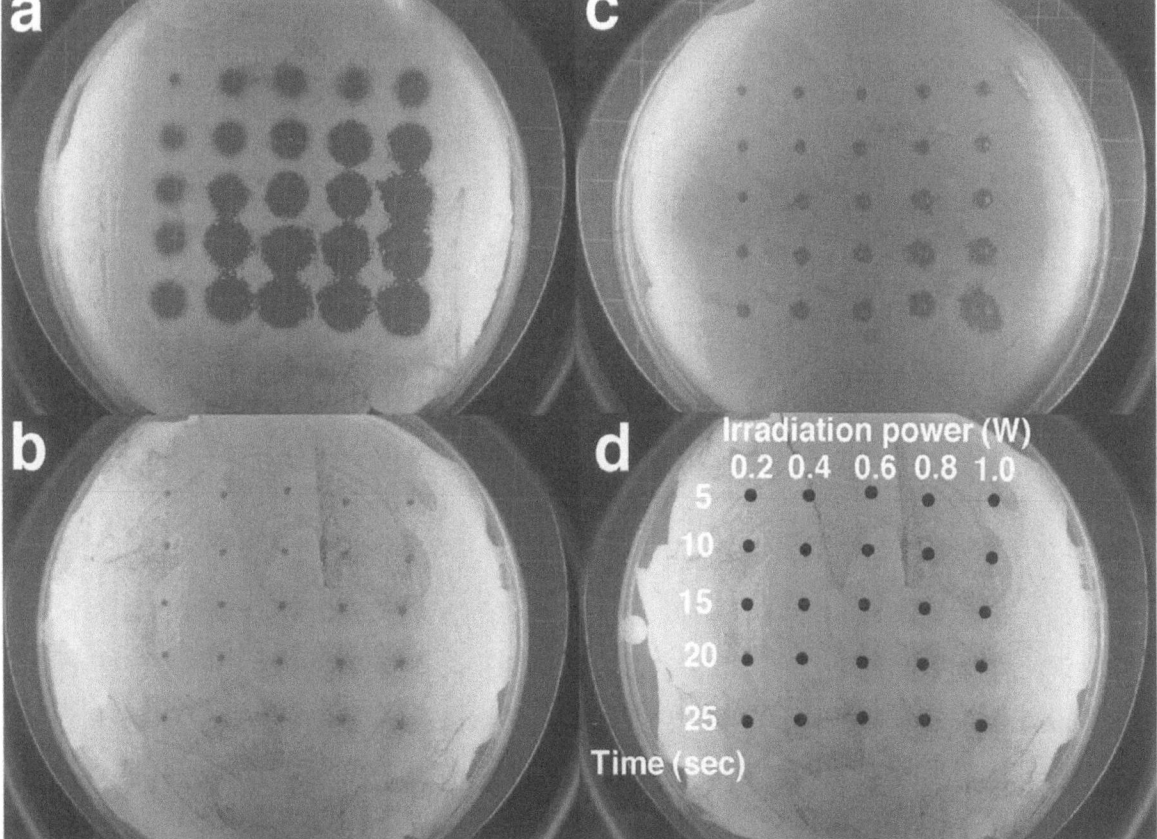

Fig. 2. Photographs of the growth inhibition circles of methicillin-resistant *Staphylococcus aureus* on heart infusion slant agar following laser irradiation with the addition food color at three different concentrations. **a** 1 mg/ml, **b** 0.1 mg/ml, **c** 10 mg/ml. **d** Scheme identifying the growth inhibition circles at each level of irradiation power (W) and duration (s)

bactericidal effect between 10 min and 30 min (data not shown), and the diameter of the bacterial inhibition circle was smaller in bacterial solutions washed twice than in those not washed (Table 2). This result showed that food color was neither taken up into the bacterial cell nor strongly bound to the bacterial wall, and it was comparatively loose at least up to 30 min.

As for bactericidal effect at the three different concentrations (0.1, 1.0, 10 mg/ml), Red no. 3 at 1.0 mg/ml showed the greatest efficiency. This indicated that with Red no. 3 at 1.0 mg/ml, laser light which reached the surface of the bacteria was absorbed effectively in the food color adherent to the bacterial wall without being absorbed into food color scattered around the bacteria. By contrast, in the case of Red no. 3 at 10 mg/ml, the laser light was more absorbed into the food color scattered around the bacteria and did not reach the surface of the bacterial wall sufficiently. In the case of Red no. 3 at 0.1 mg/ml, molecules of food color were not present around the bacterial wall, so the laser light was only slightly absorbed; most of it passed straight through.

In the future, the mechanisms of the bactericidal effects of argon laser need to be elucidated by observing changes in protein and enzyme activity in the cytoplasm and developing new types of dyes which attach to the bacterial cell strongly and absorb laser light efficiently without any toxic effects on the living body.

References

[1] Borzelleca J, Capen C, Hallagan J (1987) Lifetime toxicity/carcinogenicity study of FD & C Red no. 3 (erythrosine) in rats. Food Chem Toxicol 25:723–733
[2] Klein E, Fine S, Ambrus J, Cohen E, Neter E et al (1965) Interaction of laser radiation with biological systems. III. Studies on biologic systems in vitro. Fed Proc 24:104–110
[3] Martinetto P, Gariglio M et al (1986) Bactericidal effects induced by laser irradiation and haematoporphyrin against gram-positive and gram-negative microorganisms. Drug Exp Clin Res 12:335–342
[4] Okazaki T (1995) Mechanism of bactericidal effect by argon laser. J Jpn Soc Laser Med 16:7–15
[5] Okamoto H, Iwase T et al (1992) Dye-mediated bactericidal effect of He-Ne laser irradiation on oral microorganisms. Lasers Surg Med 12:450–458
[6] Schultz R, Harvey G, Fernandez-Beros M et al (1986) Bactericidal effects of the neodymium:YAG laser: In vitro study. Lasers Surg Med 6:445–448

Experimental Photodynamic Laser Therapy for Rheumatoid Arthritis Using Photosan-3, 5-ALA-Induced PPIX and BPD Verteporfin in an Animal Model[1]

C. Hendrich · G. Hüttmann · G. Dröge · J. Seara · T. Gomille · C. Lehnert · S. Houserek · W. E. Siebert

Introduction

Photodynamic therapy (PDT) is the activation of a dye (photosensitizer) by means of light which evokes a cytotoxic effect using oxygen [6, 32]. Descriptions of photoactive effects have been known for nearly 100 years, while systematic examination of the substances that are of therapeutic use today began in the 1950s [4]. Different substances do work in different ways, but the principal physicochemical process is the absorption of photons by the photosensitizer, leading to singlet and triplet oxygen states which are highly energetic. The following transfer of energy and charge evokes activated states of oxygen that are very reactive chemically and damage membranes and proteins [5]. The substantial cytotoxic effect is probably that of the singlet oxygen which is formed locally at the area of irradiation [33]. The specialty of PDT compared to other therapeutic methods is its double selectivity: there is only an effect if the photosensitizers are concentrated in the tissue aimed at and we have a sufficient photon density on account of the irradiation. Because of the low toxicity in the dark, there are no systemic side effects apart from photosensitizing of the skin.

The first generation of today's established photosensitizers are the derivatives of hematoporphyrin (HpD) and a cleaned fraction of the HpD, which has a larger portion of the operative porphyrin dimers and is distributed under the names Porfimer Sodium (formerly Photofrin II) and Photosan-3. Because its degradation in tumorous tissue takes longer than in other tissues, it allows selective destruction of tumors after 48–72 h. The disadvantage of these preparations lies in the above-mentioned sensitizing of the skin, which lasts up to 1 month and makes repeat use of PDT more difficult. The composition of Porfimer Sodium and Photosan-3 was not absolutely standardizable, which led to the development of second-generation photosensitizers characterized by a definite chemical structure. This development aimed not only at enhanced selectivity and faster degradation, but also improved absorbance of the substances which were located more in the red spectral range. Some of the new chemical compounds that seem to be of clinical use are the benzoporphyrin derivative BPD Verteporfin, zinc-II-phtalocyanin and the 5-aminolevulinic acid-induced protoporphyrin IX [15, 23, 24]. 5-Aminolevulinic acid (ALA) has an exceptional position here because as an amino acid it is not photodynamically active itself, but causes an endogenous concentration of the potent photosensitizer protoporphyrin IX (PPIX) in certain cells [24].

In order to achieve the greatest possible deep effect of PDT, red light between 600 and 800 nm is used for stimulation, which is able to enter very deeply into human tissue. In principle there is no need for laser light to stimulate the photosensitizers, but the intensities needed for endoscopic irradiation of the hollow organs cannot be coupled to a light conducting fiber or endoscopic optics by means of a conventional light source. Dye-lasers pumped by argon ions emit monochromatic light at more than 3 watts, which can be applied without problems endoscopically because of its parallel nature. Besides this, the monochrome nature of the laser allows easy calculation of the effective light dose. The exact wavelength is chosen for each sensitizer corresponding to its absorption maximum in this range. High-output laser diodes promise to become a low-price alternative to these lasers.

Up to now the main field for photodynamic methods of therapy was oncology [14]. Porfimer Sodium has been licensed in Canada for the treatment of superficial tumors of the urinary bladder and in the Netherlands for the treatment of bronchial and esophageal tumors [6]. A license in Japan relates to the treatment of early state carcinomas of the lung, esophagus, stomach, and the uterine cervix [16]. Several international studies involve Porfimer Sodium and the second-generation sensitizers [18, 19].

[1] Supported by research grant 0706903A5 from the Federal Ministry of Research and Technology as part of the "Photodynamic Laser Therapy" collaborative study and by the kind gift of BPD Verteporfin and cylinder diffuser tips from QLT Phototherapeutics Inc., Vancouver, Canada.

In contrast to this the nononcologic use of PDT is restricted to a small number of areas such as the treatment of psoriasis [2, 6], the avoidance of restenosis after angioplasty [7], and treatment of endometriosis [31] or of neovascularization of the eye [25]. As a further use, since 1989 our working group has been experimenting in the use of PDT to treat rheumatoid arthritis (RA) [27]. Using laser with thermic methods has shown to be helpful in the aftertreatment of arthroscopic synovectomy [17, 19, 26]. For the small joints which are almost always involved in RA no suitable minimally invasive technique is available at present. Because of the histological characteristics of RA, such as synovial cell hyperplasia, hypervascularization, and lymphoplasmacellular infiltrations, the synovium seems to be the ideal working point for the PDT [9]. For small joints, the laser with its fiber system allows the greatest possible miniaturization of instruments. This study shows the present-day state of the techniques and possibilities of PDT in relation to RA.

Methods and Results

Animal Model

In order to examine the in vivo pharmacokinetics and effect of PDT a suitable animal model was used. The animal model of IgG-induced arthritis is an adjuvant arthritis where human IgG aggregated by heat is used as an antigen. A synovitis which histologically meets the criteria of the proliferative phase of RA shows in the induced joint [3, 22]. Among other phenomena, joint effusion, a broadening of the lining cell layer, and enormous hypervascularization occurs. The cellular infiltration shows some germinal center-like structures. Induction of the arthritis is successful in 90–95 % of the animals in which an intracutaneous test allows a prediction. With this animal model we have a reproducible method for the induction of synovitis, which is the basic prerequisite for a systematic examination of the pharmacokinetics and pharmacodynamics of photosensitizers. The histologic changes in the comparable animal model of ovalbumin arthritis are not so great [29].

PDT with Photosan-3 in the Animal Model

To test this method of treatment in vivo, a series of rabbits was treated intravenously or intraarticularly with Photosan-3 after successful induction of arthritis. Irradiation was performed either 24 or 4 h later with a dye-laser pumped by argon ions at a wavelength of 630 nm. Laser application was over a single 400-μm fiber in the upper recess, which was inserted by means of an 18-gauge needle. The end of the fiber was roughened over a length of 2 cm, which guaranteed even radial spreading into the inner joint. After they had been kept in the dark for 1 week the animals were sacrificed and then examined. The macroscopic examination exposed a brown-reddish discolouring of the synovial tissue without showing changes on the surface of cartilage, menisci, or ligaments. The histologic examination showed massive bleeding in some parts of the preparations, above which the synovial tissue was raised. In the major part of the joint the synovia was already demarcated, and surrounding the remaining villous stroma there was a vast enclosure of hemosiderin. In contrast to this the morphology of the cartilage, the menisci, and the ligaments showed no change whatsoever [11]. These changes were seen independently of the method of application; nonetheless, after giving Photosan-3 intravenously the effect was less [8, 10]. Comparable studies by an American group using the animal model of ovalbumin arthritis also confirmed the selective effect of Porfimer Sodium on the synovia. However, the effect seen was less, which may be due to the animal model of ovalbumin arthritis used, and also to the fact that light application was by means of a plane-ground fiber which had no additional diffraction body, so that the irradiated area in the joint was much smaller [30].

Kinetics of 5-ALA-induced PPIX

The prolonged sensitizing of the skin is a disadvantage of first-generation photosensitizers. In contrast to this, ALA-induced PPIX degrades rapidly, within 24 h, and may be applied systemically and intraarticularly. In order to answer the question of whether inflamed synovial tissue is sensitized by ALA and to determine the most suitable application method and time, the distribution of PPIX in different tissues of the joint was studied in the animal model of IgG-induced arthritis. After three different durations of application (2, 4, and 24 h) tissue samples were taken from the rabbits and worked up to cryostatic cuts. The PPIX content was quantified using a fluorescence microscope equipped with a special, highly sensitive CCD camera [1, 12]. After both intravenous and topical application, significant fluorescence from the sensitizer showed in the synovia after no more than 2 h; after 24 h it had disappeared completely. In addition to the lining cell layer and the media of the vessels, a vast formation of PPIX showed particularly surrounding the inflamed infiltration. In contrast to this, in bradytrophic tissue like cartilage or the meniscus, fluorescence was not seen before 24 h, located in the lacunas of the chondrocytes [13]. Systemic application showed higher selectivity in concentrating in the inflamed synovia rather

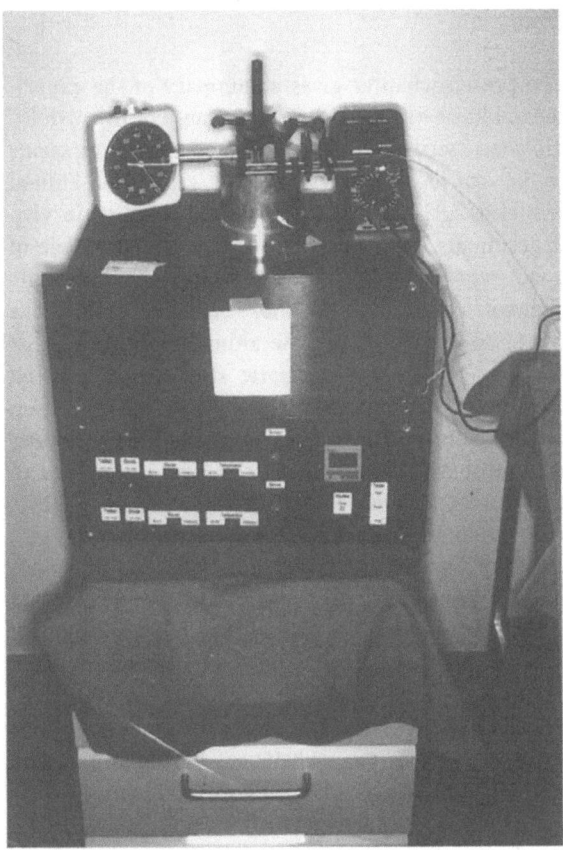

Fig. 1. Diode laser with a wavelength of 690 nm for photo-dynamic laser therapy (PDT) (Medical Laser Center, Lübeck, Germany)

than the regular synovia. The PPIX formed in the epidermis was completely degraded after 24 h, so that cutaneous sensitizing is no longer to be expected at this time [13]. However after therapy 4 h after intravenous or 2 h after intra-articular application of 5-ALA no necrosis of the synovial membrane whatsoever showed. Recent publications indicate a possible apoptotic effect of 5-ALA-induced PPIX [31]. Whether such an effect can be evoked in the arthritis model employed here is the subject of further study.

Systemic Therapy with BPD Verteporfin

One idea concerning systemic immunomodulation by means of PDT was pursued using the photosensitizer BPD Verteporfin [21]. After systemic application in an SLE mouse model, BPD concentrated preferentially in activated lymphocytes which showed a larger number of IL-2 receptors or HLA-DR antigens. These cells could be destroyed by means of whole body irradiation before cutaneous concentration of BPD. In the mouse model significant improvement was achieved both clinically and histopathologically [21]. The transdermal irradiation in use here employed a conventional light source.

In contrast to immunomodulation, BPD given at a higher dose and in combination with higher light energy can cause necrosis of the synovial membrane. In the rabbit arthritis model already mentioned, intravenous application of 2 mg BPD Verteporfin (kindly provided by QLT Phototherapeutics Inc., Vancouver, Canada) per kg bodyweight and sensitization lasting 3 h was studied. Irradiation was by a specially developed diode laser with a wavelength of 690 nm (Fig. 1) instead of the dye laser pumped by argon ions; it was applied by a "cylinder diffuser" fiber tip (QLT Phototherapeutics Inc; Fig. 2) which was

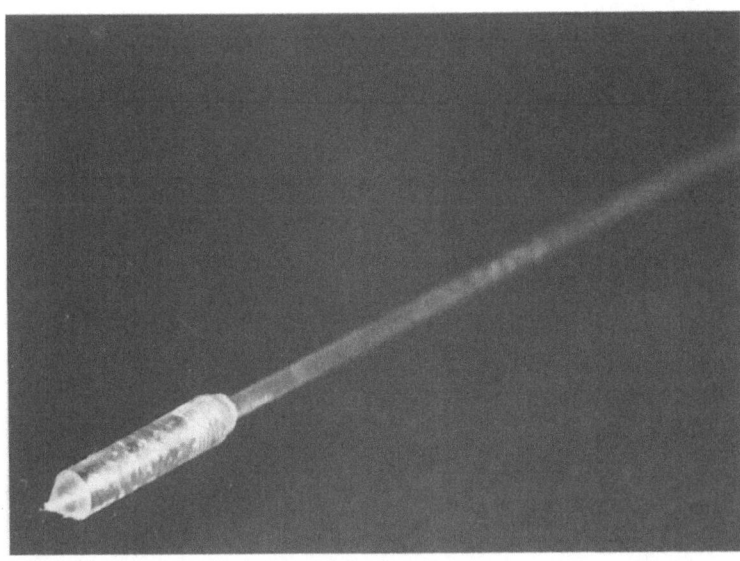

Fig. 2. Cylinder diffuser (QLT Phototherapeutics Inc., Vanvouver, Canada). The design of the fiber tip allows an even cylindrical light distribution profile

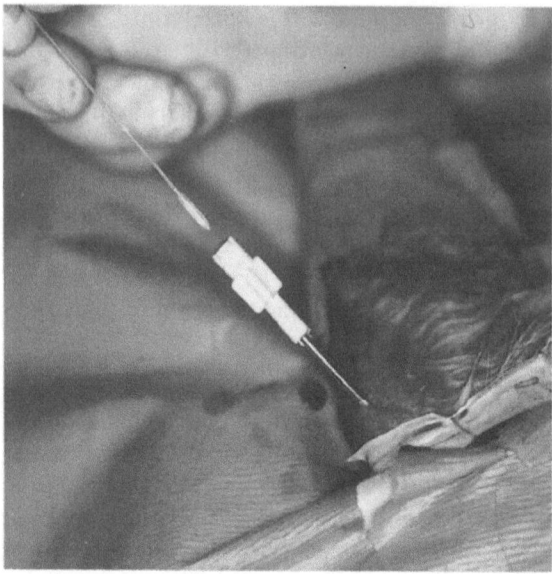

Fig. 3. A ODT procedure in an arthritic rabbit knee joint. The cylinder diffuser fiber tip is inserted over an 18-gauge needle into the upper recess of the knee joint

inserted over an 18-gauge needle into the upper recess of the knee joint (Fig. 3). A light dose of altogether 180 J was applied. After 1 week a vast zone of selective necrosis of the synovial membrane was seen in the irradiated area (Fig. 4) both macroscopically and microscopically, whereas the bradytrophic joint structures showed no change whatsoever.

Discussion

The present chapter gives a summary of the experimental basis of a PDT for RA. Because of the histologic characteristics of RA, inflamed synovium seems to be an ideal target for PDT [28]. The animal model of IgG-induced arthritis was used for in vivo experiments. First this model gives the advantage of good reproducibility, and, secondly, the histologic changes correspond to those in the proliferative phase of RA. Above all, the animal model allows us to carry out pharamcokinetic studies. Thus, using fluorescence spectroscopy, a selective concentration of the photosensitizer PPIX was seen after administration of ALA in the lining cell layer, the media of the vessels, and, especially, surrounding the cellular infiltration between 2 and 4 h after injection [12, 13]. No significant concentration of the substance in the bradytrophic joint structures could be detected earlier than after 24 h, so that 2–4 h after the injection the photosensitizer is selective for the inflamed tissue.

Selective sensitization of the synovia was also determined for the substance Porfimer Sodium, which is comparable to the Photosan-3 employed by our group [30]. In agreement with this, we saw selective hemorrhagic demarcation of the synovial tissue after PDT with Photosan-3, while the bradytrophic joint structures showed no changes either macroscopically or microscopically [8, 11]. A similar effect was also ascertained after intravenous application of BPD Verteporfin. While Photosan-3 risks cutaneous photosensitization, the second-generation photosensitizers stay in the body for a shorter time. Studies

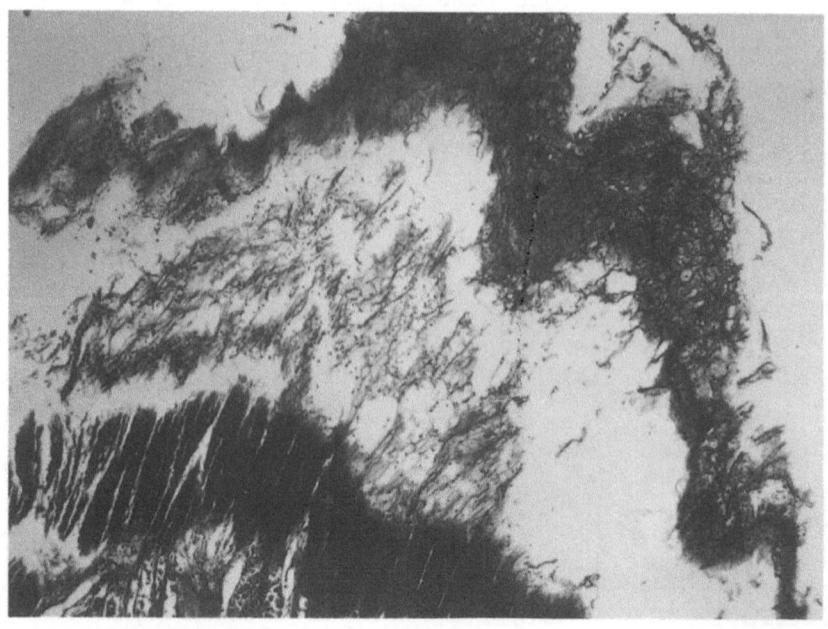

Fig. 4. Microphotograph of the synovia in IgG-induced arthritis in rabbit after PDT with BPD Verteporfin (Azan, × 200). The necrotic synovial tissue is demarcated from the underlying joint capsule tissue

of ALA-induced PPIX demonstrate favorable pharmacokinetics, although a final assessment of the therapeutic effect is not possible yet [11, 13]. In an SLE animal model, in the case of BPD a directly immunomodulating effect was observed after transdermal irradiation which might also be of use for treating RA [21]. In addition, BPD with an excitation wavelength of 690 nm has the advantage of deeper light penetration for this reason, so that present BPD seems promising for clinical use. The ability to use low-price laser diodes as demonstrated in this paper, which at present seems to suffice at least for small joints, is a further advantage of BPD. On the other hand, before clinical use, technical improvements in the field of laser application are needed in order to guarantee even illumination of small and very small joints [11]. In the field of dermatology, lasers are in some cases replaced by monochromatic lamps. Whether transdermal application with conventional light sources is sufficient or not remains to be investigated [28].

In conclusion, PDT seems to be a new and promising method of therapy for chronically inflammatory joint diseases. The potential of PDT has already been demonstrated in animal tests. Here it combines high selectivity with minimal invasiveness and the possibility to be used in small joints. Using the substance BPD Verteporfin in combination with a high-output diode laser with a wavelength of 690 nm and improved application methods, it is thinkable that the step from animal tests to clinical use for RA could be taken within the medium-term future.

Summary

The principle of photodynamic laser therapy (PDT) of rheumatoid arthritis (RA) is based upon concentrating a photosensitizer specifically in the inflamed synovium. Subsequent activation of the photosensitizer by means of a laser leads to a cytotoxic effect. An animal model of IgG-induced arthritis in rabbits was used. In this model the photosensitizers Photosan-3, 5-ALA-induced PPIX, and BPD Verteporfin were tested. Using Photosan-3 and BPD Verteprfin, appropriate laser irradiation lead to total selective demarcation of the synovium. In contrast to this, bradytrophic tissues such as cartilage, meniscus, and ligamentous structures showed no change either macroscopically or microscopically. In the animal model PDT combines high selectivity with a minimally invasive character and the ability to be used in small joints. Because of these properties, PDT fulfills the ideal requirements of a future minimally invasive treatment for chronic inflammatory joint disease.

References

[1] Bedwell, J, MacRobert A, Phillips D, Bown S (1992) Fluorescence distribution and photodynamic effect of ALA-induced PPIX in the DMH rat colonic tumour model. Br J Cancer 65:1818–824

[2] Boehncke W, Sterry W, Kaufmann R (1994) Treatment of psoriasis by topical photodynamic therapy with polychromatic light. Lancet 343:801

[3] Burmester G, Locher P, Koch B, Winchester R, Dimitriu-Bona A, Kalden J (1983) The tissue architecture of synovial membranes in inflammatory and non-inflammatory joint diseases. Rheumatology Int 3:173–182

[4] Dougherty T, Henderson B, Schwartz, S, Winkelman J, Lipson R (1992) Historical perspective. In: Dougherty T, Henderson B (eds) Photodynamic therapy: basic principles and clinical applications. Marcel Dekker, New York, pp 1–18

[5] Dubbelman T, Prinsze C, Penning L, van Steveninck J (1992) Photodynamic therapy: membrane and enzyme photobiology. In: Dougherty T, Henderson B (eds) Photodynamic therapy: basic principles and clinical applications. Marcel Dekker, New York, pp 37–46

[6] Fisher A, Murphree A, Gomer C (1995) Clinical and preclinical photodynamic therapy. Lasers Surg Med 17:2–31

[7] Grant W, Hopper C, Buonaccorsi G, Speight P, MacRobert A, Fan K, Bown S (1995) Photodynamic therapy of arteries: preservation of mechanical integrity. SPIE 2371:465–469

[8] Hendrich C, Diddens H, Lehnert C, Hüttmann G, Dröge G, Siebert W (1995) Photodynamische Lasertherapie für die chronische Polyarthritis. Lasermedizin 11:73–77

[9] Hendrich C, Diddens H, Nosir H, Siebert W (1995) Treatment of rheumatoid arthritis using photodynamic therapy? SPIE 2371:592–595

[10] Hendrich C, Diddens H, Seara J, Siebert W (1995) Photodynamic therapy for rheumatoid arthritis – a new therapeutic approach. Lasers Surg Med S7:32

[11] Hendrich C, Hüttmann G, Diddens H, Seara J, Siebert W (1996) Experimental basis of photodynamic laser therapy for rheumatoid arthritis. Orthopäde 25:30–36

[12] Hüttmann G, Lehnert C, Seara J, Hendrich C, Siebert W, Birngruber R, Diddens H (1995) Photodynamische Therapie von chronischer Polyarthritis in einem Tiermodell. Lasermedizin 11:86

[13] Hüttmann G, Hendrich C, Birngruber R, Lehnert C, Seara J, Siebert W, Diddens H (1997) Protoporphyrin IX distribution after inta-articular and systemic application of 5-aminolevulinic acid in healthy and arthritic jounts. SPIE 2675:228–242

[14] Jocham D, Baumgartner R, Beyer W, Feyh J, Haeussinger K, Huber R, Goetz A (1992) Clinical application of photodynamic therapy: German collaborative studies. In: Dougherty T, Henderson B (eds) Photodynamic therapy: basic principles and clinical applications. Marcel Dekker, New York, pp 303–322

[15] Kennedy J, Pottier R (1992) Endogenous protoporphyrin IX: a clinically useful photosensitizer for photodynamic therapy. J Photochem Photobiol B: Biol 14:275–292

[16] Levy G (1994) Photosensitizers in photodynamic therapy. Semin Oncol 21:4–10

[17] Lübbers C, Siebert W (1996) Die arthroskopische Holmium:YAG-Laseranwendung im Vergleich zu konventionellen Verfahren am Knie: Zwei-Jahres-Ergebnisse einer prospektiven randomisierten Studie. Orthopäde 25:64–72

[18] Marcus S, Dugan M (1992) Global status of clinical photodynamic therapy: the registration process of a new therapy. Lasers Surg Med 12:318–324

[19] Marcus S, Golub A, Shulman D (1995) Photodynamic therapy using 5-aminolevulinic acid-induced photosensitization: current clinical status. SPIE 2371:24–30

[20] Möller K, Lind B, Schramm U, Trautmann C, Hohlbach G (1992) Holmium-laser synovectomy of the knee for rheumatoid arthritis. Lasers Surg Med 12:382–389

[21] Ratkay L, Chowdhary R, Neyndorff H, Tonzetich J, Water-field J, Levy J (1994) Photodynamic therapy: a comparison with other immunomodulatory treatments of adjuvant-enhanced arthritis in MRL-pr mice. Clin Exp Immunol 95:373–377

[22] Reichel W, Weber K (1986) The stabilizing effect of syno-vectomy on the synovial membrane in arthritic rabbit knees. Arch Orthop Trauma Surg 105:11–17

[23] Richter A, Meadows H, Jain A, Canaan A, Lecy J (1995) Kinetics of cellular uptake and retention of the benzopor-phyrin derivative (BPD): relevance to photodynamic ther-apy. SPIE 2325:189–197

[24] Schieweck K, Capraro H-G, Isele U, van Hoogevest P, Ochs-ner M, Maurer T, Batt E (1994) CGP 55847, liposome-deliv-ered zinc(II)-phthalocyanine as a phototherapeutic agent for tumors. SPIE 2078:107–118

[25] Schmidt-Erfurth U, Hasan T, Gragoudas E, Michaud N, Flotte T, Birngruber R (1994) Vascular targeting in photo-dynamic occlusion of subretinal vessels. Ophthalmology 101:1953–1961

[26] Siebert W (1992) Laseranwendung in der Arthroskopie. Orthopäde 21:273-288

[27] Siebert W, Wirth C (1989) Laser in der Orthopädie. Bier-mann, Zülpich, pp 55–72

[28] Siebert W, Cain C, Hendrich C, Steinmetz M, Muschter R, Wirth C (1991) Arthroskopische laserpotenzierte Syno-viorthese (ALSO) - eine Möglichkeit zur photodyna-mischen Therapie der chronischen Polyarthritis? In: Sie-bert W, Wirt C (eds) Laser in der Orthopädie. Thieme, Stuttgart, pp 113–116

[29] Trauner K, Gandour-Edwards R, Shortkroff S, Bamberg M, Sledge C, Hasan T (1995) Photodynamic synovectomy with benzoporphyrin derivative in a rabbit model or rheuma-toid arthritis. Lasers Surg Med suppl 7:44

[30] Trauner K, Gandour-Edwards R, Shortkroff S, Sledge C, Nishioka N, Hasan T (1995) Photodynamic synovectomy with Photofrin in a rabbit model of rheumatoid arthritis. Lasers Surg Med Supplement 7:32

[31] Überriegler K, Banieghbal E, Krammer B (1995) Subcellu-lar damage kinetics within co-cultivated W38 human fibro-blasts following 5-aminolevulinic acid-induced protopor-phyrin IX formation. Photochem Photobiol 62:1052–1057

[32] Unsöld E, Jocham D (1988) Grundlagen photodynamischer Therapieverfahren. Chirurg 59:76–80

[33] Unsöld E, Steinmetz M (1991) Photodynamische Lasrther-apie (PDT). In: Siebert W, Wirth C (eds) Laser in der Orthopädie. Thieme, Stuttgart, pp 107–113

[34] Wyss P, Tromberg B, Wyss M, Krasieva T, Schell M, Verns M, Tadir Y (1994) Photodynamic destruction of endome-trial tissue with topical 5-aminolevulinic acid in rats and rabbits. Am J Obstet Gynecol 171:1176–1182

Bone Healing After Erbium:YAG Laser Osteotomy of Sheep Tibia

W. E. Siebert · M. Stanke

Introduction

Ever since Maiman constructed the first working laser system in 1968 [7], physicians have been studying the laser and the possibility of utilizing its transectin properties in medicine. In industry, the ability of the laser to cut through hard materials has been exploited for many years. By contrast, the medical field has been slow in employing the laser's transectin qualities, due to its thermic effect on biological tissues. In early trials, laser osteotomy of bony tissues caused carbonization and crystallization of the cut edges and hindered the healing process. More recent findings on the effect of lasers on biological tissues show that laser systems have been developed that are capable of treating bone and cartilage without any notable thermic damage [15, 18]. One of these systems is the erbium:YAG laser, an infra-red emitting solid body laser. Several in vitro and in vivo studies have been conducted on the effect of the Er:YAG laser on bone. These studies agree on the good transecting qualities and the minimal thermic damage in Er:YAG laser osteotomy [10, 11, 17, 20].

Up to now studies have been conducted on small animals with results which cannot be directly extrapolated to humans. Further studies are necessary, e.g., using a large animal model, to determine whether laser osteotomy is feasible for therapy in humans. Our study of total osteotomy of the tibia bone in sheep was intended to fill this gap.

Materials and Methods

Twenty-seven adult female Merino sheep (average weight 59 kg) were examined medically and divided into the following groups:

Group A: 6 animals, conventional osteotomy, final radiological follow-up after 8 weeks
Group B: 7 animals, conventional osteotomy, final radiological follow-up after 12 weeks
Group C: 6 animals, laser osteotomy, final radiological follow-up after 8 weeks
Group D: 7 animals, laser osteotomy, final radiological follow-up after 12 weeks

The 27th animal was kept in reserve and, after one animal died in group D, was placed in this group and treated accordingly.

A prototype Er:YAG laser, developed by MBB Medizintechnik, Ottobrun, was used for osteotomy. The wavelength applied was 2.94 μm; full width at half maximum (FWHM) was 180 μs (given value); repetition rate was 4 Hz; spot size (focal) was 0.4 mm.

The energy of a single pulse was between 750 and 800 mJ and was monitored before and after each operation. Energy density was approx. 470 J/cm^2. The laser beam was moved over the corticalis by a digital stepping-motor advance unit and produced homogenous and standardized incisions. Advance unit velocity was 0.1 mm/s. The laser energy was guided to the bone through a reflecting six-axis flex-arm (manufactured by Zeiss) and focused by a lens ($f = 15$ cm). During the osteotomy procedure we flushed the laser focus area with N$_2$ Gas (200 kPa) via a cannula (inner diameter 0.5 mm).

Once the operation field was marked (angle to tibia axis approx. 35°) The "saw animals" (groups A and B) were treated with conventional osteotomy using an oscillating saw (Aeskulap, thickness 0.5 mm). During the sawing process the area was flushed with a 0.9% saline solution. In the laser groups the tibial rim was focused on with the help of a HeNe pilot laser. Osteotomy was performed at a constant velocity using the advance unit. Subsequent osteosynthesis was carried out according to AO principles. We used a seven-hole 3.5 DC plate; the middle screw hole was left empty to simplify subsequent evaluation.

After surgery the sheep were kept in suspension frames for 10–14 days to protect the operated area and ensure healing. The use of such a suspension frame is appropriate because the result of the animals' loading would otherwise not be reproducible [4, 7]. In comparison to other immobilizing methods such as casts, this method simplifies observation and care of the animals; furthermore pain and discomfort are also reduced.

After a 14-day period the animals were X-rayed and transferred in groups of two or three to straw-filled pens. Each animal was X-rayed at least once more during the study.

In order to evaluate the bone healing process over time, we conducted a polychromatic sequence marker analysis with intravital dyes, which are stimulated by ultraviolet light. We used the following dyes:

- Xylenol-orange-tetra sodium salt (90 mg/kg) after 2 weeks in the 8-week groups (A and C) and after 3 weeks in the 12-week groups (B and D)
- Calcein-green (10 mg/kg) after 4 weeks in the 8-week groups (A and C) and after 6 weeks in the 12-week groups (B and D)
- Tetracycline (Reverin; Hoechst) (30 mg/kg) after 6 weeks in the 8-weeks groups (A and C) and after 9 weeks in the 12-week groups (B and D)
- Alicarin complex (30 mg/kg) after 8 weeks in the 8-weeks group (A and C) and after 12 weeks in the 12-week groups (B and D)

After 8 or 12 weeks, respectively, the animals were killed by intracardial T61 injection and both tibiae were removed. The tibiae were immediately frozen (–18 °C) for later processing. The operated tibiae were carved into smaller pieces with a water-flushed diamond saw (Conrad WOCO 50p) and subjected to biomechanical examinations.

For analysis of biomechanical tensile strength we used a DIN 51221 universal testing machine. This machine is driven by a recirculating ball screw and also adapted to a computer-assisted dynamometer which allows a maximum measuring force of 1000 N and a resolution of 0.01 N. For the graphic data output, an online *xy* recorder was connected; an additional printer was used for the numerical data output. The bone samples were examined according to the DIN 50114 standard for flat tensile testing. This records the tensile strength at which mechanical discontinuity of the sample occurs. The maximum tensile strength attained is computed by the testing machine with the input data and recorded as tensile strength (N/mm^2).

The complex preparation of the bone chips for fluorescence microscopy was done according to the method by Katthagen [6]. Horizontal and vertical bone samples were collected from all animals for histological examination. Haversian tranformation, bony union, carbonization, fluorescence, and callus formation were evaluated. We used a Carl Zeiss microscope with a mounted reflecting fluorescence light unit. A Hg high-pressure steam lamp HBO 50 was the light source, to which the following **dividing stimulation** color filter combinations were connected:

G 365 – FT 395 – LP 420; BP 436 – FT 460 – LP 470; G 436 – FT 510 – LP 520; G 546 – FT 580 – LP 590.

Owing to the number of animals our statistical evaluation is semiquantitative.

Results

Out of 27 sheep, 24 could be evaluated. One animal died due to an anesthesiological incident; two sheep were excluded from evaluation because of premature loading and material breakage in the osteotomy region.

Light and Fluorescence Microscopy

Six anmials were evaluated in each group. At least two longitudinal and five transversed samples were collected (in reference to the longitudinal axis of the bones). Numerical randomization of all samples meant that we had no knowledge of which group a sample belonged to during histological examinations. Afterwards the results were decoded and evaluated.

After saw osteotomy, initial production of collagenic tissue in the osteotomy gap was observed. Osteoid tissue was then produced to bridge the gap, inducing mechanical immobilization for the subsequent healing process. During the 3rd week, and especially from the 4th through the 6th week, stabilizing minerals were incorporated in the healing region. In the 6th week the first active osteones, which bond the gap, were observed. The number of osteones increased in the 9th week and after 12 weeks the edges of the gap were no longer identifiable in some samples. In one 8-week sample we observed a zone of altered fluorescence as a sign of thermal damage. This did not occur in any other 8- or 12-week sample. Callus formation was minor to moderate after 8–12 weeks.

The healing process after Er-YAG laser osteotomy was quite different. Although the sequence of healing was more or less the same, the process was delayed. After 8 weeks the gap was still filled with collagenic tissue; little osteoid tissue was present. Mineralization commenced during the 9th week through the 12th week. Haversian transformation of the corticalis began during the 6th week and continued until the 9th week, but started to bridge the gap no earlier than the 9th week or later. Zones of altered fluorescence were still visible during the 8th week. They continuously decreased in size but still had a width of 80 µm during the 12th week. Microfractures and carbonization, signs of thermal damage, were visible on the edges of the gap during the 8th through the 12th week, obstructing the haversian processes. Accumulation of osteoid tissue occurred 4 weeks later and mineralization 5 weeks later than after saw osteotomy.

In sum, the onset of the healing process following laser osteotomy was delayed and occurred at a slower pace.

Radiologic Evaluation

Standardized X-rays of the sheep tibia (13 mAs, 55 kV) in two planes were taken directly postoperatively and at regular intervals following osteotomy.

The radiological evaluation of the healing process offers only a rough estimation, because errors may occur owing to technical inaccuracies, implant overlapping, and differences in animal position. However, the overall results showed that bone consolidation in the laser groups was incomplete in comparison to that in the saw groups. This is due to technical difficulties during surgery with the laser (precise focusing) and influences the outcome of osteotomy and osteosynthesis. Although we endeavored to stabilize and immobilize the animals, they could still move about and load the operated extremity. After 4 weeks, none of the X-rays showed signs of total bone healing. After 8 weeks no sign of an osteotomy gap was observed in 4 animals from the saw group. Callus formation as a sign of incomplete healing was observed in the remaining 20 animals. After 12 weeks all animals in both the laser and the saw groups showed some degree of consolidation.

Although radiographs do not allow precise evaluation of bone healing, our results indicated increased callus formation after laser osteotomy in this large animal model.

Biomechanical Evaluation

Only samples taken from the 12-week animals were included in the biomechanical examination because other studies showed that after 8 weeks stability in both laser and conventionally treated animals is insufficient for tensile strength analysis [4]. We analyzed a few samples from 8-week animals, but stability was inadequate.

Four samples per tibia and animal were taken, giving a total of 48 samples (6 laser animals, 6 saw animals). For control, samples from the healthy untreated contralateral tibiae were analyzed.

We emphasize that only a small part of the cortical bone was analyzed. Healthy bone is composed of many overlapping, diagonal, horizontal and vertical lamellar structures that provide stability. A few samples could not be analyzed. The main problem was that the fraising process for the removal of the tibial samples had a negative effect on stability. For this reason all samples were examined macroscopically with a magnifying glass and were photographed prior to biomechanical analysis. Nineteen out of 48 samples were discarded; 16 samples from 4 saw-osteotomized animals and 13 samples from 5 laser-osteotomized animals could be analyzed. The results are given in Figs. 1 (saw osteotomy) and 2 (laser osteotomy).

After 12 weeks the average tensile strength was 38.2 N/mm^2 in the saw group and 23.7 N/mm^2 in the laser group. The biomechanical measurements agree with the radiological, macroscopic and histological evaluations with regard to the delayed healing after laser osteotomy. The difference between the biomechanical findings is not large; a few values of the laser group samples were just as high as some in the saw group. All in all, though, the biomechanical results do suggest that healing is delayed after laser osteotomy compared to saw osteotomy.

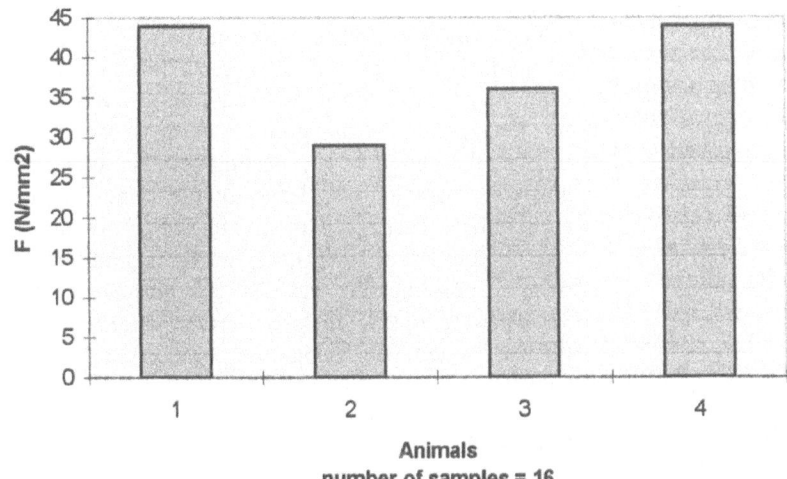

Fig. 1. Biomechanical tensile strength analysis: Results of saw osteotomy group B after 12 weeks

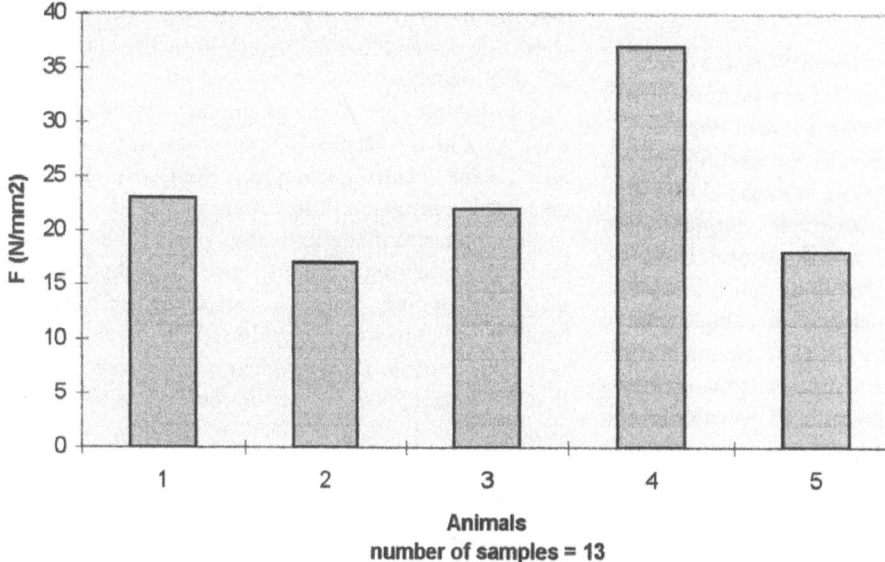

Fig. 2. Biomechanical tensile strength analysis: Results of laser osteotomy group D after 12 weeks

Discussion

Only a few studies have reported on laser treatment for bony tissue. This may well be due to the many problems that occur when applying laser energy to "laser-antagonistic" tissues. The first studies were conducted with the CO^2 laser, which was constructed for industrial use rather than biological application. In the last few years, laser systems with parameters (wavelength, pulse rate, etc.) optimized for applications in the medical field have been developed.

The results of our preliminary studies on pulsed Er:YAG laser osteotomy in the rabbit model showed the Er:YAG laser to be the most promising system for laser osteotomy procedures. The results for ablation rate, cutting velocity and bony healing were comparable to those seen with conventional methods of treating bone [17]. The aim of the present study was to use the Er:YAG laser in a complete osteotomy procedure with subsequent osteosynthesis in a larger animal in order to evaluate its clinical viability.

The sheep osteotomy model has been well established by many studies [12, 14, 19]. A postoperative period of 12 weeks is considered to be sufficient for complete bone healing and loading. Furthermore, polychromatic sequence marker analysis has been shown to be useless when the time span between each dye sequence exceeds 3 weeks [4]. On the basis of our previous studies, the healing process following laser osteotomy might be assumed to be shorter than or at least comparable to that after saw osteotomy. Taking account of all possible errors, the results of our study of Er:YAG laser osteotomy do not support this assumption.

Histology

Histological evaluation showed healing after laser osteotomy to be delayed compared to healing after saw osteotomy. It is questionable whether this delay can be attributed solely to thermic damage, identified by fluorescence. Mechanical damage to the bone – observed as numerous microfactures – should also be considered. However, this damage could also be attributed to the ablation process which occurs during a laser pulse, denoted by a perceivable bang. This process is not yet fully understood.

No fluorescence microscopy or animal experimental studies exist as to the clinical applicability of laser osteotomy using a short-pulse laser with a near-infrared emitting range of 2–3 μm. Our findings of altered fluorescence zones and delayed healing indicate that the high energy and pulse rate values of the Er:YAG laser that are necessary for adequate tibia osteotomy in sheep, may cause more severe thermic damage than in our previous study of osteotomy in the rabbit model. The healing process after saw and laser osteotomy is basically the same. In our experiments, thermic damage after laser osteotomy was notably less than in other previous studies; the delay in bone healing was also less pronounced [1, 3]. We were unable to alter certain parameters of the laser system which might have optimized the outcome.

Biomechanics

Of the few who have studied the Er:YAG laser, only Nelson et al. recommend biomechanical tensile strength tests for clinical evaluation of the thermic effect on bone stability after osteotomy [10]. Biomechanical tensile strength tests can only evaluate a small part of the entirety of the three-dimensional bone construction that makes up healthy bone. Complete healing of this three-dimensional structure takes up to 1 year, so that conclusions drawn from biomechanical tests can only pertain to a small part of the bone, not to the whole of it. Dinkelaker and Claes and Mutschler found maximal values for tensile strength (approx. 35 N/mm^2) that were similar to our results [2, 4]. The mineralization process found was also similar, but only a few osteones were found in the defect zone after 12 weeks. Our results for tensile strength of healthy controls and samples with simple drill hole defects after 12 weeks concur with the findings of Dinelaker (122.6 ± 16 N/mm^2 and 25 N/mm^2 respectively) [4]. However, the difference between the saw and laser groups in the latter study is not as pronounced in our study. Unfortunately, direct comparison of the results is not possible because Dinkelaker started biomechanical evaluations 8 weeks after surgery, at a point where bone healing is incomplete. However, Dinkelaker's 16-week results are no higher than our 12-week results. Our biomechanical evaluations also indicate that Er:YAG laser osteotomy delays the bone healing process compared to conventional methods.

Radiology

Radiological examination after orthopedic surgery is a standard clinical procedure for evaluation of healing processes, especially in complex cases. The radiographic appearance does not always correlate with the attained stability, but an experienced physician is still able to obtain valuable information from it as to the healing process.

During the 12-week postoperative period we took X-rays of the sheep directly after surgery and at 4, 8 and 12 weeks. Some animals showed notable callus formation. None of the laser-osteotomized animals displayed complete callus-free healing. These results, which agree with those of other experimental studies [4, 5], may be due not only to the premature loading by the animals but also to the periosteal process in the gap area caused by the laser osteotomy. Matter et al. observed the formation of callus after screwing osteosynthesis plates onto sheep tibia even without prior osteotomy [8].

The significance of callus formation has been interpreted differently over the past 50 years. Despite callus formation, some studies have found primary bone healing in the osteotomy gap [9, 16, 19]. We conclude that callus formation in all laser-osteotomized animals is a sign of healing. Whether increased callus formation is due to agitation of the osteotomy gap and to the chosen animal model or whether it is due to a particular laser-induced effect must be evaluated in further studies. It is possible that laser application causes callus formation as an initial response in an area of thermic damage where instant primary bone healing cannot occur. This effect could be utilized for callus distraction after laser osteotomy.

Clinical Outlook

Although the Er:YAG laser is a viable instrument for bone transection, our study shows that laser-assisted osteotomy has its limits, especially in bones with thick corticalis. The results of laser osteotomy of thinner bone are comparable to those of saw osteotomy [17]. One future use of the laser could be in surgery of smaller bones, e. g., in orthodontics. However, the endoscopic optical fibers that would be needed for this have not yet been developed.

The callus formation observed after laser osteotomy could be advantageous in callus distraction of longer tubular bones. The distraction could be conducted using a self-distracting marrow nail or an external fixator. Because it would reduce trauma to soft tissue and periosteum, laser osteotomy could deliver cosmetically good results.

Laser endoscopic bone tissue ablation, which is almost athermic, is already applied in otorhinolaryngology and neurosurgery [17].

Laser osteotomy is a minimally invasive procedure. After technical improvements, further positive results can be expected.

References

[1] Biyikli S, Modest M (1987) Energy requirements for osteotomy of femora and tibiae with a moving CW CO2 Laser. Lasers Surg Med 7:512–519
[2] Claes L, Mutschler W (1981) Quantitative investigations on newly-built bone in defects. Arch Othop Trauma Surg 98: 257–261
[3] Clauser C (1986) Comparison of depth and profile of osteotomies performed by rapid superpulsed and continuous wave CO laserbeams at high power output. J Oral Maxillofae Surg 44:425–429
[4] Dinkelaker F (1989) Die CO$_2$-Laser Osteotomie: Voraussetzungen und Möglichkeiten anhand einer tierexperimentellen Studie an Kaninchenradius und Schafstibia. Thesis, Free University of Berlin
[5] Hutzschenreuter P, Perren S, Steinmann S (1969) Some effects of rigidity of internal fixation on the healing pattern of osteotomies. Injury 1:77–83
[6] Katthagen B, Bechtel U (1985) Technik der unentkalkten Knochenhistologie und -histomorphometrie. MTA 34:164–172
[7] Maiman T (1960) Stimulated optical radiation in ruby. Nature 6:493–494
[8] Mater P, Brennwald J, Peren S (1974) Biologische Reaktion des Knochens auf Osteosyntheseplatten. Helv Chir Acta [Suppl 12] 44:5–44
[9] Müller M, Perren S (1972) Callus und primäre Knochenheilung. Monatsschr Unfallheilkd 75:442–454

[10] Nelson J, Orensein A, Liaw L-H, Berns M (1989) Mid-infrared erbium:YAG laser ablation of bone: the effect of laser osteotomy on bone healing. Lasers Surg Med 9:362–374
[11] Nuss R, Fabian R, Sarkar R, Puliafito C (1988) Infrared laser bone ablation. Lasers Surg Med 8:381–391
[12] Perren S, Cordea J (1977) Die Gewebedifferenzierung in der Frakturheilung. Unfallheilkunde 80:161–164
[13] Rahn B (1976) Die polychrome Sequenzmarkierung des Knochens. Nova Acta Leopoldina 44:249–255
[14] Rahn B, Gallinaro P, Baltensperger A, Perren S (1971) Primary bone healing. J Bone Joint Surg 53A:793–796
[15] Reichel E, Schmidt-Kloiber H, Schöffmann H, Dohr G, Eherer A (1987) Interactions of short laser pulses with biological structures. Optics Laser Technol 19:40–44

[16] Schenk R, Willenegger H (1977) Zur Histologie der primären Knochenheilung. Modifikation und Grenzen der Spaltheilung in Abhängigkeit von der Defektgröße. Unfallheilkunde 80:155–160
[17] Siebert W (1990) Laser-Osteotomie mit experimentellen Lasersystemen. Thesis, Hanover Medical College
[18] Sliney D (1985) Laser tissue interactions. Clin Chest Med 6:203–208
[19] Willenegger H, Perren S, Schenk R (1971) Primäre und sekundäre Knochenbruchheilung. Chirurg 42:241–252
[20] Wolbarsht M, Esterowitz L, Tran D, Levin K, Storm M (1986) A mid-infrared (2.94 μm) surgical laser with an optical fiber delivery system. Lasers Surg Med 6:257–269

Development of Laser Endoscope for Coagulation and Incision

Y. Hashishin · U. Kubo

Introduction

As is well known. Nd:YAG laser endoscopes with a 1-μm wavelength are superior for coagulation, but not very good for incision, as the Nd:YAG laser cannot make a clean cut. Some surgeons hope to excise stomach tumors by endoscopy. One solution how to do this is introduced in this paper.

The water absorption and the guiding systems involved are shown in Fig. 1. A quartz glas fiber is a very useful guiding system, ideal for laser power delivery in the region from 300 nm to 2 μm. Quartz glass fiber is available for delivery in seven lasers shown in Fig. 1, including the Nd:YAG laser. The laser power guiding systems have two serious problems in medical use. The first is that, in the infrared region over 2 μm and the ultraviolet region below 300 nm, many guiding systems are still in development. The second is that the guiding systems for high peak power laser delivery are not yet available for all wavelengths. So, if you need the laser beam for incision, the Ho:YAG laser with a 2-μm wave-length is the best, beacuse the Ho:YAG laser has strong water absorption in the region which is available for delivery through the quartz glass fiber. The Er:YAG laser has the strongest water absorption of all lasers [1, 6] but the quartz glass fiber cannot deliver the Er:YAG laser. We proposed a laser endoscope to consist of fibers that can deliver both Nd:YAG and Er:YAG lasers.

Laser Drilling of Soft and Hard Biotissues

It was confirmed that the Er:YAG laser is superior for incision. Figure 2 shows a comparison of four lasers, a KrF excimer laser with a 245 nm wavelength, an Er:YAG laser, a pulsed CO_2 laser, and a pulsed Nd:YAG laser, drilling through beef [1, 6]. The beef was exposed to laser beams with a focusing beam diameter of 0.5 mm with 5 pps repetition. It is clear that the Er:YAG laser drills deepest among the four lasers.

It was also confirmed that the Er:YAG laser is able to cut through the hard biotissues. Test results in the

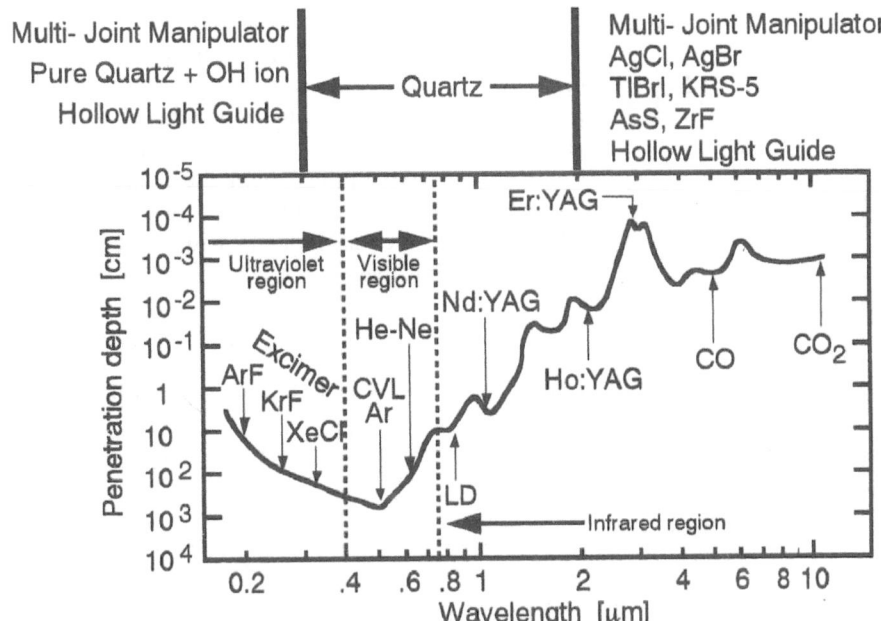

Fig. 1. Water absorption capacities of the different guiding systems plotted against wavelength

Table 1. Transmittance and delivery energy of the Er:YAG laser through the delivery systems

Delivery system	Core or hollow size	Transmittance (%/m)	Delivery energy (mJ/pulse)
Fluoride glass fiber (ZrF$_4$) [5]	450 μm Ø	90	400
	200 μm Ø	90	60
Chalcogenide glass fiber (As$_2$S$_3$) [5]	500 μm Ø	75	120
Quartz glass fiber (SiO$_2$) [2]	400 μm Ø	2.86×10^{-18}	–
Circular hollow waveguide (Pl/Ag) [4]	700 μm Ø	85	400
Rectangular hollow light guide (Al) [6]	0.5 × 8 mm	75'	170

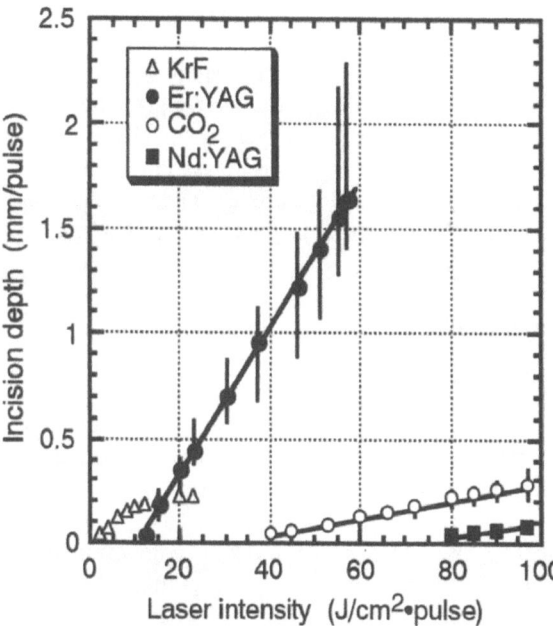

Fig. 2. Laser drilling of beef

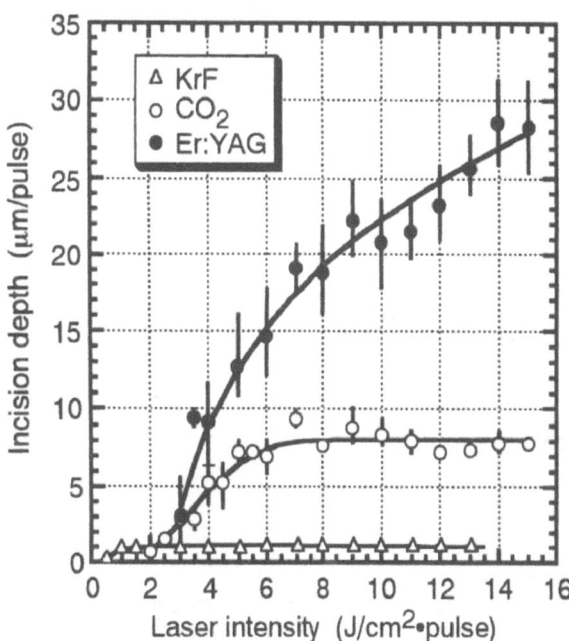

Fig. 3. Laser drilling of cow thighbone

case of a cow thighbone are shown in Fig. 3 [1, 6]. The bone was exposed to laser beams with a focusing beam diameter of 1.0 mm with 2 pps repetition. The Er:YAG laser incised the bone deepest among the three lasers tested, although the bone was water-poor biotissue.

Delivery Systems for the Er:YAG Laser

Which kind of delivery system is best for the Er:YAG laser? We tested fluoride glass fiber, chalcogenide glass fiber, quartz glass fiber, circular hollow wave guide and a rectangular hollow light guide as shown in Table 1 [2, 4–6]. It was clear that quartz glass fiber could not deliver the Er:YAG laser. The transmittance and delivery energy of the fluoride glass fiber was 90 % and 400 mJ/pulse, respectively – the highest of the five delivery systems at present. However, since the core part of the exit end melts when soaked in water, it is necessary for fluoride glass fiber to be waterproofed [2, 6]. In the end, we selected the fluoride glass fiber of the five for Er:YAG laser delivery.

Guide Lasers Through the ZrF$_4$ or SiO$_2$ Fiber

The Er:YAG laser and Nd:YAG laser are not visible light beams. Laser endoscopes using these lasers need a guide light beam to reveal the object. We tested five lasers as shown in Table 2. Every laser could be delivered through both the fluoride glass fiber and the quartz glass fiber. The guide laser was selected out of the visible lasers with regard to the color of the objective.

Table 2. Transmittance of the guide lasers through ZrF$_4$ and SiO$_2$ fibers (%/n)

Laser	ZrF$_4$ fiber	SiO$_2$ fiber
Diode (red), 670 nm	95.4	92.6
He-Ne (red), 633 nm	97.1	96.4
He-Ne (orange) 598 nm	95.1	87.6
He-Ne (green), 543 nm	97.5	95.4
LD-YAG-SH (green), 532 nm	97.4	88.6

Trial Laser Fiber and Laser Endoscope

We designed two types of laser endoscope with both coagulation and incision ability [3]. These laser endoscopes are noncontact irradiation systems. One of the two types has two fibers as shown in Fig. 4. The Nd:YAG laser with continuous-wave mode is used for coagulation, the Er:YAG laser with pulse mode for incision. The Nd:YAG laser is delivered through quartz glass fiber and the Er:YAG laser through fluoride glass fiber. The other type has four fibers as shown in Fig. 5. Three quartz glass fibers are used to deliver the Nd:YAG laser and one fluoride glass fiber to deliver the Er:YAG laser. The three quartz glass fibers surround the one fluoride glass fiber. The Er:YAG laser cannot stop hemorrhage, so when the Er:YAG laser cuts the diseased parts and the cut bleeds, the Nd:YAG laser is used to stop the bleeding.

We have made up these two types of laser fibers. The core diameters of their fibers are about 0.6 mm. If high laser power is needed, a thick fiber is selected; if flexibility and a small-size laser endoscope are needed, a thin fiber is selected. The fiber diameter depends on the purpose of the treatment. The sapphire lenses in the end of the laser fiber protect against water and smoke.

The prototype laser endoscope consists of four channels. The "forehead" part is the endoscope, which consists of illumination fibers and detective image fibers. One of the "eyes" is the smoke and water suction or gas blower. The other of the "eyes" is the solution blower. The "mouth" part is the laser fiber. The diameter of this laser endoscope is 15 mm. If this is too large, we can make a smaller size, down to around 10 mm at present.

Conclusion

A utility laser endoscope with coagulation and icision ability has been made up. Once high-power laser diodes transmitting Nd:YAG and Er:YAG lasers are made, compact and easy-handling laser endoscopes will begin to appear early in the 21st century.

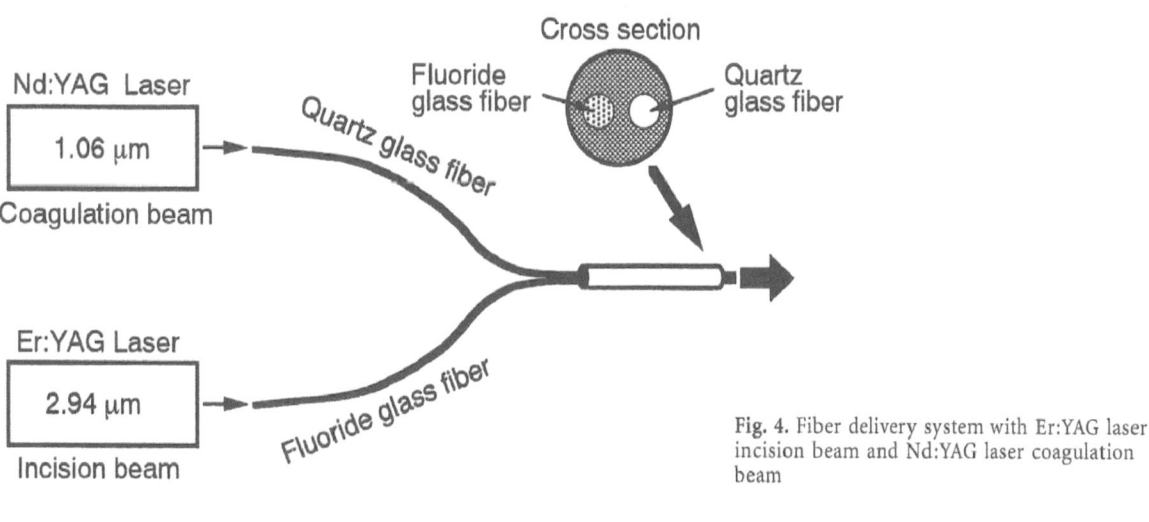

Fig. 4. Fiber delivery system with Er:YAG laser incision beam and Nd:YAG laser coagulation beam

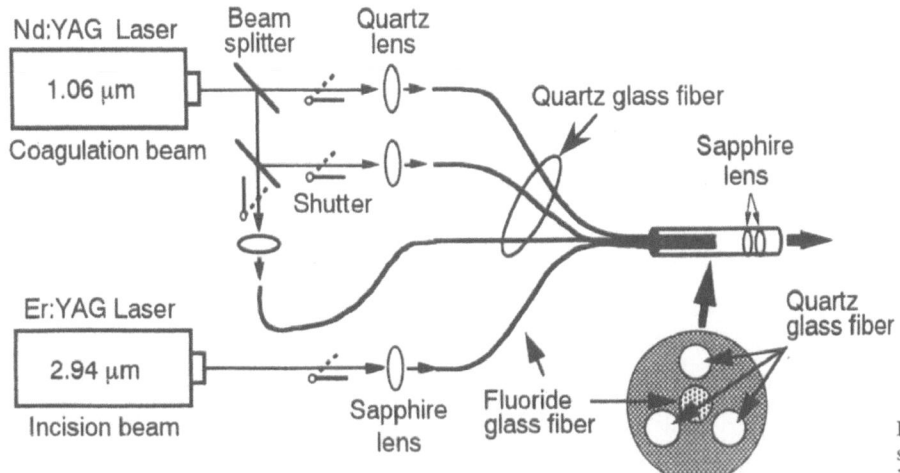

Fig. 5. Bundle fiber delivery system with Er:YAG laser incision beam and Nd:YAG laser coagulation beam

Summary

Nd:YAG laser endoscopes with a 1.06-µm wavelength are better for coagulation but cannot be used for incision. The Er:YAG laser with a 2.94-µm wavelength is better for incision than the CO_2 laser with a 10.6-µm wavelength. The characteristics of laser coagulation and laser incision using both the above lasers in soft (beef, gelatin, etc.) and hard biotissues (bone, tooth, etc.) were examined. New laser endoscope systems using Nd:YAG and Er:YAG lasers were developed. The delivery system for the Nd:YAG laser is conventional quartz glass (SiO_2) fiber. The Er:YAG laser cannot be delivered through quartz glass fiber, so fluoride glass (ZrF_4) fiber is used for Er:YAG laser delivery. Trial laser endoscopes were made.

References

[1] Hashishin Y, Shimoyama Y, Takeda A, Mochiziki T, Kuvo U (1992) Biotissue incision by Er:YAG, pulsed Nd:YAG and pulsed CO_2 lasers. J Fac Sci Technol Kinki Univ 28:173–179
[2] Hashishin, Y, Shimoyama Y, Mochiziki T, Kubo U (1993) Development of Er:YAG laser power delivery systems. J Fac Sci Technol Kinki Univ 29:133–141
[3] Hashishin Y, Ohuchida T, Tsubokura M, Kubo U (1996) Development of laser endoscope for coagulation and incision. Proc. 17th Annual Meeting Japan Society of Laser Medicine, 401–494 [In Japanese]
[4] Kato Y, Osawa M, Kubota S, Miyagi M, Abe S, Aizawa M, Onodera S (1995) Loss charactersitics of polyamide-coated silver hollow glass waveguide for Er:YAG laser light. Digest of Technical Papers in 15th Annual Meeting Laser Society Japan, p. 308 [In Japanese]
[5] Kubo U, Hashishin Y, Tanaka H, Mochizuki T (1991) Infrared delivery systems for Er:YAG laser. SPIE Infrared Fiber Optics III 1591:141–145
[6] Kubo U, Hashishin Y, Tanaka H, Mochizuki T (1992) Development of optical fiber for medical Er:YAG laser. SPIE Optical Fibers Med VII 1649:34–40

III Arthroscopy

Preface to Lasers in Arthroscopy

Arthroscopic surgery is a well-established standard procedure for diagnosis and therapy of joint disorders. Although the laser has been utilized as an assisting tool during arthroscopic procedures for several years, its advantages and disadvantages are still under avid discussion. The following contributions, written by experts in the field of laser-assisted arthroscopy, demonstrate their profound knowledge of lasers in knee and shoulder arthroscopy as well as other joints. Prospective studies and experimental laboratory studies on new possibilities will be described. There is still a lack of prospective, randomized double-blind studies; however, the days of frustration with the use of impracticable laser systems with unsuitable wavelengths are long gone. In 1984 Robert Metcalf stated that "lasers have no advantage in arthroscopic surgery".

Almost 10 years later, in 1993, AANA (the Arthroscopy Association of North America) wrote, "AANA recognizes that the use of lasers in arthroscopic surgery is an alternative to mechanical techniques."

A variety of promising applications will be discussed in the following chapters along with possible pitfalls and complications. MRI modifications after holmium:YAG laser arthroscopy and soft tissue shrinkage and other intriguing applications in shoulder surgery will also be addressed. Photodynamic-assisted tissue welding in meniscus repair procedures, which has been successful in recent experimental studies, is described. It is my hope that those who are interested in arthroscopic laser surgery will benefit from the information given in the following chapters.

W. E. Siebert

Holmium:YAG Laser-Assisted Arthroscopy Versus Conventional Methods for Treatment of the Knee

Two-Year Results of a Prospective Study[1]

C. Lübbers · W. E. Siebert

Introduction

Since the 1980s, arthroscopic surgery has become a well-established technique for the treatment of knee disorders and is, of course, the subject of continual research, development, and improvement. Arthroscopic treatment of diseases, especially chondromalacia, has produced unsatisfactory results [22, 24]. Furthermore, studies have been conducted on iatrogenic cartilage damage caused by the application instruments [6, 12] and retrospectively on the complications [3, 30].

The use of lasers has been researched as a possibility for the improvement of arthroscopic techniques. Laser systems allow the use of very small, but powerful instruments, which would be theoretically ideal for arthroscopic surgery. With this in mind, several reseach centers have developed laser systems and studied their applicability in arthroscopy [5, 14, 17, 19, 26, 31, 33]. Not all systems proved to be similarly successful due to varying physical criteria and technical deviations.

Based on experimental results, further improvement of the laser, and clinical applications, several clinical studies were conducted in the 1980s to prove the validity of laser arthroscopy [7, 8, 20, 21]. The results of these are in part very encouraging and justify continuing development and clinical use.

Recently, research groups, especially Siebert and his team, have been conducting experimental and single case studies on the holmium:YAG laser [2, 4, 16, 28, 29]. Of all laser systems currently available, the holmium:YAG laser seems to be the most suitable one for arthroscopic surgery. The following study is a guideline for surgical instrumentation and technique.

Patients and Methods

From April 1991 to August 1993, the results of 320 arthroscopic knee operations were statistically analyzed. The laser collective was composed of 100 patients (56 men, 44 women). The comparison group of 180 patients (122 men, 90 women) were treated with conventional mechanical methods. The higher number of conventional operations was due to the fact that laser arthroscopy was not conducted routinely at the beginning of the study.

The following five groups of knee disorders were treated: meniscal lesion, chondromalacia, rheumatoid synovialitis, patellofemoral pain syndrome (latera), and combined meniscal-cartilage injury. Laser patients of the last group were treated for both disorders, whereas in the conventional collective, one group of patients underwent combined surgery, while the other was treated only with meniscectomy without condromalacia treatment. Fig. 1 shows the distribution of patients. Those patients with an isolated knee disorder or combined meniscal/cartilage disorder without a further clinically relevant ligamental instability were included in the study.

The patients were admitted to the hospital and examined 1 day prior to surgery. Diagnosis was confirmed and the appropriate surgery done. Postoperative follow-ups were conducted on the day of discharge, 5–8 weeks (average 6.2 weeks), 1 year, and 2 years after surgery.

A pulsed holmium:YAG laser (Coherent, Palo Alto, Calif.) with a wavelength of 2100 nm was used during arthroscopic surgery. Energy is transferred to the intra-articular structures through a flexible quartz fiber. A 30° hand piece was used in 90 % of the operations; otherwise, a 70° laser hand piece was used as it is more advantageous, especially during lateral release procedures. During surgery of meniscal lesions, i.e., meniscectomies, 32 W were applied. Homogenous, stable edges and rims were formed when using the laser even after degenerative tears.

During the surgical treatment of chondromalacia, low repetition rates and joule value parameters were chosen so that no more than 6.4 W were produced. A defocused mode was chosen during procedures using higher values. During surgery, the occurrence of thermic tissue damage was avoided, which

[1] This chapter was published in: Knee Surg Sports Traumatol Arthrosc (1997) 5:168–175.

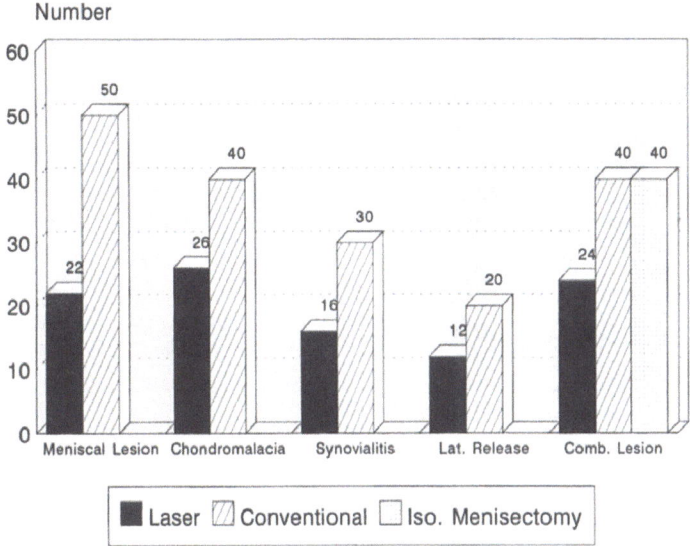

Fig. 1. Distribution of patients and surgery in the five disorder groups and surgery

Total = 320, Laser = 100, Conventional = 180

can be macroscopically detected by a light brown tissue discoloration.

The data were registered according to the Lysholm score modified by Klein and the IKDC knee follow-up questionnaire [11, 13, 16]. Patients were also examined clinically. Changes in the scores and a difference in compared scores indicate surgical success. Statistical analysis was conducted according to the t-test for unbound values; error probability, $\alpha = 0.05$ [10].

Results

There is only a slight difference in age between the laser collective (40.2 years) and the conventional collective (40.6 years). The youngest patient was 16 years old, and the oldest 71 years. Approximately 66 % of the operations were conducted in the right knee in both collectives. The duration of knee pain and complaints before surgery, as described by the patients, was similar in both collectives. Furthermore, the results of preparatory surgery were also comparable.

Meniscal Lesion

Only those patients suffering from degenerative or traumatic meniscal injury were included in this group. Patients with other knee disorders were excluded, except those with chondromalacia grade I by Fründ and/or local synovialitis. There was 77.3 % medial meniscal injuries in the laser collective and 69.2 % in the conventional collective. Also, 4.5 % of the laser collective and 6 % of the conventional collective received treatment to both medial and lateral meniscii (Fig. 2).

Average operating time was 32.4 min for laser surgery and 34.3 min for conventional surgery.

Only 27.3 % of laser patients needed a tourniquet, whereas it was necessary in 64 % of conventional operations.

The average length of hospitalization of 3.1 days for the conventional collective was slightly lower than for the laser collective (3.8 days). After at most 6 weeks, all patients in both collectives could return to work.

During hospitalization, no severe effusions occurred in either collective. After at least 6 weeks, postoperative puncture was necessary in 9.1 % of the laser collective and in 14 % of the conventional collective.

After 2 years, the subjective scores of both collectives showed improvement in over 90 % of the patients. Furthermore, the modified Lysholm score increased highly significantly to 89.3 points in the

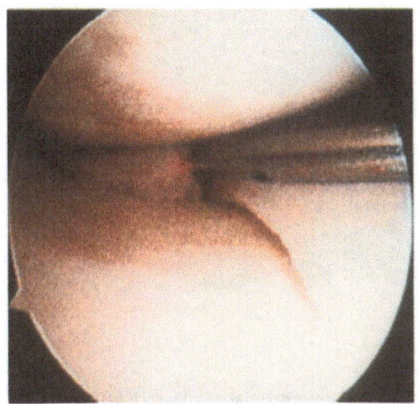

Fig. 2. Meniscal resection of posterior horn using the laser

Points

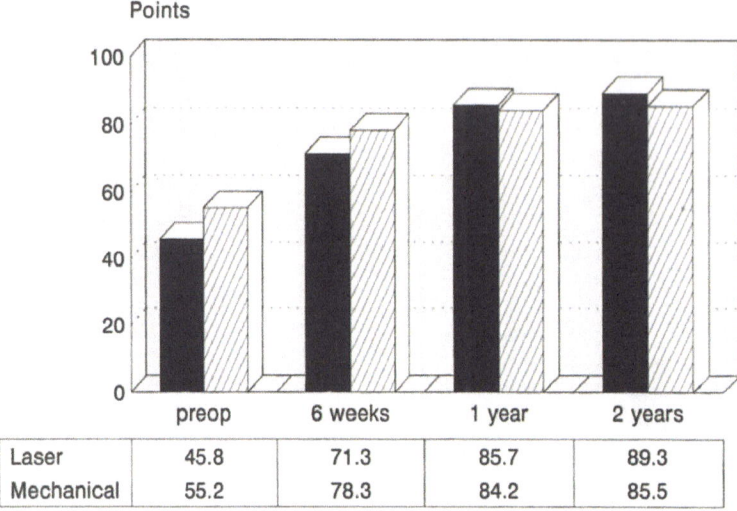

	preop	6 weeks	1 year	2 years
Laser	45.8	71.3	85.7	89.3
Mechanical	55.2	78.3	84.2	85.5

■ Laser ▨ Mechanical

Fig. 3. Meniscal lesion/Modified Lysholm score

laser collective ($P < 0.0002$) and to 85.5 in the conventional collective ($P < 0.0004$) (Fig. 3). No significant difference could be found between the laser collective and the conventional collective.

Chondromalacia

Patients suffering from chondromalacia grade II or III by Fründ in at least one knee compartment and who had undergone no cartilage shaving therapy were included in this group. No other knee disorders were allowed except for local synovialitis and loose bodies. Over 65 % of the patients in both the laser and conventional collective suffered from chondromalacia grade III (Fig. 4).

Comparison of operation time revealed hardly any difference: 53.5 min for the laser collective. 52.9 min for the conventional collective. A notable difference between the collectives was found in the use of a tourniquet: 15.4 % in the laser collective, 75 % in the conventional collective.

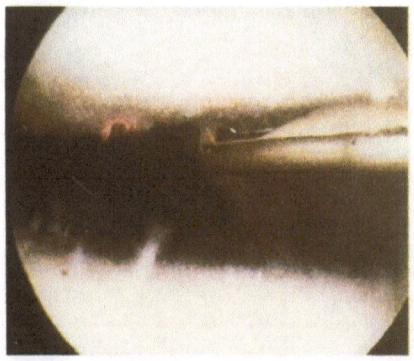

Fig. 4. Tangential chondromalacia laser treatment of the retropatellar surface

The average length of hospitalization was shorter for the laser patients (5.8 days) than for the conventional collective (7.7 days).

After 2 years, all laser patients had returned to work, whereas 18.8 % of the conventional collective were still on sick leave.

Blood loss was significantly lower in the laser collective (34.6 ml) than in the mechanical collective (96.3 ml, $P < 0.009$).

The occurrence of severe effusions in the treated knee was much higher in the conventional collective: 25 % needed postoperative puncture during hospitalization vs none in the laser collective. During the follow-up period, it was noted that 43.5 % in the conventional and 15.4 % in the laser collective had been punctured.

The patients were given analgesic medication if necessary. During hospitalization, a higher number of conventionally treated patients received medication (87.5 % in the conventional collective, 61.5 % in the laser collective). During the follow-up period, this value had notably decreased to 7.7 % in the laser collective, but only to 62.5 % in the conventional collective.

After 2 years, 84.6 % of the laser patients were satisfied with the results of surgery in comparison with 43.8 % in the conventional collective.

The Lysholm score was increased only slightly in the conventional collective ($P < 0.084$), whereas the increase was highly significant ($P < 0.004$) in the laser collective. The initial preoperative Lysholm scores were practically identical in both collectives. After 2 years, a 13.7 point difference between the laser and conventional collective was found (Fig. 5).

Although an overall improvement was attained in both collectives, especially in the laser collective, it

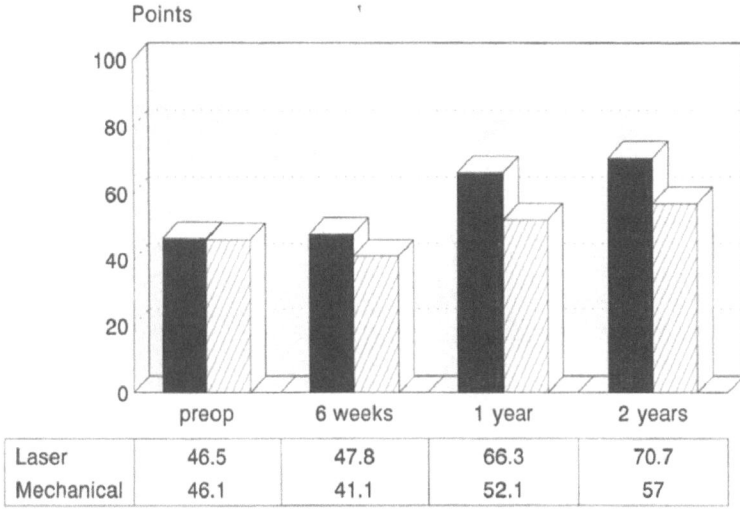

Points	preop	6 weeks	1 year	2 years
Laser	46.5	47.8	66.3	70.7
Mechanical	46.1	41.1	52.1	57

■ Laser ▨ Mechanical

Fig. 5. Chondromalacia/Modified Lysholm score

was necessary to conduct further surgery on three conventionally treated patients (two total knee arthroplasties, one tibia head valgization). One patient in the laser collective received a unicompartmental knee replacement.

Combined Cartilage and Meniscal Lesions

Only those patients suffering from a traumatic or degenerative meniscal lesion and also from chondromalacia II or III in at least one knee compartment were included in this group. Further knee injuries led to exclusion except for local synovialitis and loose bodies. The chondromalacia in all laser patients and in half of the patients in the conventional collective was treated with cartilage shaving. The other half of the conventional collective received conventional meniscectomy without chondromalacia therapy.

Only a slight difference in average operating time was found: 56 min for combined conventional surgery, 52 min for isolated conventional meniscectomy, 48.8 min for laser surgery. Average length of hospitalization was practically the same for all groups: 5.8 days for the laser collective, 5.8 for combined surgery, 5.2 days for isolated meniscectomy. After 2 years, only 8.3 % in the laser collective and 5 % in the isolated meniscectomy collective were still on sick leave. Altogether 20 % of patients in the combined conventional group were unable to work at that time.

Observation of the Redon drainage during hospitalization showed that blood loss in the laser patients (26.3 ml) was significantly lower in comparison with the combined conventional collective (86.5 ml, $P < 0.004$) and the isolated conventional collective (71 ml, $P < 0.005$).

During hospitalization, puncture was necessary in 10 % of the isolated meniscectomy patients and unnecessary in the other two groups. The 2-year follow-up results show that 16.7 % in the laser collective, 20 % in the combined conventional collective, and 15 % in the isolated meniscectomy collective had been punctured.

During hospitalization, only 41.7 % of the laser patients were given analgesic medication in comparison with 70 % in the combined collective and 75 % in the isolated collective. All values were reduced after 2 years: 16.7 % in the laser collective, 25 % in the combined collective, and 15 % in the isolated collective.

After 2 years, all of the patients in the laser collective were satisfied with the results and showed an improved status. A similar status was described by 75 % in the meniscectomy collective but by only 55 % in the combined conventional collective.

A significant increase in the Lysholm score was found ($P < 0.01$) for the combined collective, a highly significant increase ($P < 0.003$) for the isolated collective and ($P < 0.001$) for the laser collective (Fig. 6). The initial Lysholm score was practically identical in all three collectives. After 1 year, a significant difference ($P < 0.06$) beween both conventional collectives was found. After 2 years, this difference was no longer significant. The 2-year Lysholm score in the laser collective was significantly higher than in the combined conventional collective ($P < 0.02$). There was no significant difference between the laser collective and the isolated meniscectomy collective.

One total knee arthroplasty was necessary in the combined conventional collective.

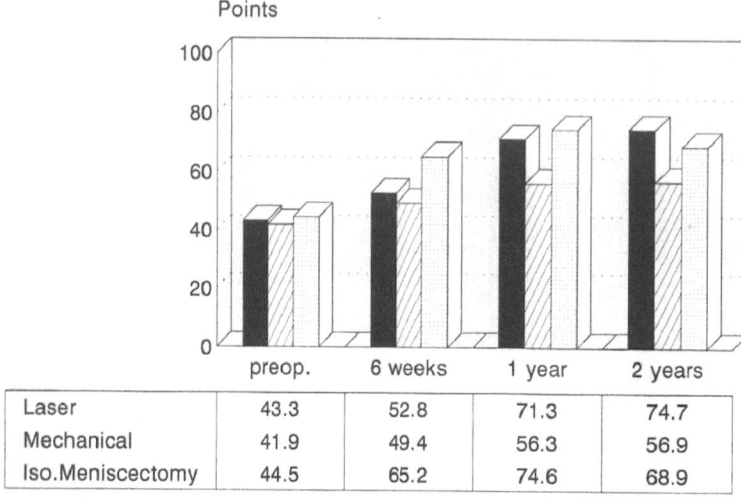

Points	preop.	6 weeks	1 year	2 years
Laser	43.3	52.8	71.3	74.7
Mechanical	41.9	49.4	56.3	56.9
Iso.Meniscectomy	44.5	65.2	74.6	68.9

■ Laser ▨ Mechanical ☐ Iso.Meniscectomy

Fig. 6. Combined meniscal and cartilage lesion/Modified Lysholm score

Rheumatoid Synovialitis

Only those patients suffering from synovialitis caused by chronic polyarthritis were included in this group. Degenerative meniscal disorders were included and treated. Severe chondromalacia was also included, but not treated.

Only a slight difference in operating time was found between the laser collective (83.1 min) and the conventional collective (78.3 min). A marked difference was found in the use of a tourniquet. Whereas it was used in only 25% of the laser procedures, it was necessary during each conventional synovectomy.

The hospital stay for the laser patients was slightly shorter (7.9 days) than that for the conventional collective (9.4 days).

There was a significant difference in blood loss according to the Redon drainage. Whereas laser patients lost only 94.6 ml, the conventional patient lost an average of 244.7 ml ($P < 0.01$).

After 2 years, 87.5% of the laser collective and 80% of the conventional collective had returned to work.

No patient in the laser collective needed puncturing during hospitalization, whereas it was necessary in 13.3% in the conventional collective. No further puncturing was conducted in either collective according to the 2-year follow-up results.

After 2 years, all of the laser patients described an improved status. The same status was found in 80% of the conventional collective.

The Lysholm score increased by a highly significant amount in the laser collective ($P < 0.001$) and

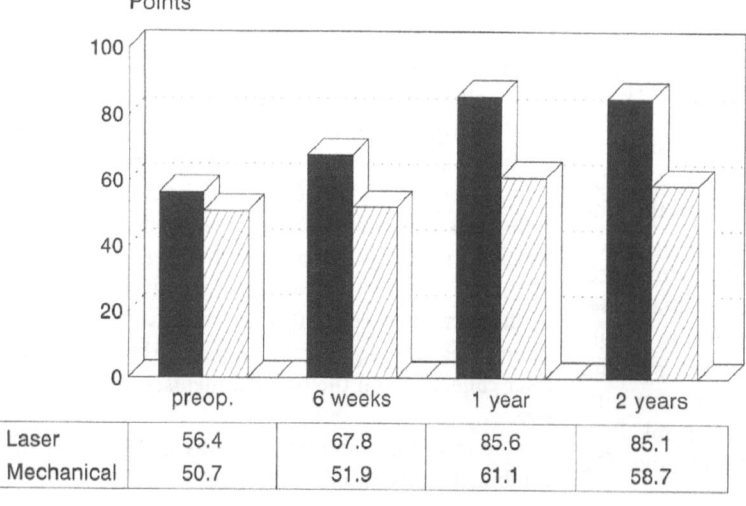

Points	preop.	6 weeks	1 year	2 years
Laser	56.4	67.8	85.6	85.1
Mechanical	50.7	51.9	61.1	58.7

■ Laser ▨ Mechanical

Fig. 7. Rheumatoid synovialitis/Modified Lysholm score

nonsignificantly in the conventional collective (Fig. 7). Preoperatively, the Lysholm score was not significantly different when comparing both collectives. After 2 years, the score for the laser collective was significantly higher than that for the conventional collective ($P < 0.004$).

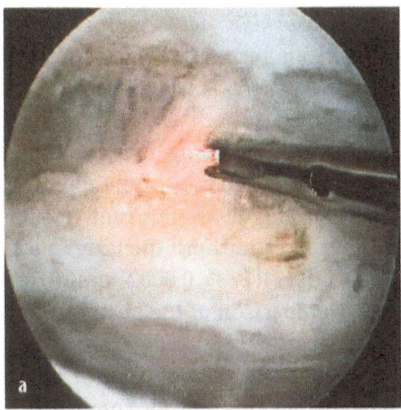
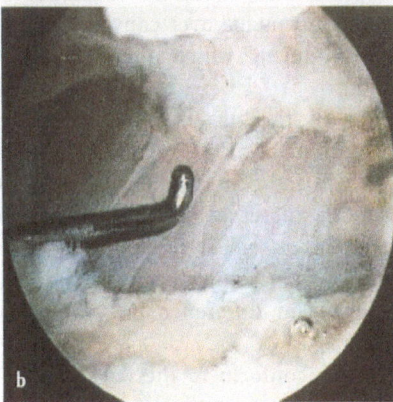

Fig. 8. Lateral retinacular release **a)** during treatment with the laser **b)** after treatment without intraarticular bleeding

Lateral Release

This group included patients suffering from patellofemoral pain syndrome with a patella lateralization grade II or III, without severe articular damage. Chondromalacia grade I was included, but not treated. The patients were treated with lateral retinacular release (Fig. 8).

Duration of surgery was similar in both collectives: 43.4 min for the laser procedure, 40.5 min for the conventional surgery. A tourniquet was applied in all conventional operations and in only 33.3 % of the laser operations.

The average length of hospitalization was practically identical: 9 days for the laser collective, 8.7 days for the conventional collective.

Average blood loss according to the Redon drainage was similar: 53.3 ml in the laser collective, 58 ml in the conventional collective.

The laser patients recovered more quickly, and all had returned to work within the 2-year follow-up period.

No severe effusions occurred in the laser collective during hospitalization or the follow-up period. Of the patients in the conventional collective, 10 % underwent puncturing in the clinic. This value did not increase during the follow-up period.

The 2-year results show an improved status in 70 % in the conventional collective and 91.7 % in the laser collective.

The total Lysholm score increased significantly in both collectives (laser $P < 0.03$; conventional $P < 0.02$) over the initial scores (Fig. 9). A comparison of the Lysholm score of both collectives showed no significant preoperative difference. After 6 weeks, only the score for pain was significantly improved in the laser collective ($P < 0.001$).

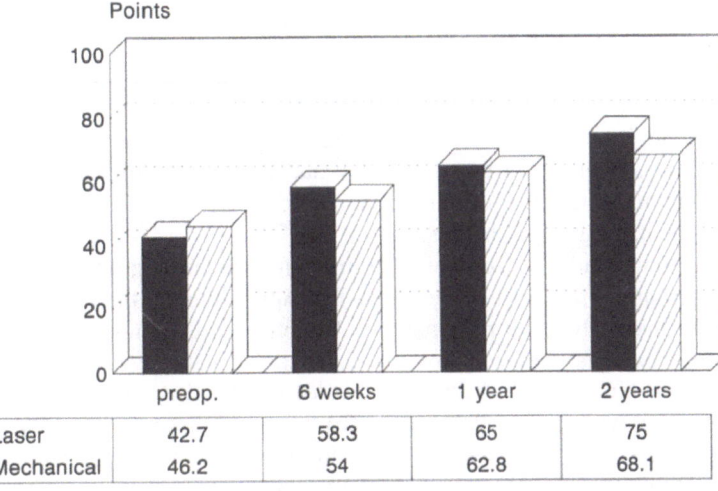

	preop.	6 weeks	1 year	2 years
Laser	42.7	58.3	65	75
Mechanical	46.2	54	62.8	68.1

■ Laser ▨ Mechanical

Fig. 9. Lateral release/Modified Lysholm score

Discussion

The patient's status was stringently and prospectively registered during a 2-year period. For documentation, standard questionnaires were adapted and combined with crucial questions that pertain specifically to laser medicine [11, 13, 16].

Altogether 320 patients were pre- and postoperatively registered and can be considered a homogenous collective. By distributing the patients into five different groups of knee disorders according to strict inclusion criteria, direct comparison became possible. The comparability of these groups was confirmed by the similarity of the preoperative modified Lysholm score in all groups.

Observations that arthroscopic laser therapy is a lengthy procedure because of the low capacity of the available laser systems could not be confirmed by this study [25]. Other publications report that through routine laser use, operating times are only slightly prologed [1, 7. 8. 27, 29]. In this study, laser surgery times were hardly longer and even shorter for laser treatment of combined lesions. This is due to the high ablation rate and the flexibility of the holmium:YAG laser. Only one application instrument is used, and it remains in the joint during the total duration of surgery. A change-over of instruments is unnecessary.

A major advantage to using a holmium:YAG laser system for arthroscopic procedures is its excellent hemostatic ability. The need for a tourniquet is drastically reduced in comparison with conventional surgery. Total postoperative blood loss (Redon drainage) was significantly reduced in laser patients of the three disorder groups. Furthermore, due to the holmium:YAG laser's ability to coagulate blood directly, visibility is highly improved. This is advantageous especially for those surgical procedures, such as synovectomy and lateral release, during which higly vascularized tissues are treated. This positive effect was also confirmed by analysis of the need for postoperative puncture and the occurrence of effusions. No puncturing was necessary in any laser patient during hospitalization, whereas it was done in many conventionally treated patients. Comparison of the follow-up values for puncture rate showed an increasing similarity between the conventional and laser collective for meniscectomy and combined lesions. In all other disorder groups, the puncture rate for the laser patients was markedly lower than for conventionally treated patients. Furthermore, within the follow-up period, no puncturing was necessary in any laser patient of the synovectomy and the lateral release groups. These results show that, when used correctly, the holmium:YAG laser is a moderate and subtle instrument for arthroscopic surgery, with several advantages over conventional methods.

Analysis of the patients' need for pain-relieving medication showed that during hospitalization, the laser patients of all groups needed fewer analgesics and antiphlogistics than the conventionally treated patients. Also during the follow-up period, laser patients took less medication and often only sporadically when needed. These results confirm that laser-assisted arthroscopy is a less traumatic procedure, from which patients recuperate more quickly.

Alongside the general and subjective evaluation, objective and standardized analysis of the surgery results was procured by using the Lysholm score as modified by Klein. Evaluation in the meniscal lesion group showed a highly significant postoperative increase in the scores for both the laser and the conventional collectives ($P < 0.0002$ and $P < 0.0004$, respectively). Comparison of the postoperative scores of both collectives showed no difference.

Keeping this and the other results for the meniscal lesion group in mind, it can be concluded that the laser offers no advantage over conventional methods for procedures during which only meniscal tissues are removed.

Evaluation of the postoperative Lysholm score in the chondromalacia group revealed no significant increase in the conventional collective. On the other hand, the increase in the total postoperative score in the laser collective is highly significant ($P < 0.004$). Comparison between the two collectives shows a significant difference for several, but not all, parameters.

These results conform to the few clinical studies on cartilaginous laser application [2, 4, 7, 15, 22, 29]. On the other hand, there are several experimental studies with contradictory results [7, 9, 18, 20, 23, 28, 32]. Because the laser was applied very carefully and tangentially in an unfocused system in this study, unlike in some experimental studies with negative results, comparison is not possible.

Based on the results of this study, laser systems can be recommended for treatment of chondromalacia. The rapid progression of cartilage destruction can be temporarily halted, but unfortunately due to the characteristics of this disease, the effect may not be permanent.

The results of the combined lesion group give support to the above findings. Although the increase in the postoperative Lysholm score is moderately significant for the conventional collective, it is highly significant for the laser collective ($P < 0.01$ and $P < 0.001$, respectively). Furthermore, the score for the laser collective in total ($P < 0.02$) and for several parameters is significantly improved in comparison with the conventional collective.

Keeping the findings of the meniscal lesion and chondromalacia groups in mind, it can be summarized that the score improvement in the conventional collective is due to the successful treatment of the meniscal lesion with mechanical methods. On the other hand, the total score in the conventional collective lags behind the laser collective, due to the inferiority of the conventional therapy for chondromalacia.

Further proof can be found in the evaluation of the third collective, in which the meniscal lesion, but not the chondromalacia, was treated conventionally. The postoperative score was significantly improved in comparison with the initial score ($P < 0.03$). Furthermore, the Lysholm score for several parameters in the isolated meniscectomy collective is significantly better than in the combined conventional collective and only slightly worse than in the laser collective. After 2 years, the Lysholm score in the isolated meniscectomy group decreased by 5.7 points, which may indicate that only short-term improvement can be achieved in comparison with conventional treatment. Furthermore, the grade of chondromalacia was even lower in the isolated meniscectomy collective than in the laser or combined conventional collective, which could lead to better results. On the other hand, the initial Lysholm scores were not significantly different.

The most apparent difference in results was found in the rheumatoid arthritis group. The postoperative score of the conventional collective did not increase significantly at any time, whereas the postoperative score in the laser collective was highly significant, not only in comparison with the initial score ($P < 0.001$) but also in comparison with the conventional collective ($P < 0.003$). The results did not change over the 2-year follow-up period and can be considered a long-term effect. These observations also agree with other studies on clinical laser application [8, 20, 29]. One reason for this very promising effect on rheumatoid synovialitis could be the influence of the laser on the deeper lying stratum subsynoviale, an effect which cannot be produced by conventional shaver synovectomy. Furthermore, laser treatment may cause an unknown effect that restores the synovia and/or delays the continuation of the disease.

The postoperative scores in the group of patellofemoral pain syndrome, in which patellar lateralization was treated with lateral release, were significant in both the conventional ($P < 0.02$) and the laser collective ($P < 0.003$) in comparison with the initial scores. The comparison between both groups shows better results for the laser collective, which are statistically significant only for the 6-week follow-up score. Due to the different surgical techniques of the lateral release procedure, direct comparison is not possible. The concern that uncontrolled postoperative bleeding can occur with formation of a hemarthrosis that could lead to open surgery is unfounded.

A further effect caused by the holmium:YAG laser at low energy settings (10 W), which can improve lateral retinacular release is tissue shrinking. This effect, which has been developed and improved upon in the last few years, causes collagenic tissue in the medial retinaculum and medial capsule to contract, enabling the patella to return to a more central position. This concept is already being used for elongation of the anterior cruciate ligament and for laser-assisted capsular shift (LACS) operations in the shoulder.

No notable complications, especially necrosis, occurred during laser surgery in this study. We presume this is due to the careful, but efficient surgical method. On the other hand, the occurrence of significant iatrogenic cartilage damage, especially in smaller joints, was observed a few times in the conventional group, although these operations were conducted by expert surgeons.

Unfortunately, the equipment for laser surgery is still more expensive than for established conventional methods. Through increased clinical use and budgetary measures, a decrease in cost is certainly possible.

In our opinion, the advantage of laser instruments lies in the effective combination with mechanical instruments and in the possibility to treat small and/or hard-to-reach joints (shoulder, elbow, hand). The laser seems to be advantageous for the treatment of chondromalacia. Up to now only limited therapeutic possibilities – in part offering only uncertain success – were available for treatment of this disease (conservative therapy, chondroprotectiva, conventional arthroscopy, osteotomy). Younger patients especially benefit through laser-assisted joint stabilizing procedures in the lateral release procedure.

The results of this study are based upon a rather small and varied collective. Further studies of single diseases are necessary to gather more information on the effectivity of lasers in arthroscopy. Although more improvements of the laser instruments themselves can be expected, the holmium:YAG laser is already an excellent tool for arthroscopic surgery. As with any other surgical instrument, it is imperative to use laser systems correctly and with care. Sufficient education and training with experienced surgeons and education centers is absolutely mandatory. Unqualified clinical use of laser systems is inappropriate and must be prevented. Only qualified surgeons will be able to exploit the beneficial effects of laser systems.

References

[1] Bickerstaff R, Wyman A, Laining R, Smith T (1991) Partial meniscectomy using the Neodym:YAG laser. An in vitro study. Arthroscopy 7:63–67

[2] Brillhart A (1991) Arthroscopic laser surgery. Am J Arthrosc 1:5–12

[3] DeLee J (1985) Complications of arthroscopy and arthroscopic surgery: results of a national survey. Arthroscopy 1:214–220

[4] Dillingham M, Fanton G (1990) The use of the Holmium:YAG-laser in operative knee arthroscopy – a double blind prospective study using a new arthroscopically guided laser system. Arthroscopy 6:152–153

[5] Glick J (1984) Use of the laser beam in arthroscopic surgery. In: Casscells S (ed) Arthroscopic diagnostic and surgical practice. Lea & Febiger, Philadelphia, pp 181–183

[6] Glinz W (1989) Die 'verschwiegenen' Schäden bei der Arthroskopie. In: Contzen H (ed) Komplikationen bei der Arthroskopie. Enke, Stuttgart, pp 14–21

[7] Grifka J (1993) Arthroskopische Therapie der Gonarthrose in Abhängigkeit vom Grad der Chondromalazie. Arthroskopie 6:201–211

[8] Grifka J, Schreiner C, Löhnert J (1994) Frühergebnisse der Nd:YAG-Laser-Synovektomie bei detritusinduzierten Synovialitiden. Arthroskopie 7:154–157

[9] Hohlbach G, Müller K, Schramm U, Baretton G (1989) Experimentelle Ergebnisse der Knorpelabrasion mit dem Excimer-Laser. Histologische und elektronen-mikroskopische Untersuchungen. Z Orthop 127:216–222

[10] Imich H (1974) Medizinische Statistik. Schattauer, Stuttgart

[11] Klein W (1988) Die maschinelle arthroskopische Chirurgie der Gonarthrose. Indikation, Technik, Nachuntersuchungsergebnisse. Arthroskopie 1:109–115

[12] Klein W, Kurze V (1986) Arthroscopic arthropathy: iatrogenic arthroscopic joint lesions in animals. Arthroscopy 2:163–168

[13] Krämer K, Maichl F (1993) Scores, Bewertungsschema und Klassifikationen in der Orthopädie und der Traumatologie. Thieme, Stuttgart

[14] Kroitzsch U, Laufer G, Egkher E, Wollenek G, Horvath R (1989) Experimental photoablation of meniscus cartilage by excimer laser energy. A new aspect in meniscus surgery. Arch Orthop Trauma Surg 108:44–48

[15] Lane G, Mooar P (1991) Holmium:YAG laser arthroscopic debridement. Lasers Surg Med O [Suppl 3]:53

[16] Lysholm J, Gillquist J (1982) Evaluation of knee ligament surgery results with special emphasis on use of a scoring scale. Am J Sports Med 10:150–154

[17] Miller D, O'Brien S, Amoczyky S, Kelly A, Fealy S, Warren R (1989) The use of the contact Nd:YAG laser in arthroscopic surgery: effects on articular cartilage and meniscal tissue. Arthroscopy 5:245–253

[18] Müller K, Lind B, Karcher K, Hohlbach G (1994) Holmium laser versus mechanische Knorpelabtragung. Vergleichende Untersuchung am Arthrosemodell bei Kaninchen. Langenbecks Arch Chir 379:84–94

[19] Philandrianos G (1985) Le laser à gaz carbonique en chirurgie arthroscopique du genou. Presse Med 14:2103–2104

[20] Puhl W (1994) Experimentelle Untersuchungen zur fraglichen Schädigung des Gelenkknorpels durch Laser-Abrasions-Arthroplastiken. Orthop Mitt 3:120–122

[21] Raunest J, Löhnert J (1989) Arthroskopische Synovektomie unter Anwendung des Neodym:YAG-Laser. Chirurg 60:782–787

[22] Raunest J, Löhnert J (1990) Arthroscopic cartilage debridement by excimer laser in chondromalacia of the knee joint. Arch Orthop Trauma Surg 109:155–159

[23] Raunest J, Sager M, Derra E (1994) Experimentelle Befunde zur Knorpelablation und Abrasionsarthroplastik mit thermisch und gepulsten UV-Lasern. Arthroskopie 7:174–181

[24] Schnid A, Schmid F, Tiling T (1988) Elektron microscopic findings after cartilage shaving. In: Müller W, Hackenbruch W (eds) Surgery and arthroscopy of the knee. Springer, Berlin Heidelberg New York, pp 426–432

[25] Schreiner C (1994) Laser in der Arthroskopie. Arthroskopie 7:148–153

[26] Schultz R, Krishnamurthy S, Thelmo W, Rodriguez J, Harvey G (1985) Effects of varying intensities of laser energy on articular cartilage. A preliminary study. Lasers Surg Med 5:577

[27] Siebert W (1992) Laseranwendung in der Orthopädie. Orthopäde 21:273–288

[28] Siebert W, Kohn D, Klanke J, Wirth C, Scholz C, Müller G (1990) Rasterelektronenmikroskopische Untersuchungen zur Oberflächenbearbeitung von Knorpelschäden mit dem Neodym-YAG-Laser, dem CO_2-Laser, dem Excimer-Laser, dem Erbium-Laser, dem Holmium-YSSG-Laser und diversen motorgetriebenen Instrumenten. In: Glinz W, Kieser C, Munzinger U (eds) Arthroskopie bei Knorpelschäden und bei Arthrose. Enke, Stuttgart, pp 82–91

[29] Siebert W, Saunier J, Gerber B, Lübbers C (1994) Ho:YAG-Laser in der arthroskopischen Chirurgie des Kniegelenkes. Arthroskopie 7:182–192

[30] Small N (1986) Complications in arthroscopy: the knee and other joints. Committee on Complications of the Arthroscopy Association of North America. Arthroscopy 2:253–258

[31] Smith C, Marschall G, Snyder S (1984) Comparisons of tissue effects of surgical scalpel, an electrocautery apparatus, and a carbon dioxide laser system when used for making incisions into the menisci of New Zealand rabbits. Lasers Surg Med 3:305

[32] Trauner K, Nishioka N, Patel D (1990) Pulsed holmium-yttrium-aluminium-garner (Ho:YAG) laser ablation of fibrocartilage and articular cartilage. Am J Sports Med 18:316–320

[33] Whipple T, Caspari R, Meyers J (1982) Arthroscopic meniscectomy by carbon dioxide laser vaporization in a gas medium. 29th annual meeting of the Piedmont Orthopaedic Society, Sea Island, Ga., USA, 6–10 May. Orthop Trans 6:136

Use of Holmium Laser in Patellofemoral Instability

P. GUILLEN-GARCIA

Introduction

The procedure known as capsular retractile surgery (CRS) is a potentially useful alternative to the various techniques used today to correct joint instability, particularly glenohumeral, and also patellofemoral instability (PFI).

Four years ago we noticed [1] together with Fanton and Dullingahn, that capsular tissue of the shoulder shrinks with holmium laser at low wattage (10–14 W). The CRS technique is performed under arthroscopy, so that shrinkage of the capsular tissue can be confirmed by direct arthroscopic visualization. Histologic studies have confirmed shortening of the collagen fibers, provided that 60 °C (corresponding to 16 W) is not exceeded.

When satisfactory results of CRS in shoulders were documented in 1993, we first started to use this technique in PFI using an arthroscopic approach [2]. Young patients with clinical signs clearly indicating PFI, X-ray studies, and CT scans in relaxation and co-traction of the quadriceps supporting the diagnosis, were selected after other meniscal, ligamentous, or inflammatory conditions had been ruled out and conservative management based on cold, nonsteroidal anti-inflammatory drugs, rest, and physical therapy had failed.

This contribution reports 35 cases of PFI treated with this technique with a 40-month follow-up; this follow-up period is probably insufficient and monitoring will continue. Only one relapse has occurred so far, with a Q angle $> 20°$. A histological study of synovial membrane treated with laser at 10, 12, 20, and 35 W is also reported.

Arthroscopic Technique

Arthroscopy is done via usual portals. We prefer only two portals, the external and the internal infrapatellar and, after documenting PFI by direct arthroscopic visualization (Fig. 1), the laser handle is inserted medially and the whole external flap sectioned at 20–35 W (this cuts, destroys, and coagulates the area) (Fig. 2). The patella thus becomes loose laterally or externally and is more easily displaced medially. Then the lens is moved medially, the laser laterally, and the handle laced perpendicular to the medial capsular or flap. A 10- to 12-W mark is then made and shots are applied to the medial capsule. The capsule shrinks, becomes rigid and whitish, and the patella is displaced medially (Fig. 3).

If the patient shows any other condition, it is resolved if possible during the same surgical procedure, particularly the patellar cartilage at 14–16 W only. A soft bandage is applied with ambulation. Physical therapy occurs at 15 days and the patient may return to sport after 3 months.

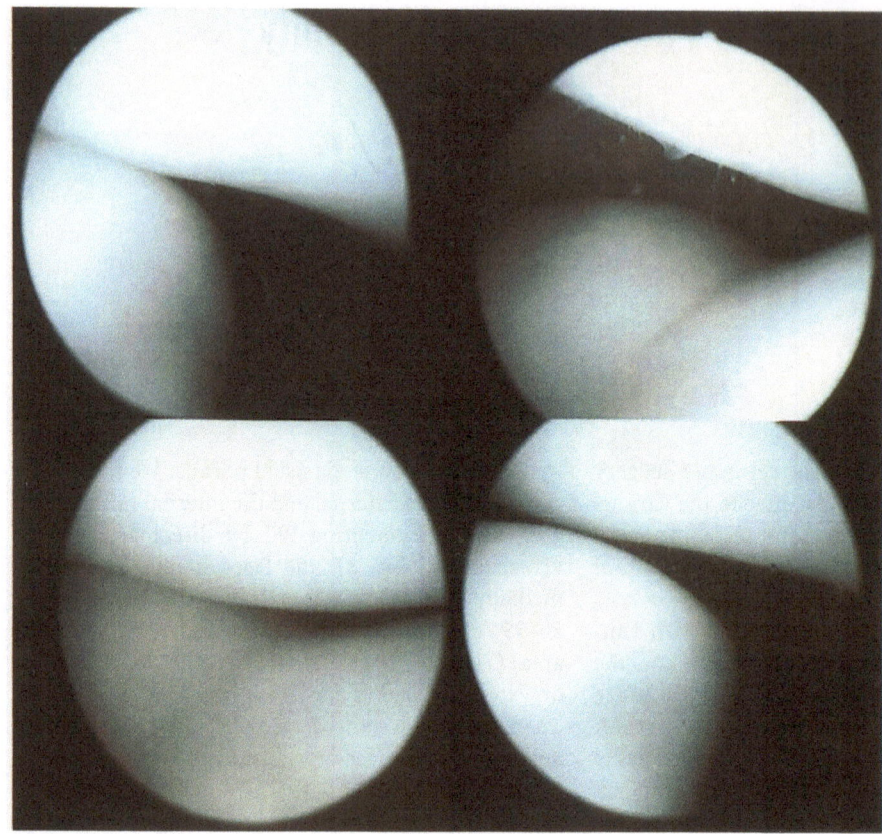

Fig. 1. Patellar subdislocation shown in knee flexion-extension under arthroscopy

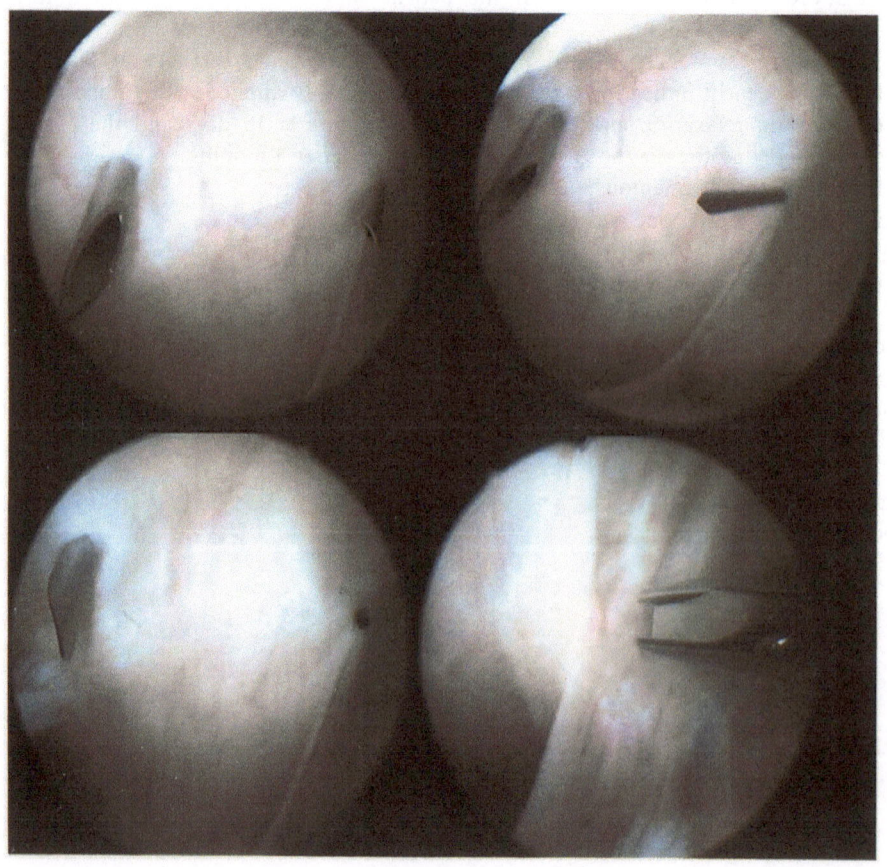

Fig. 2. With percutaneous needles, the lateral capsule is perforated, thus delimiting the area of the lateral flap to be sectioned with laser

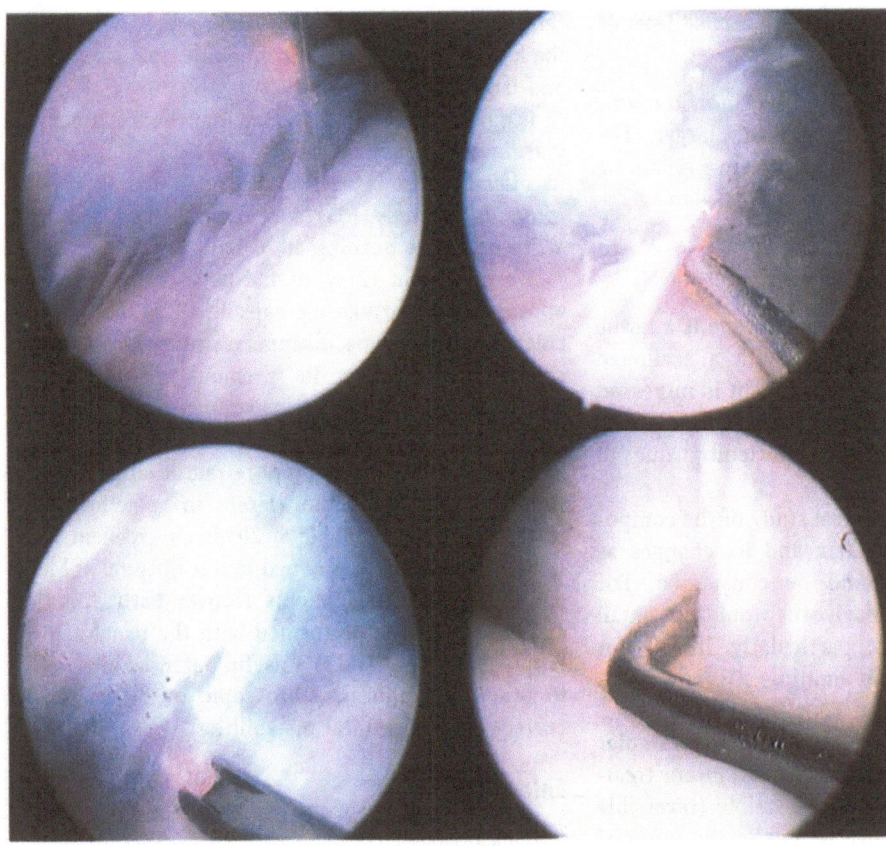

Fig. 3. Shrinkage surgery of the medial capsule of the knee by arthroscopy with 10 W

Patients

We have operated on 35 patients for PFI using a Holmium laser 2.1, with 2.5 years follow-up in all cases. We already have 31 additional patients, but the follow-up is shorter in these cases. Of the 35, 29 are male and 6 are female. Nineteen were school children and sixteen were athletes at the time of injury. They were young, with normally aligned or somewhat valgus knees ($Q < 15°$) and minimum recurvatum. In 21 patients the right knee was affected and in 14 patients the left. Eight patients were aged 12 years, five were 13, three were 14, five were 17, eight were 18, five were 22, and one was 23 years old. The last was the one who relapsed; he had undergone lateral meniscus arthroscopy previously and had a Q angle $> 20°$. In all subjects, conservative therapy had failed, and they had suffered at least three patellar subluxations.

Histological Study

We have left for the end the histological study performed by Dr. A López Bravo, which we detail due to its interest and because we think that it opens up new ways for the application of laser.

The area sectioned in the lateral flap was delimited by needles placed in the capsule from outside, thus ensuring that the area is adequately relaxed. We also placed two needles in the medial capsule, accurately defining the area to be shrunk.

Medial Capsular Membrane Treated with Holmium Laser AT 10 W

The vessels appear stained blue, which is due not to the nuclei, but to the ground substance. This corresponds to perivascular "mucoid" edema, with blue-staining features due to changes in the biochemical features of the mucopolysaccharides of the ground substance. Nothing else of interest is seen.

Medial Capsular Membrane Treated with Holmium Laser AT 12 W

Perivascular edema persists, but areas of a much more vivid, intense orange color and with no fibrillar appearance are seen. They suggest that "there was a previous drawing which was slightly erased". This is a thermal focal lesion, which appears to be scattered in the specimen. Small scars are seen.

Medial Capsular Membrane Treated with Holmium Laser AT 20–35 W

A complete thermal lesion is seen; the previous isolated lesions (thermal) are now much larger. The structure has been lost almost completely. Everything corresponds to a large scar from thermal damage.

Conclusions

We thought that if the synovial membrane is a tissue more or less "creased" (at least with a scalloped "epithelia" edge), if the fluid component is increased through the edema caused by the laser technique, the first observation would be a shortening due to "uncreasing of the scallop".

We think that a histochemical study of the components of the connective matrix and its changes as compared to controls should be considered. For instance, the study of proteoglycans would not entail many technical problems, particularly if kits for staining with alcian blue at multiple pHs are available.

It would seem that the edge in the perivascular edema corresponding to the synovial membrane treated with 10 W would always be reversible (reversible *ad integrum*). The focal burn lesions in the synovial membrane treated at 12 W, would probably be reversible leaving a collagen scar which after all is a component of the synovium and is, therefore, morphologically reversible *ad integrum*; that is, synovial edema with functional scars permitting a permanent retraction. Finally, in the capsule treated at 20–35 W, the lesions are very significant, with extensive burns, and irreversible.

It must therefore be inferred that there is a narrow margin for applying laser (10-12-20 W), ranging in effects from perivascular edema (reversible *ad integrum*) at only 10 W, to edema plus scar at 12 W, to extensive burning at 20 W.

We think that 12 W should be used for a scar to appear which shrinks the capsule when the perivascular mucoid edema disappears, since at 10 W the capsule will recover its previous length in 2–4 weeks. Of course, the extensive burn leaves no scar, but dead tissue.

We will end by noting that retractile surgery of the capsule with holmium laser in patellofemoral instability with a Q angle < 20° is an excellent technique that we have developed in our hospital at Majadahonda (Madrid). Patients recover early function and mobility. It is performed with the usual arthroscopic techniques and is a useful potential alternative to other techniques, arthroscopic or otherwise, to correct patellofermoral instabilities.

References

[1] Guillen-Garcia P (1994) 2.1 μm holmium:YAG arthroscopic laser partial meniscectomy in Athletes: 100 cases. Arhtorcopic Laser surgery. Clinical Applications. Brillhart AT (ed), Springer-Verlag
[2] Guillen-Garcia P (1996) Use of holmium laser in patellofemoral instability. SICOT 96 Amsterdam, poster 447

Laser Abrasion Multiple Puncturing (LAMP) in Osteoarthritis of the Knee

Kwon-Ick Ha · Seung-Ho Kim

Introduction

Since the beginning of the era of arthroscopy in orthopaedics when the efficacy of operative arthroscopy was acclaimed by many great surgeons, laser has been a subject of continuous debate, although it has been increasingly used by many orthopaedic surgeons around the world. As laser equipment evolves and laser surgical techniques continue to develop, the number of laser operations in this field will grow continuously.

Treatment for osteoarthritis of the knee joint has long been a challenging task for orthopaedic surgeons. Especially, sclerotic lesions on the femoral or tibial articular surface have been the focus of many surgical and experimental trials. Historically, many surgical attempts have been made on the sclerotic lesions seen in degenerative arthritis.

The conventional open surgery treatments for degenerative knee joint disease include debridement procedures. The Magnusson "house-cleaning" arthroplasty consisted of synovectomy, meniscectomy, articular shaving, sometimes condylar drilling, and osteophyte resection [10]. Pridie and Insall reported on the effects of joint surface resection into cancellous bone for articular lesions [6, 7, 12]. The exposure of cancellous bone is referred to as "spongialization", named by Ficat after the exposed spongy bone. Abrasion arthroplasty of grade IV eburnated chondral lesions using motorized instrumentation was introduced by Johnson in 1981 [8, 9]. He stated that the abrasions should extend only 1 or 2 mm into the adjacent degenerative cartilage to provide subsequent biological adherence to solid tissues. The effect of condylar drilling and abrasion arthroplasty is that pluripotent cells from the marrow or intracortical vessels can give rise to chondrocytes, which in turn lay down the cartilage matrix to form fibrocartilage on sclerotic lesions. But the arthroscopic technique of multiple drilling has some limitations. It is sometimes difficult to do the drilling on the round condylar surface using drills or Steinmann pins. Abrasion arthroplasty also has technical drawbacks: control of the abrasion depth is not easy, and because of the obliquity of both the tibial and the femoral condyle, the use of motorized instruments is not feasible. Laser is an alternative tool for condylar drilling and abrasion arthroplasty.

Choice of Laser

Laser has been thought of as a precise nontraumatic light-beam scalpel that can be delivered arthroscopically into the tight recess of the knee joint, in which no instrument has been able to avoid inadvertent articular cartilage damage. There are a few different types of lasers which were once used in the orthopaedic field.

The carbon dioxide (CO_2) laser came into use in the early 1980s. Because it is highly absorbable by water and cannot be transmitted through standard fiberoptic glass fibers, CO_2 laser is no longer used in arthroscopic surgery. The next enthusiasm was the noncontact neodymium:yttrium-aluminum-garnet (Nd:YAG) laser. This has in turn fallen out of favour because ablation depth cannot be controlled precisely and diffusion of the heat produced by the continuous wave irradiation produces unacceptable zones of damage. Similarly, visible wavelength lasers, such as argon ion and frequency-doubled Nd:YAG laser, require pigmented chromophores for absorption and do not allow effective resection of less pigmented joint tissues.

Recently, a pulsed near-infrared laser based on the rare earth element holmium has been developed which operates at a wavelength of 2.1 μm. Its output can be transmitted through readily available quartz fibres and it may be used in a saline environment. Because water is the absorbing medium, it always produces the same effect independent of tissue pigmentation or type. In addition, the Ho:YAG is truly a pulsed laser. Each energy pulse acts independently, and the cooling effect between pulses in a fluid medium greatly limits the possible tissue damage.

Pulsed delivery of laser energy has been definitively shown to reduce laser-induced tissue injury. Each tissue pulse removes a constant amount of tissue, providing the greatest control of ablative power and depth of penetration with minimum damage to the adjacent tissue. This allows delivery of high energy levels without carbonization.

Basic Concepts

The concept of drilling through eburnated bone to stimulate reparative cartilage formation was originally described by Pridie in 1959 [12]. He recommended a more systematic approach to joint debridement in which the extent of the surgical procedure was based on the arthrotomy findings. He described fibrous-like reparative cartilage filling and covering one-quarter-inch cortical drill holes through the femoral condyle.

Laboratory animal studies were performed in an attempt to confirm Pridie's findings. In a study of rabbit knee joints, Mitchell and Shepherd found that small multiple drill holes made in the subchondral bone stimulated repair from large areas of the articular surface [11]. They found that repair tissue grew from the drill holes and spread over the exposed bone. Initially, large areas of repair tissue that had the appearance of hyaline cartilage began to **fibrillate** and deleriorate within 1 year. These experiments were the first to show abrasion or perforation with fibrous cartilaginous tissue. Excessive loading, however, inhibited or prevented cartilage repair and repair tissue lacked the proteoglycan concentration found in normal cartilage.

Abrasion arthroplasty of grade IV eburnated chondral lesions using motorized instrumentation was introduced by Johnson in 1981 [8]. This procedure is essentially an extension of the Pridie procedure with the exception that in abrasion arthroplasty, a superficial subchondral bone, approximately 1–3 mm thick, is also removed to expose interosseous vessels. Theoretically, the resulting hemorrhage exudate forms a fibrin clot and allows the formation of fibrous repair tissue over the eburnated bone. This immature repair tissue should be protected from excessive loading after the procedure for a minimum of 6–8 weeks. There has been disagreement as to the drill depth and whether debridement of the sclerotic lesion should be intracortical or cancellous. This is concluded from the work of Hjertquist and Lemberg, who reported that cartilage tissue of mature appearance develops only if debridement is superficial enough to maintain a cortex [5].

Abrasion of relatively large areas of the femoral condyle and tibial plateau in osteoarthritic knees in humans has resulted in the formation of fibrocartilage repair tissue. In some patients, this fibrocartilaginous tissue lasts up to 4 years. In Johnson's series, collagen typing was performed and in only one case out of eight did biopsy specimens show any type II

collagen typical of hyaline cartilage. In this particular case, small samples were taken and the specimen "could have included hyaline cartilage at biopsy junctions". All other specimens had type I and III collagen, which are dissimilar to the collagen found in normal hyaline articular cartilage.

It is generally agreed that in an embryo the mesenchymal stem cell is a pluripotent progenitor cell which divides many times and whose progeny eventually give rise to skeletal tissues: cartilage, bone, tendon, ligament, marrow stroma, and connective tissue. Effective methods of repairing significant cartilage defects must provide cells that can migrate, proliferate, and differentiate in the chondral sites and produce and maintain a cartilage matrix. Furthermore, a mechanical and biologic environment that promotes synthesis, assembly, and maintenance of articular cartilage matrix must exist.

Because adult articular cartilage does not heal and the regenerative tissue is a fibrocartilage, not a hyaline cartilage, it lacks normal amounts of proteoglycan. Therefore, this regenerative fibroartilage theoretically should have a difficult time transferring compressive loads and cannot be expected to survive in an abnormal mechanical environment. Experimental evidence has emphasized the necessity of full-thickness condylar perforation into cancellous bone as a means of stimulating tissue response.

Equipment and Laser Setup

Standard equipment for arthroscopic surgery of the knee joint necessary for the laser abrasion multiple puncturing (LAMP) operation includes a 3.5-mm arthroscope, video camera, light source, and arthroscopic instruments. Currently, holmium:YAG laser is widely used for arthroscopic surgery and the most current version of the holmium:YAG laser has a laser console, a touchscreen control panel, a footswitch, and a fiberoptic delivery system. The laser energy setting for LAMP operation is very important to minimize inadvertent side effects of laser which include thermal necrosis of the bone, iatrogenic injury of articular cartilage and meniscal tissue, and possible avascular necrosis.

Experimental study for thermal necrosis of human bone is limited up to 250 µm in our study regardless of the laser energy level. Currently, it is unclear whether holmium:YAG laser can produce avascular necrosis of the femoral or tibial condyle. Average power for laser abrasion is 5–10 W for the femoral condyle and 10–15 W for the tibial condyle.

Operative Technique

All operative procedures were done with the patient in the supine position with or without tourniquet. The Infra Tome, a laser handpiece (1.7 mm in tip diameter), was introduced through the standard anterior arthroscopic portals. Usually straight, 30° curved and 70° side-firing handpieces were used. After appropriate debridement procedures such as partial meniscectomy, chondroplasty, synovectomy, and osteophyte removal as indicated, the laser handpiece was held closely on the sclerotic lesion. The average laser power was approximately set to minimum abrasion (ablation) possible (MAP), which is usually 5 W. The laser handpiece was swept slowly over the lesion, moving it back and forth. Superficial necrotic cortical bone was sculpted to a thickness of 1-2 mm and intracortical vessels were exposed.

After completion of cortical abrasion, the inflow system was turned off and the outflow opened to reduce intra-articular pressure. Streaming of blood from the abrasion area was noted. Sometimes the tourniquet was needed to be released to facilitate confirmation of bleeding. In poorly bleeding areas, multiple puncturing was performed by laser until satisfactory bleeding from the puncture holes was achieved.

Postoperatively, patients were instructed to use crutches with toe-touch weight bearing on the operated leg for 6 weeks. During that time, they were encouraged to do stationary bicycle exercises.

Clinical Experience

LAMP was performed on a total of 127 condyles with grade IV sclerotic lesions in 87 osteoarthritic knees in the period from November, 1994, to October, 1995. Average patient age was 58 years (range: 51–67 years). Holmium:YAG laser (VersaPulse Select, 60 W, Coherent Co., USA) with a small handpiece (Infra Tome, 1.7 mm tip diameter) was used. Average power for laser abrasion was 5–10 W (energy per pulse: 0.5–1.0 J, pulse repetition rate: 10 Hz) for the femoral condyle and 10–15 W (energy per pulse: 1.0–1.5 J, pluse repetition rate: 10 Hz) for the tibial condyle. The average power for laser multiple puncturing varied from 10 W to 25 W depending on the severity of sclerosis of the condyle.

Case Report

A 58-year-old woman had chronic pain in her right knee. She denied having had any major trauma or previous operation on the knee. Physical examination revealed moderate swelling of the right knee with patellar floating, which implied knee joint effusion. There was no instability of the knee. Range of motion of the right knee was normal, but it became painful during the end of knee flexion. Longitudinal alignment of the knee was within the normal range of values. Plain roentgenogram revealed mild joint space narrowing in the medial compartment on the Rosenberg view. Multiple osteophytes were seen at the margin of the medial tibial condyle. A LAMP operation was performed on her and a grade IV chondral lesion was noted on the inferior surface of the medial femoral condyle and posteromedial corner of the medial tibial condylar surface (Figs. 1–3).

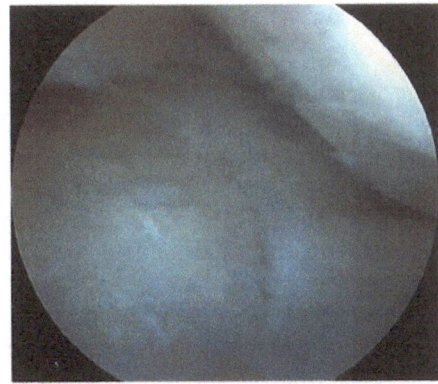

Fig. 1. Grade IV chondromalacia on the medial tibial condyle

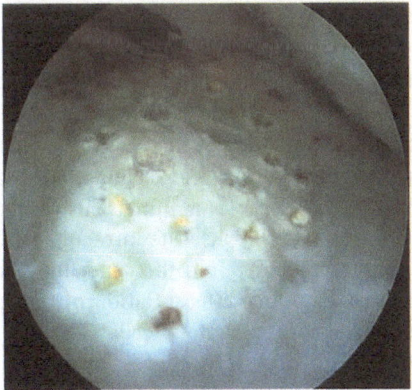

Fig. 2. Laser abrasion multiple puncturing (LAMP) procedure on the medial tibial condyle

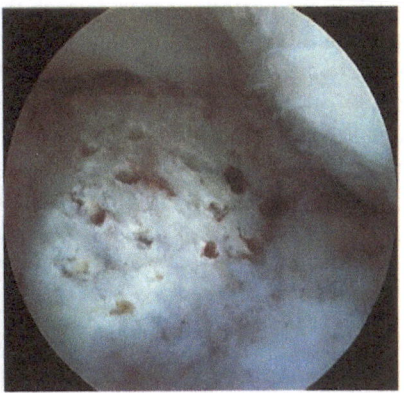

Fig. 3. Bleeding from the LAMP area

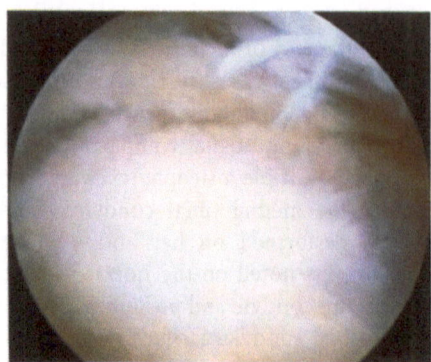

Fig. 4. Fibrocartilage resurfacing on the LAMP area

After the operation, she was allowed partial weight bearing with crutches for 6 weekks. During that period she did regular stationary bicycle exercise. Six months after the operation, she returned to our clinic and said that she was feeling better than before the operation. She permitted a second-look arthroscopy of the right knee when she had a LAMP operation of the contralateral knee and it revealed uniform covering of regenerated articular cartilage on the medial femoral and tibial condylar surface (Fig. 4). A biopsy demonstated fibrocartilagenous tissue.

Discussion

In the many attempts to stimulate fibrocartilaginous growth in the area of sclerotic lessions (grade IV chondromalacia) in osteoarthritis of the knee, two of the most frequently used procedures are abrasion arthroplasty and multiple drilling. The rationale of cortical abrasion is to expose the intracortical vessels and the drilling of holes into the cancellous bone to cause proliferation and differentiation of pluripotential cells into fibrocartilaginous cells.

However, both these procedures have some technical drawbacks. Arthroscopic surgical exposure does not facilitate a proper angle to drill a hole in the posterior area of the condyles: the obliquity of the approach to the posterior aspect is such that cortical perforation is not technically possible. Frequently, a Steinmann pin or drill bit slips and slides on the round surface of the sclerotic condyle. With abrasion arthroplasty, introduced by Lanny L. Johnson, there are also difficulties in controlling the depth of cortical abrasion, and frequently the motorized burr cannot reach the posterior area in the tight medial compartment of the knee joint without scuffing the condyle.

In our new technique, very low profile tips (1.7 mm in diameter) can easily reach the tight posterior aspect of the knee joint without injuring the normal structure. Due to the coherence, a unique characteristic of laser, the beam can be focused over only the lesion area, which in turn protects the normal tissue, such as meniscus and healthy articular cartilage, from the iatrogenic injury that can occur during abrasion arthroplasty and multiple drilling using conventional instruments. Surgical time is significantly reduced by this LAMP operation; less than 1 min is required for a lesion 1 cm in diameter. The energy setting for the LAMP procedure should start from the minimum abrasion possible (MAP) range to avoid possible osteonecrosis and thermal damage of the condyle.

Although the benefits of the LAMP procedure still need to be proven, this is a new, simple, and easy technique which can be performed on sclerotic lesions of the osteoarthritic knee joints.

References

[1] Bert J (1993) Role of abrasion arthroplasty and debridement in the management of osteoarthritis of the knee. Orthopaedics 19:725–739
[2] Caplan A (1991) Mesenchymal stem cells. J Orthop Res 9:641–650
[3] Dillingham M, Price J, Fanton G (1993) Lasers in orthopedic surgery: holmium laser surgery. Orthopaedics 5: 563–566
[4] Fanton G, Dillingham M (1992) The use of the holmium laser in arthroscopic surgery. Semin Orthop 7:102–116
[5] Hjertquist S, Lemberg R (1971) Histologic audiographic and micro-chemical studies with spontaneously healing osteochondral articular defects in adult rabbits. Calcium Tissue Res 8:5
[6] Insall J (1967) Intraarticular surgery for degenerative arthritis of the knee: a report of the work of the late K. H. Pridie. J Bone Joint Surg Br 49B:211
[7] Insall J (1974) The Pridie debridement operation for osteoarthritis of the knee. Clin Orthop 101:61–67
[8] Johnson L (1981) Diagnostic and operative arthroscopy of the knee and other joints. Mosby, St Louis
[9] Johnson L (1986) Arthroscopic abrasion arthroplasty: historical and phatological perspective, present status. Arthroscopy 2:54–69
[10] Magnuson P (1941) Joint debridement: a surgical treatment of degenerative arthritis. Surg Gynecol Obstet 73:1–9
[11] Mitchell N, Shepard N (1976) Resurfacing of adult rabbit articular cartilage by multiple perforations of the subchondral bone. J Bone Joint Surg Am 58:230
[12] Pridie K (1959) A method of resurfacing osteoarthritic knee joints. J Bone Joint Surg Br 41B:618
[13] Reed E, Abbott S (1994) Arthroscopic laser surgery using the Coherent VersaPulse Select holmium laser. In: Allen T, Brillhart A (eds) Arthroscopic laser surgery. Springer, Berlin Heidelberg New York, pp 81–88
[14] Richards R Jr, Lonergan R (1994) Arthroscopic surgery for relief of pain in the osteoarthritic knee. Orthopaedics 7:1705–1707
[15] Trauner K, Nishioka N, Patel D (1990) Pulsed Ho:YAG laser ablation of fibrocartilage and articular cartilage. Am J Sport Med 8:316–320

Chondroplasty Using the Holmium:YAG Laser

O. Şahap Atik

Arthroscopic techniques have revolutionized the treatment of intraarticular pathologies [6, 9]. Nevertheless, although these techniques are minimally invasive, even expert surgeons have referred to the problems of iatrogenic damage [10, 11]. Current mechanical and motorized instruments are relatively large and can cause trauma to the articular surfaces in joint spaces (Figs. 1, 2).

The developments in lasers and delivery systems have led to the increased use of laser in arthroscopic surgery [1-4, 12, 13, 18. 19]. Laser probes are smaller but more powerful than conventional instruments.

A prospective, randomized clinical study was conducted to compare arthroscopic chondroplasty using the holmium:YAG laser versus conventional instruments.

Patients

One hundred and two degenerative knees were randomized into the laser group (50 patients) or to the conventional instrumented group (52 patients). In all patients chondromalacia was either grade II or grade III according to Outerbridge [14]. Both groups were comparable with regard to age, sex, and complaints.

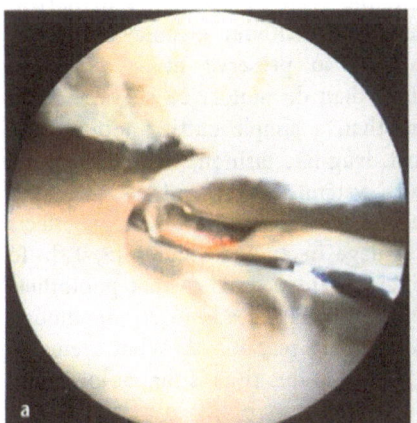 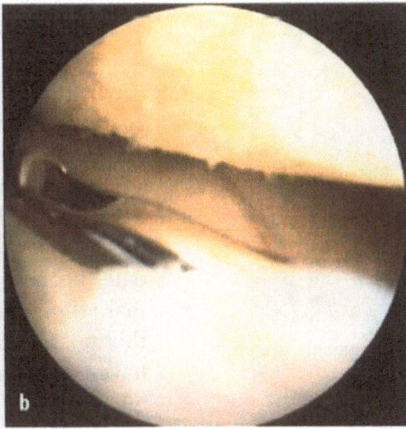

Fig. 1a,b. Chondromalacia of femoral condyle and chondroplasty using laser. Precise excision and smoothing

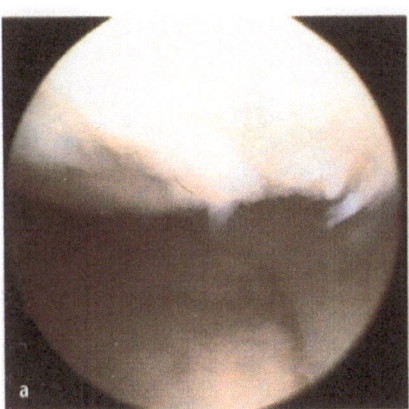 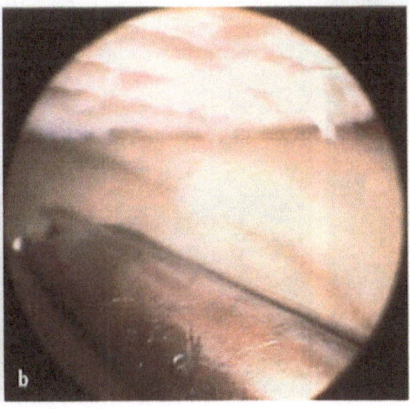

Fig. 2a,b. Chondromalacia of femoral condyle and chondroplasty using shaver. Excessive excision and rough surface

Technique

Arthroscopy was performed using a three-portal technique. The 30° or side-fire handpieces were used for chondroplasty via alternating portals for safe access to the articular surfaces. Power settings for the holmium:YAG laser were 0.5–1.5 J per pulse and 5–25 Hz. To change the power density delivered to the tissue, the laser probe was moved toward or away from the articular surface. The near-contact method with the probe perpendicular to the surface and the tangential-contact method with the probe parallel to the surface were used during laser chondroplasty. Large fragments of cartilage were amputated first and the remaining tissue was smoothed applying the tangential technique. Mechanical (basket forceps, knife, etc.) or motorized instruments were used in the conventional instrumented group (Fig. 3, 4).

The patients generally had surgery under local anesthesia. No tourniquet was used in most patients.

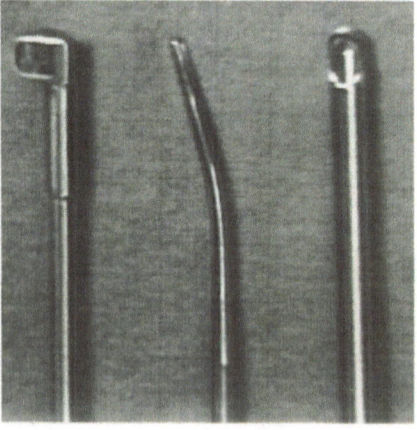

Fig. 3. Laser probe and conventional instruments used for chondroplasty

Postoperatively, a compression dressing was applied. The drainage tube was removed after 12–24 h. Physical therapy was started the next day and weight bearing begun as tolerated in both groups.

Results and Discussion

There was no serious complication in either group. Wound healing was normal. No infection, severe swelling, or severe pain was experienced. Swelling and pain were less in patients in the laser group. All patients were able to walk with weight-bearing on the 1st day following surgery. The recovery and rehabilitation periods were short and return to work was rapid (1–3 weeks). All patients had full range of motion in the postoperative period.

There was a statistically significant higher increase in Lysholm score for grade II chondramalacia patients in the laser-treated group compared to the other group.

No breakages occurred, either with the conventional instruments or with the laser probe. There was no scuffing of the articular tissue and no significant bleeding in the laser group. Ablation, homeostasis, contouring, and smoothing were more precise in the laser group.

Laser tools have a lower profile than conventional instruments and they can be inserted into narrow joint spaces and work without trauma [7, 8, 16]. Laser tools appear to preserve more remaining articular cartilage than do motorized shavers. Laser energy is more than a simple cutting tool. It can act in an almost drug-like fashion, with side effects that may have systemic repercussions [15, 22]. Laser energy has been shown to have biologic effects on articular cartilage in animal studies [5, 17]. To date, no convincing evidence exists that photothermal stimulation of cartilage leads to repair, though this possibility is being researched. What seems to have been established at this time is that at low levels

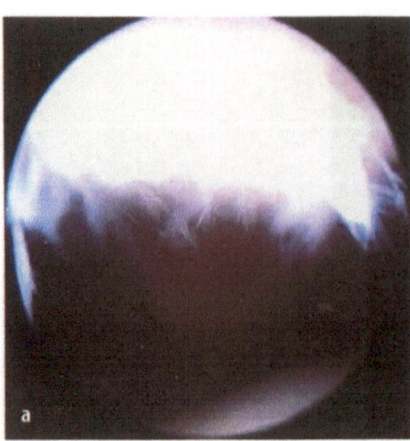

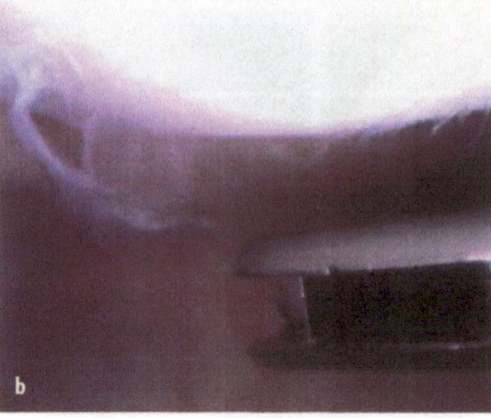

Fig. 4a,b. Chondromalacia of the patella and chondroplasty using laser probe (close-up view)

of laser energy debridement can be achieved without significant collateral damage giving cause for concern. At high levels of laser energy, cartilage cell metabolism was inhibited [20]. The ablation threshold was found by Trauner et al. [21] to be 50 J/cm^2 for hyaline cartilage.

Laser should be used in a defocused manner to ablate in chondromalacia.

The tactile feedback provided by the handpiece in direct contact with the cut surface enhances control. Visualization can be enhanced as the fragment is manipulated with the laser probe tip.

Conclusion

Fanton et al. [7] stated that "holmium:YAG laser chondroplasty yields as good or better results than mechanical chondroplasty." The present author's experience demonstrates that intraoperative and postoperative morbidity following arthroscopic chondroplasty using laser has been reduced and the results are better than those in cases in which conventional instruments were used.

References

[1] Atik OS (1994) Neodymium:YAG contact arthroscopic laser surgery. In Brillhart A (ed) Arthroscopic laser surgery. Springer, New York Berlin Heidelberg, p 183

[2] Atik OS, Sener E, Bolukbasi S, Cila E (1992) Arthroscopic laser surgery - early results. J Arthroplast Arthrosc Surg 5:1-3

[3] Atik OS, Sener E, Bolukbasi S, Cila E, Altun N, Simsek A, Baskan T (1994) Laser arthroscopy in knee injuries. J Neurol Orthop Med Surg 15:26-27

[4] Atik OS, Sener E, Bolukbasi S, Simsek A, Zuzumcugil O (1996) Arthroscopic chondroplasty using laser in knee, shoulder and ankle joints. J Arthroplast Arthrosc Surg 12:14-15

[5] Borovoy M, Zirkin R, Elson L, Borovoy M (1989) Healing of laser-induced defects of articular cartilage. J Foot Surg 28:95-99

[6] Burks R (1990) Arthroscopy and degenerative arthritis of the knee. Arthroscopy 1:43-47

[7] Fanton G, Dillingham M (1992) The use of the holmium laser in arthroscopic surgery. Semin Orthop 7:102-116

[8] Glassop N, Jackson R, Randle J, Reed S (1992) The excimer laser in athroscopic surgery. Semin Orthop 7:125-130

[9] Jackson R (1974) The role of arthroscopy in the management of arthritic knee. Clin Orthop 101:28-35

[10] Klein W, Kurze V (1988) Arthroscopic arthropath: iatrogenic arthroscopic lesions in animals. Arthroscopy 2:163

[11] Mankin H (1982) The response of articular cartilage to mechanical injury. J Bone Joint Surg 64:460-465

[12] Miller D, O'Brien S, Amoczky S, et al (1989) The use of contact Nd:YAG laser in arthroscopic surgery. Arthroscopy 5:245-253

[13] O'Brien S, Garnic J, Jackson R, Sherk H, Smith C, Wangness C (1991) Lasers in orthopedic surgery. Contemp Orthop 9:61-69

[14] Outerbridge R (1961) The etiology of chondromalacia patella. J Bone Joint Surg 43:752-757

[15] Prodoehl J, Rhodes A, Cummings R, Meller M, Sherk H (1994) 308 nm Excimer laser ablation of cartilage. Laser Surg Med 15:263-268

[16] Raunest J, Löhnert J (1990) Arthroscopic cartilage debridement by excimer laser in chondromalacia of the knee joint. Arch Orthop Trauma Surg 109:155

[17] Shultz R, Krishnamurthy S, Thelmo W et al (1985) Effects of varying intensities of laser energy on articular cartilage. Laser Surg Med 5:577-578

[18] Sherk H (1991) Orthopedist using lasers in surgery. Am J Arthroscopy 9:7-8

[19] Siebert W (1994) Overview of arthroscopic laser surgery in Europe. In: Brillhart A (ed) Arthroscopic laser surgery. Springer, New York Berlin Heidelberg, pp 175-178

[20] Smith R, Montgomery L, Fanton G, Dillingham M, Schuman D (1994) Effects of laser energy on diarthrodial joint tissues. In: Brillhart A (ed) Arthroscopic laser surgery. Springer, New York Berlin Heidelberg, p 27

[21] Trauner K, Nishioka N, Patel D (1990) Pulsed Ho:YAG laser ablation of fibrocartilage and articular cartilage. Am J Sports Med 3:316-320

[22] Whipple T, Marotta J, May T, Caspari R, Meyers J (1987) Electron microscopy of CO_2-laser induced effects on human cartilage. Laser Surg Med 7:184

Lateral Retinacular Release Using Laser

O. ŞAHAP ATIK

Lateral retinacular release is a simple procedure with low morbidity [12]. Transection of the lateral patellar retinaculum allows a reduction of lateral compression. Lateralization of the patella due to increased tension and shortening of the lateral retinaculum – the lateral compression syndrome – is the ideal indication for this procedure [6, 9] (Fig. 1).

The traditional technique has been performed both open and arthroscopically using conventional instruments [4, 8]. Although these techniques are quite effective, intra- and postoperative bleeding and hemarthrosis are not an uncommon complication [15]. Lasers are particularly useful for those procedures in which bleeding and swelling have been a problem. They represent a significant advance for lateral retinacular release as they have almost eliminated postoperative hemarthrosis [1–3, 13, 16].

A prospective, randomized clinical study was conducted to compare laser-assisted arthroscopic lateral retinacular release with arthroscopic lateral retinacular release using conventional instruments.

Patients

Twenty-three knees with patellar subluxation and lateral compression syndrome were randomized into the laser group (11 patients) or the conventional instrumented group (12 patients). The two groups were comparable with regard to sex, age, and complaints.

Technique

Arthroscopy was performed using a three-portal technique. Under direct visualization, lateral release was carried out. The synovial layer was released first, followed by the retinacular layer (Fig. 2). Lateral release was performed through the inferior lateral portal. The laser probe was placed in the inferior lateral portal rather than approaching medially. This approach reduces the risk of skin damage.

A pump system was used to improve clearing of the small bubbles created during laser use.

A retrograde blade (sickle-shaped knife) was used in the conventional instrumented group (Fig. 3). In the laser group, surgery was done using holmium:YAG laser. The laser was set at approximately 1.5 J per pulse and 15 Hz. Generally, a 30° angled or side-fire laser probe was used.

The lateral release was begun distally and carried proximally. Patellar tracking was then checked, as was physiological centralization of the patella.

In most patients local anesthesia was utilized without tourniquet.

Lasing or shaving of fibrillated cartilage of patella was performed if necessary.

Postoperatively, a compression dressing was applied. An ice-pack was utilized locally in the conventional instrumented group. The drainage tube was removed after 12–24 h. Physical therapy was

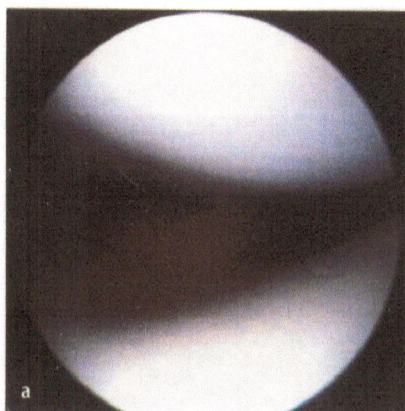
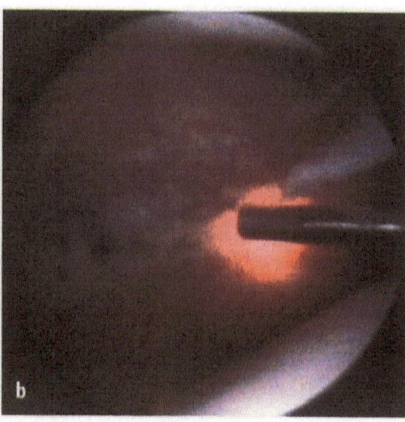

Fig. 1a,b. Patellar maltracking and lateral compression syndrome. The space between patella and femur is widened during lateral release

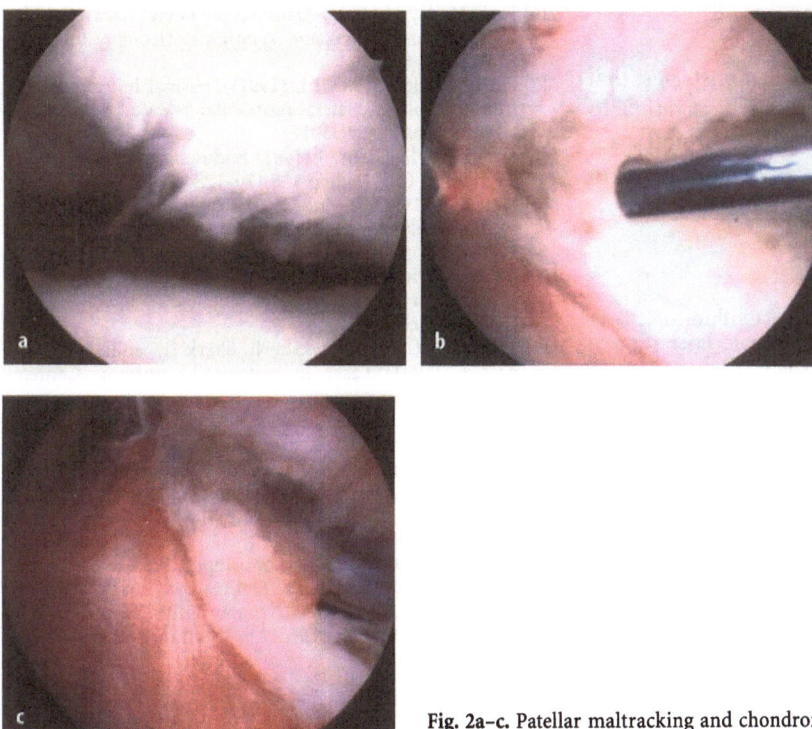

Fig. 2a–c. Patellar maltracking and chondromalacia. The synovial layer is released first, followed by the retinacular layer

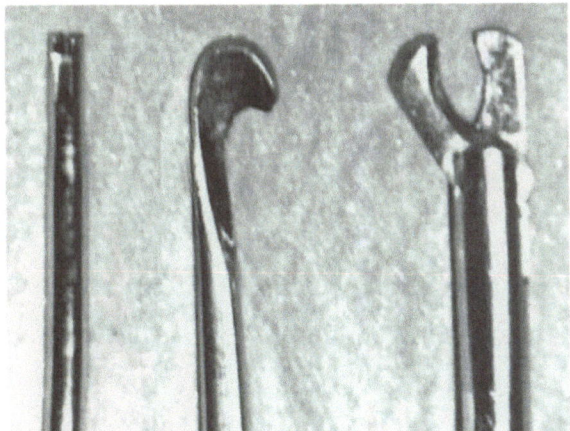

Fig. 3. Laser probe and conventional instruments used for lateral retinacular release

started the next day and weight bearing begun as tolerated in both groups.

Results and Discussion

There was hemarthrosis, mild synovitis and pain in three patients in the conventional instrumented group, whereas, in the laser group, patients had minimal swelling and pain.

Wound healing was normal and no infection was observed in either group. The complication of skin necrosis was not seen with laser.

All patients in the laser group were able to walk with weight bearing on the 1st day following surgery. All the patients in the laser group had full range of motion. However, in the other group three patients with hemarthrosis had some degree of limitation of range of motion in the postoperative period.

There was a statistically significantly higher increase in Lysholm score among patients in the laser group.

The hemarthrosis rate was zero in the laser group. This seems to be the primary reason for the significantly better range of motion and reduced consumption of pain killers. Although there are many procedures in knee surgery that have been improved with the use of laser, lateral retinacular release is probably the best of all [5, 11, 14]. During laser-assisted lateral retinacular release, there is simultaneous coagulation of bleeding vessels. As the depth of penetration is well controlled, dermal burn and skin necrosis are not seen, which are possible when electrocautery is used [7, 10].

The degree of release must be individualized to each patient. The judgement is best made with the patients under local anesthesia so that active tracking can be evaluated. As the handpiece is small and no tourniquet is used, the type of anesthesia does not affect the surgeon's ability to perform the procedure.

Conclusion

The present author's experience demonstrates that following laser-assisted arthroscopic lateral retinacular release, intra- and postoperative morbidity are reduced and the results are better than in cases in which conventional instruments are used.

References

[1] Atik OS (1994) Neodymium:YAG contact arthroscopic laser surgery. In: Brillhart A (ed) Arthroscopic laser surgery. Springer, New York Berlin Heidelberg, p 183
[2] Atik OS, Sener E, Bolukbasi S, Cila E (1992) Arthroscopic laser surgery – early results. J Arthroplast Arthrosc Surg 5:1–3
[3] Atik OS, Sener E, Bolukbasi S, Cila E, Simsek A, Baskan T (1994) Laser arthroscopy in knee injuries. J Neurol Orthop Med Surg 15:26–27
[4] Betz R, Margill J, Lonergan R (1987) The percutaneous lateral retinacular release. Am J Sports Med 15:477–482
[5] Fanton G, Dillingham M (1992) The use of Ho-Yag laser in arthroscopic surgery. Semin Orthop 7:102–116
[6] Fu F, Moday M (1992) Arthroscopic lateral release and lateral patellar compression syndrome. Orthop Clin North Am 23:601–612
[7] Lord M, Mltry J, Shall L (1991) Thermal injury resulting from arthroscopic lateral retinacular release by electrocautery. Arthroscopy 7:33–37
[8] McGinty J, McCarthy J (1981) Endoscopic lateral retinacular release. Clin Orthop 158:120–128
[9] Metcalf R (1982) An arthroscopic method for lateral release of the subluxating or dislocating patella. Clin Orthop 167:9–18
[10] Miller G, Dickason J, Fox J et al (1982) The use of electrosurgery for arthroscopic subcutaneous lateral release. Orthopaedics 5:209–316
[11] O'Brien S, Garick J, Jackson R, Sherk H, Smith C, Wangsness C (1991) Laser in orthopaedic surgery. Contemp Orthop 9:61–69
[12] Schonholtz G, Zahn M, Magee C (1987) Lateral retinacular release of the patella. Arthroscopy 3:269–272
[13] Shapiro G, Fanton G, Dillingham M, Perkash R (1995) Lateral retinacular release. Clin Orthop 310:42–47
[14] Sherk H (1991) Orthopedist using lasers in surgery. Am J Arthroscopy 9:7–8
[15] Small N (1989) An analysis of complications in lateral retinacular release procedures. Arthroscopy 5:282–286
[16] Toft J (1991) Postoperative morbidity following laser arthroscopic lateral release. Am J Arthrosc 1:23–35

Meniscectomy Using Laser

O. Şahap Atik

The commonest and most important arthroscopic operation is partial resection of a meniscus. Avulsed, torn or frayed protions of the meniscus are resected, leaving the largest and functionally effective portion. The advantages of arthroscopic surgery are reduced trauma to the joint and close examination. However, current conventional instruments can cause iatrogenic trauma [6, 7].

The steps of arthroscopic meniscectomy are as follows:

1. Identification of the lesion
2. Removal of the fragment which is less vascular, leaving a stable meniscal tissue
3. Contouring the rim

The available conventional instruments for meniscal excision are mechanical (basket forceps, knife, etc.) and motorized instruments (cutter, shaver, etc.). Lasers are useful for meniscectomy because laser handpieces can be placed into narrow joint spaces and exert their effect without mechanical trauma [1–4, 8–11] (Fig. 1, 2).

A prospective, randomized clinical study was conducted to compare arthroscopic meniscectomy using holmium:YAG laser versus conventional instruments.

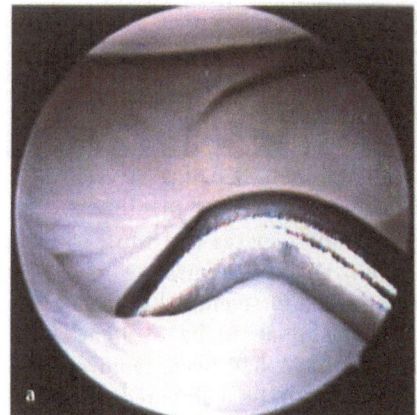
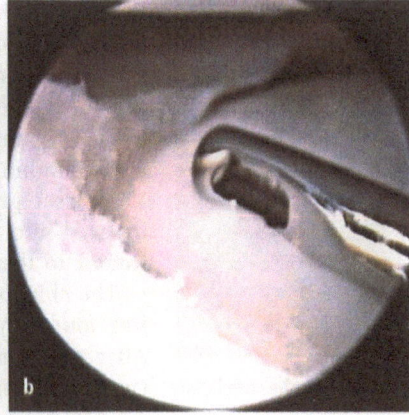

Fig. 1a,b. Partial meniscectomy using laser for radial meniscal tear. Precise excision and no damage to the adjacent healthy tissues

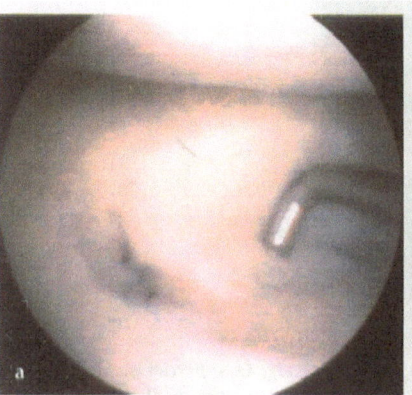
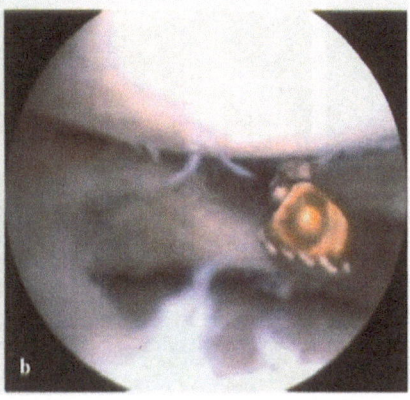

Fig. 2a,b. Partial meniscectomy using shaver for radial meniscal tear. Excessive resection and damage to the adjacent healthy tissues

Patients

Sixty-four patients with meniscal tear were randomized into the laser group (31 patients) or to the conventional instrumented group (33 patients). Both groups were comparable with regard to sex, age, and complaints.

Technique

Arthroscopy was performed using a three-portal technique.

Mechanical (basket forceps, knife) and motorized instruments were used in conventional instrumented

group (Fig. 3). Holmium:YAG laser was used in the laser group. The laser was set at 1–1.5 J per pulse and 15–25 Hz.

After cutting the meniscus, the portion to be removed was taken out of the joint with the help of a grasping forceps. For meniscal ablation, the laser probe was used in a gentle sweeping fashion, going back and forth with some pressure to the meniscus. Finally, the rim of the remaining meniscus was contoured with the laser, using low energy levels (Fig. 4).

Most of the patients underwent the surgery under local anesthesia. No tourniquet was used with local anesthesia.

Postoperatively, a compression dressing was applied. The drainage tube was removed after 12–24 h. Physical therapy was started the next day and weight bearing begun as tolerated in both groups.

Results and Discussion

There was no serious complication in either group. Wound healing was normal. No infection, severe swelling, or severe pain was observed. Swelling and pain were less in patients in the laser group. All patients were able to walk with weight bearing on the 1st day following surgery. All patients had full range of motion 1–3 weeks after surgery.

There was a statistically significantly higher increase in Lysholm score among patients in the laser group compared to the other group.

Breakage of conventional instruments or laser probe occurred in no case. Scuffing of the articular tissue was not seen. Ablation, hemostasis, contouring, and smoothing were more precise in the laser group.

As laser probes have a lower profile, they can be inserted into narrow joint spaces and work without trauma to the healthy adjacent tissues.

The ablation threshold for meniscal fibrocartilage was found by Trauner et al. to be 11 J/cm^2 [12]. After the abnormal tissue has been removed, the rim of the meniscus can be contoured with the

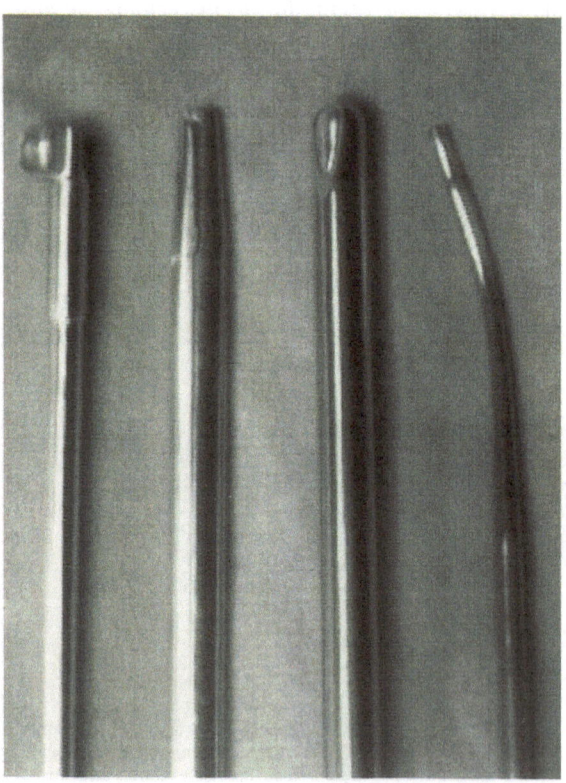

Fig. 3. Conventional instruments and laser probe used for meniscectomy

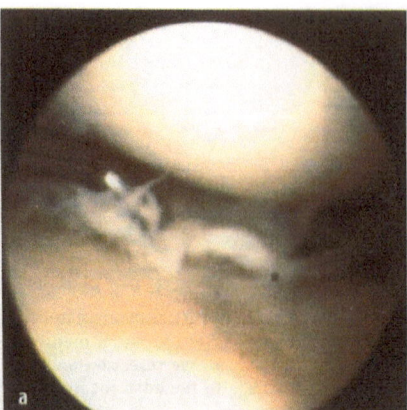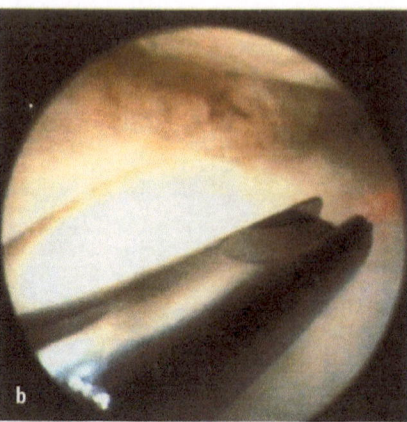

Fig. 4a,b. Partial meniscectomy using laser for degenerative tear

laser using low-level energy [5]. Direct ablation of the abnormal meniscal tissue using laser is also possible [13, 14].

Short-term clinical studies of arthroscopic partial meniscectomy using laser showed that these patients have faster postoperative recovery than did those mechanically treated. There was also a faster resolution of efffusion and diminished postoperative pain [2, 3].

Conclusion

The present author's experience demonstrates that intra- and postoperative morbidity following arthroscopic meniscectomy is reduced by the use of laser, and the results are better than in cases treated with conventional instruments.

References

[1] Atik OS (1994) Neodymium-YAG contact arthroscopic laser surgery. In Brillhart A (ed) Arthroscopic laser surgery. Springer, New York Berlin Heidelberg, p 183

[2] Atik OS, Sener E, Bolukbasi S, Cila E (1992) Arthroscopic laser surgery – early results. J Arthroplast Arthrosc Surg 5:1–3

[3] Atik OS, Sener E, Bolukbasi S, Cila E, Altun N, Simsek A, Baskan T (1994) Laser arthroscopy in knee injuries. J Neurol Orthop Med Surg 15:26–27

[4] Bickerstaff D, Wyman A, Laing R, Smith T (1991) Partial meniscectomy using neodymium:YAG laser. J Arthrosc Rel Surg 7:63–67

[5] Kroitzsch U, Laufer G, Egkher E, Wollenek G, Horvath R (1989) Experimental photoablation of meniscus cartilage by excimer laser energy. Arch Orthop Trauma Surg 108:44

[6] Klein W, Kurze V (1988) Arthroscopic arthropathy: iatrogenic arthroscopic lesions in animals. Arthroscopy 2:163

[7] Mankin H (1982) The response of articular cartilage to meniscal injury. J Bone Joint Surg 64:460–465

[8] Metcalf R, Dixon J (1984) Lasers for arthroscopic meniscectomy. Lasers Surg Med 3:366

[9] O'Brien S, Garrick J, Jackson R, Sherk H, Smith C, Wangsness C (1991) Lasers in orthopaedic surgery. Contemp Orthop 9:61–69

[10] Sherk H (1991) Orthopedist using lasers in surgery. Am J Arthrosc 9:7–8

[11] Siebert W (1994) Overview of arthroscopic laser surgery in Europe. In: Brillhart A (ed) Arthroscopic laser surgery. Springer, New York Berlin Heidelberg, pp 175–178

[12] Trauner K, Nishioka N, Patel D (1990) Pulsed Ho:YAG laser ablation of fibrocartilage and articular cartilage. Am J Sports Med 3:316–320

[13] Vangsness C, Watson T, Saadatmonesh V, Moran K (1995) Pulsed H:YAG laser meniscectomy. Lasers Surg Med 16:61–65

[14] Whipple T, Caspari R, Meyers J (1985) Arthroscopic laser meniscectomy in a gas medium. Arthroscopy 1:2

Holmium 2.1 Laser-Assisted Knee Arthroscopy: Clinical Outcome and Complications in 1000 Cases

J. A. Saunier · F. Indermühle · J Compère

Introduction

The use of laser in arthroscopy is the result of historical developments, and its evolution follows the course common to most new technologies, with particular relevance to the concept of minimally invasive surgery. The gradual introduction of new laser beams such als neodymium, holmium, and erbium – the latter still at the experimental stage – has allowed the development of fiberoptics and made it possible to use these lasers in arthroscopy surgery.

The concept of minimally invasive surgery is a result of technological progress, and is social change. Surgeons and those working in related specialties have become conscious of the importance of reducing operative trauma, of simplifying and reducing the time of postoperative care and rehabilitation.

The acceleration of human activities and professional obligations have reduced the amount of time that can be devoted to individual health and rehabilitation. The importance of sport accidents and of rapid rehabilitation of athletes have contributed to improved knowledge of trauma pathology and to more effective specific treatments. Endoscopy and arthroscopy play an important role in minimally invasive surgery and influence diagnostic and therapeutic procedures. The development and use of laser in arthroscopy is just one link in this evolutionary chain.

Being orthopedic surgeon and trauma sport specialists, we were particularly involved in these developments and decided to apply laser technology to our patients from 1992. We now present our clinical experience with knee arthroscopy.

Requirements for Laser in Arthroscopy

There are no universal lasers in medicine or surgery. Thus, the choice of a laser for arthroscopy must satisfy certain specific criteria. For each wavelength, the lasers action depends on the medium in which it is used and on the constituents of the tissue target. The laser beam must also be easily conveyed to the site of action. Last but not least, it should have no side effects of any kind [7, 29].

The requirements for laser in arthroscopy are:
1. Transmission by optic fibers. The efficiency of transmission together with its miniaturization makes it particularly valuable.
2. Surface effect, ablative and hemostatic. The ablative effect must be well controlled; the cutting effect should provoke no bleeding.
3. Compatibility with the medium. Certain lasers, e. g., CO_2, are completely absorbed by water and thus are totally ineffective.
4. No pigment action. Joint tissues being white, the laser should be active in the absence of pigment, unlike ophthalmological lasers.
5. Side effects, if any, should be controllable and reduced.
6. Superiority to traditional instruments. Technology and costs must be justified by better use and results.

In 1996 only the holmium:YAG 2.1 met these criteria [10].

Materials and Methods

Our series contains 1000 patients, 651 men, 349 women, aged from 14 to 89 years, average 38 years. Seventy-six percent were less than 40 years old; thus, the patient population was fairly young. Follow-up time was 12–60 months for the first patients (average 34.2 months) (Fig. 1).

There were 1550 lesions in total, i. e., 1.6 per patient: 38 % were torn medial meniscus, 17 % carti-

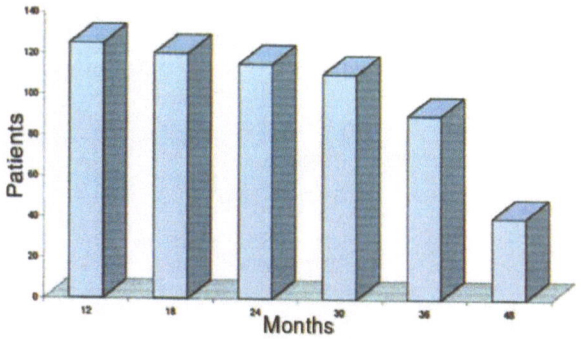

Fig. 1. Follow-up times among our 600 patients

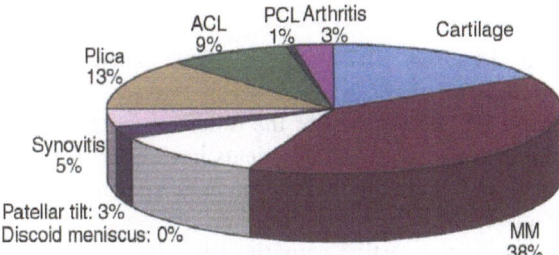

Fig. 2. Distribution of diagnoses of 930 lesions. *ACL*, anterior cruciate ligament; *PCL*, posterior cruciate ligament; *MM*, medial meniscus

laginous lesions, 11 % lateral meniscus lesions, and 13 % symptomatic plicae (Fig. 2). One hundred thirty-eight patients had a fresh or chronic tear of the anterior cruciate ligament and six a chronic tear of the posterior cruciate ligament.

Ablative surgery (meniscectomy, chondroplasty, resection of plica) and reconstructive surgery should be considered separately. One hundred sixteen of 138 patients with lesions of the anterior cruciate ligament were treated with ligament plasty, the other 22 were left untreated. Of the posterior cruciate ligament lesions, only two were reconstructed.

The diagnostic distribution is appropriate to a young and to some extent athletic population. Operative time varied from 30 to 210 min (average 49 min). With ablative treatment, performed in 882 patients, operative time was no more than 60 min (average 39 min). In all operations lasting more than 60 min reconstructive surgery was performed (Fig. 3).

Our patients undergo regional or general anesthesia or, in a few cases, local anesthesia. The incisions are classical, anterolateral (for arthroscope), anteromedial (for instruments) and, if necessary, either superolateral or superomedial for drainage. A tourniquet is used only in fresh cases where hemarthrosis disturbs the view of the joint cavity. This is certainly an important advantage of laser surgery. In reconstructive surgery, the tourniquet is used more often,

but only in limited cases such as bone drilling because of significant bleeding.

The Versapulse 30° probe was used in 90 % of the cases, and a 70° probe in the remaining 10 %. The latter is the principal instrument indicated for dealing with lateral release. Of course, the arthroscope is then inserted through the anteromedial incision, the probe through the anterolateral. The 70° probe is not recommended for chondroplasty because its action is too perpendicular, which is not the case with the 30° probe. We ourselves have no experience with 0° and 15° probes.

Results and Discussion

Our interest was centered on immediately postoperative parameters:
- Mobility
- Effusion
- Duration of hospital care
- Duration of use of crutches
- Delay of return to sport

Mobility

At 6 h after surgery, 680 patients (68 %) had active quadriceps motion and flexion up to 90°. Rehabilitation of patients who had undergone reconstructive surgery being naturally slower, the percentage in the other cases alone would be 76 %.

On day 5 after surgery, 658 patients had recovered symmetrical movements of the knees (66 %). Leaving reconstructive surgery out of account, the percentage rises to 87 %.

Effusion

Two hundred fifty patients, all presenting with chondromalacia, had preoperative effusion. Postoperatively, 250 patients had short-term effusion. In the longer postoperative term, 33 patients (3 %) had persistent effusion.

Duration of Hospital Care

After nonreconstructive surgery in 882 patients, 829 (94 %) returned home on the same day as the operation. Fifty-two of the remaining 53 patients left the next day and the last on the 2nd postoperative day.

After reconstructive surgery, the hospital stay was obviously longer. In Switzerland it is still not customary to undertake such an operation as an outpatient procedure. Insurance issues are involved, so this parameter does not really indicate very much. Most of these patients left hospital between the 4th and the 5th postoperative day (average of 4.5 days) (Fig. 5).

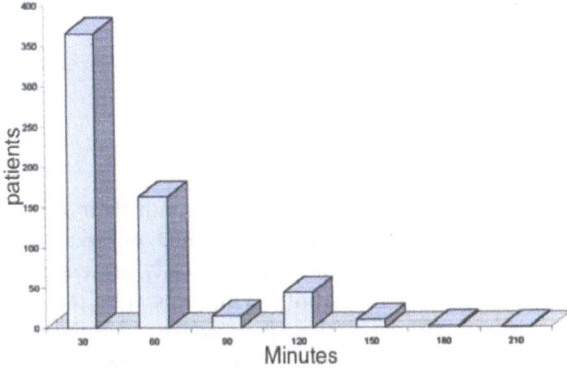

Fig. 3. Distribution of operative time

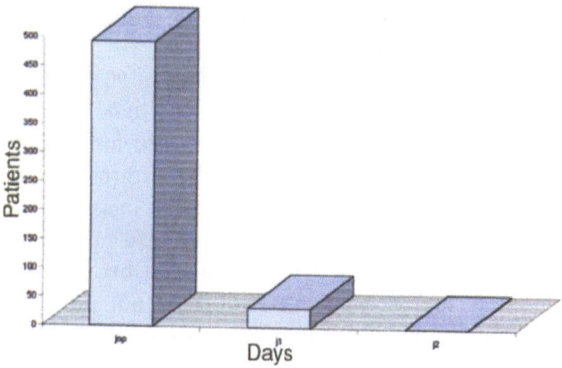

Fig. 4. Patients' return home after nonreconstructive surgery. *jop,* Day of operation; j^1 next day after surgery; j^2 2 days after surgery

Return to Sports

Four hundred fifty-eight of 1000 patients were involved regularly in sport preoperatively. Figure 7 shows the distribution of the different sport. Soccer was the most played. All patients having reconstructive surgery were among the 458 sportmen and women.

Return to sporting activities lay between the 15th and the 18th day (Fig. 8). The average was 48 days. For ablative surgery (340 patients) the average was 22 days, and for reconstructive surgery (118 patients) it was 120 days. However, 25 of the 118 patients with reconstructive surgery never recovered sufficiently to practice sport seriously again.

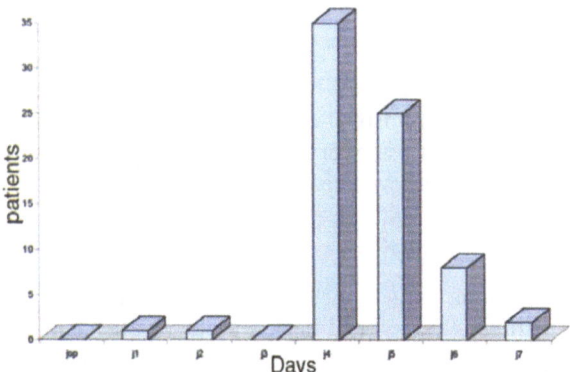

Fig. 5. Patients' return home after reconstructive surgery. *jop,* Day of operation; j^1–j^7, days 1–7 after surgery

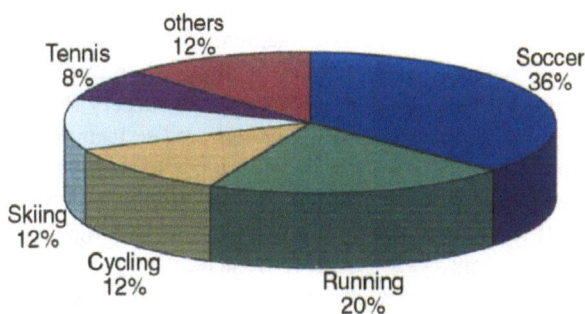

Fig. 7. Distribution of sports participarted in by patients

Crutches

Two hundred thirty-three patients left hospital without crutches, and for the remainder the number of days with crutches varied from 1 to 45 (average 8 days). Leaving patients with reconstructive surgery out of account, the average falls to 5 days for 882 patients (Fig. 6).

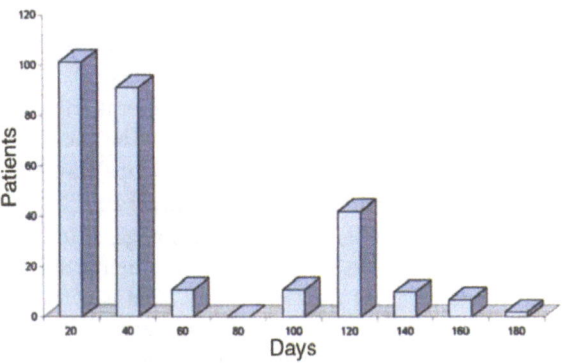

Fig. 8. Days to return to sport after surgery

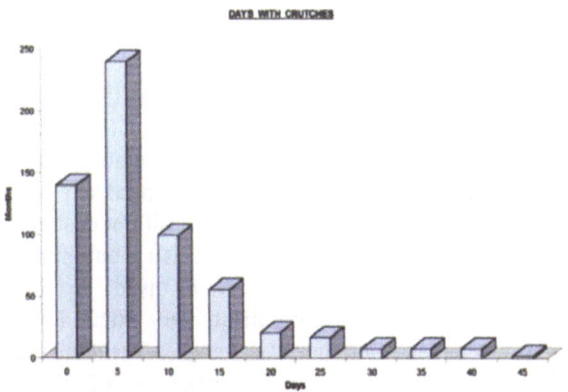

Fig. 6. Days with crutches after surgery

Failures

Sixty-one patients were dissatisfied with their surgical treatment. Twenty-six complained of persistent pain, 20 of effusions which were already present preoperatively, and 15 of both symptoms. The reasons for these failures were inappropriate indication for surgery, cartilaginous lesions, or pre-existing osteoarthritis.

Complications

We encountered 11 complications in 1000 patients:
- 7 arthroscopes damaged by laser
- 3 cases of arthrofibrosis after reconstruction of the anterior cruciate ligament
- 1 case of subtotal bone necrosis of the medial femoral condyle

Damage to the arthroscope

Direct exposure of the arthroscope irremediably destroys the optic fibers. This incident occurs of course more often in the learning period, but the risk remains, especially when performing laser arthroscopy in small joints such as ankle and elbow. We destroyed five arthroscopes in this way, without any damage to the patient. Once the instrument was changed, the operation proceeded quite normally. In two cases the cause was probably deflection of the laser beam by another intra-articular instrument, e. g., a rinsing cannula. Such a reflection of the beam is extremely rare and carries no danger to the patient because of the characteristics of holmium:YAG 2.1, which does not act at a distance of more than a few millimeters.

Arthrofibrosis

Arthrofibrosis can be considered a well-known complication of reconstructive surgery of the knee. It usually occurs if the operative indication is inappropriate or surgery is inappropriately timed or performed as on emergency, or if the joint has limited motion and the femoral and/or tibial tunnels are not rightly positioned. In our series, this complication occured in the first 30 cases when we still proceeded with semiarthroscopic ligament plasty requiring an open approach through the patellar tendon. Moreover, in two patients the positioning of the tunnels was not entirely successful. Arthrofibrosis has completely disappeared from our series since we became very critical about deciding on the time of operation, isometric placement and maintaining a totally arthroscopic approach. Thus the laser beam cannot be considered as a cause of arthrofibrosis. No scientific evidence suggests that laser could provoke arthrofibrosis, and no report in the literature sustains such a hypothesis.

Laser by itself has not fundamentally modified our ligament reconstruction results. However we emphasize that the debridement, preparation of the intercondylar notch, and resection of any associated meniscus lesions can be done more precisely and more quickly with the laser than in a conventional prodecure. The use of bone-patellar tendon-bone transplant and, most importantly, an exclusively intra-articular arthroscopic procedure coupled with absence of immobilization and Shelbourne's principles of re-education has given complete satisfaction and allowed a simpler postoperative course and better quality of rehabilitation [28].

We have now shifted the age limit for ligament plasty since three patients between 50 and 55 years of age have been operated on to the entire satisfaction of the patients, with results comparable with those of the lower age group. Thus we think that with modern operative and rehabilitation procedures it is possible, in certain cases, to give less weight to age in the operative indications for ligament plasty. In the three patients just mentioned, the relevant factors were: subjective and objective instability, willingness of the patient, and the patient's desire to continue a sport that puts the meniscus at risk by submitting the knee to rotational forces, e. g., tennis, squash, skiing. Although we have never been confronted with indications in patients older than 55 years, we should not recommend a ligament plasty in such cases.

Aseptic Osteonecrosis of the Medial Femoral Condyle

We unfortunately had one case of aseptic necrosis of the medial condyle. A 74-year-old female patient twisted her right knee 2 weeks before our first examination. She complained of pain and had a hemathrosis and flexum of the knee. Preoperative X-rays showed no osteoarthritis and MRI revealed a torn medial meniscus. Apparently the patient had no previous history of complaints in this joint. We proceeded arthroscopically to subtotal meniscectomy preceded by chondroplasty of the medial femoral condyle to allow a better view of the meniscus. Laser was used as usual for both chondroplasty and meniscectomy. Energy use was 15 W with a 30° probe applied tangentially to the joint surface. The postoperative course was particularly unfavorable with pain and eventual collapse of the condyle. Six month later a total knee prosthesis was implanted. After this unfortunate case we, of course, were highly interested in aseptic avascular bone necrosis of the medial condyle and particularly on the influence that both arthroscopy and laser could have on its development. Laser is often criticized for being a dangerous instrument in that regard without definite proof.

The idea that part of the human body could die while the rest remained alive was first introduced by Hippocrates. He gave the name "sphacelus" to the gangrene following garroting of a limb.

In the eighteenth century Hunter was the first to succeed in distinguishing living from dead bone and descriptions of bone necrosis were published thereafter, but all related to septic cases. It was only with Pasteur that the difference between septic bone necrosis and other form of such necrosis gradually became clear. Axelhausen was the first, at the beginning of this century, to use the term "aseptic necrosis", taking advantage of the discovery of X-rays, and he suspected it could be an ischemic lesion. Phemister developed the concept of bony infarct and proposed boring the necrotic femoral head. During the 1960s the spread of radionuclide scanning became of prime importance in the diagnosis of necrotic phenomena [16, 17, 20].

In 1968 aseptic bone necrosis of the internal femoral condyle was for the first time described and differentiated from osteochondritis dissecans by Ahlbäck.

The condition is caused by the breakdown of subchondral bone in the weight-bearing zones. Necrosis may also appear in the lateral condyle as in the tibial plateau. The etiology of the lesion being uncertain, the latter has been designated by several different names, such as idiopathic, spontaneous, or avascular. However, the currently most accepted hypothesis cites hyperpressure resulting in ischemia in a nonexpandable tissue. This theory could explain necrosis in cases of corticoid treatment and alcoholism by the growing of fat cells. In cases of trauma, microfractures inducing necrosis and penetration of synovial fluid into weakened osteoporotic subchondral bone in the elderly have been postulated [1, 12, 16, 17].

Despite all this, the origin of many cases of necrosis remains unexplained. Necrosis of the medial femoral condyle appears more frequently in females aged over 70, with or without trauma. Sudden pain and pseudolocking suggesting meniscus lesions are the key signs. In the absence of trauma of documented meniscus lesion, immediate arthroscopy rarely seems adequate and we prefer clinical monitorings of the course accompanied by symptomatic therapy without weight bearing. The course and prognosis depend on the size and position of the lesion. For lesions out of the weight-bearing zones the prognosis is favorable and usually conservative treatment suffices. Operative treatment, such as bone drilling, osteotomy, or prosthesis, appears to be the only appropiate measure in lesions that are larger or situated in weight-bearing areas [16].

Norman and Baker [22] recommend early arthroscopic meniscectomy in case of torn meniscus in order to avoid stress on the edge of the meniscal fragment, thus perhaps preventing aseptic necrosis in particularly vulnerable patients.

Santori et al. [27] described the development of aseptic necrosis in two patients after arthroscopic meniscectomy. Like others, they attributed this development to excess stress on the cartilage after resction of the meniscus.

It used to be generally considered that partial arthroscopic meniscectomy would reduce the risk of osteoarthritis, which was a common finding in total meniscectomies performed by arthrotomy. This, however, is only partially true, Rangger et al. [24] having proved that even after very sparing meniscectomy, the risk persisted. Again, these authors underline stress phenomena in the development of postmeniscectomy osteoarthritis. Some stress fractures have also been discovered [9, 24, 25].

Very recently, Muscolo et al. [21] reported eight cases of femoral condylar necrosis after conventional arthroscopy and related it to this stress phenomenon.

In 1990, Brahme et al. [6] published an important article in Radiology, reporting that 7 of 611 patients who underwent arthroscopic meniscectomy developed asymptomatic necrosis confirmed by MRI. The authors consider this necrosis to be due more to the increase of stress on both cartilage and subchondral bone than to some unknown disastrous arthroscopic action.

Transitory algodystrophy accompanied by bone necrosis and cured by lumbar sympathectomy has also been described [12].

Continuing unexplained condylar necrosis after ligament plasty (increased stress, ischemia?) has also been reported [4].

From the most recent literature it appears that the etiology of aseptic idiopathic or avascular necrosis of the medial femoral condyle remains unknown, but that ischemic phenomena and/or stress within the bone certainly influence the process [1, 16, 24].

Necrosis appears more likely in females of more than 70 years of age, and a history of trauma is often discovered in this disease.

As regards laser, six cases of bone necrosis were described by Garino et al. [14] after laser meniscectomy. In five cases a neodymium:YAG laser was used and in one case probably a holmium laser. These cases are reported by an author who does not use laser beam in arthroscopy.

Rozbruch et al. [26] recently reported medial tibial plateau necrosis after a neodymium:YAG laser-assisted meniscectomy in a 25-year-old woman.

Drucker et al. [11] reported 4 cases of MRI-documented necrosis among 558 holmium 2.1 laser-assisted surgical arthroscopies, versus 3 cases of MRI-documented necrosis among 2700 conventional arthroscopies.

Fink et al. [13] reported one case of femoral bone necrosis after laser arthroscopy.

Thus, of 500,000 Ho:YAG-2.1 arthroscopic procedures performed so far, bone necrosis has followed in 7 cases.

Two cases of cartilaginous lesions after holmium 2.1-assisted meniscectomy have been presented by Thal et al. [32]. One patient suffered from a sprained knee and the other had already undergone arthroscopic cartilage shaving (with a shaver). The authors attribute the cartilaginous lesions to laser, unfortunately without the slightest proof. In the first case there was trauma, and it is well known that traumatic vascular lesions may ultimately injure cartilage whatever the type of arthroscopic procedure performed. The follow-up in the second case is of only 3 months, whereas a 5-year interval separats the first two arthroscopies. Thus it is impossible to state that this patient is healed and that there will not be a third relapse, in which case, it will be difficult to incriminate the laser. Moreover we have just demonstrated the unfortunate influence of meniscectomy on load distribution whatever the type of instrument used to remove the meniscus. Thus, in this publication, there is no persuasive argument to support the assertion that laser beam is the prime cause of cartilaginous lesions, which can result from a variety of other causes.

Various experiments have proved that laser beam can provoke osteonecrosis when the beam is aimed directly perpendicularly at the bone surface in the same way as a drill [8]. This is easily explained and depends on two factors: the type of laser and the way it is handled. Laser, in continuous mode which is absorbed by cellular pigments and where penetration is deep, can easily cause necrosis if directed perpendicularly to the bone surface in the same way as a drill. This is especially true of neodymium when misused. On the other hand, pulsed-mode holmium, which is not absorbed by pigments, will hardly produce such lesions if the beam is directed tangentially to bone surfaces. Acoustic damage could be responsible for some damage, claim some authors. This would be the result of the creation of an air-bubble.

Asshauer and Delacrétaz have demonstrated that judicious and tangential use of the probe allows this so-called "Moses effect" to be minimized to the point where it would probably be innocuous [2, 3, 18].

In a randomized study, Paulos compared patients operated on using holmium laser with those operated on using conventional instruments. Postoperative MRI was performed to look for abnormal temperature elevations. No statistically significant differences were found between the two groups [23].

No recent, properly conducted clinical study has shown laser to be more dangerous than conventional instruments, particularly as regards the risk of necrosis, provided of course that the operator observes norms for wavelength, energy settings, directional impact of the probe, and, naturally, the indications for surgery. We agree with Brillhart when he says "No case of significant avascular necrosis, chondrolysis or hemarthrosis has been reported with proper Ho:YAG laser use" and "laser does not cause bone necrosis, surgeons do!" [8].

Table 1. Comparison of complications in two series of laser-assisted arthroscopy of the knee

Complications	Small [31], 1879 patients	Present series, 600 patients
Hemarthrosis	+	−
Infection	+	−
Anesthetic-related	+	−
Instrument failure	+	+
Arthrofibrosis	+	+
Other	+ (which?)	+

+, Occurred; −, did not occur.

Returning to our 74-year-old female patient, it is to be emphasized that recent trauma, meniscal tear, effusion, and preexisting chondropathy are largely sufficient factors to engender postoperative necrosis, the latter not being related to laser energy when used in the proper manner.

Lastly, in regard to complications we compared Small's 1994 series of 1879 patients [31] with ours (Table 1). The percentage of complications is much the same in both series (Small, 1.8 %; Saunier, 1.1 %). Other series report more complications with conventional surgical arthroscopy. We can confirm that our series is a totally surgical one with no diagnostic arthroscopy.

At present therefore, we may conclude that in terms of complications laser beam considerably reduces the risk of hemarthrosis and that so far there are no known complications specific to laser when properly used.

Advantages of Holmium 2.1 Laser

There is no doubt that holmium 2.1 laser has four advantages:
- Ease of use. The probe is thinner than any other instrument, motorized or not, and fulfills on its own several functions otherwise performed by forceps or resectors or miniaturized scissors. Thus the in-and-out manipulations during the operation are much reduced. In addition, tasks impossible for conventional arthroscopy become easy, e.g., remodeling or welding. After a learning curve of about 50 cases, the manipulation involved becomes simple and will certainly be preferred to conventional instruments, which will still be selected from time to time for special problems.
- Rapidity. Although much less than the maximum of 60 W is applied, laser meniscal resections particularly in the posterior part, resection of plica, and debridement, are performed in less time than in conventional surgery.
- Hemostasis. Section and resection are performed under spontaneous and immediate hemostasis.

Coagulation of a blood vessel may also be carried out at a distance with defocalization of the beam, e. g., in fresh lesions. The use of a tourniquet is now rather the exception, e. g., in fresh hemarthrosis or when drilling in fresh bleeding bone. Of itself, hemostasis is a major and indisputable advantage of laser, having a beneficial effect on operative time reducing the risk of thrombosis. The latter is already much reduced in arthroscopy compared to arthrotomy. If this is true for ablative arthroscopy, it should be even more so in more serious arthroscopic procedures such as ligament reconstruction, shoulder capsular shift in cases of recurrent dislocation, acromioplasty, arthrodesis of the ankle, etc. Therefore, to have such an efficient instrument as laser at our disposal for hemostasis is without any doubt great progress.

- Ease of postoperative recovery. Most appreciated by our patients was the reduction of postoperative pain and inflammatory phenomena, allowing rapid recovery of mobility and an easier return to normal life, professional activities, or sports. There is of course no "magic" in laser, merely a synergy of the advantages described in the three points above.

A number of comparative studies of conventional versus laser arthroscopy by other authors come to the same conclusions concerning the advantage of laser:

- Kunz compares 76 patients operated on by laser to 74 operated on by conventional arthroscopy. Time in hospital, functional knee scores, time work, and time to return to sports were studied. The results were all significantly better in laser-operated patients [19].
- In a European multicenter study published by Siebert et al. [30] it became apparent that better results were obtained in laser-operated patients after treatment of synovitis, meniscal tears associated with cartilaginous lesions, and lateral release. There was no significant difference in results after resection of meniscal tears alone. Very surprisingly, this series showed that the results remained better even after 1 year. Until now, the advantages of laser had been considered relevant essentially in the immediate postoperative period.
- In a study of 100 conventional and 100 laser arthroscopies reported by Walker [33], the results in the laser group were statistically significantly better in regard to pain, reduction of effusion, and mobility. Two cases of deep venous thrombosis and two arthrofibrosis occurred in the conventional arthroscopy group, and two damaged scopes in the laser.

- Atik compares the Lysholm score in 102 patients suffering from chondromalacia grade II and III treated with conventional arthroscopy or laser [5]. The laser-operated patients had a statistically significant better Lysholm score.
- Guten and Kenney [15] reported that in a series of 40 patients operated on by laser or with conventional instruments, the results were reduction by
  - 40 % of the pain
  - 40 % of the use of nonsteroidal anti-inflammatory drugs
  - 30 % of effusion
  - 4 days of time with crutches, and
  - 10 days of time to return to sport

in patients treated by laser.

Conclusions

The concept of minimally invasive surgery has been a major challenge in the last 20 years. Among the pioneering specialties there is no doubt that endoscopy and arthroscopy are at the forefront of progress in this field. Since 1989 the holmium:YAG laser has become largely integrated into the new panoply of surgical instruments. Ease of use for the surgeon, a bloodless intra-articular field without tourniquet, and simple postoperative recovery allowing an early return to physical activities are the main advantages of this tool. To date, data reveal no complications specific to laser. However, absolute respect for its conditions of use is essential if inappropriate surgical indications and procedures, leading to treatment errors and complications, are to be avoided.

References

[1] Ahuja S, Bullough P (1978) Osteonecrosis of the knee. A clinicopathological study in twenty-eight patients. J Bone Joint Surg (Am) 60:191–197
[2] Asshauer T, Jansen T, Oberthür T, Delacrétaz G (1995) Holmium laser ablation of cartilage. Effects of cavitation bubbles. SPIE San José 95:1–6
[3] Asshauer T, Rink K, Delacrétaz G, Salathé R, Gerber B, Frenz M, Pratisto H, Ith M, Romano V, Weber H (1994) Acoustic transient generation in pulsed holmium laser ablation under water. SPIE 2134A:423–433
[4] Athanasian E, Wickiewicz T, Warren R (1995) Osteonecrosis of the femoral condyle after arthroscopic reconstruction of a cruciate ligament. J Bone Joint Surg (Am) 77:418–422
[5] Atik O (1995) Chondroplasty using holmium:YAG laser vs conventional instruments. International Musculoskeletal Laser Society and Orthopaedic Laser Soiciety of North America. Combined Scientific Meeting and International Congress 1–3 December 1995, South Lake Tahoe, Nevada
[6] Brahme S, Fox J, Ferkel R, Friedman M (1991) Osteonecrosis of the knee after arthroscopic surgery. Diagnosis with MRI imaging. Radiology 178:851–853
[7] Brillhart A (1994) Arthroscopic laser surgery, clinical applications. Springer, Berlin Heidelberg New York, pp 1–299

[8] Brillhart A (1995) Avascular necrosis, chondrolysis, hemarthrosis, synovitis and arthroscopic laser surgery. International Musculoskeletal Laser Society and Orthopaedic Laser Society of North America Combined Scientific Meeting and International Congress, 1–3 December 1995, South Lake Tahoe, Nevada

[9] Delbart P, Lafourcade D, Calmet G, Perringerard Y (1994) Pathologie méniscale, arthroscopie justifiée, complications (algodystrophie puis nécrose du plateau tibial interne). Rhumatologie 46:51–54

[10] Dillingham M, Fanton G (1990) The use of the holmium-YAG laser in operative knee arthroscopy – a double blind prospective study in using a new arthroscopic guided laser system. Arthroscopy 6:152

[11] Drucker M, Forman M, Venuto R, Weinstein M, Kaplan A (1996) Osteonecrosis of the knee following conventional and laser assisted arthroscopy. Presented at 15th Annual Meeting of the Arthroscopic Association of North America, Washington DC, 11–14 April 1996

[12] Dunstan D, Evans R, Somers N (1992) Bone death in transient regional osteoporosis. Bone 13:161–165

[13] Fink B, Schneider T, Braunstein S, Schmielau G, Rüther W (1996) Holmium:YAG laser-induced aseptic bone necrosis of the femoral condyle. Arthroscopy 12:217–223

[14] Garino J, Lotke P, Sapega A, Reilly P, Esterhai J (1995) Osteonecrosis of the knee following laser-assisted arthroscopic surgery: a report of six cases. Arthrosc Rel Surge 11:467–474

[15] Guten G, Kenney L (1995) Comparative study of patients' response to laser vs non-laser arthroscopic knee procedures. American Society for Laser Medicine and Surgery Abstracts p 30

[16] Hernigou P (1993) Idiopathic osteonecrosis of the internal femoral condyle, prognostic elements and role of different treatments. Rev Rhum 60:203–211

[17] Insall J, Aglietti P, Bullough P, Windsor R (1993) Osteonecrosis. In: Insall J, Windsor R, Scott W, Kelley M, Aglietti P (eds) Surgery of the knee. Churchill Livingstone, 609 633

[18] Jansen E, Asshauer T, Frenz M, Motamedi M, Delacrétaz G, Welch A (1996) Effect of pulse duration on bubble formation and laser-induced pressure waves during holmium laser ablation. Lasers Surgery Med 18:278–293

[19] Kunz M (1995) Arthroscopical laser surgery in knee. A 2-year follow-up. International Musculoskeletal Laser Society and Orthopaedic Laser Society of North America Combined Scientific Meeting and International Congress, 1–3 December 1995, South Lake Tahoe, Nevada

[20] McCarthy E (1982) Aseptic necrosis of bone, an historic perspective. Clin Orthop 168:216–221

[21] Muscolo L, Costa-Paz M, Makino A, Ayerza M (1996) Osteonecrosis of the knee following arthroscopic meniscectomy in patients over 50 years old. Arthroscopy 12:273–279

[22] Norman A, Baker N (1978) Spontaneous osteonecrosis of the knee and medial meniscal tears. Radiology 129:653–656

[23] Paulos L (1996) Laser chondroplasty and aseptic necrosis. Paper presented at Arthroscopic Surgery 1996, Scottsdale, Arizona, 17 January 1996

[24] Rangger C, Klestil T, Gloetzer W, Kemmler G, Benedetto K (1995) Osteoarthritis after arthroscopic partial meniscectomy. Sports Med 23:240–244

[25] Rohde H (1979) Symptoms and therapy of spontaneous osteonecrosis of the medial femoral condyle in elder patients. Arch Orthop Trauma Surg 95:81–87

[26] Rozbruch S, Wickiewicz T, DiCarlo E, Potter H (1996) Osteonecrosis of the knee following arthroscopic laser meniscectomy. Arthroscopy 12:245–250

[27] Santori N, Condello V, Adriani E, Mariani P (1995) Osteonecrosis after arthroscopic medial meniscectomy. J Arthrosc Rel Surg 11:220–224

[28] Shelbourne K, Nitz P (1990) Accelerated rehabilitation after anterior crucial ligament reconstruction. Am J Sports Med 18:292–299

[29] Sherk H (1990) Lasers in orthopaedics. Lippincott, Philadelphia

[30] Siebert W, Saunier J, Gerber B, Lübbers C (1995) Two year follow-up results of arthroscopic laser surgery, of the knee: European multicenter study. Techn Orthopaed 10:309–317

[31] Small N (1994) Complications in arthroscopy. In: Small N (ed) Complications in orthopaedic surgery, 3rd edn. Lippincott, Philadelphia, pp 1107–1122

[32] Thal R, Dänziger M, Kelly A (1996) Delayed articular cartilage slough: two cases resulting from holmium:YAG laser damage to normal articular cartilage and a review of the literature. Arthroscopy 12:92–98

[33] Walker T (1995) 2.1 Holmium:YAG arthroscopic laser surgery: prospective report of 100 cases. In: Brillhart A (ed) Arthroscopic laser surgery. Spinger, Berlin Heidelberg New York, pp 269–279

Complications of Arthroscopic Laser Surgery

A. T. Brillhart

Introduction

"Lasers do not cause complications, surgeons do." This quote represents the most important fact that needs to be recognized in avoiding complications of laser surgery. Education and subsequent understanding of arthroscopic laser systems is the most important role of the International Musculoskeletal Laser Society (IMLAS). An all-out effort to understand laser tissue effects, both short and long-term, as well as the techniques of obtaining these effects is critical. All reported complications have one thing in common: ignorance of some related aspect of laser use. This chapter highlights the reported complications, the potential hazards, the treatment of known complications, documentation and reporting, as well as methods of prevention [1]. As with any surgical instruments, arthroscopic lasers can cause complications if improperly used.

Known Complications of Arthroscopic Laser Surgery

The worst complications that have been published are associated with gas distention arthroscopy of the shoulder and knee in which the CO_2 laser was also used. The CO_2 laser itself did not cause these severe complications, but the gas distention technique did. These complications relate to the absorption and displacement of CO_2 gas that is first pressured into the joint and either embolized or directly absorbed into a body cavity. Dr. Chadwick Smith witnessed pneumothoraces in his patients when using the gas distention technique along with the CO_2 laser in shoulder cases. In the United States, the Federal Food and Drug Administration (FDA) has not approved the use of the CO_2 laser in the shoulder for this reason. Dr. Stephen Abelow has reported a case of pneumoperitoneum with the gas distention technique for CO_2 laser arthroscopy of the knee.

Five cases of avascular necrosis of bone caused by the 1.06 μm neodymium:YAG laser have been published by Garino et al. Several thousand joules of energy were used on the femoral, tibial, or patellar surfaces in knees of patients who had chondromala-

cia. As would be expected, the majority of the laser energy was absorbed by the underlying pigmented bone marrow and not the unpigmented hyaline cartilage. Fibrous and avascular necrosis of the various condyles and/or patellas resulted. Further surgery was required for worsening of symptoms in the majority of the patients.

Three published reports of avascular necrosis of bone associated with arthroscopy during which the 2.1 μm holmium:YAG laser was used for partial meniscectomies have not scientifically explained a mechanism but merely an association. This association is no different when mechanical instruments are used for partial meniscectomy and avascular necrosis is noted postoperatively. Documentation of laser energy being used on the condylar surfaces as part of the procedures was never qualified nor quantified. Amazingly, preoperative MRI studies to document that the problems did not exist prior to laser applications were not provided. A more detailed study was recently presented at the Annual Meeting of the Arthroscopy Association of North America in which avascular necrosis seemed to be more commonly associated with laser use than when mechanical tools were used for partial meniscectomy. The rate of increase was not alarming and could be inaccurate in light of a new report on the same association with mechanical tools. It is interesting to note that the authors pointed out that the overall complicational rate was higher when mechanical tools were used than when lasers were used. No quantitative nor qualitative data were presented to reveal how much or whether any laser energy was used in all of the cases on the condylar surfaces in this study also.

Treatment of Arthroscopic Laser Complications

Intraoperative air embolism can represent a life-threatening emergency. Air embolism must be recognized by the anesthesiologist and treated by his protocols. The insufflation device must be disconnected and the operation terminated immediately. The extremities should be elevated above the heart and head. If a tourniquet has not been used consideration should be given to applying one. The patient should be monitored in the intensive care unit by a critical care specialist and neurologist for at least 48 h. Appropriate X-rays of the head, chest and abdomen should be obtained. Respiratory support may be required. Overall, the best treatment is prevention. Residual permanent neurological problems can result. Pneumothoraces are treated best by a pulmonary specialist or general surgeon. Again, recognition is the responsibility of the anesthesiologist. The operation and insufflation must be abandoned immediately when and if this problem is recognized. Avascular necrosis of bone has many treatments available, none of which are 100 % reliable. The most common treatment is to keep the patient on crutches, nonweightbearing, until clinical and radiographic healing of bone is seen. With rapid progression and collapse of the condyle, replacement arthroplasty may be considered. Osteotomies, bone grafting, and allografts have unpredictable results. Patellectomy is an option if the patella is involved. A recent report of bone grafting with an arthroscopic-assisted procedure is interesting.

Documentation and Reporting

There are eight parameters that should be recorded in each operative note of an arthroscopic laser procedure. These parameters are often overlooked by inexperienced surgeons, authors, and reporters of anecdotal complications. Without the complete list for each case, it is impossible to form scientific conclusions on cause and effect. Patient outcomes are not reliable unless the information is available. The proper operating note, case report, and patient result should mention these parameters. Simply recording that a laser has been used is no different than stating that a surgical procedure was carried out with a knife and leaving out further details. How the laser was used is essential. How laser energy is used in an arthroscopic procedure cannot be understood completely without understanding these parameters:
1. Laser device and its wavelength
2. Delivery system
3. Energy settings
4. Total energy used
5. Tissue type
6. Arthroscopic medium
7. Technique of the surgeon
8. Surface area of the tissue
These parameters will allow the investigator to understand the approximate fluence or amount of energy per square millimeter. Energy fluence equals energy per pulse over area or spot size, which equals joules per square millimeter [EIA = energy/pulse area (spot size) = I/mm^2]. If too much energy is used, necrosis may be anticipated. If too little energy is used, no effect may be expected. Ignoring this information eliminates scientific critique.

Potential Hazards

By far and away the vast majority of complications that could arise from arthroscopic laser surgery have never been reported. The potential hazards are much greater than when mechanical tools are used. Foot pedal clutter can lead to inadvertent firing of the laser. This can set the drapes on fire and burn the patient. The CO_2 laser and the 1.06-µm neodymium:YAG laser have a nominal hazard zone far greater than the useful distance between the probe tip and tissue. This is also true to a lesser degree of the 2.1-µm holmium:YAG laser. Therefore, all arthroscopic lasers should not be fired outside the joint. Eye injury is a concern if protective eyewear is not worn. The CO_2 laser beam can damage the cornea. The 1.06-µm neodymium:YAG laser beam can damage the retina. The 2.1-µm holmium:YAG laser can damage the cornea and somewhat beyond. The helium-neon laser can also damage the eye. Eyewear is specific to each individual laser. The protective goggles and glasses are not usually interchangeable. The patient, surgeon, and assistants, as well as all others within the operating room, should wear protective eyewear. An extra pair of goggles should be placed on the entrance to the room.

Endoscopic equipment damage is rare but can occur if the laser beam is directed into the endoscope. Inadvertent tissue effects, immediate and delayed, can occur if the surgeon misdirects the laser beam or exposes the target tissue to too much energy. Plume, or laser smoke, is copious when the CO_2 laser is used and a suction device is required for evacuation. Plume is produced by all lasers. As with electrocautery, undesirable particles of tissue and even viral particles can be transmitted through plume. Such effects from infrared laser such as the 2.1-µm holmium:YAG laser have never been reported. They are not as much of a concern as they are with the high-energy, shorter wavelengths of the ultraviolet lasers. Nevertheless, no mutagenic effects have ever been reported with the use of the 0.038-µm excimer laser. Bright and shiny objects found within the joints, such as the surfaces of polished metal total knee replacements, reflect laser beams and can promote complications if this is not considered. Reflectance is a factor when consideration is given to avoid inadvertent tissue damage, fire, eye damage, and other undesired effects. The surgeon should not view the laser beam directly through the endoscope with the naked eye because the laser beam can be reflected or directly transmitted to this eye from the lens.

Safety and Institutional Controls

The institution in which arthroscopic lasers are used is responsible for establishing and enforcing policies that ultimately protect the patient and the personnel involved. These policies should be based on American National Standards Institute (ANSI) standards and govermental regulations, and most of all common sense. The institution and the surgeon should contact organizations such as the International Musculoskeletal Laser Society (IMLAS) and the Orthopaedic Laser Society of North America (OLSNA) for information on how to formulate these policies if questions arise. The subject has been addressed extensively in the text edited by the present author. *Arthroscopic laser surgery: clinical applications* (Springer, New York, 1995). The following is reprinted from that text:

Composition of a Laser Safety Committee

The committee should be composed of, but not limited to, the following members:
Chief of medical advisory board or designee
Director of nursing
Laser safety officer
Chief of anesthesia or designee
Biomedical engineer
Administration or financial representative
Surgeon from each department utilizing a laser

Duties of the Laser Safety Committee

The duties of the laser safety committee should be as follows:
1. To review, no less often than annually, laser safety policies and standards of practice.
2. To be responsible for coordinating ongoing activity as to the laser(s) in the center (i.e., credentialing, education requirements, maintenance, reviewing of standards to ensure they are current).
3. To ensure that (a) the standards address, as a minimum, restriction of those allowed to use the laser clinically; and (b) they have attended a laser workshop with a minimum of 4 h CME-approved (CME, Continuing Medical Education) credit. The workshop should include hands-on experience, laser basic sciences, laser safety, and equipment operation (must submit course outline).
4. To ensure that each physician requiring laser privileges has the necessary credentials that are wavelength- and procedure-specific. This physician must be credentialed in the basic laser procedures, but this certification does not credential the surgeon for similar procedures that do not require use of the laser.
5. To ensure that the credentialed surgeons be reviewed by the laser safety committee at the time of recredentialing for continued use of the laser. (Credentialed individuals who have not used the laser or attended an updated hands-on workshop between review periods require proctoring until the laser safety committeee deems the reinstatement application appropriate.)
6. To assist in the final decision as to the model purchased when a new laser is required.
7. To review and act on all incidents and accidents.
8. To meet no less than quarterly and maintain a permanent record of its proceedings, actions, reports, findings, and recommendations to the credentialing and risk management committees. A quorum of at least 50 % of the members must be present.

Laser Safety Officer

The laser safety officer, under the general direction of the director of nursing, directs, organizes, and coordinates all activities of the laser program. The laser safety officer functions as facilitator of nursing practice for quality patient care. The following is a list of typical responsibilities of the laser safety officer:
1. Supervises and evaluates, during training, the staff of the laser program
2. Assesses and evaluates the quality of care delivered and determines action to be taken in regard to staffing patterns and staff development needs; maintains, evaluates, and reports quality ensurance indicators
3. Coordinates the activities of the laser program within the operating room
4. Collaborates with director of nursing and the schedule coordinator to meet the needs of the physician, patient, and institution
5. Identifies learning needs of the staff; plans, develops, coordinates, implements, and evaluates teaching tools for individual and group education and support
6. Initiates and recommends policies and procedures necessary to achieve safe and appropriate use of the laser and the objectives of the laser program
7. Serves on the laser committee and functions as the laser resource person to physicians and staff members
8. Reviews, reports, and evaluates laser statistics to note trends as requested
9. Assists with laser procedures as needed
10. Remains current in the field of laser surgery
11. Ensures the appropriate medical surveillance of all workers, including eye examinations
12. Ensures that all workers are adequately trained
13. Maintains the laser log

Laser Safety Policy

The following rules and regulations must be observed by all physicians utilizing a laser and by all employees and any other individuals present during the demonstration or utilization of laser equipment. A copy of the rules and regulations should be issued to each individual directly or indirectly involved in the use of the laser.

1. When the laser is in use, the operating room staff directly involved in the procedure must wear a gown, gloves, laser mask, and protective eyewear. Laser-specific protective eyewear must be worn by all personnel within the room. Patients who are awake must wear a laser mask to eliminate contact with the smoke plume.
2. Patients undergoing laser procedures on the head and neck must have their eyes lubricated with a water-based artificial tear solution, taped closed, and covered with a moist eye pad or proper, specific eyewear. Eye pads should be kept moist throughout the procedure. Patients with local or regional block anesthesia must wear eyewear specific to the laser being used.
3. The laser is not used in the presence of flammables or explosives [i.e., anesthetics, preparation solutions, degreasing agents, combustible drying agents, or methane (intestinal gas)].
4. The master control key for the laser is retained by the laser safety officer(s) or designee who shall limit access to only those personnel qualified to use or operate the laser. The key is removed from the laser when it is not in use and is kept in the locked operating room medication room key cabinet.
5. A sign is posted on each operating room door leading into the room when the laser is in use. The sign states the type and class of laser, its maximum output, and the aiming beam and its output. Appropriate eye glasses are put with the sign on each door.
6. All physicians desiring to use the laser clinically must have been granted privileges by the institution's credentialing committee. A list of credentialed physicians is maintained at the surgical schedule desk along with the surgeon's privileges files.
7. The laser safety officer(s) or designee must be present whenever the laser is in operation. The laser safety officer/designee has full authority to supervise and control the laser. The laser safety officer/designee functions only as the laser operator during a procedure. Circulating duties are delegated to a registered nurse. The laser safety officer must be an insitution employee.
8. The laser machine remains off when not in use.

9. During the laser operation, the machine is placed on Standby when adjusting the power meter or when using other instrumentation (i.e., cautery, bipolar, or dissection). A verbal exchange must be undertaken between the laser surgeon and the laser operator at all times when there is a change in settings or power and regarding all other machine adjustments.
10. The operating surgeon controls the laser foot pedal with no other foot pedal(s) to operate.
11. All instrumentation and contiguous tissue are covered with moist sponges, towels, or cottonoids.
12. Those instruments that cannot be covered are brushfinished or ebonized if laser beam reflectance is a danger.
13. During oral, nasopharyngeal, or laryngotracheal surgery, the endotracheal tube, if used, must be a special laser-shielded tube. Cuffs are inflated with dyed saline and padded with moist cottonoids. (*Caution: Laser-shielded tubes can be used only when the laser is in pulsed mode and under 20 W power.*) Any visible reflective surface shall be covered with moist cottonoids. *A polyvinylchloride tube must never be used.*
14. Suction tubing to evacuate smoke and fluid from the operative site is attached to a suction canister in conjunction with a smoke evacuator or in-line filter.
15. Specifically manufactured laser facial masks should be worn by all personnel during laser operations to prevent inhalation of laser plumes.
16. Only medical-grade gases are purchased for use with the laser. The supplying company must provide written assurance of the purity of the gas and assume responsibility for any laser tube damage resulting from impure gases.
17. The laser safety officer, schedule coordinator, or director of nursing has the authority to shut down the laser in event of malfunction of the laser or associated equipment or noncompliance with the institution's policy and procedures for laser use.
18. Procedure- and wavelength-specific precautions must be observed.
19. A baseline funduscopic eye examination, including a macular evaluation, is required of all laser personnel and physicians.

10.6-μm CO$_2$ Laser Policy

WARNING: The 10.6-μm CO$_2$ laser is potentially hazardous if not properly used. The emergent beam can burn the skin or eyes or ignite clothing of the operator, bystanders, or patient. Do not use volatile sterilizing agents on the operative field, as a flash *fire may occur. Heat generated by the laser may cause the glass to fragment. Eye protection is usually required, and adequate venting of vaporized tissue is essential to avoid exposure to potential toxic agents produced in the plume.*

Use of the 10.6-μm CO_2 laser is restricted to physicians and staff members properly trained or credentialed. The purpose of these limits is to provide for patient safety during the use of the laser, personnel safety during use of the laser, and proper care and handling of the laser.

1. Only personnel qualified to use and operate the laser should have access to the laser key. The key is removed when the laser is not in operation and is kept locked in the operating room medication room key cabinet.

2. The laser safety officer or designee, trained in the proper care and handling of the laser, is assigned to each case.

3. The laser operator is responsible for documenting, on the operating room/laser record, the type of laser used.

4. A log is maintained and kept at the operating room control desk. The laser operator is responsible for recording the following information on each case:
   (a) Patient information (label)
   (b) Physician performing laser treatment
   (c) Type of procedure
   (d) Wattage, seconds, and mode used
   (e) Microscope/lens used, if applicable

5. Preoperative, intraoperative, and postoperative safety checklists are completed by the nurse for each procedure and maintained in the laser logbook.

6. All personnel, including the anesthesiologist, should wear laser safety eye protection with appropriate wavelength and optical density. Contact lenses, half-glasses, and sunglasses are not sufficient. Protective eyewear is not necessary for physicians using the microscope.

7. Additional goggles are kept at ready access outside the laser surgery room for personnel entering the laser area.

8. The patient's eyes should be covered with moist eye pads, which are kept moist throughout the procedure. When performing surgery under local or regional block anesthesia, the patient should wear protective eyewear.

9. Signs are posted on all doors entering the room, stating, "Laser surgery in progress."

10. The laser beam should not be aimed at any personnel, and personnel should not look directly into the 10.6-μm CO_2 or 0.632-μm helium-neon light source.

11. When the laser is not in use, the laser safety officer/designee switches the laser to Standby mode. If the laser is not in use for a substantial length of time, it should be turned off.

12. The laser should not be used in the presence of flammable anesthetics.

13. Alcohol solutions should not be used as a preparatory agent.

14. Whenever the laser is used near the area of the endotracheal tube special precautions must be observed: the laser endotracheal tube must be used as per the manufacturer's instructions.

15. All sponges on the field are moistened when the laser is used. Drapes close to the surgical site are covered with moist lap pads or moist towels.

16. Guard against the laser beam coming into contact with reflective instruments.

17. Extra suction should be available for the plume of smoke from vaporization of tissue. The suction bottle port exiting to the wall vacuum should be connected with a filter, available from the suction canister manufacturer. A heavy-duty smoke evacuator may be necessary for vaporization of large areas. Laser masks should be worn when the laser is in use.

18. The rectum must be packed with wet sponges when laser surgery is performed in the perineal area: methane gas is flammable, and a burn could occur.

19. The laser team is responsible for the cleaning, maintenance, and storage of laser instruments and equipment. After the operation is completed, return the arm to its proper position and secure the arm in its holder.

20. Surgical consent must be obtained from the patient, specifying the laser surgery to be performed.

21. Comply with the institution's policy for laser safety at all times.

22. Direct the laser beam at a target board to ensure location and quality of the focal spot. Use the built-in calibrations, if available. Check to ensure that connectors in the articulated arm are properly attached and secure.

23. Use the focusing head that has the shortest focal length applicable for each procedure. This practice minimizes any specular (mirror-like) reflections, because the reflected beam diverges more rapidly.

24. Do not use cautery with this laser.

25. Wear flame-retardant surgical clothing. Check that laundering does not change flammability characteristics. (Fabric softener is known to impair flame-retardation treatments.)

26. Maintain the plume exhaust nozzle within 10 cm of the site of the laser vaporization at all times; surgical masks must be worn.
27. Biomedical engineering representatives should be called if technical difficulties arise.
28. The surgeon and anesthesiologist should be aware of the risk of a gas embolus, and know how to recognize and treat it.
29. When gas insufflation is used, all operators must be trained on proper technique.
30. The gas insufflation device must be in proper working order before use. The biomedical engineer must inspect this device periodically.

1.06-μm Neodymium:YAG Laser Policy

WARNING: The 1.06-μm neodymium:YAG laser is potentially hazardous if not properly used. The emergent beam can burn the skin or eyes or ignite clothing of the operator, bystanders, or patient. Do not use volatile sterilizing agents in the operative field, as a flash fire may occur. Heat generated by the laser may cause the glass to fragment. Eye protection is usually required and adequate venting of vaporized tissue is essential to avoid exposure to potential toxic agents produced in the plume.

Follow these precautions to minimize the hazards to the eyes of bystanders from the direct and reflected beams of this laser:

1. If the patient is not positioned in the beam path, the beam should be directed toward the wall. Refelcted beams should strike a nearby wall behind the laser operator.
2. Do not allow persons without eye protection behind or at the side of the laser operator during laser treatment.
3. One or more pairs of eye protection (optical density of at least 5 at 1.06 μm) should be readily available at all times.
4. To avoid unauthorized use of a laser not in use, remove and secure the keyswitch master control key.
5. Only authorized persons knowledgeable in the use of the laser should operate the laser.
6. Post a laser warning sign at the closed door during laser operation.
7. If technical difficulties arise, contact the biomedical engineering representative.
8. Only contact lenses approved by the chief of service should be used with the laser.

1.44-μm Neodymium:YAG Laser Policy

WARNING: The 1.44-μm neodymium:YAG laser can be potentially hazardous if not properly used. The emergent beam can burn the skin or eyes or ignite the clothing of the operator, bystanders, or patient. Do not use volatile sterilization agents in the operative field, as a flash fire may occur. Heat generated by the laser may cause the glass to fragment. Eye protection is usually required, and adequate venting of vaporized tissue is essential to avoid exposure to potential toxic agents produced in the plume.

Follow these precautions to minimize the hazards to the eyes of bystanders from direct and reflected beams of this laser:

1. If patient is not positioned in the beam path, the beam should be directed toward the wall. Reflected beams should strike a nearby wall behind the laser operator.
2. Do not allow persons without eye protection behind or at the side of the laser operator during laser treatment.
3. One or more pairs of eye protection (optical density of at least 5 at 1.44 μm) should be readily available at all times.
4. To avoid unauthorized use of the laser that is not in use, remove and secure the keyswitch master control key.
5. Only authorized persons knowledgeable in the use of the laser should operate the laser.
6. Post a laser warning sign at the closed door during laser operation.
7. If technical difficulties arise, contact the biomedical engineering representative.
8. Only contact lenses approved by the chief of service should be used with the laser.

0.632-μm Helium-Neon Aiming Beam Laser Policy

WARNING: The 0.632-μm helium-neon aiming beam is not entirely safe.

1. Only authorized, trained personnel may operate the laser.
2. Do not direct the laser beam at the eye or at any reflective surfaces.
3. Secure the laser when not in use.
4. When directing the beam near the patient's face, secure eye protection over the patient's eyes.

2.1-μm Holmium:YAG Laser Policy

WARNING: The 2.1-μm holmium:YAG laser is potentially hazardous to the operator, bystanders, or patient if not properly used. The emergent beam can burn the skin or eyes and ignite clothing.

Precautions must be followed to minimize the potential hazard. The material below delineates proper use of the 2.1-μm holmium:YAG laser according to safety rules and regulations established by the institution's medical advisory board.

1. Obtain laser key, equipment, and laser.
2. Move equipment to the room in which the laser will be used.
3. Post "holmium laser in use" signs on all doors; secure additional safety eyewear on each door entering the room; and cover all windows in the room.
4. Keep operating room door closed.
5. Position the laser and plug into a 220-V outlet.
6. Put on safety glasses specific for 2.1-μm holmium:YAG laser. All personnel and the patient in the operating room must wear laser safety glasses or goggles with a minimum optical density of 4.0 at 2.1 μm to prevent accidental eye damage.
7. Open sterile items and place in the sterile field. For the sterile fiber delivery system, have a spare handpiece of the same degree available at all times.
8. Insert fiber delivery system into the fiberoptic receptacle; ensure a proper connection.
9. Turn key on. Warm up laser 30 min before the first case.
10. Select desired energy by depressing the energy/pulse increase or decrease button.
11. Select the rate by depressing the increase or decrease button.
12. Select aiming beam intensity.
13. Place the foot pedal near the surgeon's foot. Only one foot pedal at a time is to be near the surgeon's foot.
14. Press the Ready mode when the surgeon states that he or she is ready to deliver the treatment beam. Always return to Standby mode when the laser is not in use.
15. Turn key off at the end of the procedure and record the energy settings and total energy utilized in the operating room laser record.
16. Comply with the institution's policy for laser safety at all times.

Laser Credentialing of Physicians

A written policy is established for those who wish to use lasers within the institution, requiring the physician to obtain the necessary training and experience in the safe and appropriate use of lasers.

1. The physician seeking laser credentials must have staff privileges in good standing at the institution.
2. The physician must send a copy of the certificate of attendance for a laser course (4 h CME credit, to include safety, basic science, hands-on, and equipment operation training) to the chairman of the laser safety committee. The certificate should state the types of lasers involved and the number of contact hours given. Special consideration is given by the laser committee to physicians who undergo laser coursework and have gained experience during their residency or fellowship training. Appropriate documentation must be submitted to verify this experience. Clinical requirements are issued for each laser type and are not transferable to another laser.
3. Laser coursework or education programs are reviewed by the laser committee for approval of appropriateness, including those on safety, basic science, hands-on, and equipment operation.
4. The laser committee chairman contacts the physicians seeking laser credentialing to communicate that the coursework has been approved.
5. Applicants are required to meet with the laser safety officer for familiarization with the institution's lasers and equipment. They are also required to have a practice session before using the laser on patients. A preceptorship should be required.
6. The physician seeking laser credentials must contact a physician already credentialed in using that particular wavelength to precept the laser procedure (oversee the safe and appropriate use of the laser and complete a preceptor form). The laser safety officer delivers the completed form to the laser committee chairman.
7. The laser committee chairman submits the copy of the laser coursework and the preceptor form(s) to the director of administrative services for filing in the physician's folder. The specialty department chairman is notified to process the physician's request for privileges, and the credentials committee is told to make recommendations on which the governing board can act at their next scheduled meeting.
8. The credentials committee/medical advisory board action is forwarded to the governing board for final approval. The physician receives a written communication from the executive director as to the status of the laser credentialing approval. A copy of this letter is kept in the physician's file in the administrator's office.
9. The laser credentialing status is documented in the laser credentialing file of the institution by the laser committee chairman.
10. Preceptors are credentialed, experienced laser surgeons who observe, guide, and certify the applicant's acceptable performance. They report their findings, good or bad, to the laser safety committee. They have the authority to stop laser usage at any time during the preceptorship.

Applicant: I understand and have reviewed the policies and safety procedures for the laser surgery privileges for which I now apply.

Wavelength:
- ☐ 10.6 µm CO_2
- ☐ 2.1 µm holmium:YAG
- ☐ 1.06 µm neodymium:YAG
- ☐ 1.44 µm neodymium:YAG

Name: _____
(Please Print)

Specific Procedure _____

Office Address _____

_____

_____

_____ Signed _____
Date   Applicant

_____   _____
Date   Laser Section Representative

_____   _____
Date   Laser Safety Chairman

Signature _____ Date _____

Having satisfied above requirement, the applicant must demonstrate to his/her department chairman, in a minimum of three (3) procedures, his/her ability to operate in a safe and effective manner.

Certification of Laser Education

Laser course (attach CME certification copy and course outline)

_____   _____
Date of 1st   Preceptor Signature

Name _____

_____   _____
Date of 2nd   Preceptor Signature

Program Director _____

_____   _____
Date of 3rd   Preceptor Signature

Location _____

Date _____

I believe this applicant has demonstrated adequate proficiency in this procedure and so recommend unrestricted privileges.

I have read all safety rules of the institution and will follow them.

Final approval

_____ Approved _____
Preceptor for   Laser Section
Last Procedure   Representative

_____
Signature

_____   _____
Date   Laser Safety Chairman

Preceptor Form

A separate preceptor form is required for each laser type requested. In specialties in which adjunctive instrumentation for therapy is required, certification of training and documentation of experience with such instruments must be provided.

_____   _____
Date   Medical Advisory Board
                Chairman

_____   _____
Date   Governing Board
                Chairman

Fig. 1. Laser privilege form

Investigational Requirements

To use a laser that is not market-approved by the US FDA for a specific procedure, the laser-credentialed physician must petition the institutional review board (IRB) of the institution for consent for the procedure. The IRB reviews and grants approval to perform the procedure if all of the specified criteria have been met. The IRB routinely monitors the status of each investigational protocol to continue the investigation.

Physician Annual Credentialing Review Policy

The purpose of the annual physician review is to provide a means of reviewing physician laser utilization and to monitor laser credentialing status on an annual basis.

1. Each laser-credentialed physician's utilization is noted, based on statistics for the previous fiscal year.
2. Physicians with fewer than three laser procedures recorded are designated "low users." The laser committee then contacts each physician to determine the reason for the low utilization.
3. The laser committee reviews the analysis and recommends corrective measures to increase utilization and to help physicians who are "low users" to remain proficient in the laser's use.

Forms Used

Laser privilege form (Fig. 1, see page 129).

Requirements of the Laser Safety Committee for the Credentialing of Laser Privileges

The applicant must have received minimum laser surgery training from a recognized 4-h CME, including laser basic science, laser safety, hands-on experience, and equipment operation. This training may be waived based on documentation of residency training or previous experience and proficiency with appropriate credentialing at another institution (documentation to be attached).

Regulation of Vendors

Vendors, rental agents, and manufacturing representatives should obviously not be allowed to perform arthroscopic laser surgery on patients. Their exact role depends on many factors, but it must be defined by the rules and regulations for laser use of the institution. The ultimate responsibility for their action and safety rests with the institution. The institution must not believe that the vendor is justified in assuming responsibility of the hospitals and ambulatory surgical centers.

Appropriate and Inappropriate Uses of Arthroscopic Laser Systems

In the United States the FDA determines the safety of specific arthroscopic laser devices and delivery systems and approves their marketing for specific procedures on specific tissues (US Department of Health and Human Services, 1988). The FDA states it does not approve the lasers but does approve the marketing of the lasers. Each manufacturer is required to go through an approval process that includes limited, controlled clinical trials. A 510(k) Approval can be obtained by competitive manufacturer's if the FDA determines that the competitive manufacturer's device is essentially similar to an already approved device. Each manufacturer has a list of procedures and tissues for which their arthroscopic laser systems are approved. The surgeon must be aware of these specific indications prior to use. Use of arthroscopic laser systems outside the United States obviously requires a different approval process relative to the specific country in question. Each surgeon must be referred to his or her specific governmental regulatory body for approval. Beyond US federal approval, state regulatory agencies generally follow federal guidelines (US Department of Health and Human Services, 1983). Nevertheless, they should be contacted before arthroscopic lasers can be considered approved for marketing. The specific hospital or outpatient surgical center in which the arthroscopic laser system is to be used usually has the most stringent controls beyond the FDA. The hospital administration, the laser safety committee, and the operating room committee must approve the use of the arthroscopic laser systems for arthroscopy (Ball 1990; Brillhart 1991). From a medicolegal tort standpoint, the orthopedic community ultimately determines whether arthroscopic laser system use is acceptable. In the United States the American Academy of Orthopaedic Surgeons has issued a revised advisory statement in this regard. From a criminal standpoint, the FDA ist responsible for the enforcement of laws that apply to the improper use of laser systems. Each surgeon should obviously consult with these entities and an attorney if questions arise.

Current Indications for Arthroscopic Laser System Use

It is the current opinion of the author that there are two general indications for use of FDA market-approved arthroscopic laser systems (Brillhart 1992).
1. When, in the judgement of the surgeon, conventional instruments cannot cut, coagulate, or ablate tissue as safely or as well as the arthroscopic laser

2. When, in the judgement of the surgeon, the patient's outcome, immediate or long-term, will be better than when conventional instruments are used

Based on these two general indications, it is obvious that some surgeons justify arthroscopic laser use for virtually every operative arthroscopy they perform. At the other extreme, some arthroscopic surgeons are never able to justify the use of arthroscopic laser systems in their practice. As with the use of any other FDA market-approved arthroscopic instrument, the final decision to use that device rests with the judgement of the surgeon.

Definition of Inappropriate Arthroscopic Laser System Use

"Inappropriate" arthroscopic laser use should not be misconstrued to mean an absolute medical contraindication. What is inappropriate under most circumstances is not a contraindication in all circumstances. "Inappropriate" in this context means that I would not recommend use of the arthroscopic laser system, under the given circumstance.

In my opinion there are 11 circumstances in which use of arthroscopic laser systems should be considered inappropriate.

1. Use of a laser system that is not FDA market-approved, or an untested arthroscopic laser system, device, or probe, used in other than a approved research setting
2. Use of an arthroscopic laser system by an unauthorized individual or a surgeon untrained or noncredentialed for the specific arthroscopic laser system, except under qualified supervision for approved training purposes
3. Use of a faulty arthroscopic laser system, including reusing nonreusable disposable probes
4. Use of an arthroscopic laser system by a surgeon who does not comply with established rules and regulations
5. Use of an arthroscopic laser system in an unapproved or unsafe environment, especially in an unprepared office environment
6. Use of an arthroscopic laser for purposes of financial gain only and no patient benefit
7. Use of an arthroscopic laser for an instrument in an untested procedure other than in an approved research setting
8. Use of an arthroscopic laser without consideration to resultant pathology created from inadvertent tissue damage, including effects not desired because of unacceptable depth of penetration and delayed effects
9. Use of an arthroscopic laser system for surgery on an uninformed patient
10. Use of an arthroscopic laser system with a guarantee to the patient of unrealistic or "larger than life" results
11. Use of an arthrocopic laser system by a physician who is not skilled in arthroscopy (especially gas arthroscopy and the use of the 10.6-μm CO_2 laser), except under supervision for training purposes

Agencies currently involved in establishing regulations, guidelines, or advisory statements of laser use in the United States are as follows (US Department of Health and Human Services 1983, 1988; American National Standards Institute 1988; Ball 1990; Brillhart 1991; Sliney and Trokel 1993):

American Academy of Orthopaedic Surgeons (AAOS)
6300 North River Road
Rosemont, IL 60018-4262, USA
Tel. (+1) (708) 823-7186

American National Standards Institute (ANSI)
1430 Broadway
New York, NY 10018, USA
Tel. (+1) (212) 354-3300

American Society for Laser Medicine and Surgery (ASLMS)
813 Second Street, Suite 200
Wausau, WI 54401, USA
Tel. (+1) (715) 845-9283

Association of Operating Room Nurses (AORN)
10170 E. Mississippi Avenue
Denver, CO 80231, USA
Tel. (+1) (303) 755-6300

Food and Drug Administration (FDA)
Center for Devices and Radiological Health (CDRH)
1390 Piccard Drive
Rockville, MD 20850, USA
Tel. (+1) (301) 427-1307

Joint Commissions of Hospital Accreditation Organization (JCHAO)
1 Renaissance Boulevard
Oak Brook Terrace, IL 60181, USA
Tel. (+1) (708) 916-5600

Occupational Safety and Health Administration (OSHA)
200 Constitutional Avenue NW Rtr N 3647
Washington, DC 28210-0001, USA
Tel. (+1) (202) 523-6148

United States Department of Health and Human Services
200 Independence Avenue SW
Washington, DC 20201-0000, USA
Tel. (+1) (202) 475-0257

International Musculosketal Laser Society (IMLAS)
Wilhelmshöher Allee 345
34131 Kassel, Germany

Orthopaedic Laser Society of North America
(OLSNA)
c/o Dr. Stephen P. Abelow
212 Elks Point Rd. St. 200, P.O. Box 11889
Zephyr Cove, NV 89448, USA
Tel. (+1) (795) 588-3636; Fax. (+1) (775) 588-1299

The proper application of arthroscopic laser energy is the responsibility of the surgeon. This begins with selecting the laser wavelength for the operation. The temptation to use a specific laser device just because it is available must be avoided. The first decade of laser use has advanced laser arthroscopy beyond this problem. At the time of this writing the 2.1-μm holmium:YAG laser is the most popular laser used for arthroscopic laser surgery. Use of other laser systems including the 1.06-μm neodymium:YAG and the CO_2 laser must be limited to those surgeons who are specially trained and are familiar with their application. Far more clinical information exists with the use of 2.1-μm holmium:YAG laser.

Surgical technique for applying the 2.1-μm holmium:YAG laser is truly a matter of experience. A comprehensive understanding of energy technique is needed. Table 1 outlines a guideline for the settings of the 2.1-μm holmium:YAG device for most common procedures; however, the guidelines do not include a method to avoid applying too much energy. This is the most vulnerable point for the inexperienced surgeon. It is also the most significant gap in teaching. Table 1 presents, for the first time, guidelines that should be helpful in determining the amount of energy for safe laser use.

As a rule any procedure requiring more than 12 000 joules of energy is exceptional.

Table 1. Recommended surgical parameters for laser-assisted musculoskeletal arthroscopy

Salvage chondroplasty of entire partellar surface	2 000 J
Partial meniscectomy, degenerative tear	6 000 J
Lateral release	6 000 J
Minor synovectomy, knee	5 000 J
Major synovectomy, knee	12 000 J
Labral debridement, shoulder	4 000 J

Success of Arthroscopic Laser Surgery

As one recent report seems to indicate, the overall complication rate with laser arthroscopy appears to be as good if not better than that when mechanical tools are used. The recent attempts to incriminate the 2.1-μm holmium:YAG laser as a unique cause of avascular necrosis of bone have only resulted in the discovery that this phenomenon occurs with significant frequency when mechanical tools are used for partial meniscectomy. The witnessing of avascular necrosis caused by the 1.06-μm neodynium:YAG laser was not unexpected and has been warned against in the past years. The difference between the two laser systems and their tissue effects is obvious in that the 2.1-μm holmium:YAG laser beam penetrates less than 500 μm beyond the ablative zone, whereas the 1.06-μm neodymium:YAG laser beam penetrates as much as 5 mm beyond and this laser energy is absorbed predominantly in the subchondral marrow. Most arthroscopic laser surgeons now agree that the 2.1-μm holmium:YAG laser is the best for arthroscopic laser surgery at this time. It has not been associated with the technical complications of the CO_2 laser or the expense of the excimer laser nor the untoward reactions of the 1.06-μm neodymium:YAG laser. Over one half of a million arthroscopic laser probes have been sold and procedures performed with the 2.1-μm holmium:YAG laser with excellent results. With the advent of new procedures such as capsular shrinkage in the shoulder for instability and triangular fibrocartilage debridement in the wrist, arthroscopic laser surgery continues to increase in usage yearly. With the focus on this one system, arthroscopic laser surgery has become less complex and is now routine in the practice of thousands of orthopedic surgeons. It is reliable and safe when used in the correct environment and in the proper way by a trained surgeon.

References

[1] Brillart AT (ed) (1994) Arthroscopic laser surgery. Clinical applications. Springer, Berlin Heidelberg New York

MRI Modifications After Ho-2.1 Laser Knee Arthroscopy

J. A. Saunier · P. Kindynis · E. Juillerat · F. Indermühle

Introduction

Since its introduction in 1990 as a new tool in arthroscopic surgery, the Ho-2.1 laser has been used in more than 500 000 procedures. Most of the advantages of this laser use are related to its small size and hemostatic effect, and also the fact that it can be used as an "all-in-one" device for resection arthroscopy. These properties are unique and specific to the Ho-2.1 laser arthroscopic device.

However, controversies exist concerning the cost, efficiency, and adverse secondary effects of laser in the joint tissues, especially in subchondral bone. In our own experience of 1000 cases, we have observed one case of subchondral bone necrosis in a 74-year-old woman, which persuaded us to investigate this special point of interest. To assess the safety of the laser and to observe the modifications of the subchondral bone that occur after laser irradiation, we performed MRI studies before and after 50 surgical knee arthroscopies.

Materials and Methods

Fifty patients (31 male and 19 female) aged from 13 to 76 years old (mean age 47 years) underwent Ho-2.1 laser knee arthroscopy. The diagnoses were as shown in Fig. 1. Most torn menisci were degenerated and in 24/42 cases associated with medial condyle chondromalacia (grade II–IV, Outerbridge classification). "Others" included plicas, anterior cruciate ligament (ACL) tears (which were not reconstructed), synovitis, and ganglia.

Preoperatively, all patients underwent MRI (1.5 T, SignaHorizon superconductor and, since August 1996, Echospeed, GE Medical Systems, Milwaukee, Wis.).

To assess bone signal, two sequences were used:
1. Coronal T1 interleaved sequence, TR 200–400, TE 10–20, $512 \times 256 \times 256$ matrix 1.5–2 Nex.
2. Coronal T2 fat-suppressed FSE, contiguous slices, 4 mm thickness, TR 3500, TE 102, 256×128 matrix, 2 Nex.

The surgical treatment consisted of resection exclusively, with no bone drilling and no ACL plasty.

We performed 50 meniscectomies, 15 chondroplasties, and 7 other procedures, such as plica removal, synovectomy, and cyst resection (Fig. 2). No device other than the Ho-2.1 laser was used. Laser parameters as follows:
- Up to 40 W (20 Hz, 2 J) for synovectomies, plicae resection and meniscectomies.
- Up to 10 W (10 Hz, 1 J) for chondroplasies.

Most procedures were with a 30°-oriented probe. In chondroplasties, the 30° probe was used exclusively and was held tangentially to the chondral surface.

MRI was carried out again 4–8 weeks postoperatively (mean 6.2 weeks) with the same settings as preoperatively to asses any modification of bone signal and observe any adverse effect of the laser such as necrosis. The literature on the subject was also reviewed.

DIAGNOSIS

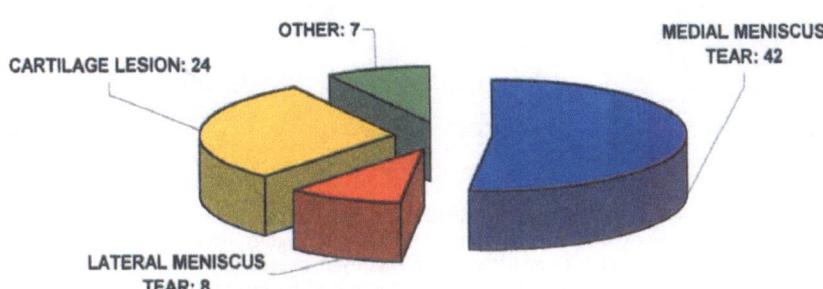

OTHER: 7

CARTILAGE LESION: 24

MEDIAL MENISCUS TEAR: 42

LATERAL MENISCUS TEAR: 8

Fig. 1. Diagnoses in 50 patients undergoing Ho-2.1 knee arthroscopy

TREATMENTS

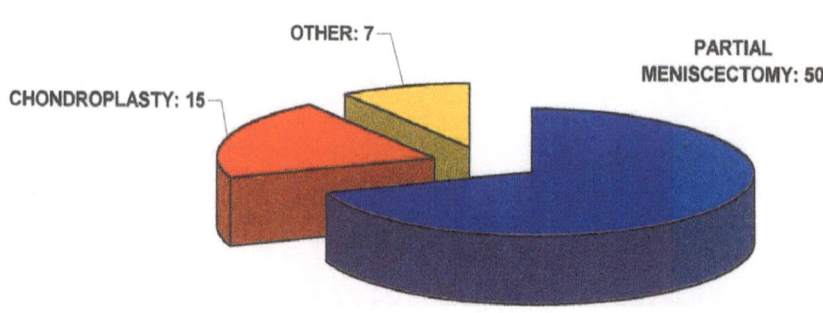

Fig. 2. Treatments given to 50 patients using Ho-2.1 knee arthroscopy

Results

Thirty-one patients (62 %) had a normal preoperative MRI, according to bone signal, without taking in account the intra-articular soft tissue lesions described above, and a normal postoperative MRI.

Eleven (22 %) patients presented edema or a hypodense signal preoperatively, which remained identical at the follow-up MRI in seven cases, reduced in three, and aggravated in one. This one, a 74-year-old woman, had an abnormal preoperative signal on the medial femoral condyle and the anterior tibial spine, which increased in the postoperative MRI. A second MRI had been done 6 months later, showing degenerative osteoarthritis (Figs. 3–5).

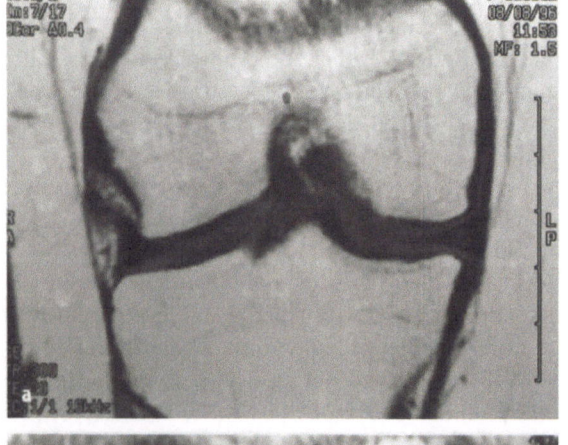

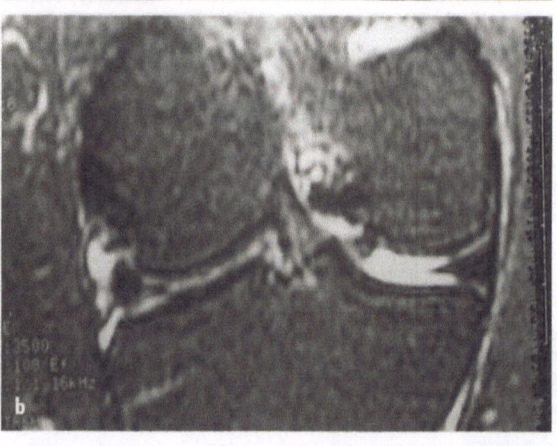

Fig. 3a, b. Patient 1 **a** Abnormal preoperative T1-weighted (**a**) and T2-weighted fat saturation MRI images in a 74-year-old woman, demonstrating slight mirror subchondral edema of the medial compartment and edema of the lateral tibial spine

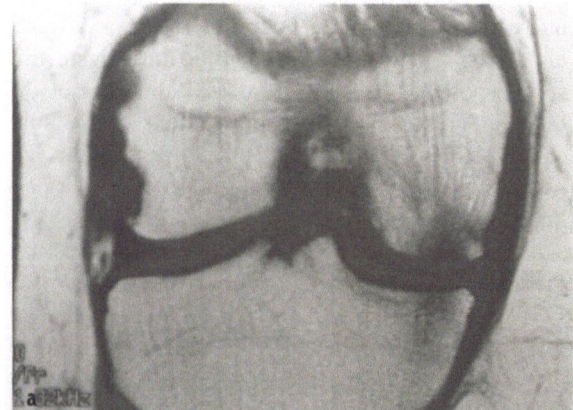

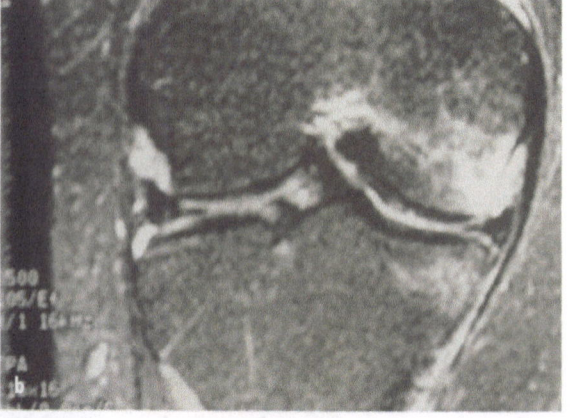

Fig. 4a, b. Patient 1. Two months after laser meniscectomy, the subchondral edema has slightly decreased in the medial compartment and slightly increased in the lateral tibial spine. **a** T1-weighted, **b** T2-weighted fat saruration MRI

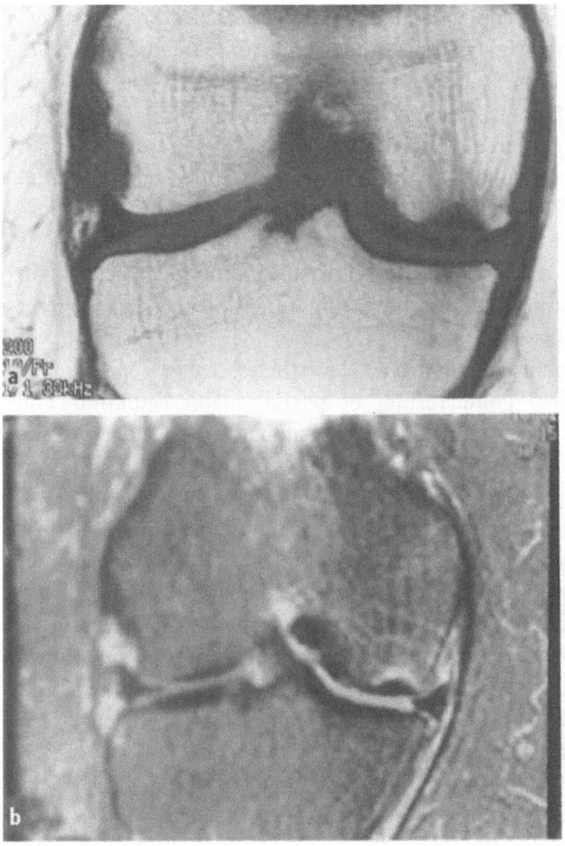

Fig. 5a, b. Patient 1. Degenerative arthritis 7 months after laser meniscectomy. a T1-weighted image demonstrates a mirror subchondral hyposignal of the medial compartment with flattened articular surface of the medial condyle and a tiny marginal osteophyte. b T2-weighted fat saturation image demonstrates hypointense subchondral sclerosis with subchondral cysts surrounded by marrow edema, typical of degenerative arthritis. Increased subchondral edema of the tibial plateau is also noticed

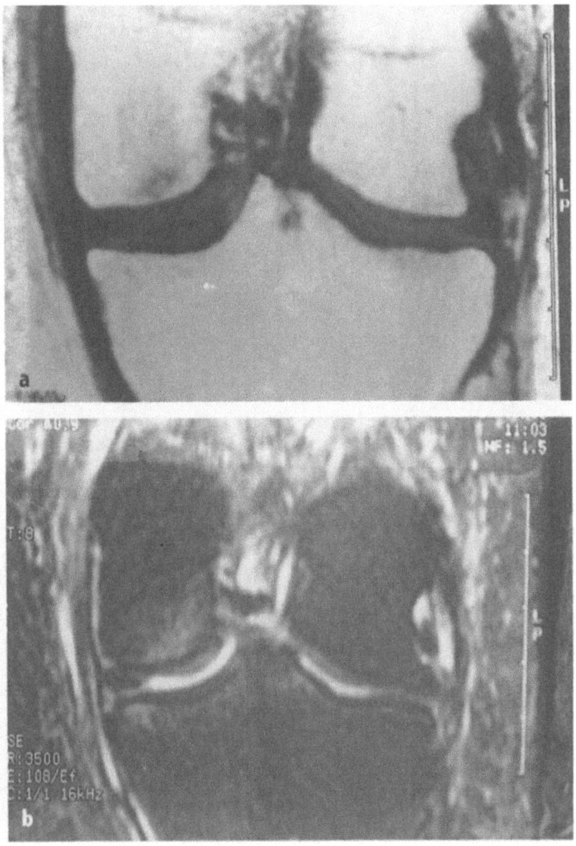

Fig. 6a, b. Patient 2. Normal preoperative MRI: a T1-weighted and b T2-weighted fat saturation images in a 60-year-old woman

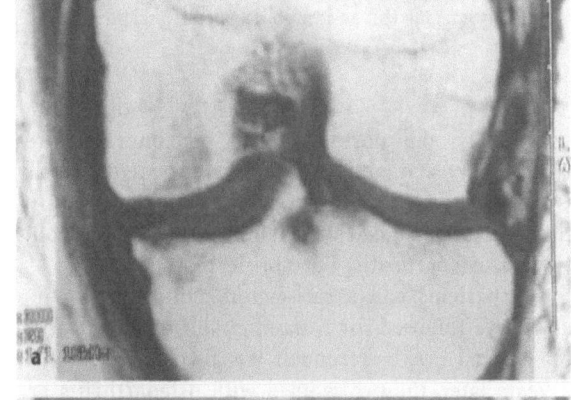

Eight patients (16 %) with a normal preoperative MRI had an abnormal postoperative one. In seven cases, we observed a slight edema or reflex sympathetic dystrophy signal; the clinical course was uneventful. In the last aggravated case, a 60-year-old woman developed a "mirror edema" and inflammation at follow-up which remained the same at further follow-up 3 and 5 months later and finally evolved into osteoarthritis (Fig. 6–8).

Only two of these last eight patients underwent chondroplatsy to remove large and unstable flaps.

There was no mean age difference between the three groups of patients.

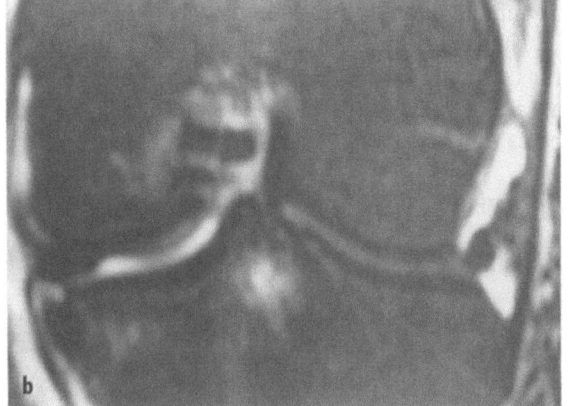

Fig. 7a, b. Patient 2. Abnormal MRI 2 months after laser meniscectomy: subchondral mirror edema of the medial compartment; hypointense on T1-weighted imaging (a) of the medial compartment, hypointense on T1-weighted imaging (a) and hyperintense on T2-weighted fat saturation imaging (b)

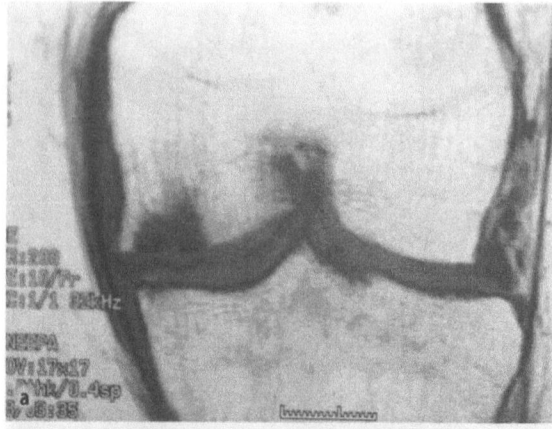

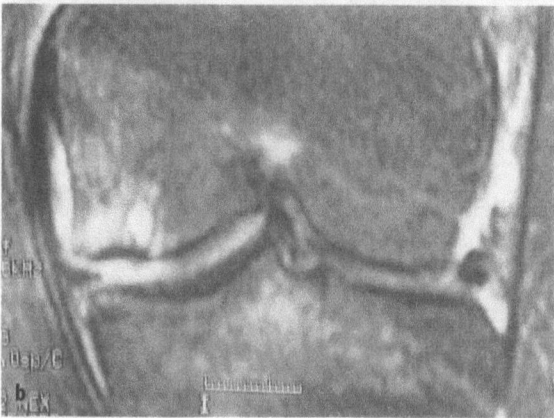

Fig. 8a, b. Patient 2. Degenerative arthritis, 5 months after laser meniscectomy: diminution in size of the subchondral edema on T1-weighted imaging (a) with increasing subchondral bone sclerosis shown by a hypointense signal on T2-weighted fat saturation imaging (b), as seen in degenerative arthritis

Thus, in 41 (82%) patients MRI was normal pre-operatively and postoperatively or abnormal pre-operatively and unchanged postoperatively. Only two patients (4%) showed significant aggravation of the MRI bone signal, with failure to heal and evolution to osteoarthritis, but not necrosis.

All patients had a satisfactory clinical follow-up and were followed for 6 months, during which time no clinical event presented. We also observed that, 2 years later, the two women with osteoarthritis are asymptomatic.

This study demonstrates bone signal abnormalities that may be observed preoperatively are not always aggravated postoperatively. There are even cases in which these abnormalities disappear.

Discussion

Biomechanical Aspect of the Meniscus

Formerly regarded as a development remnant, the meniscus is now recognized as an important structure of the knee joint. Its partial or complete removal

has biomechanical consequences leading to over-stressing of the other joint components, especially in the subchondral bone, and there are also biochemical changes [21]. In 1986 Radin and Rose [34] compared joint failure to heart failure, in which mechanical factors play a role, and established that the progression of cartilage lesions requires stiffness of the subchondral bone.

Baratz et al. [5] reported that the meniscus has an important weightbearing function and that contact stresses increase in proportion to the amount of meniscus removed. Nevertheless other reports confirm good results of partial meniscectomies. The problems are especially emphasized in older people, in whom poor results are reported in relation to articular cartilage condition [7, 8, 21–23].

Newman et al. [31] recommended early arthroscopic meniscectomy in cases of torn meniscus in order to avoid stress on the edge of the meniscal fragment, thus perhaps preventing aseptic necrosis in particularly vulnerable patients. Jackson and Rouse [22] concluded that a partial meniscectomy could reduce the pain arising from a torn meniscus, even in osteoarthritis.

It was generally considered that partial arthroscopic meniscectomy would reduce the risk of osteoarthritis, which was a common finding in total meniscectomies by arthrotomy. This statement is only partially true, Rangger et al. [35] having proved that even after very sparing meniscectomy, the risk persisted. Thus, again, the present authors emphasize the stress phenomenon in the development of post-meniscectomy osteoarthritis. Some stress fractures have also been discovered.

Aseptic Osteonecrosis of the Medial Femoral Condyle

Ahlbäck et al. [1] reported aseptic bone necrosis of the medial femoral condyle for the first time in 1968. This relates to the breakdown of subchondral bone in the weightbearing zones. Necrosis may also appear in the lateral condyle as in the tibial plateau. The etiology of the lesion remains uncertain, but at present the most current hypothesis implicates hyperpressure resulting in ischemia in an inexpandable tissue.

Necrosis of the medial femoral condyle appears more frequently in female subjects over the age of 70, with or without trauma [15].

Very recently, Reddy and Frederick [36] demonstrated the difference in blood flow between the medial and the lateral femoral condyle, which could explain, at least partially, why necrosis occurs more frequently in the medial femoral condyle than in the lateral one, and Johnson et al. [26] observed cartilage alteration and necrosis of osteocytes after so-called bone bruise on MRI.

Conventional Arthroscopy and Bone Necrosis

The hypothesis that conventional arthroscopy can provoke aseptic necrosis has been documented by several publications. In 1991, Brahme et al. [10] confirmed by MRI seven cases of reported asymptomatic necrosis among 611 patients who underwent arthroscopy. The authors attribute the etiology of these necroses more to the increase of stress on both cartilage and subchondral bone than to some unknown disastrous arthroscopic movement. Most of the patients were over 50 years of age.

Delbart et al. [12] reported one case of tibial bone necrosis after arthroscopic meniscus removal, followed by reflex sympathetic dystrophy. Santori et al. [38] described the development of aseptic necrosis in two patients after arthroscopic meniscectomy. They also cited excess of stress on the cartilage after resection of the meniscus as the reason for this development.

Very recently, Muscolo et al. [30] reported eight cases of femoral condyle necrosis after conventional arthroscopy and pointed to a stress phenomenon. Al-Kaar et al. [2] and Prues-Latour et al. [33] reported on nine cases of femoral condyle no necrosis after arthroscopy with preoperative and postoperative MRI; one of these cases is our own laser-related case. Drucker et al. [14] reported three cases of MRI-documented necrosis among 2700 conventional arthroscopies (see below). Fritschy et al. [17] reported 40 cases of femoral condyle necrosis after conventional arthroscopy in a European multicenter study.

Laser Arthroscopy and Bone Necrosis

Adverse effect and thermal injuries have been claimed after laser irradiation. Ith et al. [21], in fresh resected menisci, showed collateral thermal tissue damage up to 1 mm with the Ho laser, and Bernard et al. [6], in an experimental study in pigs, showed acceptable thermal lesions in resected menisci immediately postoperatively, but extension of the damage 2–12 weeks later. Asshauer et al. [3, 4] studied the acoustic shock wave in pulsed laser very precisely and showed how to reduce this risk with appropriate settings and a tangentially oriented probe.

Hendrich et al. [19], in a specific MRI study, ruled out the possibility of significant thermal damage due to Ho laser when used at settings appropriate for cartilage laser surgery.

Some authors report necrosis after laser arthroscopy. Six cases of bone necrosis were described by Garino et al. [18] after laser meniscectomy. In five cases a Nd:YAG laser was used and in one case probably a Ho laser. Rozbruch et al. [37] recently reported

a case of medial tibial plateau necrosis after a Nd:YAG laser-assisted meniscectomy in a 25-year-old woman. Fink et al. [15] reported two cases of femoral bone necrosis after Ho-2.1 laser arthroscopy. A third case showed MRI signs of bone necrosis, but no clinical evidence later on, even at arthroscopy.

Drucker et al. [14] reported 4 cases of MRI-documented necrosis among 558 Ho-2.1 laser-assisted surgical arthroscopies, versus 3 MRI-documented cases of necrosis among 2700 conventional arthroscopies. In the laser cases, the authors reported that in the cases where MRI necrosis occurred the laser settings were 56 % higher than the average setting in the other cases.

Janzen et al. [24] reported two cases of osteonecrosis after Nd:YAG laser meniscectomy. Two cases of cartilaginous lesions after Ho-2.1 laser-assisted meniscectomy were reported by Thal et al. [40], but there was no true relationship between the lesion and the laser. Bonutti et al. [9] presented three cases of femoral condylar necrosis and one case of chondral slough after Ho-2.1 laser-assisted chondroplasty. All four patients were women aged over 50 years. No complications occurred with lateral release or meniscectomy.

Thus, the review of the literature together with our own case show that, when one speaks of bone necrosis after Ho laser use, one is speaking about 11 cases in the world.

In a randomized study, Paulos et al. [32] compared patients operated on with a Ho-2.1 laser to those operated on with conventional instruments. Postoperative MRI was performed to search for abnormal temperature elevations. No statistically significant differences were found.

In a similar study, Sherk et al. [39] failed to find MRI evidence of necrosis after laser arthroscopy, while the MRI study by Kishimoto et al. [25] found no bone abnormalities after Ho-2.1 laser meniscectomy.

It is very important to distinguish the cases operated on with a Nd:YAG laser from those operated with a Ho laser. The Nd:YAG laser, because of its wavelength properties, can penetrate much more deeply into the surrounding tissues than the Ho-2.1 laser, which has a much better surface-limited effect. Thus, when talking about "lasers" it is of the highest importance to specify the wavelength and the power setting being considered. Because of these important physical differences, we disagree with Dr. A. Frank [16], who stated that, because there have been similar numbers of cases of bone necrosis after Nd:YAG and Ho:YAG laser treatment (7 vs 8) reported in the literature, these two lasers carry similar and important risks of bone necrosis. To the contrary Janecki et al. [23] demonstrated the innocuousness of the Ho laser in 504 chondroplasties in which no alteration was seen on postoperative MRI. It is also important to note that in this series the preoperative MRI revealed eight cases of femoral condyle necrosis, which remained unchanged postoperatively. Drez et al. [13] stated that the Ho-2.1 laser cannot produce a higher incidence of necrosis than conventional arthroscopy so long as safe parameters are used. Thus, we cannot find any report in the literature which clearly proves any necrotic effect of the Ho-2.1 laser when properly used with settings that are appropriate to the tissue to be removed.

Nevertheless, it is important to be aware of added risks in treating cartilage, especially in older women. The cartilage must be preserved as much as possible, whatever device is used. The power settings of the Ho laser should lie between 10 and 15 Hz and between 0.8 and 1 J; the beam must be directed tangentially with a 15° or 30° probe, never 70°. Finally, we consider that the Nd:YAG laser is contraindicated for this procedure.

No recent, properly conducted clinical publication has shown laser beam to be more dangerous than conventional instruments, particularly in regard to the risk of necrosis, as long as the operator observes the norms of wavelength, energy settings, directional impact of the probe, and, naturally, the indications for surgery.

We agree with Brillhart [11] when he states. "No case of significant avascular necrosis, chondrolysis or hemarthrosis has been reported with proper H:YAG laser use," and, "Laser does not cause bone necrosis, surgeons do!"

Conclusion

Partial arthroscopic meniscectomy is most often a successful operation. Nevertheless, one must keep in mind that it causes biomechanical modifications in the joint, especially in people older than 40 with cartilage lesions. The few cases of femoral condyle necrosis reported after arthroscopy are probably due to stress and vascular impairment.

In some cases, preoperative MRI can reveal an abnormal bone signal. Any postoperative bone signal modification must be compared with the preoperative MRI to assess what role the surgical procedure may have had.

MRI after laser arthroscopy showed some modifications, in a few cases, but not true bone necrosis. From a clinical point of view, all our patients showed improvement after the procedure, even thoses cases where osteoarthritis evolved.

The Ho-2.1 laser is a safe and useful tool when the appropriate settings are used, i. e., settings that are specific to the target tissue, with tangential direction of the probe, and with minimal chondroplasty performed. There is no scientific evidence that this tool can cause more bone necrosis than any other, conventional one.

References

[1] Ahlbäck S, Bauer G, Bohne W (1968) Spontaneous osteonecrosis of the knee. Arthritis Rheum 11:705–733
[2] Al-Kaar M, Garcia J, Fritschy D, Bonvin J (1997) Osteonécrose aseptique du condyle fémoral interne après méniscectomie par voie arthroscopique. J Radiol 78:283–288
[3] Asshauer, T, Rink K, Delacrétaz G, Salathé R, Geber B, Frenz M, Pratisto H et al (1994) Acoustic transient generation in pulsed holmium laser ablation underwater. SPIE 2134A:423–433
[4] Asshauer T, Rink K, Delecrétaz G (1994) Acoustic transient generation by holmium-laser-induced cavitation bubbles. J Appl Phys 76:5007–5013
[5] Baratz M, Fu F, Mengato R (1986) Meniscal tears: the effect of meniscectomy and of repair on intraarticular contact areas and stress in the human knee. A preliminary report. Am J Sports Med 14:270–274
[6] Bernard M, Grothues-Spork M, Hertel P, Moazami-Goudarzi Y (1996) Reactions of meniscal tissue after arthroscopic laser application: an in vivo study using five different laser systems. Arthroscopy 12:441–451
[7] Boe S, Hansen H (1986) Arthroscopic partial meniscectomy in patients aged over 50. J Bone Joint Surg Am 68B:707
[8] Bonamo J, Kessler K, Noah J (1992) Arthroscopic meniscectomy in patients over the age of 40. Am J Sports Med 20:422–429
[9] Bonutti et al (1997) American Academy of Orthopaedic Surgeons Annual Meeting, San Francisco
[10] Brahme SK, Fox JM, Ferkel R, Friedman M (1991) Osteonecrosis of the knee after arthroscopic surgery: diagnosis with MRI imaging. Radiology 178:851–853
[11] Brillhart A (1995) Avascular necrosis, chondrolysis, hemarthrosis, synovitis and arthroscopic laser surgery. Techn Orthop 4:346–351
[12] Delbart P, Lafourcade D, Calmet G, Peringerard Y (1994) Pathologie méniscale, arthroscopie justifiée, complications (algodystrophie puis nécrose du plateau tibial interne). Rheumatologie 46:51–54
[13] Drez et al (1998) Symposium on bone necrosis after arthroscopic surgery. American Academy of Orthopaedic Surgeons Annual Meeting, New Orleans
[14] Drucker M, Forman M, Venuto R, Weinstein M, Kaplan A (1996) Osteonecrosis of the knee following conventional and laser assisted arthroscopy. 15th Annual Meeting of the Arthroscopie Association of North America, Washington DC, 11–14 April 1996 (Abstract 81).
[15] Fink B, Schneider T, Braunstein S, Schmielau G, Rüther W (1996) Holmium:YAG laser-induced aseptic bone necrosis of the femoral condyle. Arthroscopy 12:217–223
[16] Frank A et al (1998) 8th ESSKA Meeting, Nice, 29 April-2 May 1998
[17] Fritschy et al (1998) 8th ESSKA Meeting, Nice, 19 April-2 May 1998
[18] Garino J, Lotke P, Sapega A, Reilly, Esterhai J (1995) Osteonecrosis of the knee following laser-assisted arthroscopic surgery: a report of six cases. Arthroscopy 11:467–474
[19] Hendrich C, Jakob P, Breitling T, Berden A, Krenn V, Haase A, Siebert W (1996) MRI measurement of the temperature distribution in cartilage following laser therapy. Orthopäde 25:17–20
[20] Insall J, Aglietti P, Bullough P, Windsor R (1993) Osteonecrosis. In: Insall J, Aglietti P, Bullough P, Windsor R (eds) Surgery of the knee. Churchill Livingston, Edinburgh, pp 609–633

[21] Ith M, Pratisto H, Staübli H, Altermatt H, Frenz M, Weber H (1996) Side-effects of laser therapy on cartilage. Sport Exerc Injury 12:207–209

[22] Jackson R, Rouse D (1982) The results of partial arthroscopic meniscectomy in patients over 40 years of age. J Bone Joint Surg [Br] 64B:481–485

[23] Janecki C, Perry M, Bonati A Bendel M (1998) Safe parameters for laser chondroplasty of the knee. Laser Surg Med 23:141–150

[24] Janzen D, Kosarek F, Helms C, Cannon W Jr, Wright J (1997) Osteonecrosis after contact neodymium:yttrium aluminium garnet arthroscopic laser meniscectomy. Am J Roentgenol 169:855–858

[25] Kishimoto et al (1998) 4th International Musculoskeletal Society Meeting, Kyoto, 5–7 November 1997

[26] Johnson D, Urban W, Caborn D, Vanarthos W, Carlson C (1998) Articular cartilage changes seen with magnetic resonance imaging: detected bone bruise associated with acute arterior cruciate ligament rupture. Am J Sprts Med 26:409–414

[27] Lanzer W, Komenda G (1990) Changes in articular cartilage after meniscectomy. Clin Orthop 252:41–48

[28] Lotke P, Lefkoe R, Ecker M (1981) Late results following medial meniscectomy in an older population. J Bone Joint Surg Am 63:115–119

[29] Matsusue Y, Thompson M (1996) Arthroscopic partial medial meniscectomy in patients over 40 years old: a 5 to 11-year follow-up study. Arthroscopy 12:39–44

[30] Muscolo D, Costa-Paz M, Makino A, Ayerza M (1996) Osteonecrosis of the knee following arthroscopic meniscectomy in patients over 50 years old. Arthroscopy 12:273–279

[31] Newman A, Daniels A, Birks R (1993) Principles and descision making in meniscal surgery. Arthroscopy 9:33-51

[32] Paolas L et al. (1996) Laser chondroplasty and aseptic necrosis. Paper presented at Arthroscopic Surgery 1996, Scottsdale, Ariz, 17 January 1996

[33] Prues-Latour V, Bonvin J, Fritsch D (1998) Nine cases of osteonecrosis in elderly patients following arthroscopic meniscectomy. Knee Surg Sports Traumatol Arthrose 6:142–147

[34] Radin E, Rose R (1986) Role of subchondral bone in the initiation and progression of cartilage damage. Clin Orthop 213:34–40

[35] Ranger C, Klestil T, Gloetzer W, Kemmler G, Benedetto K (1995) Osteoarthritis after arthroscopic partial meniscectomy. Am J Sports Med 23:240–244

[36] Reddy A, Frederick R (1998) Evaluation of the intraosseous and extraosseous blood supply to the distal femoral condyles. Am J Sports Med 26:415–419

[37] Rozbruch S, Wickiewicz T, DiCarlo E, Potter H (1996) Osteonecrosis of the knee following arthroscopic laser meniscectomy. Arthroscopy 12:245–250

[38] Santori N, Condello V, Adriani E, Mariani P (1995) Osteonecrosis after arthroscopic medical meniscectomy. Arthroscopy 11:220–224

[39] Sherk H et al (1996) 3rd International Musculoskeletal Laser Society Meeting, Kyoto, 5–7 November 1997

[40] Thal R, Dänziger M, Kelly A (1996) Delayed articular cartilage slough: two cases resulting from halmium:YAG laser damage to normal articular cartilage and a review of the literature. Arthroscopy 12:92–98

Laser Surgery on the Menisci

J. Raunest

Morphology of the Menisci: Implications for Clinical Laser Application

The menisci of the knee joint are fibrocartilaginous, crescent-shaped wedges interposed between the femoral condyles and the tibial plateau, thus serving a "socket function" which contributes to stabilizing the joint irrespective of its degree of flexion. They seem to be well adapted to their functional demands as the majority of collagenous fibers are dispersed circumferentially so as to transform varying vertical compressive loads into circumferential tensile strain to be absorbed by the collagenous fibers (Fig. 1). However, some of these fibers are orientated radially, particularly on the meniscal surfaces (Fig. 2). Disturbances in this complex arrangement caused by trauma or degeneration may result in a typical fibrillation of the meniscal edge and surface, which tends to progress as the arc-like configuration favors the disintegration of fibers [7].

In accordance with the geometric properties of the meniscus, vertical load applied during a gait cycle leads to regions of positive and negative shear forces, creating a boundary area in which radial strain develops on loading. This region corresponds to a special fiber arrangement called "middle perforating bundles" and coincides with the areas in which degenerations and ruptures can be observed most frequently. Occasionally, these bundles are visible macroscopically (Fig. 3).

Arterial perfusion of the menisci is provided by the middle genicular artery and the medial and lateral inferior genicular artery, which form an arterial network running in the parameniscal zone parallel to the outer circumference. Radially orientated vessels intrude upon the peripheral portion of the meniscus and create a microvascularized zone [43]. On the basis of morphological examinations performed by Scapinelli, three zones of the meniscus are to be distinguished according to their degree of vasculature [2]:

Zone I: avascular central area which constitutes three-quarters of the inner width of the meniscus

Zone II: microvascularized portion consisting of the peripheral rim

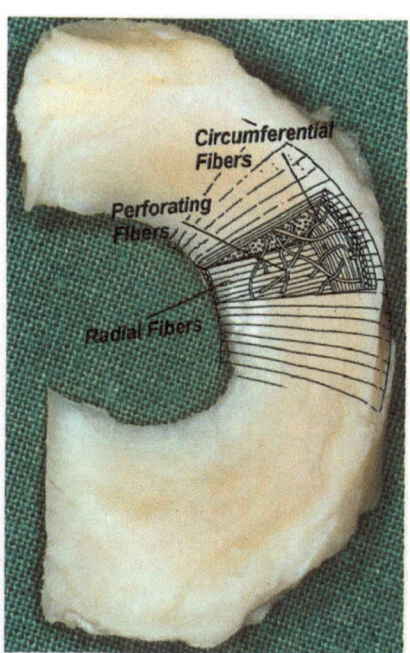

Fig. 1. Microscopic arrangement of the different fibers in the meniscus

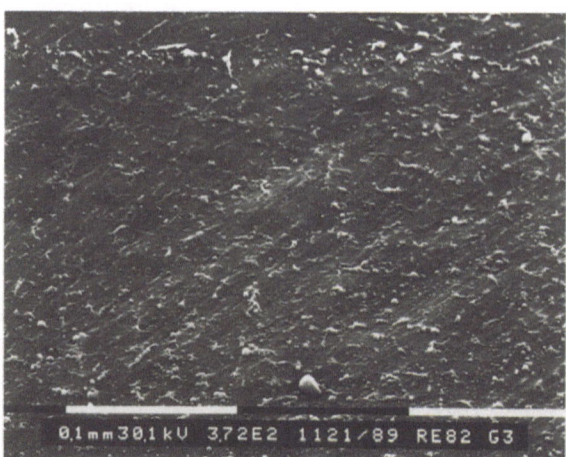

Fig. 2. Morphology of the radial fibers on the meniscal surface (SEM, × 276)

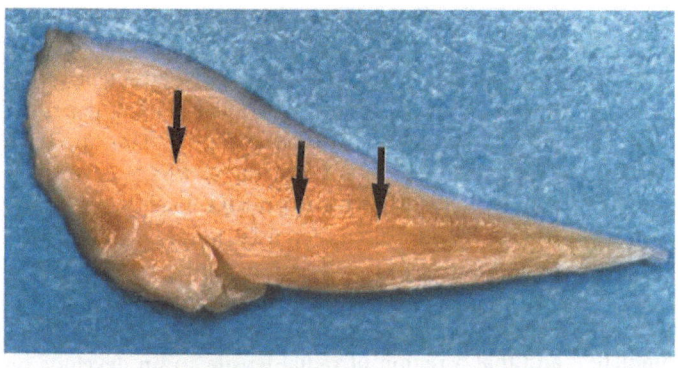

Fig. 3. Typical configuration of the collagenous fibers in the central part of the meniscus arranged as "middle perforating bundles"

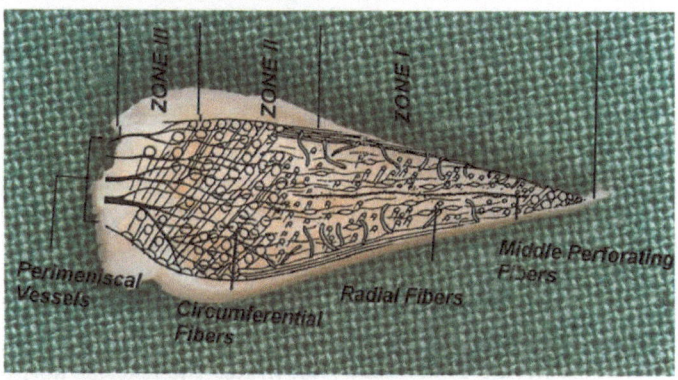

Fig. 4. Cross-section of the meniscus showing the classification of the three zones according to their degree of blood supply

Zone III: meniscocapsular junction bearing the perimeniscal arterial arc (Fig. 4).

This morphological differentiation leads to clinical implications with regard to the differential indications for meniscus resection and repair.

The changes in the main matrix components of the menisci with aging and degeneration consist in a decline of the collagen content, which increases from birth to the 3rd decade of life, then remains steady, and finally decreases towards the 7th and 8th decades. The most obvious changes are found in the noncollagenous matrix proteins, which decrease from a 22% concentration in neonates to 8% between the ages of 30 and 70 years [25]. On light microscopy these areas are characterized by an accumulation of myxoid material (Fig. 5). The specific content of water differs significantly between normal areas and regions of degeneration, allowing detection with the help of magnetic resonance imaging [12] (Fig. 6).

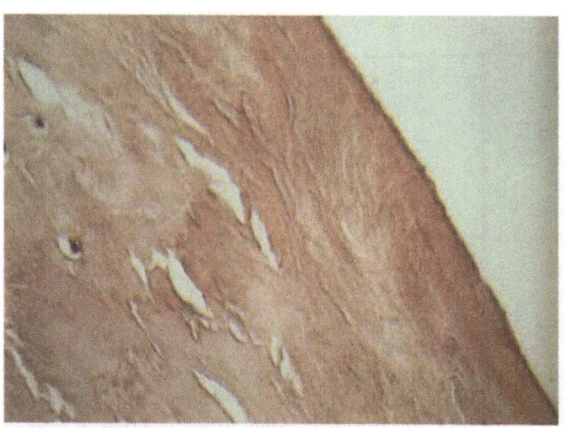

Fig. 5. Myxoid degeneration of the meniscus. (LM, × 68)

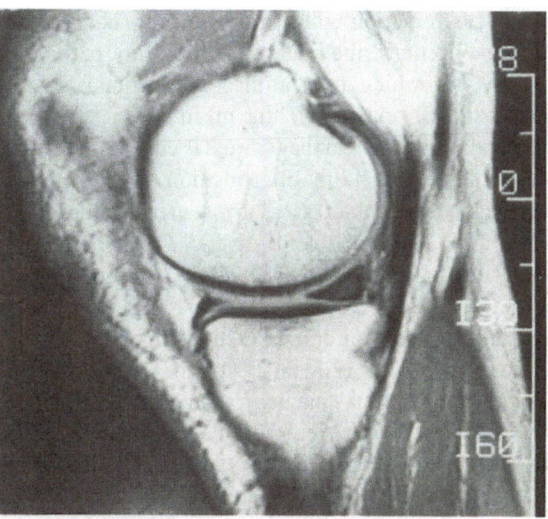

Fig. 6. Magnetic resonance image showing increased signal intensity in the area of the middle perforating fibers

Biomechanical Considerations

The knee joint possesses features characteristic of both a ginglymus and a trochoid joint, permitting extension and flexion as well as some rotation movement around the longitudinal axis of the leg. Rolling motions occur during the first 20° flexion; above that the motion is basically gliding. The knee joint is most stable at full extension, when rotational movements do not occur. The complex interplay of rolling and gliding motions prevents the femoral condyles from impinging on the posterior tibial plateau at complete flexion. Along with bony structures and the cruciate ligament complex, the knee joint menisci are central units in the control of joint kinematics. There is no evidence to suggest that these structures are undergoing phylogenetic regression [21, 45].

The complex functions of the menisci are not entirely confined to providing resistance to compression, but comprise:
- congruity of femur and tibia
- load transmission
- shock absorption
- stress reduction
- maintaining joint stability
- controlling extremes of flexion and extension
- articular cartilage lubrication and nutrition

The geometric structure and the material characteristics of the menisci provide unimpaired performance as stabilizers and transmitters of load as well as significantly reducing peak loads between tibia and femur during weight bearing. From experimental studies using cadaveric specimens it has been estimated that the lateral meniscus transmits 75 % of the axial load of the lateral joint compartment and the medial meniscus absorbs 50 % of the load applied to the medial compartment [15]. Due to the geometric properties of the femoral condyles and tibial plateau, meniscus resection will result in incongruence, leading to circumscribed areas exposed to pathologic peak loads which may induce chondromalacia and arthrosis. On extension, the mean contact areas of femoral and tibial cartilage are 2.9 cm^2 medially and 4.7 cm^2 laterally [26]. Interposition of the menisci increases the contact areas by a mean value of 3.7 cm^2 and 2.2 cm^2, respectively. Correspondingly, experimental studies and clinical reports have shown that meniscectomy may lead to loss of articular cartilage integrity and impaiment of joint stability [8]. According to experimental studies performed by Hehne et al., partial meniscectomy results in a 12 % loss of contact area, and subtotal or total resection in a loss of 46 % and 75 %, respectively [18]. The characteristic orientation of the collagenous fibers within the meniscus serves to dissipate tensile stresses on the long axis of the knee by converting the vertical com-

pressive loads into circumferentially orientated stresses [31]. With regard to their anchorage in the anterior and posterior areas, radial displacement of the menisci induced by compressional loading generates circumferential hoop stresses (Fig. 7). This approach shows that the internal stresses, which develop in response to varying compressive loads, are mainly translated into circumferential tensile strain that is absorbed by the collagenous fibers. The analysis also indicates that a horizontal boundary exists between areas of positive and negative shear strains, and that a region of radial tensile strain develops on mechanical loading. The cross-sectional shape, integrity of meniscal stability, and elastic modulus of the meniscal tissue may be decisive factors determining their biomechanical properties [19, 56].

In a gait cycle the menisci move backward during flexion, thus following the contact areas of tibial and femoral cartilage. This mechanism is facilitated by a close relationship between the quadriceps, popliteus, and semimembranous muscles and the meniscal function. In a synergistic action, contraction of the semimembranous and popliteus muscles pulls the meniscal attachments posteromedially and posterolaterally as the knee joint flexes. The anterior horns and the midparts of the menisci are exposed to strain

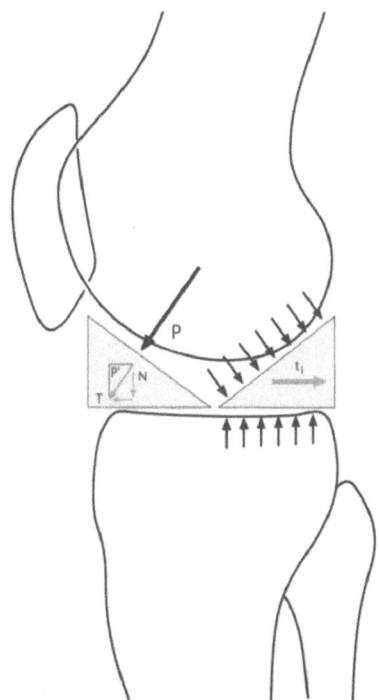

Fig. 7. Biomechanics of the menisci according to Kummer [31]. Loading of the knee joint leads to a compressive force P directed perpendicularly to the meniscal surface. P consists of two components: a tangential component T and an axial component N. The wedge-shaped configuration of the meniscus translates various compressive forces into a number of tangential forces t_i which create a circumferential tensile strain

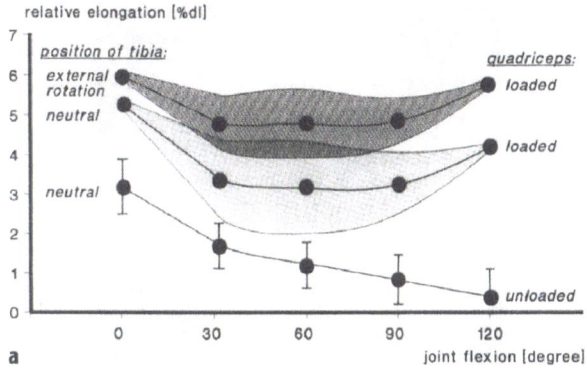

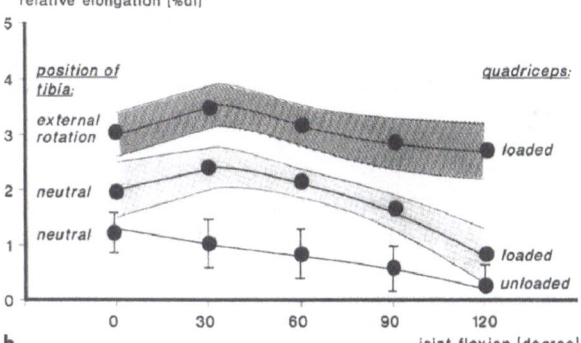

Fig. 8a, b. Stress and strain behavior of the anterior (**a**) and porterior (**b**) horns of the meniscus under conditions of weight bearing and external rotation of the tibia

forces, while the posterior horns are simultaneously compressed (Fig. 8). Due to its more spherical shape and less rigid attachment to capsular structures, especially in the area of the popliteal hiatus, the lateral meniscus has more mobility than the medial side.

While gliding and translation mechanisms are performed in the meniscotibial joint, in the meniscofemoral compartment flexion and extension are characteristic. At full extension the menisci rest in their most anterior position, which in combination with relaxation of the meniscotibial ligaments allows external rotation of the tibia in relation to the femoral condyles, creating the typical "screwed-home" mechanism with the anterior horns of the menisci acting as a block to further extension. Likewise, in full flexion the posterior horns are driven far posteriorly to assist in blocking any further flexion.

Most likely the menisci contribute to lubrication, by reducing the joint space available where fluid can pool and by decreasing contact stress. McConail et al. reported that the friction coefficient within the knee joint increases by 20 % following meniscectomy [34]. Furthermore, the semilunar cartilage serves to compress the nourishing synovial fluid into the articular cartilage by bearing a considerable shear of the load transmitted across the knee joint.

Indications for Resection, Reconstruction, and Repair

Today conventional meniscus surgery is based upon clearly defined indications which also relate without restrictions to laser surgery. Laser surgery is not indicated in cases where reconstruction or conservative therapy promises success. Depending on the morphology of the lesion and the degree of pre-existing degeneration, partial meniscectomy or a subtotal/total resection can be performed with the help of laser energy. Furthermore, laser surgery offers some advantage over conventional instruments by welding the fibrillated meniscus surface, thus providing a completely new way of tissue interaction.

Partial Meniscectomy

This technique consists of tissue removal up to the plane of the lesion (Fig. 9). The extent of resection depends on the prevalence of tissue degeneration. Horizontal cleavage tears especially are accompanied by an extended area of myxoid degradation which could form the basis for further ruptures if limited resection is carried out. Because of the typical three-dimensional arrangement of the collagenous fibers within the meniscus, the resection rim may transform into an area of fibrillation which promotes further degeneration and a recurrence of symptoms. In addition, large remnants of the posterior horn would also disturb joint mechanics and cause further ruptures and incarceration. From experimental and clinical studies there is evidence that partial meniscectomy carries a reduced risk of degenerative arthritis compared to subtotal or total resection [3, 60]. Therefore partial meniscectomy can be regarded as method of choice in both laser and conventional meniscus surgery.

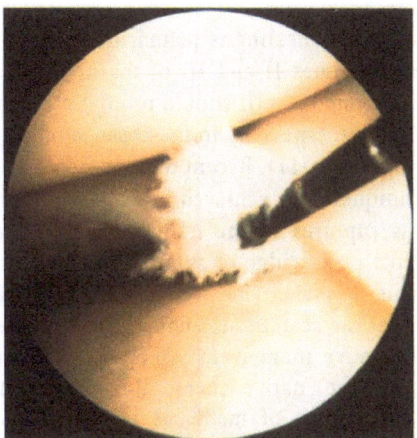

Fig. 9. Typical flap rupture in the posterior part of the meniscus: indication for selective flap resection

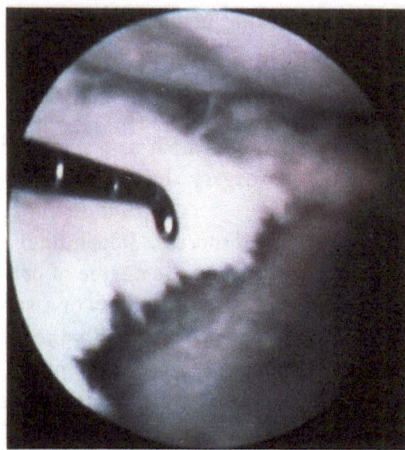

Fig. 10. Degenerated meniscus presenting fibrillations up to the meniscosynovial junction and multiple ruptures: indication for subtotal meniscectomy

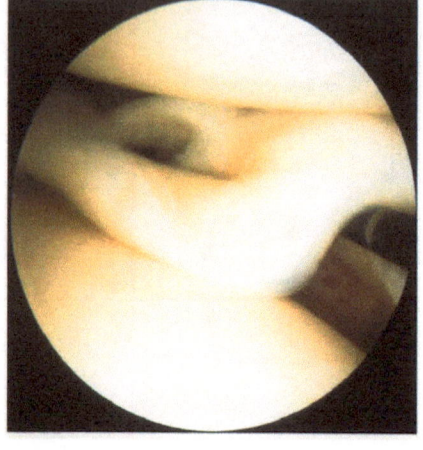

Fig. 11. Longitudinal rupture running over zone II of the meniscus. No significant degenerations present: indication for meniscal repair

Subtotal and Total Meniscectomy

In total meniscectomy the whole meniscus is excised, including the peripheral vascular zone. In subtotal meniscectomy the meniscocapsular junction is preserved. Clinical observations prove beyond doubt that the meniscus can regenerate from the well-vascularized peripheral zone [3]. However, differing histological structures and inadequate size of the regenerated structure indicate that this "pseudoregenerate" cannot achieve the full function of a healthy meniscus. Typical indications for subtotal resection are extended meniscal tears that cannot be repaired, especially in combination with severe degeneration, symptomatic discoid meniscus, and degenerative meniscus lesions in cases with advanced degenerative arthritis [6, 60]. As to the promotion of degenerative arthritis that follows subtotal excision of the meniscus, this procedure is only appropriate if no other operative options are available (Fig. 10).

Reconstruction, Meniscal Suture

The potential of healing is primarily confined to the vascularized zones II and III of the meniscus. Thus a lesion of zone II or III should prompt a reconstructive procedure, especially in the absence of degenerative changes (Fig. 11). Recent developments in operative techniques have achieved healing even of central meniscus ruptures in the nonvascularized areas by fibrin clots or a bridge of synovial tissue sutured in the meniscal cleft. However, animal experiments proved that the scar tissue achieved with these additional operative maneuvers offers lower mechanical resistance than native meniscal tissue. With the increasing success of meniscus reconstruction, the decision regarding laser-assisted resection must be weighed carefully in every individual with an eye to

the chances of reconstruction. On the other hand, recent developments in laser surgery offer first options to achieve successful tissue repair with the help of laser welding, so that the indication for laser surgery, confined so far to meniscus resection, is likely to be extended to meniscus repair [13, 42, 61].

Conservative Treatment

Indications for conservative, i.e., nonoperative, treatment are short longitudinal ruptures (≤ 1 cm) in the peripheral zone of the meniscus, short radial ruptures (≤ 0.5 cm) arising from the central margin, and circumscribed fibrillations of the meniscus rim. Recent research confirms that healing of these lesions can be promoted by laser-assisted tissue welding [20]. However, further in vivo studies are necessary before this procedure can be recommended as a routine method in clinical practice.

Shortcomings of Conventional Meniscus Surgery

Although developed to a high state of art, arthroscopic surgery of the menisci faces a number of technical problems and operative shortcomings that cannot be solved by an improvement of conventional instruments. Compared with open meniscectomy, arthroscopic techniques have offered a way of selective meniscal resection which exclusively affects the degenerated and ruptured tissue areas, preserving a maximum of healthy structure. Due to the narrowness of the joint space, especially in the posterior compartment where most meniscal derangement occurs, iatrogenic lesions to the hyaline cartilage next to the meniscus area to be resected by mechanical instruments are a common complication in

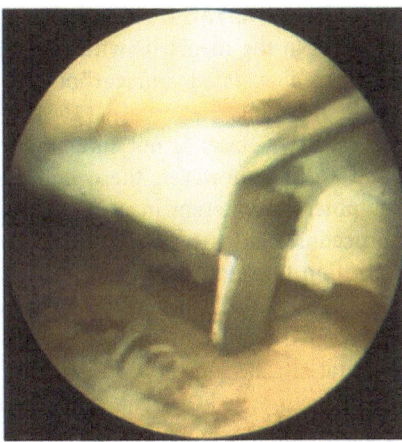

Fig. 12. Possible iatrogenic lesion to the hyaline cartilage during meniscectomy using an arthroscopic knife

meniscus surgery (Fig. 12) [17]. In their prospective clinical study Klein et al. found an 11.8 % rate of iatrogenic chondral lesions in arthroscopic surgery [29]. This entity, described as "arthroscopic arthropathy", is therefore common with arthroscopic surgery [28]. Experiences gained from experimental studies and clinical observations indicate that partial thickness defects of the hyaline cartilage created as adverse side effects of arthroscopic surgery have no significant tendency towards regeneration, so that the advantages of a minimally invasive arthroscopic procedure are – at least in part – reduced by the considerable risk of a permanent lesion to the hyaline cartilage surfaces [14].

Following arthroscopic surgery the configuration of the meniscal resection rim usually remains rough and fibrillated (Fig. 13). The specific arrangement of the collagenous bundles within the meniscal structure gives rise to further fibrillation, leading to degenerative changes and radially orientated rup-

tures. Although experimental investigations indicate that the meniscus has some regenerative properties, allowing a certain degree of remodeling and even the development of a pseudoregenerate arising from the meniscocapsular junction [3], clinical observations from control arthroscopies show the fibrillated resection borderline as the origin of further degeneration and rupture.

Compared with conventional surgery, laser energy offers some completely different qualities of tissue interaction that may contribute to a solution of the problems described above. Because of the relatively small dimension of the lightguides introduced to the meniscus the risk of iatrogenic joint lesions can be significantly reduced from that with conventional mechanical instruments, even within the limitations of a very narrow joint space. Furthermore, the ability of laser energy to induce welding of the collagenous fibers largely protects the meniscus rim from further fibrillation, thus stabilizing the collagenous network and reducing the risk of initiating degenerative arthritis [39, 49].

Laser Systems for Meniscus Surgery

Several laser systems have been used so far in the field of arthroscopic meniscus surgery. Figure 14 relates these laser types to their respective spectral ranges of emission. With regard to the predominant characteristics of laser tissue interaction, two basic principles can be distinguished: *ablation*, which creates tissue defects without any significant thermal alteration in the resection borders, and a *thermal* principle of tissue interaction that leads to coagulation and welding of the meniscal surface.

The optical properties of articular tissue determine the quality and effectiveness of laser tissue interaction in dependence on the specific laser output characteristics. Reflection, transmission, scattering, and absorption are the basic principles of reaction when laser light is directed onto any tissue structure [9, 46].

Ultraviolet lasers such as the 308 nm XeCl excimer laser are absorbed by specific components of protein molecules due to a photochemical mechanism which leads to bond breaking in tissue proteins, converting them to a gaseous plasma. This mode of

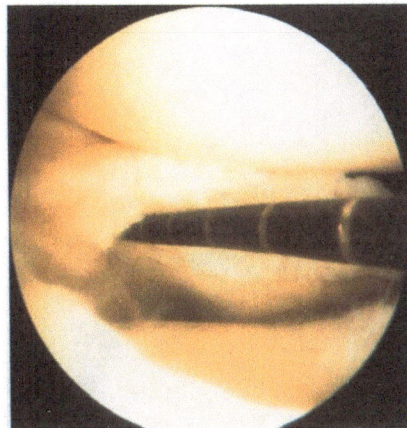

Fig. 13. Fibrillated resection rim following conventional arthroscopic resection

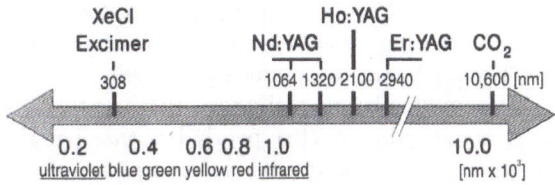

Fig. 14. Laser systems used for arthroscopic meniscectomy

operation contrasts with the photothermal mechanisms of infrared lasers, which depend on the conversion of light to heat through absorption phenomena. The maxima of absorption in human menisci are at 280 and 340 nm wavelengths, attributable to the presence of tryptophan and hydroxypyridinoline, respectively. The tissue effects of the XeCl excimer laser on fibrocartilage have been evaluated by Dressel et al., Kroitzsch et al., and Raunest et al. [10, 31, 39]. As the laser beam is delivered fiberoptically by 600 to 1000 μm lightguides, the practicability of its use in arthroscopic meniscectomy is excellent. There is basically no relevant photothermal effect with its use, and the fibrocartilage surfaces remaining after ablation are smooth and well delineated [10]. However, the relatively low amount of energy that can be delivered through a fused silica fiber restricts ablative effectivity and makes the excimer laser unsuited for meniscectomy in clinical practice. Another concern with regard to excimer lasers is the possibility of a mutagenic effect. As studies have proved so far, at least the 308 nm spectral range does not reveal any adverse consequence. The ArF and KrF excimer lasers, emitting at 193 nm and 248 nm, have no clinical importance in meniscal surgery bearing an increased risk of mutagenicity [30].

Mid-infrared and far-infrared lasers, such as the 2100 nm Ho:YAG laser, the 2940 nm Er:YAG laser, and the 10 600 nm CO_2 laser, are primarily absorbed by tissue water, which converts light energy to heat. With the power density exceeding the ablation threshold of tissue, these lasers are able to ablate and cut tissue. The Er:YAG and CO_2 lasers are well absorbed by water in the meniscus so that the ablation threshold is very low. The emission band of the Ho:YAG laser does not correspond directly to the typical water absorption peaks; however, this laser proved to be an excellent tool for cutting and ablation of fibrocartilage, provided that appropriate laser output characteristics above the typical ablation threshold for fibrocartilage are used. Under these conditions the Ho:YAG laser prevents thermal energy from spreading into the adjacent tissue and avoids adverse thermal side effects on the meniscal tissue [53]. In contrast, studies employing the CO_2 laser for meniscectomy revealed a considerable spread of thermal energy into the adjacent tissues, resulting in an extended transitional zone of protein denaturation [51, 57, 59]. The Er:YAG laser is quite effective for cutting and ablating meniscal tissue. Widespread clinical application is limited by the necessity of using an extremely rigid ZnCl lightguide which is too fragile for routine use [22, 46].

Near-infrared lasers, such as the 1064 nm Nd:YAG laser, are absorbed relative poorly by water but are absorbed by tissue chromophores and pigments. As fibrocartilage has a low content of chromophores,

the coninuous-wave Nd:YAG laser induces extended thermal changes in the meniscus with a transitional zone presenting coagulated and carbonized tissue. In relation to meniscus surgery the 1064 nm continuous-wave Nd:YAG laser is not suitable for tissue ablation and cutting; however, there may be some therapeutic potential inherent in using this laser for welding procedures at energy densities far below the carbonization threshold [4].

To avoid extensive thermal injury, contact Nd:YAG lasers have been designed for meniscus surgery. A sapphire crystal attached to the tip of the lightguide converts light energy to heat. The fiber then functions as a heater probe which cuts and ablates fibrocartilage with a significantly reduced extent of thermal damage, even when the laser is used in continuous-wave mode [35].

Morphology of Laser-Assisted Meniscectomy

The nature of tissue ablation or coagulation employing laser energy varies widely with the wavelength, delivery system, energy density emitted, and the operating mode of the laser. For this reason, morphometrical data obtained from in vitro studies published so far are not directly comparable owing to their inhomogeneity with regard to experimental set-up. Despite these shortcomings, Table 1 tries to compile morphometric data based upon a metaanalysis of the literature so as to gain some idea about the extent and variety of transitional zones. Most investigators agree that the formation of transitional zones is the most important adverse effect associated with laser-assisted meniscal surgery, so a minimum of denatured tissue area is desirable [6, 10, 11, 35, 49]. However, results obtained from in vivo experiments indicate that this transitional zone may have some important effect in restricting of further tissue fibrillation by welding the surface of the meniscal ablation area.

Fibrocartilage exposed to XeCl excimer laser energy presents conical tissue defects (Fig. 15). The

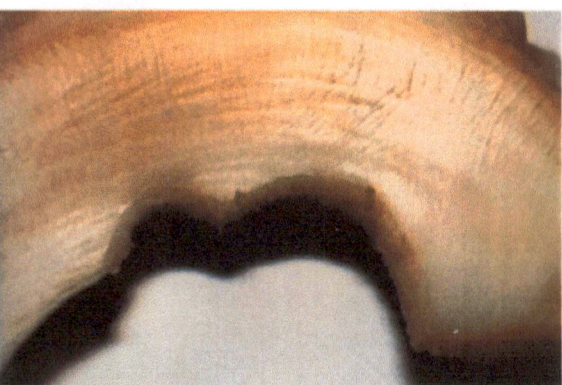

Fig. 15. Specimen of the meniscus following partial resection with the help of a XeCl excimer laser

Table 1. Transitional zones associated with various lasers at different energy settings

Laser	Output characteristics	Diameter of transitional zone	Reference
KrF excimer	400 mJ/pulse	17.5 μm	[31]
XeCl excimer	2 J/cm^2	24 μm	[46]
XeCl excimer	17 mJ/pulse	96 μm	[55]
XeCl excimer		45 μm	[23]
XeCl excimer	40 mJ/mm^2, 20 ns pulse width,	lateral 18 μm,	[40]
	40 Hz repetition rate	basal 21 μm	[40]
Nd:YAG	30 W, 1064 nm, continuous wave	870 μm	[46]
Nd:YAG	25 W, 1064 n, sapphire tip	191 μm	[46]
Nd:YAG	17 W, continuous wave	678 μm	[55]
Nd:YAG	21 W/mm^2, continuous wave	800 μm	[40]
Ho:YAG	1.3 J/cm^2	552 μm	[46]
Ho:YAG	15 W	1100 μm	[55]
CO$_2$	20 W, continuous wave	447 μm	[46]
CO$_2$	20 W, continuous wave	402 μm	[55]
CO$_2$	20 W, pulsed	350 μm	[55]

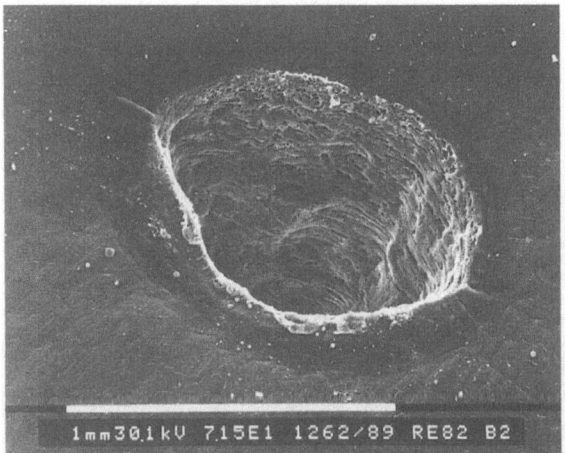

Fig. 16. Ablation crater in the fibrocartilage created by XeCl excimer irradiation (SEM, × 53)

Fig. 17. Higher magnification of the crater wall in Fig. 16. The stumps of the collagenous fibers are covered with amorphous material, indicating a welding effect of laser energy. (SEM, × 276)

area of maximum energy density corresponds to the deepest point in the cut profile. At light microscopy level, the tissue boundaries are smooth and well-delineated without irregularities or tissue fibrillations. Depending on the total energy deposited on the tissue, the pulse width, and the repetition rate, a small transitional zone characterized by an increased eosinophilia can be recognized. The diameter varies with the laser output characteristics, with the repetition rate as the most critical factor [38]. In some instances an aggregation of amorphous material can be found at the bottom of the ablation crater, which might consist of tissue remnants and ablation products. Scanning electron microscopy shows clear-cut tissue defects in the meniscal specimens. The exposed collagenous fibers are covered by amorphous material, indicating some potential for sealing activity. Similarly, the entrance of the laser-induced crater is surrounded by a margin of amorphous tissue (Figs. 16, 17). Although the quality of tissue alterations induced by excimer lasers on the menisci are identical for

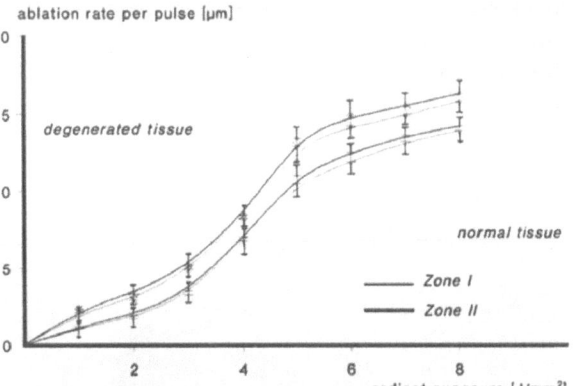

Fig. 18. Ablation curve of the meniscus following XeCl excimer irradiation. The amount or tissue ablation is significantly greater in degenerated tissue than in normal fibrocartilage. Furthermore, a difference in ablation efficency can be noted between zone I and zone II of the meniscus

both degenerated and healthy tissue and for the different anatomical zones, there are some significant differences in regard to the ablation rate which are illustrated in Fig. 18 [6, 10].

On light microscopy, menisci exposed to continuous-wave Nd:YAG laser irradiation present poly-
morphous lacunae and irregular borderlines. An
extended transitional zone with intramural dissocia-
tions of fibers and numerous interstitial bursts indicates considerable thermal activity. The meniscal surface exposed to Nd:YAG laser energy is characterized
by a typical zonal arrangement (Fig. 19):
- a carbonized zone
- a vesicular zone of vaporization
- a coagulated zone

Scanning electron microscopy confirms these observations. The surface of the irradiated meniscal
tissue shows bursts following interstitial vaporization
processes. Simultaneously the fibrocartilage is covered by amorphous tissue detritus (Figs. 20, 21).
When employing relatively low energy densities,
just above the threshold needed to induce macroscopically detectable laser effects, the meniscus surface
is covered with a smooth film of coagulated tissue
remnants; bursts and tissue disruptions hardly
occur at these laser parameters [39, 52].

In contrast to the free beam Nd:YAG laser, the contact tip Nd:YAG equipped with a sapphire crystal
produces a significantly reduced zone of thermal
necrosis. This device, working as a heater probe,
serves to convert the coherent energy into an intense
pinpoint heat source that converts the free-beam laser
from a coagulation instrument to a device suitable
for cutting and ablating the meniscus with excellent
precision [35, 59].

The CO_2 laser produces sharply defined cuts on
the meniscus with a borderline of laser-induced tissue damage measuring up to 450 µm. Corresponding
to observations from Nd:YAG laser meniscectomy,
the fibrocartilage shrinks markedly on laser application, which makes a precise control of the process
difficult. To minimize the degree of tissue scarring,
a pulsed CO_2 laser was introduced in meniscus surgery with the aim of permitting thermal relaxation
of the target tissue. Histological studies revealed
that the pulsed CO_2 laser produces thermal tissue
injury to a distance of 350 µm from the laser tissue
interface and also reduces surface shrinking [47, 51].

The Ho:YAG laser produces smooth tissue defects.
The transitional zones of thermal alterations in the
meniscal tissue are well controlled and do not exceed
150 µm in light microscopy sections under the condition of optimal output parameters. There is no gross
evidence of thermal injury, coagulation necrosis, or
carbonization. With regard to the laser parameters
to be employed in meniscus surgery, the pulse
width seems to be the most decisive factor in the
determination of ablation and cutting efficiency.
Morphometrical studies came to the conclusion that
a pulse width of 250 ns can be considered an optimum value for clinical application [53]. Interestingly

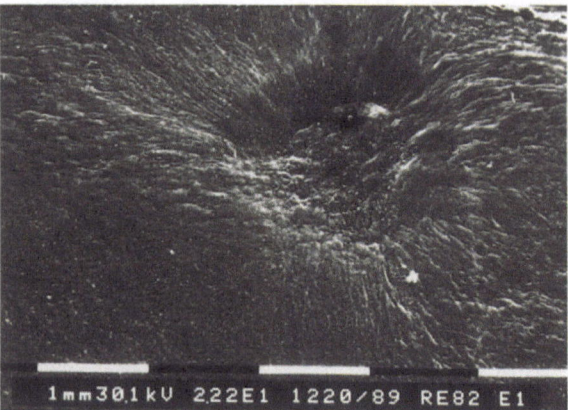

Fig. 20. Surface of the meniscus exposed to low energy Nd:YAG
laser irradiation. Smooth surface without tissue damage (SEM,
× 70)

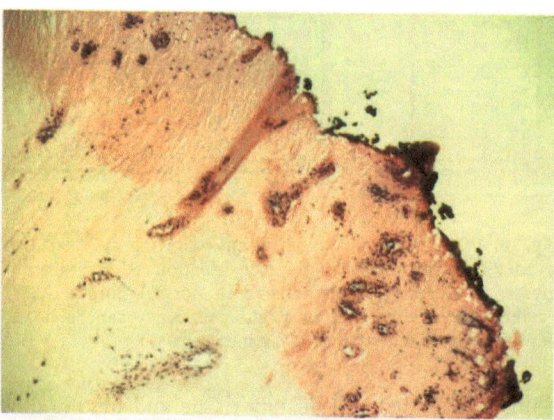

Fig. 19. Histology of the meniscus following Nd:YAG laser
irradiation, showing the typical zonal arrangement of thermal
tissue damage (LM, × 75)

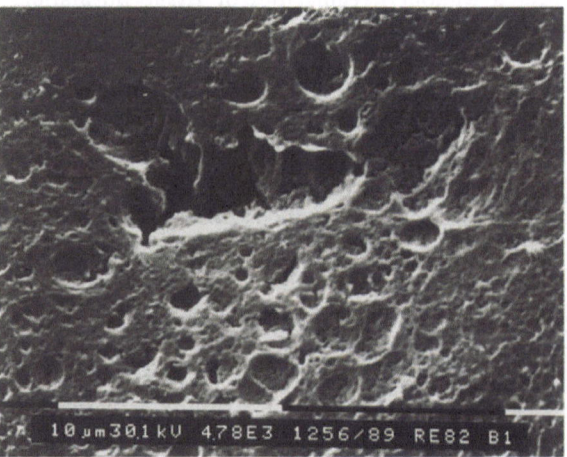

Fig. 21. Surface of the meniscus following Nd:YAG laser exposure. Numerous bursts and vaporizing cleavages indicating
thermal activity within the deep tissue layers (SEM, × 351)

the extent of the lateral damage zone is independent of the pulse width employed. The Ho:YAG laser has rapidly gained support for its use in meniscus surgery because of its practicability in clinical use combined with its effective and precise ablation characteristics [40, 50, 55].

Biomechanical Alterations

Besides considerations relating to perioperative morbidity, the long-term results of meniscus surgery depend strongly on the induction of degenerative arthritis. Experimental studies and clinical observations substantiate the hypothesis that alterations in the load transmission across the knee joint in the presence of partial or total deficiency of the meniscus lead to degeneration of the hyaline cartilage. The inhomogeneity of femorotibial pressure transmission creates regions of pathological cartilage pressure as well as areas lacking contact between the articulating surfaces, resulting in tissue degeneration from mechanical overload and insufficient nutrition [18].

As the menisci serve in the transformation of compressive loads into circumferential tensile strain, distribution of internal stresses must be regarded as a main feature of meniscal function. The histological composition and biomechanical properties of the collagenous tissue may contribute to precision of mechanical performance and to recovery of the fibrocartilage structure following deformation [32]. Although the roles of proteoglycan and noncollagenous matrix proteins in the biomechanics of the fibrocartilage are not yet precisely known, the possibility of tissue alteration at a histological and biochemical level by laser irradiation, resulting in unphysiological elasticity properties, has to be taken into account when analyzing laser – tissue interaction [15, 24].

Figure 22 represents the extent of radial stress and strain of the medial meniscus following irradiation with a XeCl excimer laser, determined with the help

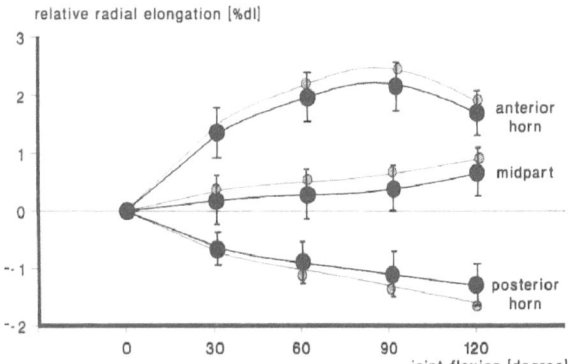

Fig. 23. Stress and strain phenomena in the meniscus following Nd:YAG laser exposure. Significantly reduced amount of radial tissue elongation due to increased rigidity. ● Native tissue, ● tissue following Nd:YAG laser irradiation

of strain gauges in an in vitro experiment employing human cadaver knee joints. Compared with nonirradiated tissue, the degree of relative radial strain during passive joint movement is reduced by a mean of 17.5 %, indicating increased rigidity of the fibrocartilage. Following Nd:YAG laser application (Fig. 23), maximum strain in the anterior horn is significantly reduced from 3.0 ± 0.3 % to 1.5 ± 0.2 %, corresponding to a reduction of compressibility in the posterior horn from 1.5 ± 0.2 % to 0.6 ± 0.1 % ($p < 0.01$).

These results lead to the conclusion that both thermal and ablative laser interaction initiate significant alterations in the biomechanical properties of fibrocartilagenous tissue which primarily increase the rigidity of the meniscus. Via a reduced femorotibial contact area and alterations in the biomechanical performance of the fibrocartilage, laser-assisted meniscectomy might have greater potential to promote earlier manifestation of gonarthrosis than conventional techniques [39]. However, further in vivo studies are necessary for a final assessment of these experimental results, especially in relation to their effect in clinical practice.

Experimental In Vivo Results

A review of the current literature gives relatively little evidence about in vivo reactions following laser-assisted meniscectomy on the basis of reliable experimental data. Whipple et al. were among the first to investigate biological response following CO_2 laser meniscectomy in a rabbit model, with special reference to the initiation of reactive synovitis by tissue degradation products [58, 59]. The results of their short-term study have demonstrated the surgical efficiency of laser application during meniscectomy with sealing and smoothing of the fibrocartilage, although the thermally altered transitional zones were not specifically addressed. As it is hard to achieve the clini-

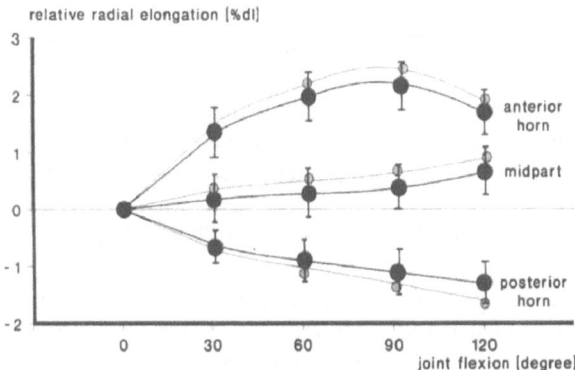

Fig. 22. Stress and strain phenomena in the meniscus following XeCl excimer laser exposure. Compared to normal tissue, a significant increase in tissue rigidity is noted. ● Native tissue, ● tissue following Nd:XECl laser irradiation

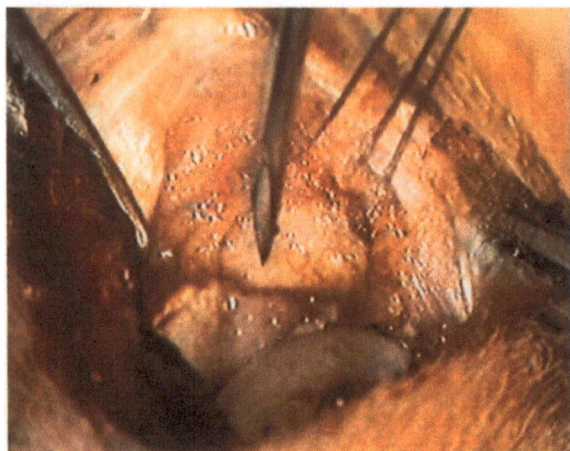

Fig. 24. Experimental laser ablation of the meniscus

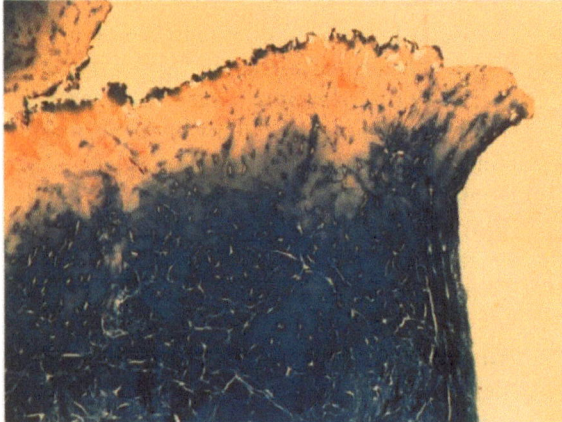

Fig. 25. Meniscus 14 days following Nd:YAG laser exposition. Extended transitional zone, superficial carbonization, and vesicular formation (LM, × 65)

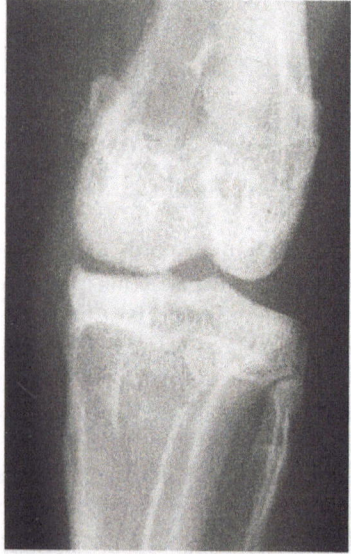

Fig. 26. Narrow medial joint space and subchondral sclerosis indicating a compartment arthrosis 6 months after laser meniscectomy in a rabbit model

cal conditions of laser-assisted meniscectomy in an animal model, these studies had some shortcomings; for example, there was no information available about the total laser energy deposited on the meniscal surface. Concerning the incidence of laser-induced synovitis, the authors came to the conclusion that ash residues within the joint cavity do not promote synovitis in the postoperative period. It is interesting to note that electrocautery produced less tissue damage than some lasers. Furthermore, some in vivo studies suggest significant healing of the coagulated fibrocartilage, which may lead to meniscal regeneration even if the tissue surface presents severe thermal necrosis.

In a controlled in vivo study employing a rabbit model we found a precise cutting profile following excimer-laser-assisted partial meniscectomy (Fig. 24). However, the application of a continuous-wave Nd:YAG laser leads to severe thermal damage with a transitional zone that increases during the postoperative period (Fig. 25). The most important finding was that both thermal and ablative lasers prevent fibrillation of the meniscal rim following partial resection, which was a common finding in the control group operated on by conventional mechanical instruments. Meniscal regeneration was not observed in any experimental group. The extent of cellular infiltration in the synovial membrane is significantly increased following Nd:YAG laser surgery, indicating reactive synovitis. In contrast, XeCl excimer laser meniscectomy leads to a significantly reduced degree of reactive synovitis, which is in agreement with some clinical observations of a reduced effusion rate and a lower intensity of pain in the perioperative phase following arthroscopic laser surgery. Radiographs performed 1–6 months following meniscectomy show greater progression of degenerative changes following laser surgery than after conventional meniscectomy (Fig. 26). These observations were confirmed by in vivo studies performed by Buchelt et al. [6]. With regard to clinical practice, these data substantiate the implication that laser surgery is superior to conventional meniscectomy in that it prevents further fibrillation of the fibrocartilage. However, early development of arthrosis may be promoted when meniscectomy is performed by thermal lasers in continuous-wave mode [38–40].

Laser-Assisted Meniscectomy in Clinical Practice

Lasers providing minimal thermal tissue alteration are most suitable for meniscal resection in clinical use, as results from morphological studies and experimental in vivo investigations indicate. Philandrianos and Smith et al. were the first to introduce the CO_2 laser as routine procedure in the arthroscopic surgery of the knee joint [37, 51]. With regard to the absorption features of the CO_2 laser, gas insufflation of the joint cavity is required to prevent absorption of the laser by the liquid distension media. Occasionally, gaseous distension media may lead to subcutaneous emphysema that resolves quickly [51]. However, some severe complications in connection with emphysema formation have been reported [16]. Furthermore, frequent postoperative effusions are observed because of the lack of lavage effect inherent in gaseous joint media. Smith et al. described a technique for CO_2 laser arthroscopy in which the jet of CO_2 gas creates a bubble on the meniscal surface, so that the laser beam passes through the gas to the target tissue without being absorbed by the liquid media used to distend the joint, largely eliminating the problems of postoperative joint effusion and emphysema formation. The authors reported having good experiences with this technique and stated that no specific complications occurred [52].

Despite modifications in the operative techniques that have led to significant improvements in CO_2-laser-assisted meniscectomy, the main problems in clinical practice remain the cumbersome light delivery device and the poor visualization of the meniscus due to bubble formation.

The use of the Ho:YAG laser in meniscectomy has been investigated by Fanton and Dillingham in a randomized clinical study [11] in which the postoperative course of a group in which a meniscal lesion was operated on using the Ho:YAG laser was compared with a group managed with conventional mechanical instruments. The authors found that the laser group seemed to do better during the first 4 weeks, especially with regard to pain, swelling, and effusion. Thereafter, no difference between the two groups was noted [32]. Although the study had some methodological shortcomings and the data presented lack statistical significance, the results may indicate that the Ho:YAG laser is a suitable tool for meniscal resection.

O'Brien et al. described their clinical experience with the Nd:YAG contact probe used for 110 partial meniscectomies [36]. They hypothesized that its main advantages are the reduced need for secondary trimming and better access to narrow joint compartments. Furthermore, the laser has eliminated the need to use multiple instruments in meniscectomy. A typical initial shortcoming common with the sapphire tips utilized was instrument breakage when the lightguide was vigorously used within the joint. The development of new ceramic tips which were much more resistant solved this problem and provided enhanced tactile feedback for the surgeon.

Finally, the XeCl excimer laser has been used for meniscectomy in clinical practice. Concerning the operative technique, advantages arise from the small diameter of the quarz fibers delivering the laser beam, allowing good access even to narrow joint compartments. However, the relative low energy density transmitted through the fibers leads to reduced ablation efficiency, which causes a time-consuming prolongation of the ablation process. Similar to experiences gained from Ho:YAG laser assisted meniscectomy, clinical data comparing this technique to conventional meniscus surgery show reduced incidence of postoperative swelling and effusion, reduced pain, and earlier return to normal function following laser meniscectomy [1].

It is important to notice that no clinical study published so far has been able to show that the long-term results of meniscus surgery are significantly improved by the use of laser energy. Therefore, further research will be necessary for a definitive judgement of the value of laser energy as a clinical tool in the surgery of the menisci.

Future Perspectives

At present, laser-assisted meniscectomy may offer some advantages over conventional surgery, but it may also carry potential risks, especially in relation to the induction of arthrosis. Before this technique can be generally recommended as a procedure for clinical routine, further research will be necessary. In this respect it should be stated that laser energy may offer some advantages over conventional meniscus surgery based upon the specific laser – tissue interaction.

These advantages include:
- tissue welding and soldering of the menisci
- promotion of cell proliferation and reparative process
- selectivity of tissue ablation by specific optical properties

As demonstrated in controlled experimental studies, laser energy provides a capacity for tissue sealing which may prevent the resection rim of the meniscus from fibrillation leading to further degeneration and rupture formation. Forman et al. have examined a method of meniscus repair by fibrin clot bonding in connection with argon ion laser irradiation [13]. Compared with the nonirradiated control group, laser-assisted fibrin-clot-bonded menisci had a 40-fold increased tensile strength following repair. These data lead to the conclusion that laser assisted tissue repair holds the rupture planes together with a biological scaffold and possibly induces reparative cell migration and proliferation.

Another feature of laser energy that might be useful in the area of meniscal repair is the ability for biostimulation. Experimental observations performed on hyaline cartilage demonstrated increased mitotic activity following low-energy Nd:YAG laser irradiation. However, the few communications on laser-induced biostimulation, some of which are contradictory, do not provide unanswerable evidence for the potential of laser energy to stimulate tissue proliferation [5, 25, 43]. Further research will be necessary to obtain precise knowledge about the capacity of laser for biostimulation and its use in meniscal repair.

Finally, optical properties of fibrocartilage may form a basis for a selective or at least preferential laser application. Data gained so far from in vitro experiments have proved that it is possible to distinguish between degenerated and healthy tissue, and between the various zones of the meniscus by utilizing specific optical properties [40]. First attempts to use these phenomena by creating a feedback system based upon clearly defined algorithms in laser fluorescence have been performed and seem to be promising in realizing the principle of selective meniscal surgery.

References

[1] Abelow S (1993) Use of lasers in orthopedic surgery: current concepts. Orthopaedics 1:551–553
[2] Arnoczky S, Warren R (1982) Microvasculature of the human meniscus. Am J Sports Med 10:90–95
[3] Arnoczky S, Warren R, Kaplan N (1985) Meniscal remodelling following partial meniscectomy: an experimental study in the dog. Arthroscopy 1:247–254
[4] Bickerstaff D, Waman A, Laing W, Smith T (1991) Partial meniscectomy using the neodymium:YAG laser. An in vitro study. Arthroscopy 7:63–70
[5] Boulton M, Marshall J (1986) He-Ne laser stimulation of human fibroblast proliferation and attachment in vitro. Life Sci 1:125–131
[6] Buchelt M, Papioannou T, Fishbein M, Peters W, Beeder C, Grundfest W (1991) Excimer laser ablation of fibrocartilage: an in vitro and in vivo study. Lasers Surg Med 11:271–279
[7] Bullough P, Munerva L, Murphy J, Weinstein A (1979) The strength of the menisci as it relates to their fine structure. J Bone Joint Surg 52-B:564–570
[8] Burke D, Ahmed A (1978) A biomechanical study of partial and total meniscectomy of the knee. Trans Orthop Res Soc 3:91–98
[9] Dew D, Supic L, Darrow C, Price G (1993) Tissue repair using lasers: a review. Orthopaedics 16:563–569
[10] Dressel M, Jahn R, Neu W, Jungbluth K (1991) Studies in fiber guided excimer laser surgery for cutting and drilling bone and meniscus. Lasers Surg Med 11:569–579
[11] Fanton G, Dillingham M (1992) The use of the holmium:YAG laser in arthroscopic surgery. Semin Orthop 7:102–107
[12] Ferrer-Roca O, Vialta C (1980) Lesions of the meniscus: microscopic and histologic findings. Clin Orthop 146:289–298
[13] Forman S, Oz M, Lontz J, Treat M, Forman T, Kieman H (1995) Laser-assisted fibrin clot soldering of human menisci. Clin Orthop 310:37–41
[14] Fuller J, Ghadially F (1972) Ultrastructural observations on surgically produced partial thickness defects in articular cartilage. Clin Orthop 86:192–205
[15] Ghosh P, Taylor T (1987) The knee joint meniscus: a fibrocartilage of some distinction. Clin Orthop 224:52–59
[16] Grunwald J (1993) Complication during arthroscopy: fatal air embolism. Complic Orthop 4:304–308
[17] Hausmann B, Forst R (1982) Nachweis einer möglichen Traumatisierung des Kniegelenkes bei der Arthroskopie. Z Orthop 120:725–728
[18] Hehne H, Riede U, Hauschild G, Schlageter M (1981) Tibiofemorale Kontaktflächenmessungen nach experimentellen partiellen und subtotalen Meniskektomien. Z Orthop 119:54–59
[19] Heish H, Walker P (1976) Stabilizing mechanisms of the loaded and unloaded knee joint. J Bone Joint Surg 58-A:87–93
[20] Henning C, Lynch M, Yearout K (1990) Arthroscopic meniscal repair using an exogenous fibrin clot. Clin Orthop 252:64–72
[21] Hertel P, Schweiberer L (1976) Die Diagnostik der Meniskusläsionen. H Unfallheilkd 121:14–20
[22] Hibst R (1992) Mechanical effects of erbium:YAG laser bone ablation. Lasers Surg Med 12:125–130
[23] Hohlbach G, Möller K, Schramm U, Baretton G (1989) Experimentelle Ergebnisse der Knorpelabrasio mit dem Excimer-Laser. Histologische und elektronenmikroskopische Untersuchungen. Z Orthop 127:116–127
[24] Hopker W, Angres G, Klingel K, Komitowski D, Schuchardt E (1986) Changes of the elastin compartment in the human meniscus. Virchows Arch Path Anat 408:575–581
[25] Ingman AM, Ghosh P, Taylor T (1974) Variation of collagenous and non-collagenous proteins of the human knee joint menisci with age and degeneration. Gastroenterology 20:212–216
[26] Karu T (1989) Photobiology of low-power laser effects. Health Phys 56:691–695
[27] Kettelkamp D, Jacobs A (1972) Tibiofemoral contact area – determination and implications. J Bone Joint Surg 54-A:349–356
[28] Klein W, Kurze V (1986) Arthroscopic arthropathy: iatrogenic arthroscopic joint lesions in animals: Arthroscopy 2:163–168
[29] Klein J, Tilling T, Steffens H, Roeddecker K (1989) Kniegelenksarthroskopie – eine problemlose Operation? In: Hofer H, Henche H (eds) Komplikationen bei der Arthroskopie. Enke, Stuttgart, pp 41–45 (Fortschritte in der Arthroskopie, vol 5)
[30] Kochevar I (1989) Cytotoxicity and mutagenicity of excimer laser radiation. Lasers Surg Med 9:440–445
[31] Kroitzsch U, Laufer G, Egkjer E, Wollenek G, Horvath R (1989) Experimental photoablation of meniscus cartilage by excimer laser energy. Arch Orthop Trauma Surg 108:44–48
[32] Kummer B (1986) Die Biomechanik des Kniegelenkes nach Meniskektomie. In: Tilling T (ed) Arthroskopische Meniskuschirurgie. Enke, Stuttgart, pp 30–34 (Fortschritte in der Arthroskopie, vol 2)
[33] Lane G, Sherk H, Mooar P, Lee S, Black J (1992) Holmium:YAG laser versus carbon dioxide laser versus mechanical arthroscopic debridement. Sem Orthop 7:95–99
[34] MacConail M (1950) The movements of bone and joints. J Bone Joint Surg 32-B:244–251
[35] Miller D, O'Brien S, Arnoczky S, Kelly A, Fealy S, Warren R (1989) The use of the contact Nd:YAG laser in arthroscopic surgery. Effects on articular cartilage and meniscal tissue. Arthroscopy 5:245–253
[36] O'Brien S, Fealy S, Miller D (1992) Nd-YAG contact laser arthroscopy. Sem Orthop 7:117–123
[37] Philandrianos G (1985) Le laser à gaz carbonique en chirurgie arthroscopique du genou. Presse Med 143:2103–2110
[38] Raunest J (1995) Laseranwendung in der Gelenkchirurgie – Experimentelle Ergebnisse zum arthroskopischen Einsatz thermischer und gepulster UV-Laser. Unfallchirurg Suppl 247

[39] Raunest J, Derra E (1995) Morphologische, biomechanische und experimentelle in-vivo-Untersuchungen zur laserassistierten Meniskusresektion. Langenbecks Arch Chir 380:12-21

[40] Raunest J, Derra E (1996) Arthroseinduktion durch Lasereingriffe. Orthopäde 25:10-16

[41] Raunest J, Schwarzmaier H (1995) Optical properties of human articular tissue as implication for a selective laser application in arthroscopic surgery. Lasers Surg Med 16:253-261

[42] Roeddecker K, Nagelschmidt M, Koebke J, Guensche K (1993) Meniscal healing: a histological study in rabbits. Arthroscopy 9:28-37

[43] Scapinelli R (1968) Studies on the vasculature of the human knee joint. Acta Anat 70:305-314

[44] Schultz R, Krishnamurthy S, Thelmo W, Rodriguez J, Harvey G (1985) Effects of varying intensities of laser energy on articular cartilage. A preliminary study. Lasers Surg Med 5:577-582

[45] Seedholm B, Hargreaves D (1979) Transmission of load in the knee joint with special reference to the role of the menisci. Eng Med 8:22-29

[46] Sherk HH (1993) The use of lasers in orthopaedic procedures. J Bone Joint Surg 75-A:768-776

[47] Sherk H, Block J, Prodoehl J, Diven J (1995) The effect of lasers and electrosurgical devices on human meniscal tissue. Clin Orthop 310:14-20

[48] Siebert W (1992) Laseranwendung in der Arthroskopie. Orthopäde 21:273-280

[49] Siebert W, Kohn D, Klanke J, Wirth C, Scholz C, Müller G (1990) Rasterelektronenmikroskopische Untersuchungen zur Oberflächenbearbeitung von Knorpelschäden mit dem Nd:YAG-Laser, dem Er:YAG-Laser, dem Ho:YSSG-Laser und diversen motorgetriebenen Instrumenten. In: Hofer H, Henche H (eds) Arthroskopie bei Knorpelschäden und Arthrose. Enke, Stuttgart, pp 82-91 (Fortschritte in der Arthroskopie, vol 6)

[50] Siebert W, Saunier J, Gerber B, Lübbers C (1994) Ho:YAG Laser in der arthroskopischen Chirurgie des Kniegelenks. Arthroskopie 7:182-191

[51] Smith C, Johansen E, Vangsness C, Sutter L, Marshall G (1989) The carbon dioxide laser. A potential tool for orthopedic surgery. Clin Orthop 242:43-50

[52] Smith C, Johansen E, Vangsness C, Marshall G, Sutter L, Bonavolet T (1992) Gas bubble technique in arthroscopic surgery. Semin Orthop 7:86-94

[53] Trauner K, Nishioka N, Patel D (1990) Pulsed holmium:yttrium-aluminium-garnet (Ho:YAG) laser ablation of fibrocartilage and articular cartilage. Am J Sports Med 18:316-320

[54] Vangsness C, Akl Y, Nelson S, Liaw L, Smith C, Marshall G (1995) In vitro analysis of laser meniscectomy. Clin Orthop 310:21-26

[55] Vangsness C, Watson T, Saadatmanesh V, Moran K (1995) Pulsed Ho:YAG laser meniscectomy: effect of pulsewidth on tissue penetration rate and lateral thermal damage. Lasers Surg Med 16:61-65

[56] Walker P, Erkman M (1975) The role of the menisci in force transmission across the knee. Clin Orthop 109:184-192

[57] Walsh J, Flotte T, Anderson R, Deutsch T (1988) Pulsed CO_2 laser ablation: effect of tissue type and pulse duration on thermal damage. Lasers Surg Med 8:108-114

[58] Whipple T, Caspari R, Meyers J (1984) Laser subtotal meniscectomy in rabbits. Lasers Surg Med 3:297-304

[59] Whipple T, Marotta J, May T, Caspari R, Meyers J (1987) Electron microscopy of CO_2 laser induced effects in human fibrocartilage. Lasers Surg Med 7:184

[60] Wirth C (1995) Meniscal surgery: resection, suture and replacement. In: Cassteleyn P, Duparc J, Fulford P (eds) European instructional course lectures, vol 2, p 110, British Editorial Office J Bone Joint Surg

[61] Wirth C, Rodriguez M, Milachowski K (1988) Meniskusnaht - Meniskusersatz. Thieme, Stuttgart

Soft Tissue Shortening with the Ho:YAG Laser: Experimental Model, Structural Effects, and Histologic and Ultrastructural Analysis[1]

M. E. BEREND · R. R. GLISSON · K. P. SPEER

Introduction

Lasers are currently utilized in many areas of orthopedic surgery [1, 2]. Due to limitations in fiberoptic and laser medium technology, however, lasers have had limited application in orthopedics [8] as their primary roles have been hemostasis and tissue ablation. The holmium:yttrium-aluminum-garnet (Ho:YAG) laser has gained popularity recently as it has been applied to spine [4, 17], knee [10], and shoulder surgery for capsular [16] cartilage and bone resection while providing excellent tissue hemostasis and controlled penetration depth. Recently, the Ho:YAG laser has been utilized to produce collagen shortening [13] and it may have potential in clinical soft tissue shortening procedures such as capsular tightening in multidirectional shoulder instability.

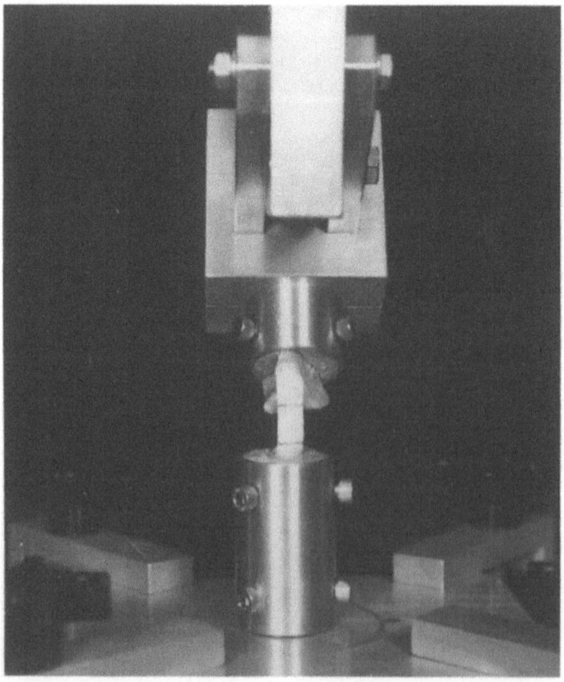

Fig. 1. Photograph of the canine infrapatellar tendon fixed to an Instron materials testing machine in the testing apparatus. Saline bath has been removed to demonstrate the orientation of the collagen fibers in the testing jig

The structural or mechanical changes which occur in collagen following lasing below ablation thresholds are unknown. These changes include the specific effects the laser has on tissue length, strength, stiffness, and energy absorption. The biology of laser-treated collagen remodeling has not been described either. The purpose of this investigation was to determine the structural properties, histologic morphology, and ultrastructural appearance of normal and lased tissue to serve as a foundation for both safe, selective, and effective clinical trials and additional in vivo laboratory studies on potential laser–tissue interactions in orthopedic surgery. This paper presents a model for evaluating the structural properties of soft tissue treated with subablation lasing with the Ho:YAG laser.

Materials and Methods

Experimental Model and Specimen Preparation

The patella-infrapatellar tendon-tibia construct was harvested from 12 skeletally mature dogs weighing 15–25 kg. The specimens were wrapped in sponges moistened with saline and frozen at −20 °C until testing. Following thawing, two K-wires were placed transversely through the patella and two screws placed in the tibia perpendicular to the metaphysis. The bones were each secured in aluminum pots with polymethyl methacrylate (PMMA). The posterior half of the tibial plateau was removed using a saw to allow for clearance in the testing apparatus during shortening and mechanical testing.

The pots were mounted on an Instron servohydraulic materials testing machine (model 1321, Instron Corp., Canton, Mass.) for mechanical properties testing (Fig. 1). The length, width, and thickness of the specimens was determined using calipers before testing. The initial length for strain calcula-

[1] This work has been presented at the American Orthopaedic Society for Sports Medicine in Toronto, Ontario, Canada, July 16–19, 1995, and at the American Orthopaedic Association Residents' Meeting in Pittsburgh, Pennsylvania, March 28–April 1, 1995

tions was defined as the length from the patellar insertion to the tibial insertion on the anterior surface of the tendon. Two transverse ink marks, 5 and 20 mm distal to the patellar insertion, were placed on the tendon, creating a 15-mm uniform lasting length (Fig. 2). On half of the specimens this area was further divided into a grid pattern with 18 equal areas (Fig. 3). The pots were placed in a testing

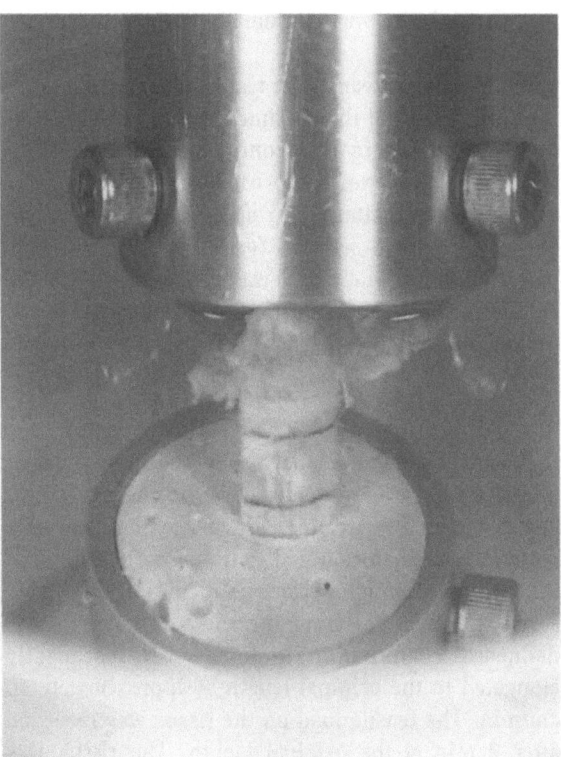

Fig. 4. Photograph of a specimen immersed in the saline bath prior to lasing

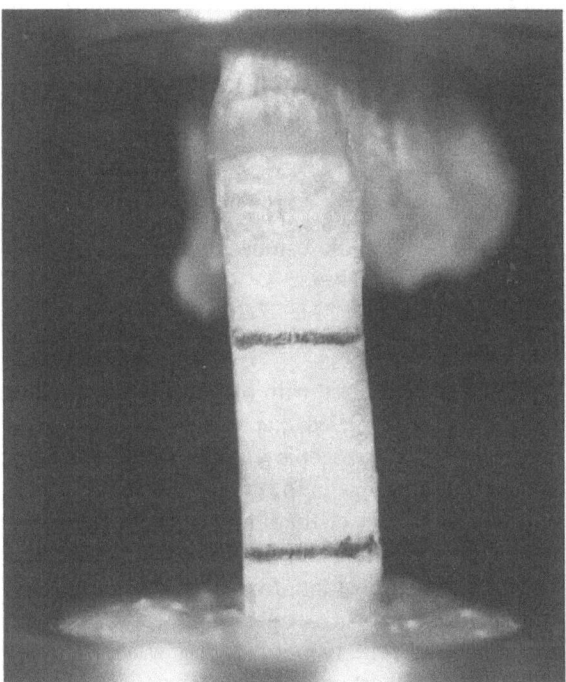

Fig. 2. Photograph of the ink marks on the anterior tendon surface defining the full-width patern lasing area

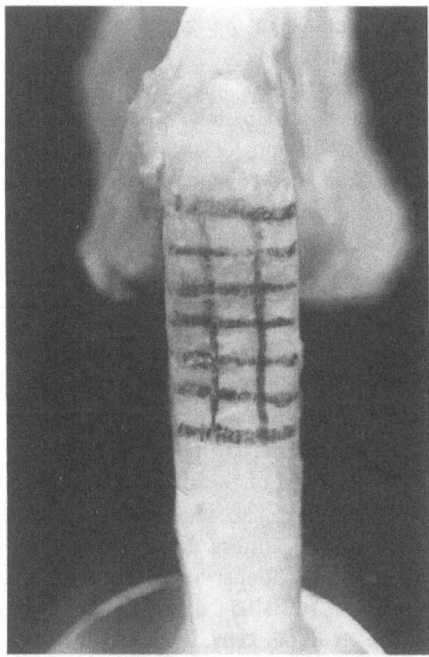

Fig. 3. Photograph of the ink marks on the anterior tendon surface defining the grid pattern lasing area

jig with the axis of displacement directed in line with the fibers of the infrapatellar tendon and perpendicular to the testing platform. The femoral port was fixed with a femoral shaft-patellar tendon angle of 30°. All tests were conducted with the entire tendon in a saline bath at room temperature (Fig. 4). Before lasing, the tissue was placed under a 0.5-N preload and preconditioned with 10 cycles of loading and unloading to 4 % strain at a rate of 1 cm/min to provide a uniform strain exposure as described by Woo et al. [26]. This set of cyclical testing served as the control for each tendon for further comparisons following lasing.

Laser Protocol

Using a 40-W Ho:YAG laser (Trimadyne Inc, Irvine, Calif., OMNIPulse 1210-40W holmium laser) with a 600-μm fiber and a 20° lasing probe, a standard lasing protocol was performed. Strict safety precautions with filtered goggles and limited access to the lasing area were employed during all testing. The probe was positioned in the saline bath perpendicular to the anterior surface of the tendon approximately 2 mm from the tissue. Energy was delivered using the following parameters: pulse repetition rate = 10 Hz, power = 10 W, with resulting J/pulse = 1. 500 J overall was delivered to each area, approximating 300 J/cm^2. As energy was delivered and the tissue shortening, tissue laxity was continually maintained under zero tension.

Two lasing patterns were tested. One pattern lased the entire width of the specimen (full-width) (Fig. 2); in this pattern energy was continuously delivered and the probe was moved in an oscillating manner ($n = 6$). The other pattern left unlased collagen fibers between the lased sections (grid) (Fig. 3); with this pattern approximately 55 J was delivered to 9 of the 18 areas. Each lased section was adjacent to an unlased section, creating a checkerboard appearance.

Mechanical Testing

Following lasing, the shortened length was determined under a 0.5-N load using the Instron LVDT. Ten cycles to 4% strain at a displacement rate of 1 cm/min were then repeated in a manner identical to the preconditioning performed before lasing. This set of strain cycles from the shortened length was defined as condition 1. The tissue was subsequently elongated to the original length at approximately 10 cm/min. The tensile load on the tissue was recorded after 2 min at the original length. The tissue was then subjected to an additional ten cycles to 4% strain at a displacement rate of 1 cm/min. The final set of cycles after lasing, shortening, and returning to the original length was defined as condition 2.

From the tenth 4% strain hysteresis cycle of each set (control, condition 1, and condition 2) the load displacement curves were analyzed to determine the length, peak load, hysteresis energy, and tangent stiffness of the tissue.

Histologic Analysis

Unlased control and lased tissues were fixed in 10% formalin at the postlasing length for 24 h. The qualitative morphologic changes in the collagen architecture were analyzed using hematoxylin and eosin, Verhoeff-van Gieson's, and Masson stains under conventional and polarized light microscopy. Axial, coronal, and sagittal sections were obtained to characterize depth of penetration, thermal injury, cellular necrosis, collagen fiber morphology, and orientation.

Electron Microscopic Ultrastructural Analysis

Longitudinal sections of control and lased tissue were fixed in 2% glutaraldehyde and processed for electron microscopic analysis using sequential tannic acid, uranyl acetate, propylene oxide, and Spur embedding medium preparations in order to obtain adequate specimen contrast. Transmission electron microscopic sections 70 nm thick were made and stained with Sato solution and examined with a Geol electron microscope (25 000×).

Statistical Analysis

Statistical analysis was performed on the data with a repeated-measures ANOVA. The data had an exponential distribution and were therefore normalized with a log-transform scale. A Student's t-test, f-test, and least-squares means comparison test were utilized to determine differences between experimental groups. A p value of 0.05 or less was considered significant and a Bonferoni adjustment was utilized for multiple comparisons.

Results

Tendon Morphology

Quantitative

The dimensions of the canine infrapatellar tendons ($n = 12$) were: thickness 1.8–2.0 mm, width 11.0–12.0 mm, and length 34.0–47.0 mm.

Qualitative

Experiments conducted with a variety of low radiant energy settings revealed that tissue shrinkage coincided with a macroscopic change in the collagen appearance. A change in the consistency, appearance, and deorganization of the linear collagen array was noted following lasing and tissue shortening. The tissue made the transition from a highly organized white collagen network of parallel fibers to a gelatinous and confluent tissue as lasing was conducted and the tissue shortened. The distance from the tissue at which the probe was maintained which produced shortening was dependent upon the radiant energy delivered. Very low radiant energy settings did not produce a change in the length until direct tissue contact was obtained.

The depth of penetration macroscopically and microscopically was approximately 30% of the 2-mm tissue thickness. The posterior unlased surface retained the white organized collagen linear network; however, it appeared wavy and foreshortened and could be likened to an accordion.

Tendon Structural Properties

Reproducible collagen shortening in the canine infrapatellar tendon with the Ho:YAG laser was achieved in this model. A representative example of shortening is shown in Figs. 5 and 6. Shortening of the lased area ranging from 41% to 68% of the original length in both patterns was tested. The changes in length, peak load at 4% strain, stiffness, hysteresis energy, and load after lasing and elongation are recorded in Table 1. There was no statistical difference between the full-width and grid patterns in the magnitude of shortening or in any of the structural properties tested ($p < 0.05$). The peak load ($p < 0.0001$)

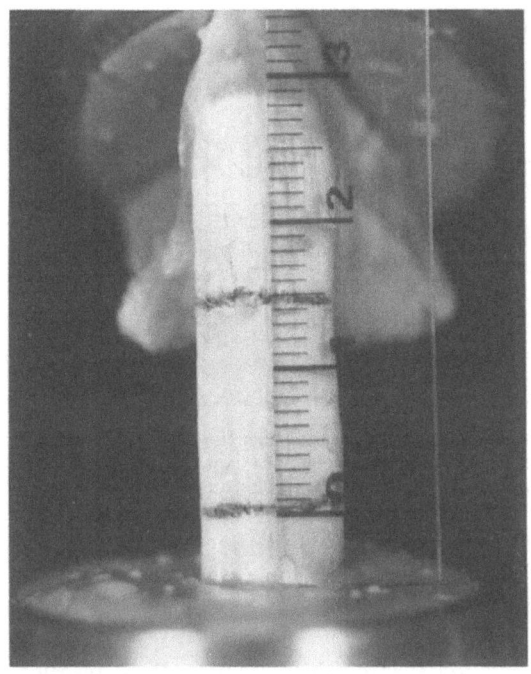

Fig. 5. Photograph of the prelasing length determination at 15 mm under 0.5 N load

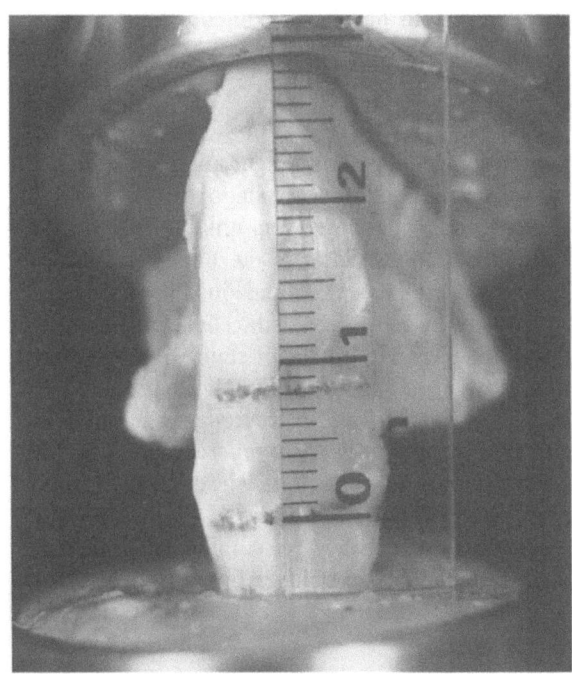

Fig. 6. Photograph of the postlasing length determination at 8.5 mm under 0.5 N load. Note the confluence and gelatinous appearance of the lased region

under a 4% strain from the shortened length was markedly decreased from controls following lasing. Once the tissue was elongated back to the original length the tendon was under a markedly increased load averaging 37 N. When subjected to a 4% strain after lasing and returning the tissue to the original length, the peak load ($p < 0.0001$) and stiffness ($p = 0.06$) were increased. The energy of hysteresis was defined as the energy lost during one 4% strain cycle and was measured as the area under the load displacement curve. The energy of hysteresis for a 4% strain from the shortened length was unchanged from controls ($p = 0.12$),

while there was a decrease in the energy of hysteresis for a 4% strain after lasing and returning to the original length ($p < 0.0009$). There was therefore a length-dependent change in the structural properties of the lased tissues, with increased stiffness in lased tissue compared to length-matched controls.

All strain cycles demonstrated the viscoelastic property of stress relaxation as the peak load decreased approximately 5%–10% from the first to the tenth cycle. Furthermore, when the shortened lased tissue was elongated to the original length, a plateau in the load on the tendon was observed

Table 1. Summary of structural properties of canine tendons undergoing Ho:YAG laser treatment[a]

	Full-width pattern ($n = 6$)	Grid pattern ($n = 6$)
Energy delivered (J/cm²)	289.0 ± 15.1	305.0 ± 19.7
Shortening (mm)	8.4 ± 1.5	7.1 ± 1.0
Condition 1 peak load (% control)	−92.7 ± 6.3	−95.0 ± 2.6
Condition 2 peak load (% control)	+239.0 ± 88.0	+210.0 ± 148.0
Condition 1 stiffness (% control)	−95.5 ± 3.2	−96.5 ± 2.4
Condition 2 stiffness (% control)	+56.3 ± 43.0	+79.2 ± 84.6
Hysteresis control[b] (%)	26.4 ± 9.8	24.5 ± 11.7
Hysteresis condition 1[c] (%)	24.3 ± 10.9	20.0 ± 23.0
Hysteresis condition 2[d] (%)	3.9 ± 3.8	4.4 ± 6.8
Load at condition 2 (N)	46.4 ± 27.7	29.4 ± 4.8

[a] Values are given as the mean and the standard deviation.
[b] Control was defined as the 4% strain cycle from the original length during preconditioning.
[c] Condition 1 was defined as the 4% strain cycle after lasing starting from the shortened length.
[d] Condition 2 was defined as the 4% strain cycle after lasing, shortening, and returning to the original length.
  + = increase; − = decrease.

after the length had been maintained for approximately 2 min.

Histologic Analysis

Conventional and polarized light microscopy demonstrated that the collagen orientation of the lased tissue was different from control unlased tissue. Lased tissue did not demonstrate the ability to polarize light (Fig. 7). An area of thermal injury was observed beneath the lased surface, with cellular necrosis, and there was increased uptake of stain when compared to controls (Fig. 8) which may indicate protein denaturing. A consolidation in the collagen bundles was observed with routine light microscopy. The posterior unlased portion of the laser-treated tendon demonstrated the foreshortened collagen fibers remaining in their wavy yet parallel array and they retained the ability to polarize light (Fig. 9).

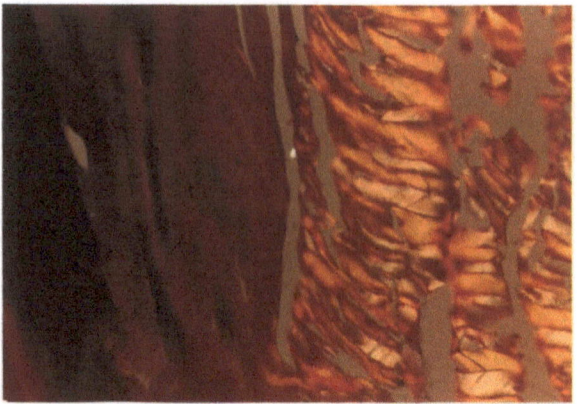

Fig. 9. Photomicrograph showing a longitudinal section of lased infrapatellar tendon under polarized light. The lased area *(left)* no longer polarizes light and the unlased posterior fibers *(right)* are foreshortened, wavy, and retain the ability to polarize light. (Verhoeff-van Gieson's stain, × 20)

Ultrastructural Analysis

Transmission electron microscopic analysis revealed a change in the morphology, striation pattern, size, and linear arrangement of the collagen fibers. There was an increase in the width of the collagen fibers from the normal collagen (Fig. 10) to approximately two times the original width following lasing (Fig. 11). There was marked loss of the striation pattern within the collagen fibers and a decrease was observed in the area of the interspaces between the collagen fibers. Consolidation, fusion, and interdigi-

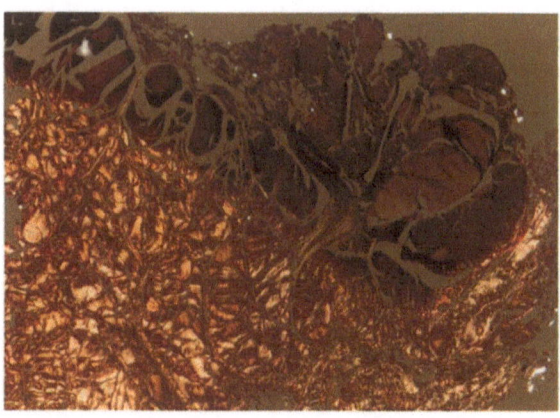

Fig. 7. Photomicrograph showing a cross-section of lased infrapatellar tendon under polarized light. The darker area *(top)* is the lased surface with consolidation of collagen bundles and loss of polarization. (Verhoeff-van Gieson's stain, × 4)

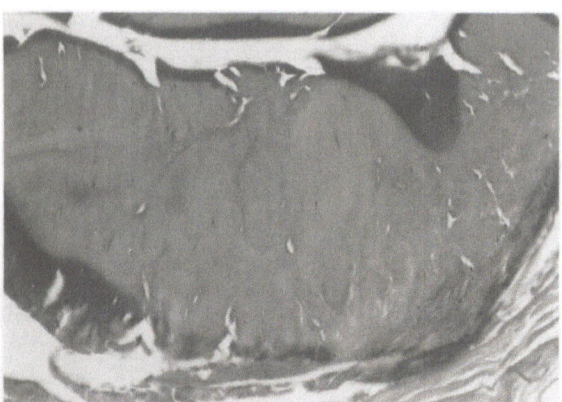

Fig. 8. Photomicrograph showing a cross-section of lased infrapatellar tendon under light microscopy with consolidation and interdigitation of the collagen fibers and cellular necrosis. (Verhoeff-van Gieson's stain, × 20)

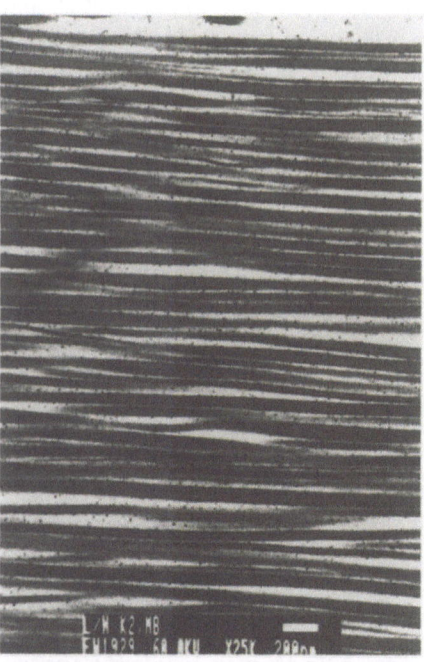

Fig. 10. Transmission electron photomicrograph of unlased control collagen with parallel oriented collagen fibers with regular periodicity to the striation pattern. (× 25 000)

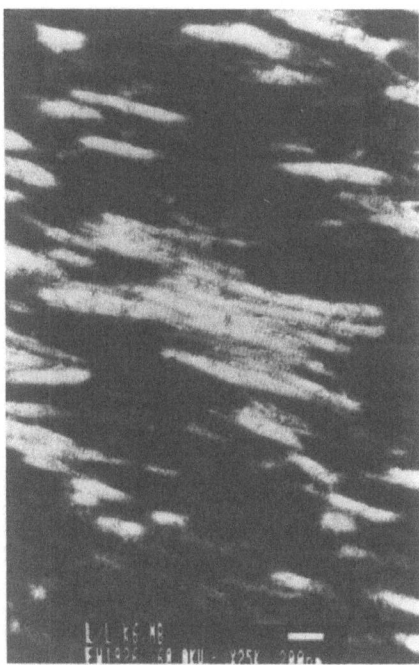

Fig. 11. Transmission electron photomicrograph of lased collagen with alterations in the parallel oriented collagen fibers and loss of the regular periodicity to the striation pattern. Interdigitation and fusion of the collagen fibers with an overall increase in the fiber size is also demonstrated. (× 25 000)

tation of the individual collagen fibers was also seen (Fig. 11).

Discussion

Lasers produce monochromatic, collimated, and coherent light energy which can be focused on musculoskeletal tissues, creating a specific laser-tissue interaction [5, 12]. The tissue absorption of the laser energy produces photothermal, photodisruptive, and photochemical effects [7]. These tissue effects may be regulated to produce a wide variety of effects including tissue ablation and collagen shortening, as described in this model, through the selection of the wavelength of lasing medium, energy output, pulse repetition rate, distance of the laser probe from the tissue, and the inherent absorptive properties of the tissue.

The Ho:YAG laser provides a near-infrared electromagnetic radiation wavelength of 2.1 μm and a feasible delivery system with flexible quartz optic fibers. Lasing is possible in a saline environment with near-direct or direct tissue contact, as needed in arthroscopy. Current technology provides laser probe tips which deliver the light energy at 0–90° from the probe while producing a controlled energy delivery with predictable tissue absorption and depth of penetration. These features make the Ho:YAG laser uniquely applicable to many

clinical and experimental procedures in orthopedics.

Numerous in vivo and in vitro effects of laser energy on tissue such as the menisci [10, 14, 18, 20, 23], intervertebral fibrocartilage [4, 17], bone [19], and articular cartilage [20–22, 24] have been demonstrated. The extent of tissue injury and thermal damage, ablation thresholds, histoligic responses, and mechanism of ablation have been examined. Anecdotes from studies using the Ho:YAG laser for ablation of fibrocartilage noted an effect of "considerable tissue shrinking" [4] and laser energy delivered to the meniscus in a noncontact fashion was noted to "curl and deform" the meniscal fragment edges [8].

Collagen buckling similar to the shortening produced in this model has been demonstrated in vitro in scleral tissues [13]. In that study Ho:YAG laser energy was utilized to induce a "buckle effect" in the collagen of the sclera designed to treat retinal detachment. The authors hypothesize that the shrinkage was induced by fusion of the collagen lamellae and collagen fiber contraction through increases in local tissue temperature from laser energy absorption in scleral water. The histologic appearance of the lased collagen fibers in our present study was similar to the appearance of the collagen fibers in scleral tissues treated with the Ho:YAG laser.

The mechanism of collagen shortening and the development of length-dependent increased stiffness observed in this investigation is not well understood. Bass et al. [2] examined the structural changes in collagen molecules which follow lasing. They demonstrated an absence of the helical structure in collagen after lasing similar to that found in heat-denatured collagen. From biochemical studies, they concluded that collagen molecules are indeed denatured by photothermal laser energy. They also showed that noncovalent interactions were created between collagen molecules after lasing.

In the 1950s, the Nobel Prize in Chemistry winner P. J. Flory [11] described the thermodynamic effects of increased temperature on collagen shrinkage. They noted that collagen shrinkage denoted a change in the characteristics of the collagen structure from a crystalline to an amorphous phase. This process may be occurring during lasing, as light energy is transformed into thermal energy in the interstitial water of the tissues tested in our experiments, resulting in a change in the configuration of the collagen and thus producing shrinkage. The direct thermal effects, or temperature change in the tissue, from the laser energy are likely to account for many of the changes in the collagen we have presented; however, the tissue temperature was not quantified in this series of experiments.

Schober et al. [15] demonstrated the loss of periodicity, increased caliber, and interdigitation of collagen fibrils after lasing which was directed toward microsurgical tissue welding. White et al. [25] reported a loss of collagen striation and swelling of collagen fibrils to 100–400 μm from normal 70 μm in collagen treated with laser energy. These findings of distinct and reproducible alterations in the collagen ultrastructure after lasing are consistent with the changes noted in our series of experiments. The loss of the ability to polarize light coupled with the changes in the collagen striations observed in this model strongly suggest a change in the collagen helical structure and linear alignment of the collagen fibers after lasing. One may hypothesize that the mechanisms described above, of laser-induced changes in collagen ultrastructure, may account for the reproducible shortening and increased stiffnes observed in the canine infrapatellar tendons lased in this study.

The canine infrapatellar tendon was selected as a substrate for this series of experiments for a number of reasons. The osseous attachments of the infrapatellar tendon to the patella and the tibia afford reliable fixation for mechanical testing and length determination. Further, the thickness of the canine infrapatellar tendon approximates that of the human inferior glenohumeral ligament [3] and is also composed of highly organized and parallel collagen bundles [9]. The tendon exhibited reproducible viscoelastic properties including stress relaxation, creep, and hysteresis under the testing conditions utilized in these experiments.

The changes in the structural properties which follow lasing observed in this study include decreased length, a decrease in the stiffness and resistance to elongation when subject to a 4 % strain from the shortened length, and a marked increase in stiffness and resistance to elongation with decreased energy of hysteresis when subjected to a 4 % strain after lasing and returning to the original prelasing length. Overall, the lased tissue demonstrated increased stiffness when at the same length as unlased controls.

The influence of in vivo initial inflammatory response, subsequent healing, and remodeling of the lased collagen when treated with subablation levels of laser energy has not been defined. The lowest threshold for the power settings which produces laser-induced shortening needs to be further clarified to allow controlled shortening with the least amount of cellular damage and collagen ablation. Furthermore, the effect of tissue tension or preload on the ability of laser energy to produce shortening requires additional investigation.

Summary

This study presents a reproducible model of collagen shortening with the Ho:YAG laser in the canine infrapatellar tendon. The laser–tissue interaction may be controlled and is uniquely suitable in an arthroscopic fluid environment. The structural properties of lased tissue reveal significantly increased stiffness compared to unlased controls which is dependent upon the strain on the tissue. Histologic analysis in vitro shows loss of orientation of collagen fibers with loss of polarization, alterations in staining patterns suggesting protein denaturing, and cellular necrosis in lased areas. Ultrastructural changes include increased collagen fiber size, loss of striations, and fusion of fibers, possibly through the creation of new noncovalent bonding between collagen fibers leading to collagen shortening and increased tissue stiffness. The Ho:YAG laser may have important relevant clinical applications in shortening collagen structures, such as the inferior glenohumeral ligament, while further evaluation of remodeling in laser-treated collagen structures needs to be examined.

Acknowledgement. The authors thank Michael Helms and Ewa Worniallo for their technical assistance.

References

[1] Abelow SP (1993) Use of lasers in orthopedic surgery: current concepts. Orthopedics 16:551–556
[2] Bass LS, Moazami N, Pocsidio J, Oz MC, LoGerfo P, Treat MR (1992) Changes in type I collagen following laser welding. Lasers Surg Med 12:500–505
[3] Bigliani LU, Pollock RG, Soslowsky LJ, Flatow EL, Pawluk RJ, Mow VC (1992) Tensile properties of the inferior glenohumeral ligament. J Orthop Res 10:187–197
[4] Buchelt M, Kutschera H-P, Katterschafka T, Kiss H, Schneider B, Ullrich R (1992) Erb:YAG and Hol:YAG laser ablation of meniscus and intervertebral discs. Lasers Surg Med 12:375–381
[5] Dew DK (1995) Laser biophysics for the orthopedic surgeon. Clin Orthop 310:6–13
[6] Dillingham MF, Price JM, Fanton GS (1993) Holmium laser surgery. Orthopedics 16:563–566
[7] Fuller TA (1987) Surgical laser: a clinical guide. MacMillan, New York, pp 1–17
[8] Metcalf RW (1987) Lasers in orthopedic surgery. In: Dixon JA (ed) Surgical application of lasers. Year Book Medical, Chicago, pp 275–286
[9] O'Brien SJ, Neves MC, Arnoczky SP et al (1990) The anatomy and histology of the inferior glenohumeral ligament complex of the shoulder. Am J Sports Med 8:449–456
[10] O'Brien SJ, Miller DV, Fealy SV, Gibne MA, Kelly AM (1992) Lasers and the meniscus. In: Mow VC, Arnoczky SP, Jackson DW (eds) Knee meniscus: basic and clinical foundations. Raven, New York, pp 153–164
[11] Oth JFM, Dumitru ET, Spurr OK, Flory PJ (1957) Phase equilibrium in the hydrothemal shrinkage of collagen. J Am Chem Soc 79:3288–3289
[12] Parrish JA (1987) Laser photomedicine: selective laser-tissue interaction. In: Dixon JA (ed) Surgical application of lasers. Year Book Medical, Chicago, pp 34–51

[13] Ren Q, Simon G, Parel J-M, Smiddy W (1993) Laser scleral buckling for retinal reattachment. Am J Ophthalmol 115:758–762

[14] Schaffer JL, Dark M, Itzkan I et al (1995) Mechanisms of meniscal tissue ablation by short pulse laser irradiation. Clin Orthop 310:30–36

[15] Schober R, Ulrich F, Sander T, Durselen H, Hessel S (1986) Laser-induced alteration of collagen substructure allows microsurgical tissue welding. Science 232:1421–1422

[16] Shapiro GS, Fanton GS, Dillingham MF, Perkash R (1995) Lateral retinacular release: the holmium:YAG laser versus electrocautery. Clin Orthop 310:42–47

[17] Sherk HH, Black J, Rhodes A, Lane G, Prodoehl J (1993) Laser discectomy. Clin Sports Med 12:569–577

[18] Sherk HH, Black JD, Prodoehl JA, Diven J (1995) The effects of lasers and electrosurgical devices on human meniscal tissue. Clin Orthop 310:14–20

[19] Stein E, Sedlacek T, Fabian RL, Nishioka NS (1990) Acute and chronic effects of bone ablation with a pulsed holmium laser. Lasers Surg Med 10:384–388

[20] Trauner K, Nishioka N, Patel D (1990) Pulsed holmium:yttrium-aluminum-garnet (Ho:YAG) laser ablation of fibrocartilage and articular cartilage. Am J Sports Med 18:316–320

[21] Trauner KB, Nishioka NS, Flotte T, Patel D (1995) Acute and chronic response of articular cartilage to holmium:YAG laser irradiation. Clin Orthop 310:52–57

[22] Vangsness CT, Ghaderi B (1993) A literature review of lasers and articular cartilage. Orthopedics 16:593–598

[23] Vangsness CT, Akl Y, Nelson SJ, Liaw L-H L, Smith CF, Marshall GJ (1995) In vitro analysis of laser meniscectomy. Clin Orthop 310:21–26

[24] Vangsness CT, Smith CF, Marshall GJ, Sweeney JR, Johansen E (1995) The biological effects of carbon dioxide laser surgery on rabbit articular cartilage. Clin Orthop 310:48–51

[25] White RA, Kopchok GE, White GH, Klein SR, Uitto J (1987) Laser vascular anastomotic welding. In: White RA et al (eds) Lasers in cardiovascular disease. Year Book Medical, Chicago, pp 103–117

[26] Woo SL-Y, Peterson RH, Ohland KJ, Sites TJ, Danto MI (1990) The effects of strain rate of the medial collateral ligament in skeletally immature and mature rabbits: a biomechanical and histological study. J Orthop Res 8:712–721

Basic Properties of Collagen Shrinkage and Laser–Collagen Interactions

M. D. Markel · K. Hayashi · G. Thabit III

Introduction

The thermal properties of collagen have been extensively studied in a variety of experimental models since the mechanism of collagen shrinkage was first proposed by Flory et al. [7–9] in the 1950s. Flory et al. [7–9] described how thermal contraction of collagen is brought about by a transition between the crystalline and amorphous phases of collagen. The investigators applied the thermodynamic theory of high-polymeric materials described by Gee [11] to collagenous shrinkage and demonstrated that the transition from a crystalline to an amorphous phase is fully analogous to that involved in the melting of other crystalline polymers. The transition to an amorphous state where polypeptide chains are disordered and randomly coiled was deduced from the disappearance of X-ray diffraction and the loss of optical birefringence of native collagen [9]. The process was described as "degradation to gelatin" or as "denaturation."

It has been shown that the thermal properties of collagen vary with the age of the animal and the environmental condition [1, 19, 30, 33]. Rosenbloom et al. [26[showed that hydroxyproline content determines the denaturation temperature of collagen using a chick tendon model. More recently, Allain et al. [1] described collagen network behavior under the influence of heat during hydrothermal shrinkage and swelling in rat skin. These investigators proposed that the onset of denaturation of collagen starts with the unwinding of the triple helix. During the course of the temperature rise, hydrolysis of the heat-labile crosslinks occurs, while the maintenance of heat-stable crosslinks is responsible for the residual tension within collagen fibrils (Fig. 1). The investigators concluded that swelling and shrinkage of collagen fibrils are secondary to unwinding of the triple helix with maintenance of heat-stable intermolecular crosslinks. Hogan et al. [19] reported a strong correlation between thermal properties of tendon and the concentration of nonreducible crosslinks. To date, the thermal properties of collagen have been explained mainly in terms of the crosslinks. A number of different methods have been used to study this parameter, including differential

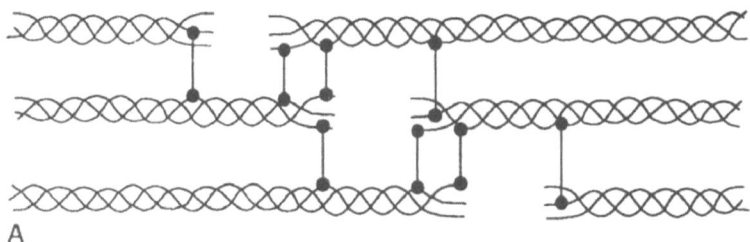

A

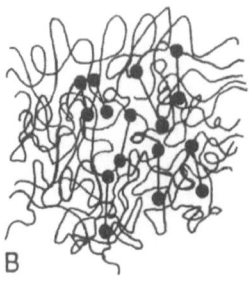

B

Fig. 1A, B. Effect of heat on the strcutural properties of type I collagen. **A** shows the native structure of collagen. In **B**, the triple helix of collagen has undergone thermal unwinding due to disruption of the hydrogen bonds between the α-chains of the triple helix. Shrinkage occurs because of the combination of thermal unwinding and the maintenance of heat-stable crosslinks during this process

scanning calorimetry, ultraviolet difference spectroscopy, isometric tension measurement, and isotonic contraction measurement [1, 5, 19, 30, 33].

Laser Tissue Welding

The joining of tissues together requires uniform heating of the tissues to approximately 70 °C [31]. At that temperature, the collagen of the tissue changes its physical properties and the tissue becomes sticky. If the temperature exceeds 100 °C, the water in the tissue vaporizes and the tissue is destroyed. Milliwatt CO_2 lasers can achieve satisfactory tissue heating in thin-walled structures such as small arteries and veins, and for this reason these lasers have been used successfully in sutureless anastomoses of small vessels and in thin-walled, hollow organs such as the fallopian tube and the vas deferens. Mechanical testing of weld strengths by measurement of the intraluminal pressure required to disrupt repair sites revealed that vascular and other tubular structures repaired with the laser are as strong as those repaired with sutures [34]. Small nerves can also be repaired with laser techniques. Campion et al. [4] found, in rabbits, that the repair of peripheral nerves with an argon laser was superior to repair with a standard epineural suture in terms of time to return of function.

The mechanism by which lasers achieve tissue welding has been debated since the technique was first described by Schober et al. [28]. In their study, Schober et al. described collagen fibrils that had lost their periodicity, were greatly increased in caliber, and were split into fine fibrillary substructures with a roughly concentric arrangement on cross section. The fibrils were closely interdigitated with each other, implying that this interdigitation was the structural basis for the laser-induced welding effect. Guthrie et al. [12] studied argon laser-fused canine veins and noted alterations in several proteins after laser welding: the putative β-chain of type V collagen, the putative γ-chain of type I collagen, a 156-kDa protein, an 82-kDa protein, and several lower molecular weight proteins. The authors postulated that their findings suggested that laser welding may occur by formation of crosslinks or by denaturation and reannealment of structural proteins. Bass et al. [3] studied rat tail tendon after tissue welding using an 808-nm diode laser. Circular dichroism studies of the welded tendon showed absence of helical structure in collagen with no evidence of covalent bonding in the tissue. The authors concluded that noncovalent interactions between denatured collagen molecules may be responsible for the creation of tissue welding. Pearce and Thomsen [25] confirmed these findings by developing a kinetic model of laser-tissue fusion processes and reported that fusion depended primarily on thermal denaturation of tissue collagen with the fibrils of apposed collagen strands apparently unraveling under sufficient heat and re-entwining during the cooling phase. Each of the above-mentioned studies confirms that laser energy can significantly alter the collagenous architecture of tissues. These studies were an important first step toward the development of the laser-assisted capsular shift (LACS) procedure for the treatment of glenohumeral joint instability.

Thermokeratoplasty

The concept of thermokeratoplasty arose from studies which demonstrated that corneal stromal collagen shrinks to approximately one-third of its original length when heated to a temperature of 60–65 °C [23, 30]. At higher temperatures, substantial additional shrinkage does not occur, but additional thermal injury and necrosis results. In the mid-1970s, thermokeratoplasty was explored as a potential therapeutic alternative to penetrating keratoplasty in patients with keratoconus [24]. Initial reports of success [10] were followed by reports of profound initial flattening but with subsequent return to preoperative topography [21]. Complications such as delayed epithelial healing, recurrent epithelial erosions, aseptic stromal necrosis and melting, and vascularization were also reported [2]. Rowsey and Doss [27] described an instrument designed to heat stromal collagen using radiofrequency waves, but the procedure produced short-lived topographic changes and was withdrawn from clinical experimentation [23]. Despite failure to achieve permanent corneal topographic changes as a result of heating the stroma, two groups in 1990 reported stable curvature changes with laser thermokeratoplasty. Seiler et al. [29] used a pulsed Ho:YAG laser to steepen corneas of blind eyes; they described hyperopic changes of up to 5 diopters that remained stable. Horn et al. [20] used a cobalt:magnesium fluoride laser that was tunable to a wavelength of 1.65–2.25 μm and described curvature changes in rabbits of as much as 8 diopters that were stable for at least 1 year. In a slightly different application, thermal tendinoplasty was evaluated in order to shrink extraocular muscle tendon for the treatment of strabismus. In this study, the investigators proposed the advantages of thermal tendinoplasty over conventional surgical techniques [6]. These studies and others indicate that lasting topographic changes can be achieved if stromal heating of appropriate magnitude and depth is accomplished [32].

Both of these bodies of research (thermokeratoplasty, tissue welding) indicate that permanent long-lasting alteration of collagenous architecture can be achieved by application of nonablative laser energy with minimal or no concomitant inflammatory response. The concept of applying laser energy to joint capsular tissue to achieve shrinkage, diminishmant of joint capsular volume, and joint stabilization in patients with glenohumeral instability is both novel and exciting. Preliminary studies conducted by our laboratory and by a collaborative group of orthopedic surgeons indicate that this application of laser energy may have important clinical ramifications.

Joint Capsular Studies

Over the past 4 years, several investigations have been performed evaluating laser-induced joint capsular shrinkage, including in vitro and in vivo rabbit studies, an in vivo sheep study [18], and an in vitro human joint capsular study in order to evaluate the potential application of nonablative laser energy for joint capsular modulation.

In Vitro Rabbit Studies

The purpose of the studies was to evaluate the effect of laser energy at nonablative energy densities on joint capsular material properties. Specifically, we evaluated the effect of three power settings (5 W, 10 W, and 15 W) on the mechanical, biochemical, histological, and ultrastructural properties of joint capsular tissue in an in vitro rabbit model.

Twenty-four mature New Zealand white rabbits were used for this experiment [13]. Animals were euthanized and two 5-×-20-mm specimens were collected from the medial and lateral portion of the femoropatellar joint of each rabbit under a dissecting microscope; thus four specimens were collected from each rabbit (right medial, right lateral, left medial, left lateral). Specimens were divided into four groups using a randomized block design: a control group and a group for each of the three laser power settings, 5 W, 10 W, and 15 W. Laser energy was applied using the Ho:YAG laser in four transverse passes across the tissue at a velocity of 2 mm/s and the distance from the tip of the handpiece to the synovial surface of the specimen set at 1.5 mm in a 37 °C tissue bath of lactated Ringer's solution.

Forty-eight specimens ($n = 12$) were mechanically tested to determine single-cycle structural properties (stiffness) and viscoelastic properties (% relaxation) before and after laser treatment. Shrinkage of the tissue and the loads required to return specimens to their original length were recorded after laser treatment. Twenty-four specimens ($n = 6$) were processed for biochemical analysis to evaluate the effect of laser energy on type I collagen content and nonreducible

crosslinking of joint capsular tissue. Collagen content was measured by hydroxyproline (Hyp) concentration and nonreducible crosslinking was measured by hydroxylysylpyridinoline (HP) concentration using high performance chromatography. Twenty-four specimens ($n = 6$) were processed for histological analysis using light mircoscopy to evaluate the effect of laser energy on the morphology of fibroblasts and collagen in treated joint capsular tissue. Twenty-four specimens ($n = 6$) were processed for ultrastructural analysis using transmission electron microscopy.

The application of laser energy resulted in 9 %, 26 %, and 36 % reduction in capsular tissue length in the 5-W, 10-W, and 15-W groups, respectively (Fig. 2). Tissue shrinkage was significantly and strongly correlated with energy density ($p < 0.0001$; $R^2 = 0.80$) (Fig. 3). Laser energy caused a significant decrease in tensile stiffness only in the 10-W and 15-W groups ($p < 0.05$) (Fig. 4). There was a significant but weak correlation between energy density and post-laser stiffness values ($p < 0.0001$; $R^2 = 0.34$). Laser energy did not change the relaxation properties of capsular tissue at any energy density when compared to prelaser values ($p > 0.05$; $\Delta = 29$ % at power = 0.8) (Fig. 5). There was no significant correlation between energy density and relaxation properties of the tissue ($p > 0.05$). The loads required to return specimens to their original length were significantly lower for the 5-W group (3.6 ± 5.1 N) than for the 10-W (15.0 ± 6.2 N) and 15-W (14.0 ± 5.2 N) groups. There was a significant correlation between

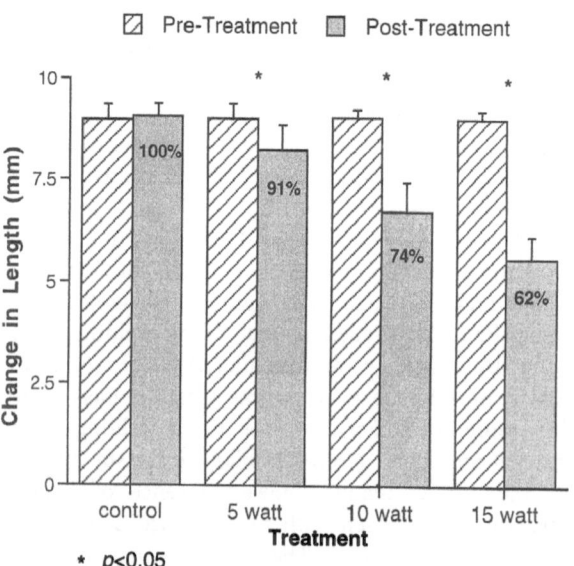

Fig. 2. Effect of laser energy on capsular shrinkage. Post-treatment length is significantly shorter than pretreatment length for each of the laser treatment groups. In addition, each of the post-treatment lengths is significantly different from each of the others ($p < 0.05$)

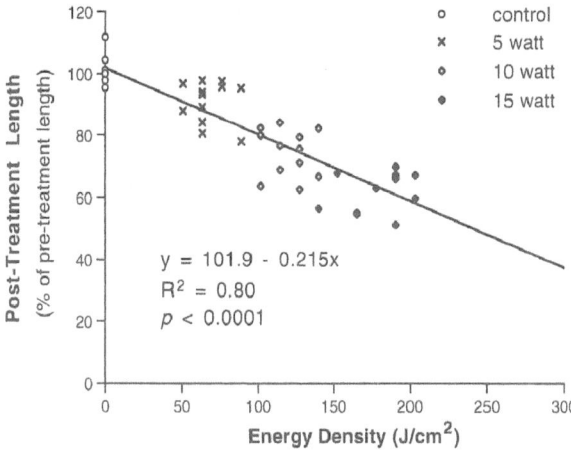

Fig. 3. Correlation between energy density and capsular shrinkage

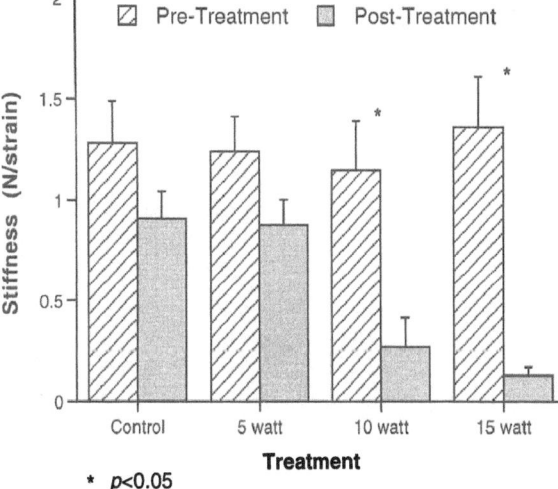

Fig. 4. Effect of laser energy on capsular stiffness. Treatment with the laser at a power setting of 10 or 15 W significantly reduced the stiffness of the joint capsule compared to pre-treatment values *(asterisk)* and compared to control and the 5-W group

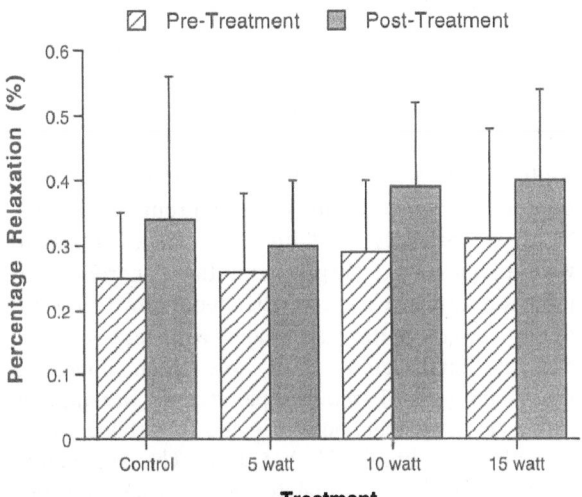

Fig. 5. Effect of laser energy on capsular percentage relaxation. Means are not different from each other ($p > 0.05$)

energy density and the load required to return the specimen to its original length ($p < 0.0001$; $R^2 = 0.58$).

Biochemical analysis indicated that application of laser energy did not cause significant alteration of collagen content and nonreducible crosslinks at any energy density [15]. There were no significant differences in collagen content among groups: 47.6 ± 10.8, 46.1 ± 5.3, 46.8 ± 9.8, and 45.9 ± 10.0 mg Hyp/mg dry weight (mean $\pm$ SD) in the control, 5-W, 10-W, and 15-W groups, respectively ($p > 0.05$; $\Delta = 20\%$ at power $= 0.8$). In addition, there were no significant differences in nonreducible collagen crosslinks among groups: 0.75 ± 0.17, 0.85 ± 0.17. 0.87 ± 0.17, and 0.87 ± 0.16 mole HP/mole of collagen (mean $\pm$ SD) in the control, 5-W, 10-W, and 15-W groups, respectively ($p > 0.05$; $\Delta = 23\%$ at power $= 0.8$).

Histological examination of the tissue revealed evidence of thermal damage of the tissue at all laser energy densities, which was characterized by fusion of collagen and pyknotic nuclear changes in fibroblasts; each progressively higher laser energy caused significantly greater morphological changes over a larger area (Fig. 6) [15].

Transmission electron microscopy revealed alteration of the collagen architecture, with significantly increased fibril cross-section for each of the treated groups compared to controls (Fig. 7) [14]. The fibrils began to lose their distinct edges and their periodical cross-striations at progressively higher energy densities. The results of ultrastructural morphometry of fibril diameter distributions revealed that each progressively higher laser energy caused a significant increase in collagen fibril diameter ($p < 0.05$) (Fig. 8). Mean fibril diameter was significantly correlated with energy density ($p < 0.0001$; $R^2 = 0.51$).

This study demonstrated that significant capsular shrinkage can be achieved with the application of nonablative H:YAG laser ernergy without detrimental effects on the viscoelastic properties of the tissue, although at higher energy densities, laser energy did lessen capsular stiffness properties. Application of laser energy did not cause significant alteration of biochemical parameters evaluated in this study; however, histological/ultrastructural analysis revealed thermal changes in the tissue and significant alteration of collagen ultrastructure.

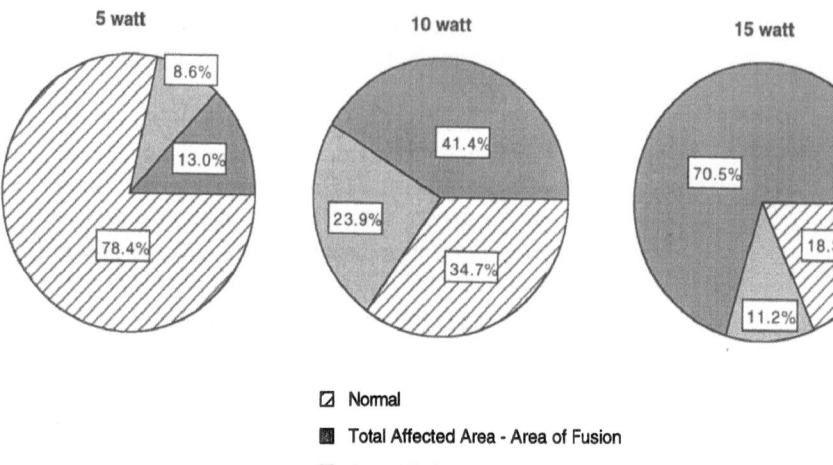

Fig. 6. Effect of laser energy on percentage area with histological alterations caused by laser energy. The percentage of area with collagen fiber fusion and the percentage of area with any change observed (% total affected area – area of fusion) were significantly different among laser-treated groups

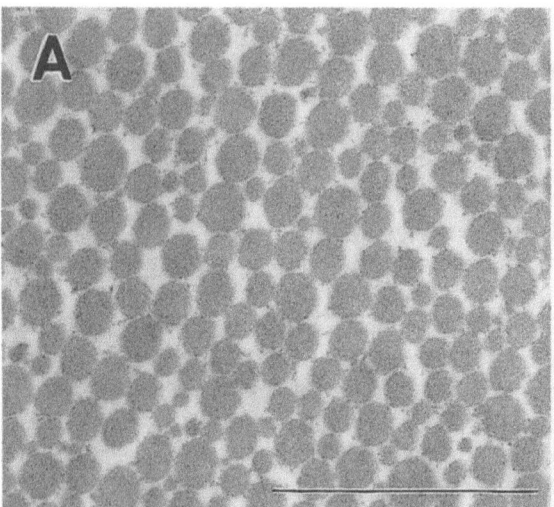
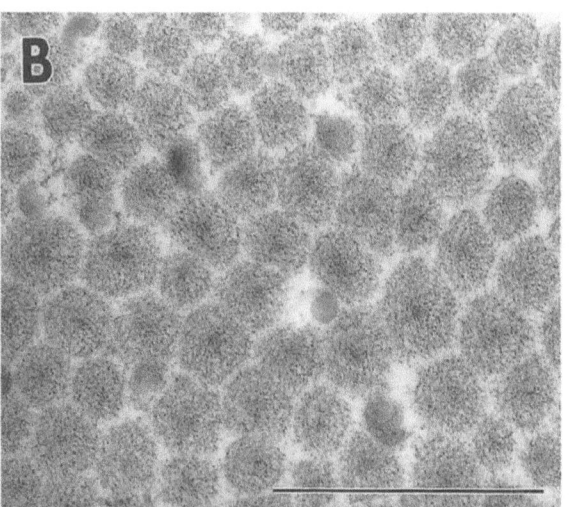

Fig. 7A, B. Transmission electron microscopy of cross-section of A control joint capsular tissue, B 10-W groups (× 24 000; *bar* = 1 μm)

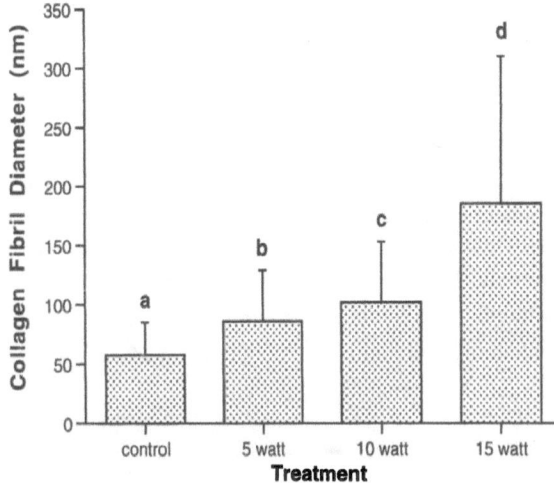

Fig. 8. Histogram of fibril diameter control, 5-W, 10-W, and 15-W groups. Means with different *letters* are significantly different from each other ($p < 0.05$)

In Vivo Rabbit Study

The purpose of this study was to evaluate the effect of nonablative laser energy on the short-term histological properties of joint capsular tissue in an in vivo rabbit model [16]. Eighteen mature New Zealand white rabbits were used in this study. Rabbits were randomly assigned to one of three groups (0, 7, and 30 days postsurgery). Both stifles of each rabbit were prepared for surgery and the femoropatellar joint was exposed via a patellar tenotomy. One randomly selected stifle was treated with laser energy, and the contralateral stifle was sham operated. Laser energy (0.5 J/10 pulses per second) was applied to the femoropatellar joint capsule in lactated Ringer's solution using the Ho:YAG laser. The laser handpiece was held approximately 1.5 mm away from the synovial surface and moved over the tissue in a paintbrush motion. Animals were euthanized at three time intervals: immediately after surgery (day 0), 7 days after surgery, and 30 days after surgery. The femoropatellar joint capsule was harvested immediately after euthanasia. Specimens were processed for histological staining with hematoxylin and eosin.

Control tissues obtained from animals euthanized immediately after sham operations showed no significant histological lesions (Fig. 9A). Laser-treated samples at day 0 showed diffuse hyalinization and fusion of collagen with nuclear karyorrhexis and nuclear streaming of fibroblasts in treated regions (Fig. 9B). Control tissues at 7 days after sham operations showed granulation tissue, mixed inflammatory cell infiltration, and fibrosis. Laser-treated tissue at 7 days after surgery revealed similar histological changes to control tissue along with fibroblast proliferation around and into acellular hyalinized collagen regions (Fig. 9C). Control tissue at 30 days after sham operations showed mature granulation tissue and regular dense fibrous connective tissue in the normal collagenous joint capsule tissue. Laser-treated tissues at 30 days after surgery showed fibrosis with cellular and disorganized connective tissue (Fig. 9D). Fused collagen regions were greatly reduced by 30 days after laser treatment as large reactive fibroblasts migrated to the site and secreted new matrix to replace the hyalinized tissue (Fig. 9D).

This study illustrates the short-term in vivo tissue response and collagen repair process following laser treatment of joint capsular tissue. Both control and laser-treated samples showed normal responses to tissue trauma resulting from the standard surgical procedure. At 7 and 30 days after laser treatment, acellular hyalinized regions of collagen are infiltrated by fibroblasts which have used the fused collagen as the framework for migration and secretion of new collagen matrix in order for tissue repair to proceed, thereby reducing the area of hyalinized collagen.

In Vitro Human Tissue Bath Study

The purpose of this study was to evaluate the effect of temperature on thermal shrinkage and histological properties of glenohumeral joint capsular tissue using a temperature-controlled tissue bath [17]. Our previous histological study revealed that the application of nonablative laser energy caused thermal alteration of collagen (fusion) and fibroblasts (pyknosis) [16]. Thermal shrinkage of collagen is a well-described phenomenon. Based on these findings, we hypothesized that the shrinkage of the tissue induced by laser is predominantly caused by the thermal effect of laser energy and is a function of temperature.

Six fresh frozen cadaver shoulders were used for this study (age 52.3 ± 4.9 years; mean ± SD). The entire joint capsule was detached from the glenoid and humerus. Seven regions of interest were dissected in a radial manner from the humeral to the glenoid edge; 10-×-30-mm specimens were collected

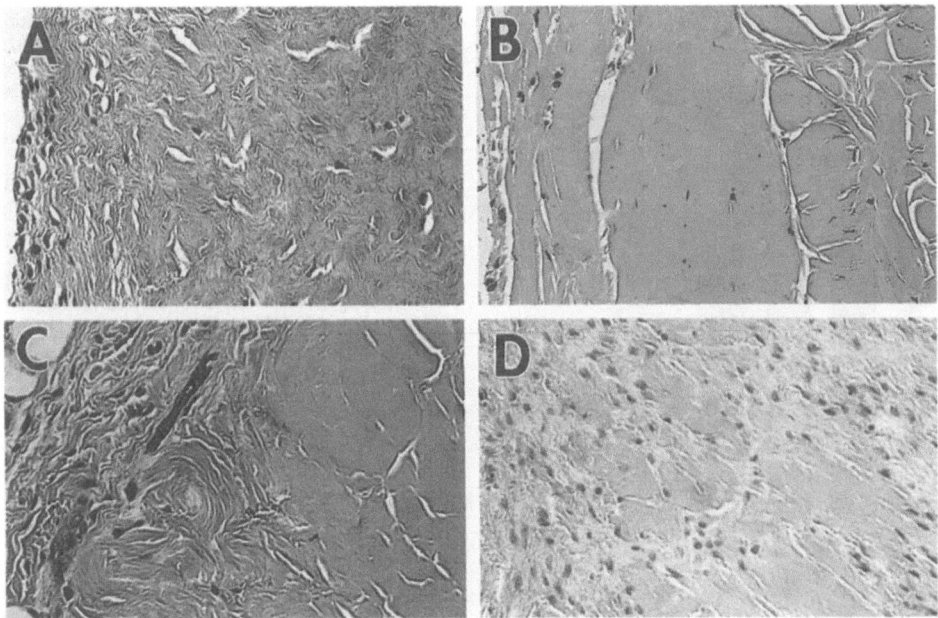

Fig. 9. A Light micrograph of control day 0 capsular tissue demonstrating normal collagen and fibroblasts. B Light micrograph of laser-treated day 0 capsular tissue demonstrating hyalinization of collagen and karyorrhexis of fibroblasts. C Light micrograph of laser-treated day 7 capsular tissue demonstrating acellular region and adjacent active fibroblasts. D Light micrograph of laser treated day 30 capsular tissue demonstrating reduced acellular regions with surrounding fibroblasts. (H & E, × 50)

from the superior, middle, inferior (anterior band, axillary pouch, posterior band), and posterior (inferior portion, superior portion) glenohumeral ligament/capsule. Specimens were assigned to one of seven treatment groups (37, 55, 60, 65, 70, 75, 80 °C) ($n = 6$). Each specimen was placed in a custom jig with a pulley system designed to provide a constant load (0.098 N) on the specimen. Following measurement of pretreatment tissue length, specimens were placed in a tissue bath heated to one of the designated treatment temperatures. Changes in tissue length were recorded for 10 min. After treatment, specimens were processed for histological analysis. A subjective scoring system was used to evaluate the effect of temperature on histological properties of collagen structure on a scale from 0 to 3 (0 = normal, 1 = mild, 2 = moderate, 3 = severe thermal alteration).

Treatments with 37, 55, and 60 °C tissue bath did not cause significant changes in tissue length (Fig. 10). Temperature treatments at or above 65 °C caused significant shrinkage when compared to 37, 55, and 60 °C groups (65 °C, 11 %; 70 °C, 41 %; 75 °C, 56 %; 80 °C, 59 %). Posttreatment lengths in 70, 75, and 80 °C groups were significantly less than pretreatment lengths. Shrinkage of the tissue started immediately after the temperature treatment and reached a maximum within 3 min in 75 and 80 °C groups. There was no significant effect of tissue region on tissue shrinkage.

Histological analysis revealed significant thermal alteration of the tissue characterized by fusion of collagen in 65, 70, 75, and 80 °C groups. Scores for collagen were significantly higher for 65, 70, 75, and 80 °C groups than for 37, 55, and 60 °C groups.

There were no significant differences in this parameter among 70, 75, and 80 °C groups.

This study demonstrated that temperatures at or above 65 °C caused significant shrinkage of glenohumeral joint capsular tissue, and that higher temperatures caused an increase in capsular shrinkage, although there was no significant difference between 75 and 80 °C groups. These results are consistent with the histological findings. To verify the effects of non-ablative laser application, studies designed to compare these tissue bath findings with the effects of laser, as well as mechanical studies, must be performed.

References

[1] Allain JC, Le Lous M, Cohen-Solal L, Bazin S (1980) Isometric tension developed during the thermal swelling of rat skin. Conn Tiss Res 7:127–133
[2] Aquavella JV, Smith RS, Shaw EL (1976) Alterations in corneal morphology following thermokeratoplasty. Arch Ophthalmol 94:2082–2085
[3] Bass LS, Moazami N, Pocsidio J, Oz MC, LoGerfo P, Treat MR (1992) Changes in type I colagen following laser welding. Lasers Surg Med 12:500–505
[4] Campion ER, Bynum DK, Powers SK (1990) Repair of peripheral nerves with the argon laser. A functional and histological evaluation. J Bone Joint Surg [Am] 72:715–723
[5] Danielsen CC (1982) Precision method to determine temperature of collagen using ultraviolet difference spectroscopy. Collagen Rel Res 2:143–150
[6] Finger PT, Richards R, Iwamoto T (1987) Heat shrinkage of extraocular muscle tendon. Arch Ophthalmol 105:716–718
[7] Flory PJ, Garrewtt RR (1958) Phase transition in collagen and gelatin systems. J Am Chem Soc 80:4836–4845
[8] Flory PJ, Spurr OK (1960) Melting equilibrium for collagen fibers under stress. Elasticity in the amorphous state. J Am Chem Soc 83:1308–1316
[9] Flory PJ, Weaver ES (1959) Helix coil transition in dilute aqueous collagen solutions. J Am Chem Soc 82:4518–4525
[10] Gasset AR, Kaufman HE (1975) Thermokeratoplasty in the treatment of keratoconus. Am J Ophthalmol 79:226–232
[11] Gee G (1947) Some thermodynamic properties of high polymers, and their molecular interpretation. Q Rev 1:265–298
[12] Guthrie CR, Murray LW, Kopchok GE (1991) Biochemical mechanisms of laser vascular tissue fusion. J Invest Surg. 4:3–12
[13] Hayashi K, Markel MD, Thabit G, Bogdanske JJ, Thielke RJ (1995) The effect of non-ablative laser energy on joint capsular properties: an in vitro mechanical study using a rabbit model. Am J Sports Med 23:482–487
[14] Hayashi K, Thabit G, Bogdanske JJ, Mascio LN, Markel MD (1996) The effect of non-ablative laser energy on the ultrastructure of joint capsular collagen. Arthroscopy 12:474–481
[15] Hayashi K, Thabit G, Vailas AL, Bogdanske JJ, Cooley AJ, Markel MD (1996) The effect of non-ablative laser energy on joint capsular properties: an in vitro histologic and biochemical study using a rabbit model. Am J Sports Med 24:640–646
[16] Hayashi K, Nieckarz JA, Thabit G, Bogdanske JJ, Cooley AJ, Markel MD (1997) The effect of non-ablative laser energy on the joint capsule: an in vivo rabbit study using a holmium:YAG laser. Lasers Surg Med 20:164–171
[17] Hayashi K, Thabit G, Massa KL, Bogdasnke JJ, Cooley AJ, Orwin JF, Markel MD (1997) The effect of thermal heating on the length and histological properties of the glenohumeral joint capsule. Am J Sports Med 25:107–112

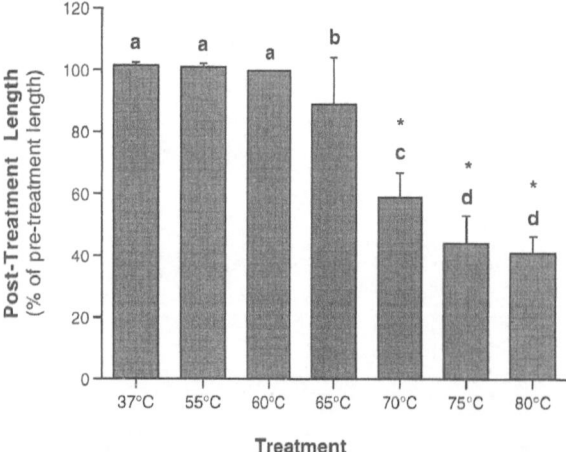

Fig. 10. Changes in length of human glenohumeral joint capsular tissue following submersion in a tissue bath at one of seven temperatures (37, 55, 60, 65, 70, 75, 80 °C). Means with different *letters* are significantly different from each other. Means with an *asterisk* are significantly different from pretreatment length ($p < 0.05$)

[18] Hayashi K, Hecht P, Vaderby R, Peters DM, Cooley AJ, Xiang Z, Thabit G III, Fanton GS, Markel MD (1998) The long term effect of laser energy on joint capsular tissue. Orthop Res Soc 23:1026

[19] Hogan DJ, King NL, Kurth LB (1990) Collagen crosslinks and their relationships to the thermal properties of calf tendons. Arch Biochem Biophys 281:21–26

[20] Horn G, Spears KG, Lopez O (1990) New refractive method for laser thermal keratoplasty with the Co:MgF$_2$ laser. J Cataract Refract Surg 16:611–616

[21] Keates RH, Dingle J (1975) Thermokeratoplasty for keratoconus. Ophthalmic Surg 6:89–92

[22] Mapstone R (1968) Measurement of corneal temperature. Exp Eye Res 7:237–243

[23] McDonnell PJ, Garbus J, Romero JL (1980) Electrosurgical keratoplasty: clinicopathologic correlation. Arch Ophthalmol 106:235–238

[24] Moreira H, Campos M, Sawusch MR, McDonnell JM, Sand B, MacDonnell PJ (1993) Holmium laser thermokeratoplasty. Ophthalmology 100:752–761

[25] Pearce JA, Thomsen S (1993) Kinetic models of laser-tissue fusion processes. Biomed Sci Instrum 29:355–360

[26] Rosenbloom J, Harsch M, Jimenez S (1973) Hydroxyproline content determines the denaturation temperature of chick tendon collagen. Arch Biochem. Biophys 158:478–484

[27] Rowsey JJ, Doss JD (1981) Preliminary report of Los Alamos keratoplasty technique. Ophthalmology 88:755–760

[28] Schober R, Ulrich F, Sander T, Dhrselen H, Hessel S (1986) Laser-induced alteration of collagen substructure allows microsurgical welding. Science 232:1421–1422

[29] Seiler T, Matallana M, Bende T (1990) Laser thermokeratoplasty by means of a pulsed holmium:YAG laser for hyperopic correction. Refract Corneal Surg 6:355–359

[30] Shaw EL, Gasset AR (1974) Thermokeratoplasty (TKP) temperature profile. Invest Ophthalmol 13:181–186

[31] Sherk HH (1993) Curent concepts review: the use of lasers in orthopedic procedures. J Bone Joint Surg [Am] 75:768–776

[32] Thompson VM, Seilter T, Durrie DS, Cavanaugh TB (1993) Holmium:YAG laser thermokeratoplasty for hyperopia and astigmatism: an overview. Refract Corneal Surg 9:S134–S137

[33] Verzar F, Zs-Nagy I (1970) Electron microscopic analysis of thermal collagen denaturation in rat tail tendons. Gerontologia 16:77–82

[34[White AA III, Pankabi MM (1990) Clinical biomechanics of the spine, 2nd edn. Lippincott, Philadelphia, pp 446-487

Effects of Laser on the Anterior Band of the Inferior Glenohumeral Ligament

C. L. SHIELDS · J. R. BRESCH · S. PARK · R. WALLER

Glenohumeral instability is a complex problem with many etiologies and treatment modalities. Conventional treatment options for shoulder laxity are etiology-dependent and include:

- Bankart repair
- Anterior capsulolabral reconstruction
- Capsular shift
- Rehabilitation
- Modification of activities

The simple goal of each of these treatment modalities is to increase stability. This is accomplished by decreasing capsular volume and increasing the tension on the glenohumeral ligaments, resulting in increased static stability through a check rein effect.

Recently, investigators have used a laser to achieve this same effect, producing very promising clinical reports [1]. Laser applications have been proposed for the treatment of individuals with multidirectional stability refractory to therapy, and – in conjunction with an arthroscopic Bankart repair – in subjects with concomitant tissue laxity [3, 4].

Unfortunately, the available literature does not adequately describe the mechanisms for the laser's effect on glenohumeral stability in human subjects, nor are there adequate outcome studies or guidelines for the use of this treatment tool. Futhermore, most of the published data that are available suffer from a lack of sound scientific methodology, consisting primarily of anecdotal reports or clinical accounts, with no consistency as to research technique used or subject populations studied. Although researchers have described the physics of laser absorption and other parameters of laser energy on living animal tissue, nothing has yet been published that specifically describes its effects on human glenohumeral ligaments. Many people are therefore sceptical regarding the use of laser in the treatment of shoulder laxity.

A study we carried out was based on the premise that, if stability is to be achieved, the laser must accomplish one or more of the following:

- Shorten the ligament
- Increase the stiffness of the ligmanet to resist translation

- Alter the healing phase in such a way as to achieve one of the above effects permanently

Our study was designed to examine only the first two outcomes. Since we chose a cadaveric tissue model for our experiment, we could not study healing properties. Our primary objective was to record the amount of force required to stretch untreated ligament, then treat the ligament with the laser to determine whether there was, in fact, shortening. If the ligament was thus shortened, we wanted to know how much force would then be needed to achieve the same degree of stretch as had been obtained in the untreated tissue. Clinically, this would represent an increase in the amount of force required to move the head out of the glenoid fossa after laser treatment.

Method

We chose to examine the anterior band of the inferior glenohumeral ligament of ten fresh frozen human cadaver shoulders. The inferior glenohumeral ligament was selected because it has been shown to be integral to normal stability [2]; we chose the anterior band because, as a reliably identifiable structure, it can be more readily isolated.

The anterior band of the inferior glenohumeral ligament was isolated, along with wedge-shaped bone blocks from the humeral head and glenoid, and the bone blocks potted in polymethylmethacrylate. With a 5-N load to remove laxity from the system, the length, width, and thickness of each specimen was measured in three locations, and the total area of the ligament was calculated. The tissue was then mounted on an MTS tensiometer machine in a special tank so that the experiment could be carried out in a bath of lactated Ringer's solution, simulating the intra-articular environment during arthroscopy. This bath is very important because the laser effects and properties are dependent on a fluid medium.

We chose to control the displacement with the MTS and measure the load required to achieve a determined length. A 5-N force was applied to the tissue at a rate of 1 %/s for five cycles to remove laxity from the system. Displacement of 10 % was then performed and the force generated was recorded (Table 1).

Simulating laxity by bringing the bone blocks closer together in the MTS machine provided very sensitive calculations of shortening. We arbitrarily chose 15 % shortening based on estimates of how much clinical shortening is achieved with open capsular shifts, as reported for other laser procedures. We chose 0.5 W at 10 Hz, a very low total energy load, to apply a forcally controlled beam that would effect collagen cross-linking without causing tissue necrosis [5, 6].

The laser was applied until visible shrinkage occurred and all laxity in the tissue was removed. With the bone blocks brought together, no force was recorded on the MTS, so that a positive force shown on the MTS would then represent removal of laxity from the system. The MTS was also used to determine the endpoint (Table 2).

The total energy applied and the total area of the ligament treated were recorded. Tissue length being load-dependent, however, we then applied a 2-N force to the treated tissue to standardize our pre- and postlaser treatment lengths. Lengths were recorded as the actual amount of shortening achieved.

Under displacement-controlled mode we then displaced the ligament 10 % and recorded the force required to reach this point. Again under displacement control, we stretched the ligament to failure at a rate of 80 cm/s and recorded the stress/strain curve, the load to ultimate failure, and the mode of failure.

Results

We found that laser energy, when applied at 0.5 W, 10 Hz in a sweeping motion to the articular surface of the anterior band of the inferior glenohumeral ligament, results in contraction of the ligament. In conjunction with this shortening, an increase in stiffness also occurs. The degree of contraction is decreased when there is a positive load on the ligament at the time of laser applications, and, under high loads, there is no lengthening without tissue injury. Clinically, this is important, since an effort must be made to decrease traction on the extremity during arthroscopy to maximize contration without tissue injury.

The initial force at 10 % displacement was averaged and showed that the (Fig. 1) average force at 110 % of initial length was 69.7 ± 20.3 N (Table 1). The average amount of contraction obtained, expressed as a percentage of change from the initial

Table 1. Mechanical qualities in the study

	Before laser treatment	After laser treatment
Force for initial length (N)	0	16.7 ± 5
Force for 10 % elongation (N)	69.7 ± 20	98.3 ± 30
Stiffness at 10 % elongation (N/mm)	20.2 ± 6.6	22.7 ± 8.9
Ultimate strength (N)	162 ± 52	157.5 ± 45

Table 2. Physical qualities in the study

Laser energy per ligament (J)	348 ± 165
Energy density (J/cm^3)	82.5 ± 26.1
Percent area treated (%)	77 ± 16
Actual shortening (%)	7.4 ± 1.8
Area shrinkage (%)	14.7 ± 4.6

length, was 7.4 ± 1.8 % (Table 2). The average area of shrinkage was 14.7 ± 4.6 %. This was proportional to the change in length, suggesting that as the length changes, so does the width: the amount of capsular volume change is apparently influenced by changes on at least two planes.

Values of the force required to displace the tissue back to its initial length, 110 % of the initial length, and the force exerted to reach the point of failure were recorded and averaged. It took 16.7 N to achieve the prelaser resting length and 98.3 N to achieve the 110 % length, an average increase of 42.5 % from 69.7 N.

We observed in every tissue the need for additional force to achieve the same amount of stretch and change in the curve, an increase in stiffness that was statistically significant. Analyzing the actual stress/strain curve, the stiffness could be calculated by taking the tangent of the slope. The mean stiffness before and after laser at failure was 20.2 ± 6.6 N/mm and 22.7 ± 8.9 N/mm, respectively, an increase of about 4 % ($p = 0.15$).

Our stiffness measurements were controlled by using the same tissue for pre- and postlaser treatment. We could not likewise control the measurement of ultimate load to failure because we lacked match-

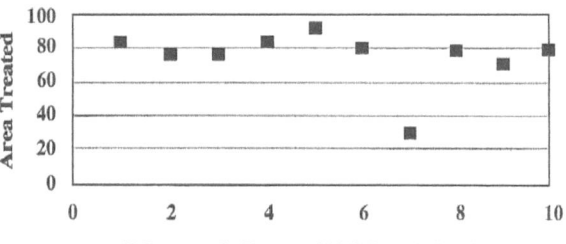

Fig. 1. Area treated vs. increase in force at 110 % length

ing controlled non-laser-treated tissue to study. For this reason we had to compare our average failure point with those recorded by other investigators. The comparative data show a similar strain failure percentage, suggesting little effect on the ultimate load to failure. Bigliani et al. [2], for example, showed a strain percentage of 34 ± 10.5% at failure for the anterior band of the glenohumeral ligament. Our postlaser strain percentage at failure was 29 ± 4.2%, suggesting little change in overall failure strain after laser application of our study at similar magnitude. Future trials will include matched pairs to permit a more accurate comparison.

In an attempt to show a linear relationship between the amount of energy applied and the degree of shortening and stiffness achieved, we plotted these variables against each other. Unfortunatly, due to the scatter of our data, we cannot conclude that there is a direct and predictable amount of shortening achieved with a specific amount of energy; the cadaver shoulder tissue exhibited varying degrees of tensile strength. The average energy applied was 348 ± 165 J (Figs. 2, 3). We obtained similar findings after correcting for total area and volume. This is not surprising, since the variance in change of length was so small. Using a larger population and varying the length, a linear relationship might be demonstrated.

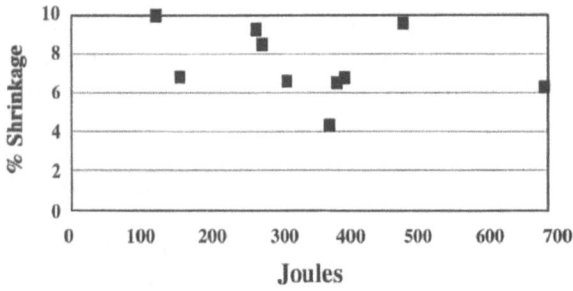

Fig. 2. Relationship between shrinkage and applied energy (J)

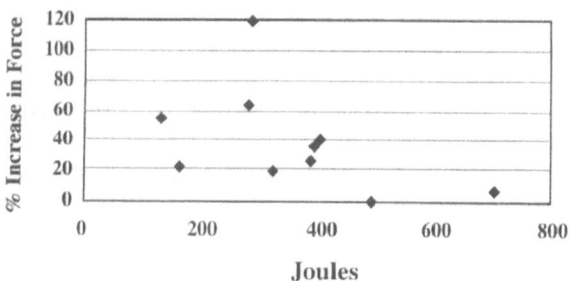

Fig. 3. Relationship between increase in force and applied energy (J)

Clonclusions

Our study supports clinical reports showing that laser capsulorrhaphy achieves improvement in laxity symptoms by decreasing capsular volume and length. This is most likely due to the changes we observed in shortening and stiffness. Additional laboratory studies are needed to provide further clinical guidelines with regard to the amount of tissue to treat and the percentage of shrinkage desired, as well as appropriate laser settings.

Further investigation is also needed to document this effect and to monitor chances during the healing process in living tissue.

References

[1] Abelow SP (1993) Use of lasers in orthopedic surgery: current concepts. Orthopaedics 16:551–556
[2] Bigliani LU, Pollock RG, Soslowsky LJ, Flatow EL, et al (1992) Tensile properties of the inferior glenohumeral ligament. J Orthop Res 10:L187–197
[3] Dillingham MF, Price JM, Fanton GS (1993) Holmium laser surgery. Orthopaedics 16:563–566
[4] Hayashi K, Markel MD, Thabit G, Bogdanske JJ, Thielke RJ (1995) The effect of laser energy on joint capsular properties – an in vitro mechanical study using a rabbit model. Am J Sports Med 23:482–487
[5] Naseff G, Foster TE, Solhpour S, Zarins B (1996) The thermal properties of type 1 collagen: the basic science of the laser assisted capsular shift. AANA (Arthroscopy Association of North Amercia) Annual Meeting, San Diego, California, April 1996
[6] Schober R, Ulrich F, Sander T, Durselen H, Hesses S (1986) Laser-induced alteration of collagen substructure allows microsurgical tissue welding. Science 232:1421–1422

The Ho:YAG Laser in Shoulder Surgery

A. B. IMHOFF

Introduction

The holmium:YAG laser emits light at a wavelength of 2.1 µm and can be transmitted through conventional optical fibers. The Ho:YAG laser has the ability to precisely and rapidly resect, cut, coagulate, vaporize and ablate cartilaginous tissues. It causes a minimal amount of thermal necrosis while providing superior hemostatic control [27, 30]. This laser can function in a saline medium and may be used in direct contact with the tissue (feedback for the surgeon); however, a *near-contact mode* with a free beam is typically utilized [16, 18].

The present author has used the Ho:YAG laser for knee arthroscopy and for endoscopic intervertebral surgery of the spine with good results since 1989 [9, 13, 19], and has therefore extended the use of this laser to arthroscopic surgery of the shoulder [11]. The arthroscopic use of the Ho:YAG laser not only makes it possible to resect concomitant lesions of the margin of the labrum, but also to debride degenerative tears in the rotator cuff. *Glenoid labral tears* are very successfully treated with laser debridement or resection. Flaps of a loose, torn labrum or degenerative labral tissue can be ablated with the laser. The Ho:YAG laser allows improved labral tissue sparing. *Partial rotator cuff teams* with associated frayed tissues can be treated with laser-assisted debridement.

Synovectomy

Synovectomies using Ho:YAG laser could be an alternative to existing therapeutic techniques in the treatment of rheumatoid arthritis and other synovial proliferative disorders such as synovial chrondromatosis [15] or pigmented villonodular synovitis (PVNS) [9, 14, 28]. Synovectomies can be easily performed because the small handpiece can reach nearly every recess of the joint. The laser dramatically decreases the intraoperative bleeding of this highly vascular tissue. Synovitis is ablated with a typical laser setting of 2.0 J.

Arthroscopic Subacromial Decompression (ASD)

Etiology of the Impingement Syndrome and Indication for ASD

Painfully restricted shoulder motion in adults can be due to many causes. It is usually the result of injury or disease of the rotator cuff, ranging from chronic tendinitis to complete rupture. Probably the most common cause of shoulder pain in adults, however, is the impingement syndrome [7,12, 17, 22, 25]. The space under the acromion is very narrow. It is bounded cranially by the coracoacromial arch which extends from the acromion and the acromioclavicular joint with the coracoacromial ligament to the coracoid process. During active abduction, the upward displacement of the greater tubercle causes the subacromial bursa and the rotator cuff to become squeezed, sandwich-like, between the head of the humerus and this coracoacromial arch. Additional constriction occurs during forced flexion and, especially, during rotation [8]. Chronic repetitive microtrauma results in injury to the rotator cuff with subsequent degeneration. The pathological findings range from bursitis, tendinitis, and fibrotic changes to partial or complete rupture of the rotator cuff [15, 21].

Many factors can cause impingement. *Extrinsic factors* include primary and secondary impingement. *Primary impingement* occurs due to an acromion of variant shape [2], os acromiale, the acromioclavicular joint [5], chronic synovitis of the subacromial bursa, and pathological thickening of the coracoacromial ligament ("outlet impingement"). *Secondary impingement* may result from upward displacement of the humeral head, caused by instability, by posterior capsular tightness, or by abnormal muscular or neurogenic control of the rotator cuff (e. g., suprascapular nerve entrapment syndrome [7, 8, 20]. Pathogenically, stretching of the capsule-ligament complex caused by overuse leads to anterior subluxation when the shoulder is in the externally rotated and abducted position [7].

Intrinsic factors include impingement due to overuse, accompanied by reduced blood supply due to squeezing in the critical zone at the distal end close to the insertion of the supraspinatus muscle [3]. This area is supplied only by anastomoses between two areas of terminal vessels. Rothman and Parke in 1965 [26] were of the opinion that the supply of blood to this area diminished with advancing age, but they were unable to demonstrate this in autopsied shoulders. Rathbun and McNab in 1970 [24] found this hypovascular area in microangiographic studies of the rotator cuff. The key factor leading to impingement syndrome is perhaps repetitive overuse of the supraspinatus muscle [23]. This type of overuse occurs primarily in overhead activities, in which the supraspinatus muscle is contracted eccentrically in order to prevent internal rotation. In the presence of muscle weakness, this ultimately leads to glenohumeral instability. The repetivie microtraumas cause small lesions of the tendons, which trigger the inflammatory process or "inflammatory cascade", as Nirschl has described [23].

There have been many reports of good results with operative treatment (open or arthroscopic) for both stage II and stage III (partial tear only) impingement syndrome refractory to conservative therapy [1, 4, 7, 21, 22, 29, 31, 33]. Since 1985, when Ellman reported his results of arthroscopic subacromial decompression (ASD), there has been growing acceptance of this technique of performing an acromioplasty, coracoacromial ligament resection and bursectomy using a motorized shaver, burr, and electrocautery [4]. As an alternative, the present author has been using the *Ho:YAG laser* in arthroscopic surgery of the knee and the spine since 1991 and in ASD since December 1992 [10]. The benefit of the laser technique is its effective coagulation of small bleeding vessels from the bursa, the undersurface of the deltoid, and the acromion. With the laser, the cicatrized subacromial bursa can be cleanly stripped away and removed while maintaining hemostasis. In these cases, the laser is utilized after standard mechanical instrumentation has removed thick areas of synovium and bursa to create a large working space for laser coagulation and resection of the coracoacromial ligament. With higher power lasers, the anterior portion of a type III acromion can be removed and ablated. After acromioplasty, the bony undersurface of the acromion is virtually "sealed" by the Ho:YAG laser [11, 12].

Surgical Technique

Glenohumeral arthroscopy proceeds subacromial decompression in order to diagnose and treat concomitant pathology. The bursectomy is performed first by means of a 5.5-mm full-radius resector introduced via the anterolateral approach. Two spinal needles are used to isolate the insertion of the coracoacromial ligament. The Ho:YAG laser is then introduced to complete the resection of the subacromial bursa under direct vision and to coagulate hemorrhagic sites and detach the coracoacromial ligament. The use of the laser engenders a relatively bloodless field, with the result that the free ends of the ligament can be resected cleanly and precisely to avoid scarring. Using a higher laser energy for bone removal, acromioplasty can be performed to remove osteophytes from the anterior acromion. Osteophytes at the insertion of the coracoacromial ligament are also resected. Special attention is given to caudal osteophytes of the acromioclavicular joint, which are smoothly resected in the same manner with the shaver and the laser. The use of the laser eliminates hemorrhaging, which frequently restricts visibility severely.

To see how much subacromial bone has to be removed, we start at the lateral acromion lasing a notch with the laser, similar to the conventional arthroscopic procedure. The energy we use is 1.5–2.0 J, 15 Hz, and 40–50 W. Evidence of thermal injury to tissue adjacent to the laser-treated sites has not been seen in our experience so far.

Prospective Study

Patients and Methods

In a prospective study, 52 patients with stage II and III impingement syndrome undergoing ASD were divided into two consecutive groups. The first 18 patients underwent conventional arthorscopic surgery using a motorized shaver and electrocautery (group S). Subsequently, 34 patients undewent ASD performed with the Ho:YAG laser (22 W) and without electrocautery (group L). Subjective, objective, and functional results were assessed using the Constant score preoperatively and postoperatively at specified intervals up to 1 year.

Results

The greatest improvement in the laser group was seen in the areas of pain with activity, pain at night, activity, and movement at 1 week and at 6 weeks. The patients in group L also exhibited significantly better values for abduction power ($p < 0.05$). There were no complications in either group. Pre- and postoperative radiographic evaluation of supraspinatus outlet views demonstrated adequate bone resection in all cases. The postoperative Constant scores for group L were significantly better: the average score increased from 54.7 to 79.8 in group L and from 50.3 to 68.7 in group S. Due to the low level of postoperative pain, the absence of adhesions, and the almost complete lack of swelling. patients in group L were able to regain the full range of shoulder motion sooner than those in group S.

Conclusion

Arthroscopic acromioplasty with the Ho:YAG laser resulted in more rapid achievement of ultimate symptomatic relief. The sealing of the undersurface of the acromion, the bursa, and the deltoid muscle constitutes one of the prime advantages of this minimally invasive technique. Arthroscopic acromioplasty with the Ho:YAG laser is an alternative to conventional ASD in patients who have stage II impingement syndrome and selected patients with selected stage III impingement syndrome. Laser ASD, however, is a technically demanding procedure.

Laser-Assisted Capsular Shift

Plastic deformation or stretching and attenuation are the common pathologic features of multidirectional instability. The aim of using the Ho:YAG laser in laser-assisted capsular shift (LACS) is to correct unidirectional and multidirectional glenohumeral instability arthroscopically. This procedure addresses shoulder instability secondary to capsular redundancy and excessive joint volume by "shrinking" tissue in the shoulder capsule.

Human tissue analysis of collagen fibrils subjected to Ho:YAG laser energy shows loss of collagen cross-strations and increased collagen cross-sectional diameter [32]. The collagen-containing tissue becomes visibly and microscopically shorter and thicker. When Ho:YAG laser energy raises tissue temperature to between 50 ° and 60 °C, denaturation and reanneling of collagen fibers occurs. Temperatures beyond this level may contribute to further tissue shrinkage, but may weaken the tissue as well.

Early results of animal studies suggest that the Ho:YAG laser energy induces visible capsular contraction with shortening of the glenohumeral ligaments and a decrease in joint volume [6]. The degree of tissue shrinkage can be controlled through energy delivery; however, overtightening of the shoulder capsule can occur. Measurements before and after the laser treatment have revealed shrinkage of the capsule by 30%–35%.

The arthrocopic procedure typically uses energy levels of 1.0 J per pulse at a repetition rate of 10 Hz (10 W). Fanton et al. [6] demonstrated excellent clinical results in 93% of their first 41 patients. The procedure resulted in minimal postoperative pain and morbidity. Younger patients appeared to have the best results, and the results appear to be stable over the 1-year follow-up. Results have not deteriorated with time and 100% of athletes have returned to their previous level of sports participation.

Summary

The holmium laser is the most widely used wavelength in arthroscopy. The holmium laser is clinically useful not only for meniscal cutting and ablation, but also for labral tear ablation in a shoulder, subacromial decompression, rotator cuff debridement, and tissue tightening (collagen shringing). Current investigation with laser tissue – photoagglutination and tissue welding – may make it possible to repair labral tear or rotator cuff tears by tissue welding with laser energy.

References

[1] Altcheck DW, Warren RF, Wickiewicz TL, Dines D, Skyhar M, Ortiz G, Schwartz E (1990) Arthroscopic acromioplasty – technique and results. J Bone Joint Surg 72A:1198–1207
[2] Bigliani LU, Morrison DS, April EW (1986) The morphology of the acromion and its relationship to rotator cuff tears. Orthop Trans 10:228
[3] Codman EA (1937) Rupture of the supraspinatus – 1834 to 1934. J Bone Joint Surg 19:643–652
[4] Ellman H (1987) Arthroscopic subacromial decompression: analysis of 1 to 3 year results. Arthroscopy 3:173–181
[5] Ellman H, Harris E, Kay SP (1992) Early degenerative joint disease simulating impingement syndrome: arthroscopic findings. Arthroscopy 8:482–487
[6] Fanton GS, Thabit GM, Thorpe WP, Dillingham MF (1994) Laser shoulder capsulorraphy – treatment of glenohumeral instability by holmium:YAG laser assisted capsular shift (LACS). Proceedings of the 3rd symposium on laser assisted endoscopic and arthroscopic interventions in orthopaedics. 27 May 1994, Balgrist, Zürich (abstract)
[7] Fu FH, Harner CD, Klein AH (1991) Shoulder impingement syndrome. A critical review. Clin Orthop 269:162–173
[8] Hawkins RJ, Kennedy JC (1980) Impingement syndrome in athletes. Am J Sports Med 8:151–158
[9] Imhoff A (1991) [Knee arthroscopy: special diagnosis and surgical techniques] Kniearthroskopie: Spezielle Diagnostik (Synovialis, Knorpelschäden) und Operationstechniken (Elektromesser, Lasersysteme). Akt Probl Chir Orthop 40:44–63
[10] Imhoff A (1993) New developments in arthroscopic joint surgery of the shoulder: arthroscopic subacromial decompression and rotator cuff debridement by holmium:YAG laser. Swiss Med 10-S:306–310
[11] Imhoff A (1994) Arthroscopic operations on the knee and shoulder – an experimental and clinical comparison of the excimer and holmium:YAG lasers. In Rehm KE (eds) [Annual Conference of the German Society for Trauma Surgery] Jahreskongress der Deutschen Gesellschaft für Unfallchirurgie e. V. Springer, Berlin Heidelberg New York, pp 529–536
[12] Imhoff A, Ledermann T (1994) Shoulder-impingement syndrome: arthroscopic subacromial decompression with holmium:YAG laser. Arthroskopie 7:158–169
[13] Imhoff A, Leu H (1991) Arthroscopic operations with the excimer laser. Initial experiences. In: Siebert WE, Wirth CJ (eds) [Lasers in orthopaedics] Laser in der Orthopädie. Thieme, Stuttgart, pp 48–53
[14] Imhoff A, Schreiber A (1988) Etiology and pathogenesis of synovitis villonodosa pigmentosa. Orthopäde 17:223–232
[15] Imhoff A, Schreiber A (1988) Synovial chondromatosis. Orthopäde 17:233–244
[16] Katzky M, Susani M, Schenk P (1992) The holmium:YAG infrared laser and the UV excimer. Effects of lasers on the oral mucosa. Laryngorhinootologie 71:347–352

[17] Kessel L, Watson M (1977) The painful arc syndrome: clinical classification as a guide to management. J Bone Joint Surg 59B:166–172

[18] Lane HJ, Sherk HH, Mooar PA, Lee SJ, Black J (1992) Holmium:YAG laser versus carbon dioxide laser versus mechanical arthroscopic debridement. Semin Orthop 7:95–101

[19] Leu H, Imhoff A, Schreiber A (1991) [Percutaneous nucleotomy with discoscopy: early results of photoablation with excimer laser] Perkutane Nukleotomie mit Diskoskopie: erste Erfahrungen mit der Excimer Photoablation. In: Sieber WE, Wirth CJ (eds) [Lasers in orthopaedics] Laser in der Orthopädie. Thieme, Stuttgart, pp 163–167

[20] Liu SH, Boynton E (1993) Posterior superior impingement of the rotator cuff on the glenoid rim as a cause of shoulder pain in the overhead athlete. Arthroscopy 9:697–699

[21] Neer CS (1972) Anterior acromioplasty for the chronic impingement of the shoulder. J Bone Joint Surg 54A:41–50

[22] Neer CS (1983) Impingement lesions. Clin Orthop 173:70–77

[23] Nirschl RP (1989) Rotator cuff tendinitis: basic concepts of pathoetiology. Instr Course Lect 38:439–445

[24] Rathbun JB, McNab J (1970) The microvascular pattern of the rotator cuff. J Bone Joint Surg 52B:540–553

[25] Rockwood CA, Lyons FR (1993) Shoulder impingement syndrome: diagnosis, radiographic evaluation and treatment with modified Neer acromioplasty. J Bone Joint Surg 75A:409–424

[26] Rothman RH, Parke WW (1965) The vascular anatomy of the rotator cuff. Clin Orthop 41:176–186

[27] Shi W, Vari SG, van der Veen MJ, Fishbein MC, Grundfest WS (1993) Effect of varying laser parameters on pulsed Ho:YAG ablation of bovine knee joint tissues. Arthroscopy 9:96–102

[28] Sibert WE, Saunier J, Gerber B, Lübbers C (1994) Holmium:YAG-Laser in der arthroskopischen Chirurgie des Kniegelenkes. Arthroskopie 7:182–192

[29] Speer KP, Lohnes J, Garrett E (1991) Arthroscopic subacromial decompression: results in advanced impingement syndrome. Arthroscopy 7:291–296

[30] Stein E, Sedlacek, T, Fabian RL, Nishioka NS (1990) Acute and chronic effects of bone ablation with a pulsed holmium laser. Lasers Surg Med 10:384–388

[31] Stuart MJ, Azevedo AJ, Cofield RH (1990) Anterior acromioplasty for treatment of the shoulder impingement syndrome. Clin Orthop 260:195–199

[32] Thorpe WP, Thabit GM, Fanton GS, Dillingham MF (1994) Treatment of glenohumeral instability by laser-assisted capsular shift (LACS). Proceedings of the 3rd symposium on laser assisted endoscopic and arthroscopic interventions in orthopaedics. 27 May 1994, Balgrist, Zürich (abstract)

[33] Van Holsbeeck E, DeRycke J, Declercq G, Martens M, Verstreken J, Fabry G (1992) Subacromial impingement: open versus arthroscopic decompression. Arthroscopy 8:172–178

Arthroscopic Treatment of Shoulder Joint Instability Using Laser-Assisted Capsular Shift

M. Kunz · K. Johann

Introduction

There are many different surgical procedures for treating shoulder joint instability. Basically, these can be divided into open and arthroscopic techniques. The arthroscopic techniques are usually a combination of capsular shrinkage and/or decrease and surgery of the damaged labrum complex.

When treating shoulder luxations, it is imperative to differentiate between the direction of luxation and the possibility of one directional or multidirectional instability. Patients with inherent instability and/or subluxations are especially difficult to treat.

Since the establishment of laser-assisted arthroscopy in orthopedic surgery, the holmium:YAG laser has been used especially for treatment of the shoulder joint because the advantages in comparison to mechanical instruments are very apparent [4]. The first report on the possibility of "tissue shrinkage using non-ablative laser energy" was published in the USA in 1993 and rapidly led to animal experiments and then to clinical use of the holmium laser for treatment of shoulder luxations. Controlled studies show encouraging preliminary results [1, 6].

In the St. Elisabeth Clinic in Saarlouis we have been conducting arthroscopic surgery with the holmium laser since 1992. During this time we have observed the possibility of capsular shrinkage when applying low-energy laser and therefore have conducted medial parapatellar capsular shrinkage procedures during lateral release surgery in order to stabilize the patella.

Based on the positive reports and experience with shoulder joint shrinkage and our own ecouraging results with laser application [2, 3, 5], we conducted the first laser-assisted capsular shrinkage (LACS) procedure for treatment of recurring shoulder luxation at the beginning of 1994. A study of five patients treated with LACS with 6-monthly follow-up examinations was conducted in order to register any complications, i.e. recurring luxations. Since the 6-monthly results were very positive, we have been performing the LACS procedure more often.

Technique

For arthroscopic surgery the patient is under general anesthesia and positioned in the beach chair. Capsular shrinkage is conducted with the holmium:YAG laser (Versapulse). Energy per pulse is 1 J with a frequency of 8–10 Hz. Laser energy is applied with an infratome via a ventral or dorsal approach. The infratome has an irradiation angle of 30° or 70°. The shrinking effect is quite rapid and causes the condyle to be pulled towards the socket, thereby decreasing the joint space. For this reason the shrinkage procedure should always begin peripherally at the distal capsular insertion point and not proximally near the socket, because the lateral capsular area would then no longer be accessible (Fig. 1). The shrinkage procedure usually follows a dotted or lined pattern; according to more recent reports the pattern has no effect on tissue reaction. Concurrent Bankart or SLAP lesions were also treated with either resection or laser application to the labrum. Since 1996, we treat Bankart and SLAP III lesions with a shoulder – anchor system (Sure-Tacs; Smith & Nephew, Hamburg). These cases are not included in this study because of the very short follow-up time.

Postoperative Treatment

After surgery the shoulder is wrapped in a modified Gilchrist abduction sling for 3 weeks. Afterwards

- ▸ general anesthesia
- ▸ beachchair-position
- ▸ anterior/posterior approach
- ▸ procedure starts distal-lateral to proximal-medial
- ▸ treatment of labrum lesions
- ▸ constant fluid pressure in joint

Fig. 1. Summary of the laser-assisted capsular shrinkage (LACS) technique

▸ **2-3 days hospitalized**

▸ **3 weeks sling immobilization**

▸ **4th-6th week physio with limited movement (AB./EL. to 90°, ER 0°)**

▸ **from week 7 physio without limitation**

Fig. 2. LACS postoperative treatment

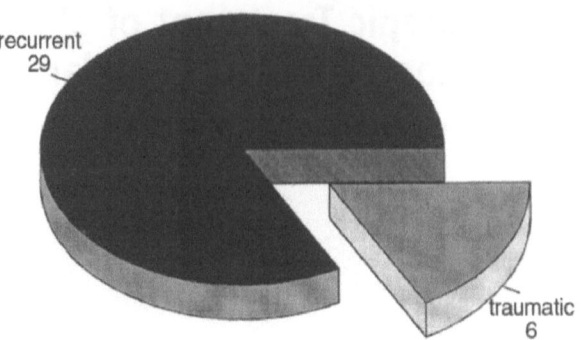

Fig. 4. Breakdown of patients according to type of dislocation ($n = 35$)

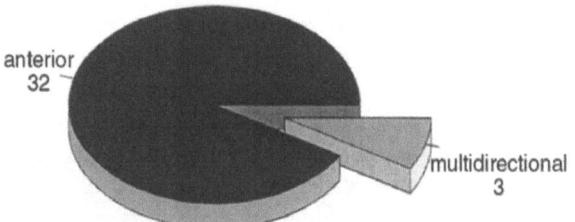

Fig. 5. Breakdown of patients according to direction of dislocation ($n = 35$)

physical therapy is administered. For the first 3 weeks movement should be restricted to the horizontal plane for abduction and elevation without rotation. After this time all movement is allowed. (The postoperative treatment is summarized in Fig. 2.)

Patient Collective

Up to now we have treated over 50 patients with the LACS technique. This particular study included 35 patients (24 male and 11 female). The average age was 27.9 years, range 16 to 43 years. The right shoulder was afflicted in 23 cases, the left shoulder in 12 cases. We treated 29 cases of recurring luxations and six fresh traumatic luxations. We found 32 ventral and three multidirectional luxations. The Hill-Sachs defect was present in 27 patients. The labrum was affected to different degrees in all cases (tears, degeneration, SLAP I). In seven cases we found old lesions, for example, Bankart lesion, which were resected. The breakdown of the patients according to sex, type of dislocation, and direction of dislocation is given in Figs. 3–5.

The follow-up period was at least 12 months, maximally 31 months, on average 2 years. Of the 35

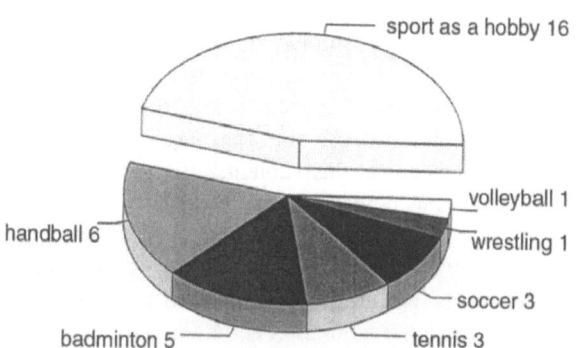

Fig. 6. Sports activity of patients in study group ($n = 35$)

patients, 19 were active athletes (Fig. 6) and involved in a shoulder-stressing sport (5 badminton, 3 tennis, 6 handball, 1 wrestling, 3 soccer, 1 volleyball). Of these patients, 9 were high-performance athletes (first and second national leagues of handball, badminton, and wrestling).

Results

No complications occurred during all operations, with no incidence of hemorrhage or thrombosis, no infections or wound-healing disorders. On average, the patients could be discharged from the hospital 2 to 3 days after surgery and continue treatment on an outpatient basis.

One incidence of dorsal luxation occurred 12 months after surgery after the patient, who had been treated for habitual ventral shoulder luxation,

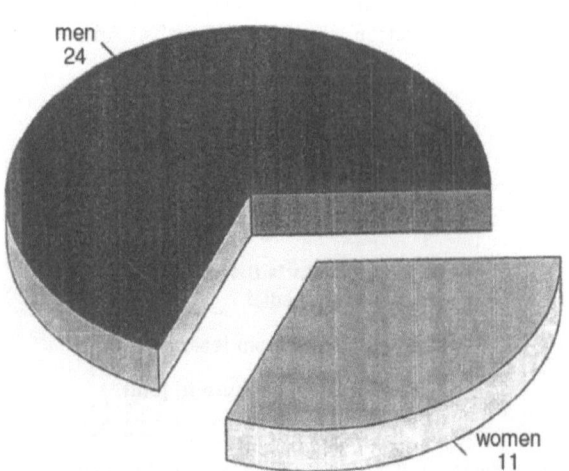

Fig. 3. Breakdown of patients according to sex ($n = 35$)

fell on his shoulder. No other cases of reluxation were observed.

On average, patients were able to return to work 7 weeks after surgery; range 2 to 12 weeks.

All athletes, including the high-performance athletes, were able to resume their former sport activities after an average of 3 months after surgery.

The shoulder joints were evaluated according to the Rowe score (1978) and the Rowe–Zarins Score (1982).

a) Rowe score (Figs. 7, 8): This score particularly evaluates stability (50 %). The postoperative score was 95.69 out of 100 points. The score was between 90 and 100 points in 34 cases which is an excellent result. In one case (a patient with multidirectional instability), the score was lower than 50.

b) Rowe–Zarins score (Figs. 9–14): This score is mainly for evaluation of movement ability (40 %) along with pain (30 %) and function (30 %). The preoperative score was 41.5 %. The average postoperative score was 94 points. Outer rotation was slightly limited (10°): in nine cases 26 patients had unlimited movement, 23 patients were absolutely pain-free, and 12 patients sometimes had slight pain during sports activities. The results for function (stability/strength) were also good.

Assessment	Number
excellent	27
good	7
fair	1
poor	0

Fig. 9. Rowe–Zarins evaluation distribution ($n = 35$)

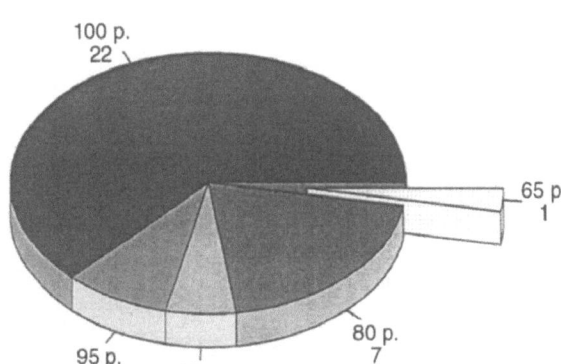

Fig. 10. Rowe–Zarins score distribution ($n = 35$)

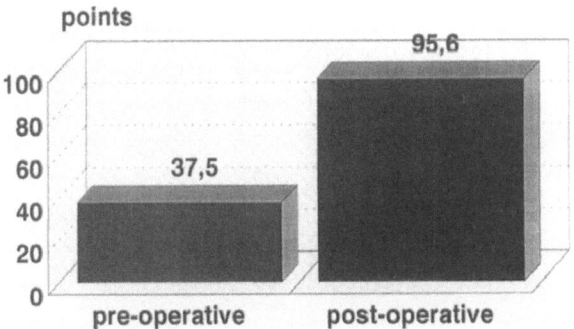

Fig. 7. Comparison of pre- and postoperative Rowe's scores ($n = 35$)

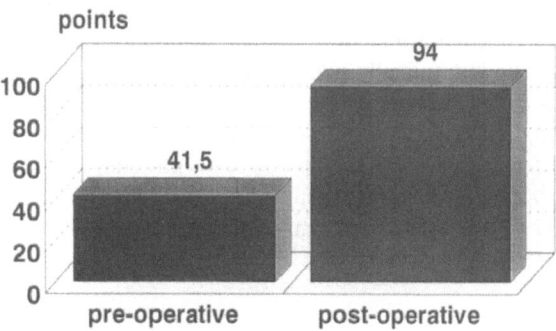

Fig. 11. Comparison of pre- and postoperative Rowe–Zarins score

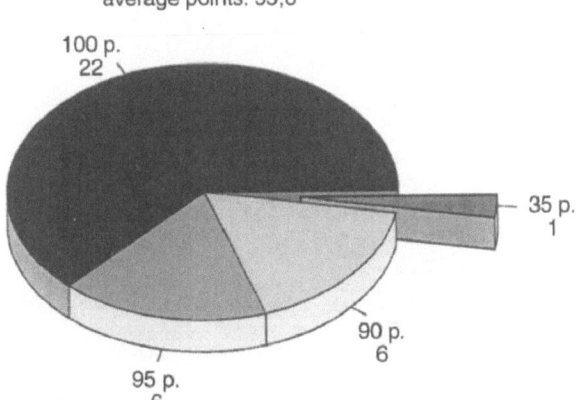

Fig. 8. Rowe's score distribution among patients ($n = 35$)

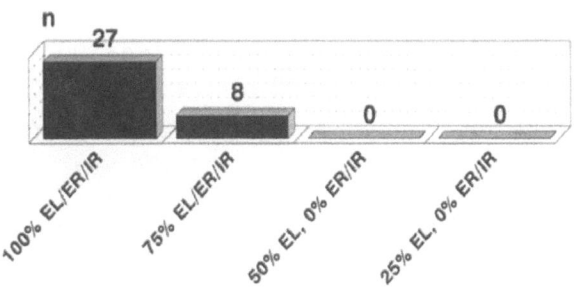

Fig. 12. Postoperative movement ability of patients according to Rowe–Zarins score

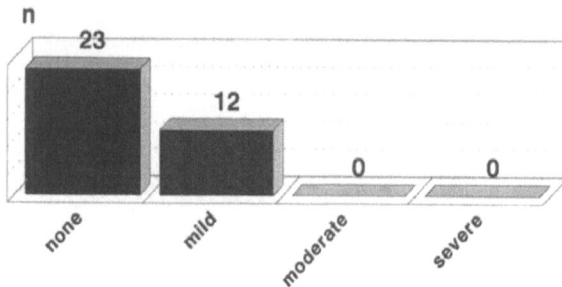

Fig. 13. Pain experienced by patients postoperatively according to Rowe–Zarins score ($n = 35$)

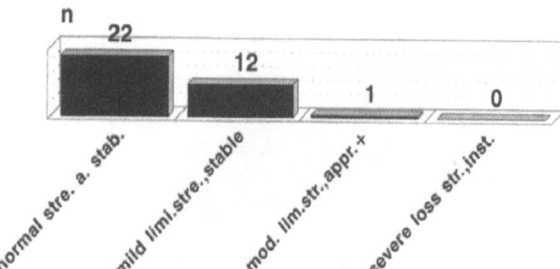

Fig. 14. Postoperative function (strength/stability) of patients ($n = 35$) according to Rowe–Zarins score

Conclusion

The postoperative results of the 35 patients who were treated with arthroscopic laser-assisted capsular shrinkage and were followed up after an average of 2 years are very good. These results encourage us to continue using this surgical technique. The technique is minimally invasive, easy on the patient and practically without complications. We have found that additional stabilization with the laser for treatment of a severe labrum defect or, nowadays, with a shoulder anchor system in case of a Bankart or SLAP III lesion is advantageous.

References

[1] Hardy P, Thabit G III, Fanton GS, Blin JL, Lortat-Jacob A, Benoit J (1996 Arthroscopic treatment of recurrent anterior glenohumeral luxations by combining a labrum suture with holmium:YAG laser-assisted capsular shrinkage. Der Orthopäde 1:91–93

[2] Hayashi K, Markel MD, Thabit G III, Bogedanske JJ, Thielke RJ (1995) The effect of non-ablative laser energy on joint capsular properties: an in vitro mechanical study using a rabbit model. Am J Sports Med 23:482–487

[3] Hayashi K, Thabit G III, Bogdaske JJ, Mascio LN, Markel MD (1996) The effect of nonablative laser energy on the ultrastructure of joint capsular collagen. Arthroscopy 12(4):474–481

[4] Imhoff A, Ledermann T (1995) Arthroscopic subacromial decompression with and without the holmium:YAG laser: a prospective comparative study. Relat Surg 11(5):549–556

[5] Markel MD, Hayashi K, Thabit G III, Thielke RJ (1996) Modulation of joint capsular tissues using the holmium:YAG laser at non-ablative energy densities: potential application to joint stabilization procedures. Der Orthopäde 1:37–41

[6] Thabit G III (1994) Treatment of unidirectional and multidirectional glenohumeral instability by laser-assisted capsular shift. Presented at the California Orthopedic Association. Squaw Creek, Nevada, May 1994

Laser-Assisted Arthroscopy of the Shoulder – What Merit Does Laser Surgery Have in Modern Shoulder Surgery?

F. P. Sommerfeld · W. E. Siebert · H.-G. Pape

Introduction

The idea that minimal invasive surgery of the shoulder is only useful as a form of keyhole diagnostics has become obsolete. Analogous to the development of knee surgery years before, shoulder surgery underwent fundamental changes in diagnosis as well as in therapy. This process was accompanied and supported by the advent of new radiological techniques (sonography, MRI, Arthro-CT, etc.). The progress made in imaging diagnostics and clinical assessments has profoundly improved the understanding of shoulder joint anatomy, pathology and biomechanics [1, 17, 21] and has led to a variety of new and more specific diagnoses which required adequate therapeutic remedies.

Alongside this newly acquired knowledge, advances in technique and methodology in shoulder surgery have been made. Especially arthroscopic techniques – with minimal operative trauma and the possibility of rapid rehabilitation – play an important role.

Initially arthroscopy was just another diagnostic tool; now arthroscopic surgery is being conducted more frequently with an increasing number of indications and is often considered to be the method of choice. This minimally invasive technique gained more and more ground, also because of methodological and instrumental improvements [15, 17, 21].

Although a variety of surgical techniques are being performed, there is still debate concerning the indications of arthroscopic interventions for treatment of the shoulder. The treatment of the various shoulder instabilities has especially been the subject of controversial discussion. Many different stabilization techniques are available, and they can basically be divided into two groups: open surgery and arthroscopic surgery.

Although there are a large number of open techniques, they have the disadvantage of being traumatic and necessitate a prolonged postoperative rehabilitation phase. However, due to their relatively low reluxation rate, open procedures are still often performed.

The initial euphoria over minimally invasive arthroscopic stabilization procedures was kept in check by the relatively high reluxation rate of up to 40 %. While emphasis was often placed on stabilization of the glenoid cavity by various anchor and suture systems, too often not enough attention was paid to capsular laxity and ligament damage. The reluxation rate remained higher than after open surgery.

Alternative minimally invasive techniques that shrink the shoulder capsule and refixate the damaged labrum-capsula-ligament complex were developed. One option – the arthroscopic shift technique – is under trial, and short-term results are now available [2, 3, 6, 15, 16, 19, 20]. As technique and instrumentation of minimally invasive procedures improve, arthroscopic surgery covers an ever increasing range of indications.

The laser along with specialized arthroscopic equipment is quite suitable for minimally invasive treatment of the shoulder joint and its very distinct anatomy [1, 3, 5, 14, 17]. The laser can cut, ablate and shrink tissue and has excellent coagulating properties. As it is applied with thin flexible fibers, it can precisely reach very small spaces with very few access points. It reduces the necessity of the intraoperative changeover of instruments and is quite simple to handle. All these properties make it an attractive tool for arthroscopic therapy of shoulder joint disorders.

The first report on the possibility to shrink tissue with the laser was made in the USA in 1993. Since then many studies have been conducted on the application of laser as a method to effectively shrink the redundant joint capsule of patients with glenohumeral instability, in an attempt to stabilize the joint – even in comparison to conventional surgery [2, 11, 15, 17, 20].

Numerous studies have now shown that the Ho:YAG laser is the most suitable laser system for arthroscopic surgery (compared to other systems, e.g., CO_2 Laser, Excimer, Nd:YAG Laser). Noteworthy experimental sutdies by Markel and Hayashi demonstrated the suitability of the Ho:YAG laser for surgery of the shoulder. Markel showed that the non-ablative Ho:YAG laser can significantly shrink joint tissue without negative changes in joint elasticity due to energy absorption in deeper-lying tissues [6, 7, 8, 9, 11, 12, 13, 14].

Using Markel's results, Hardy, Thabit and Fanton conducted arthroscopic surgery with the laser to treat shoulder instability, and achieved remarkably good results [2, 7, 8, 12, 18, 19]. Furthermore, multidirectional instability, which is quite difficult to cure, can be successfully treated with the minimally invasive LACS procedure (laser-assisted capsular shrinkage). Results obtained with this technique have additionally been shown to be long lasting.

A growing number of hospitals and medical centers are treating shoulder disorders, especially post-traumatic instability with a combination of Bankart lesion reconstruction and LACS. Encouraged by the promising results obtained in the mentioned studies, we analyzed our own experience with the method.

Our Experience

We have carried out this combined procedure since 1994. From November 1994 to December 1999 we conducted altogether 1128 shoulder arthroscopies. There were 203 patients who underwent arthroscopic surgery because of persisting shoulder instability (>3 months). Of these, 80 were female and 123 were male. The average age was 27.5 years (15–56 years). This included 16 woman and 31 men who were high-performance athletes. Out of a total of 107 patients with recurring luxations (rL, < 10 in 10 years), only 23 patients suffered from unidirectional instability without capsular laxity. Out of 69 primary luxations (pL, < 15 months), there were 23 cases with unidirectional instability without capsular laxity. We also had 27 cases of chronic subluxation (cSL).

In accordance to the studies by Markel, we used the non-ablative 2.1-µm Ho:YAG laser to treat the capsular laxity. Standard arthroscopy instrumentation and the Ho:YAG laser [10 W (1 J, 10 Hz)] with 30° and 90° fibers were used. The patients were in a beach-chair position. The LACS procedure was conducted with use of an anterior and posterior access, starting from posterior in anterior direction. In the event of staple or anchor fixation, LACS was performed subsequently. LACS without any other procedure was carried out in 102 cases and in combination with Suretac staples in 91 cases. The laser parameters were 1.0 J, 10 Hz with tissue-near application. We treated the axillar recessus through an anterior access.

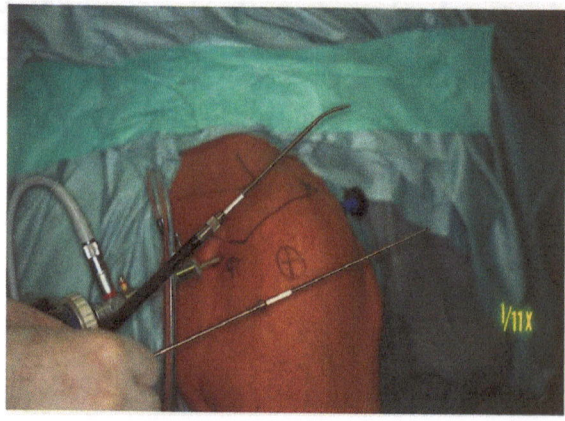

Fig. 1. View of the LACS procedure with possible surgical approaches

The rest of the capsule was treated through a posterior access.

The following is a summary of the LACS (laser-assisted capsular shrinkage) procedure and the operative technique (see also Figs. 1 and 2):

– Laser parameters: 2.1-µm Ho:YAG laser,
 1.0 J, 10 Hz
– Surgical approach: Anterior port:
 axillar recessus/anterior
 capsular region;
 Posterior port:
 rest of capsule
– Eventual staple application
– Laser shrinkage of the capsule: fish-school-like matrix

We reached 185 of the 203 patients for retrospective follow-up questioning and clinical examination. The average time for follow-up was 32 months. All patients were able to participate in sports after 5 months. Time for sick leave and physiotherapy remained under 14 weeks in all cases. Restriction of outer rotation with 90° abducted arm by more than 15° was obseved in only 15 patients (one with a notable 20° restricted range of motion). The average constant score was 91/100 for patients with chronic subluxation, 93 points for primary laxations and 88 for patients with recurring luxations. The modified Rowe score was excellent in 114 cases, good in 60 cases, fair in 11 cases. (See Table 1 for a summary of these results.)

Our complication rate was very low. Staple dislocations occurred in 6 cases (3 times after a fall). Three of these patients underwent restabilization surgery at a different hospital. One female patient underwent a second LACS procedure which led to complete stability and relief. We were able to achieve good results with excellent stability in 90 % of the patients, especially in athletes.

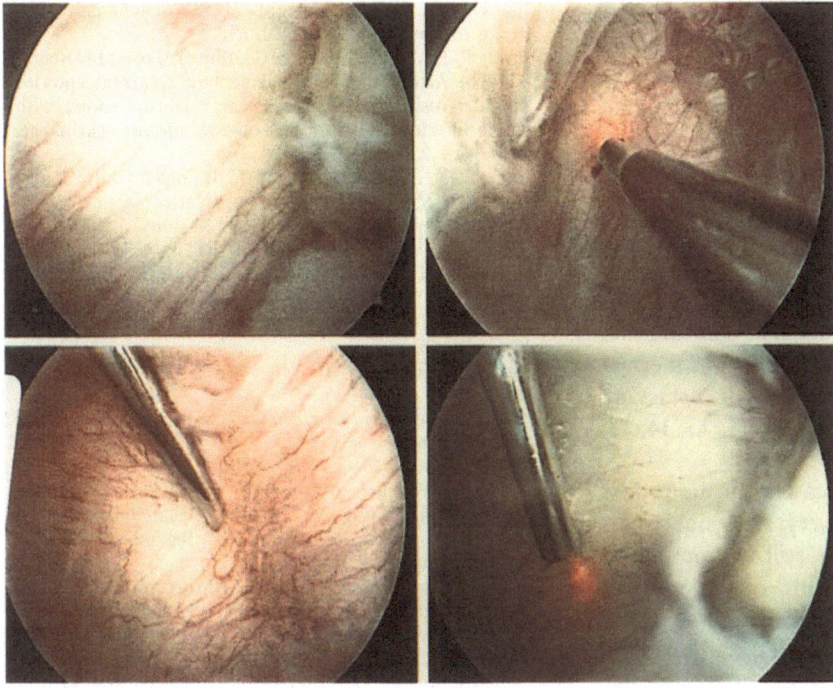

Fig. 2. Intraoperative view of the shoulder capsule including the laser

Table 1. Results after LACS (laser-assisted capsular shrinkage)

	Laxity $n = 26$ (27)	Primary luxation $n = 64$ (69)	Recurrent luxation $n = 95$ (107)
Rowe score	excellent 15 good 10 fair 1	excellent 48 good 15 fair 1	excellent 51 good 35 fair 9
Constant score	91	93	88

Altogether, 203 patients were treated. For follow-up, 185 patients were reached.

Discussion

As many studies have now shown, LACS causes collagen fibrils to shorten and thicken; this along with an increased formation of collagen within the first 30 postoperative days and proper postoperative physiotherapy, leads to long-lasting stability of unstable shoulder joints [2, 6, 12, 18, 19, 20]. Recurring luxations and multidirectional instabilities can be treated effectively with this minimally invasive method.

To effectively treat shoulder instability, it is necessary to diagnose the direction of luxation and to differentiate between uni- and multidirectional instability. Furthermore, the number of prior luxations and whether the luxation is traumatic or habitual must be established. With this information, the physician can choose the appropriate surgery. Correct diagnosis and adherence to the range of indications are imperative for choosing between open and arthroscopic surgery and can

determine the success or failure of the operation [2, 3, 6, 17, 19, 20, 21].

In our study, almost all cases of capsuloligamental laxity could be stabilized with LACS, making mechanical shift surgery unnecessary. Increased stability, decreased pain and a subjective as well as an objective improvement of function allowed the patients to return to their previous levels of activity.

The features of the LACS procedure can be summarized as follows:

– Thermal shrinkage of collagen fibers
– Targeted reduction of the capsule volume
– Uni- and multidirectional instabilities can be treated

The laser is also used as an assisting tool during subacromial decompression procedures. After Ellmann introduced the procedure of arthroscopic subacromial decompression in 1983, this method has become a standard procedure for treating "outlet impingement" syndrome. This procedure is, however, inconvenienced by bleeding, which decreases visibility of the subacromial area. The laser with its excellent hemostatic effect allows this disadvantage to be overcome, as it is possible, without changing instruments, not only to ablate tissue and seal the surface, but also to simultaneously stop the bleeding. Postoperative scarring is reduced, and rehabilitation can be started and is less painful.

The laser can also be used in synovectomy procedures for treatment of rheumatoid arthritic shoulders. The laser's good hemostatic and thermal effect in deeper-lying tissues – a kind of "thermal synoviorthesis" – can be exploited for achieving good long-term results [1, 3, 4, 5, 10, 11, 13, 14, 15, 17].

Minimally invasive procedures play an important and vital role in shoulder surgery alongside traditional open methods, which are still appropriate in certain patients. However, arthroscopic methods have now supplanted open procedures in many cases. Due to its characteristic effects, the laser is a helpful tool in arthroscopic procedures and has increased the range of indications for minimally invasive shoulder surgery. Several studies have documented the positive intra- and postoperative effects of the laser, based on its tissue-shrinking and thermal properties. More studies are necessary to prove the long-term value of these new and exciting procedures.

References

[1] Abelow SP (1997) Laser capsulorrhaphy for multidirectional instability of the shoulder. Operative Techniques in Sports Medicine 5(4):244–248
[2] Abelow SP (1993) Use of lasers in orthopedic surgery: current concepts. Orthopedics 16(5):551–556
[3] Brillhart AT (1991) Arthroscopic laser surgery. Am J Arthors 1:5–12, and Clinical applications, Springer, Berlin Heidelberg New York
[4] De Simoini C, Ledermann T, Imhoff AB (1996) Holmium:YAG laser in outlet impingement of the shoulder. Mid-term results. Orthopäde 25(1):84–90
[5] Fanton GS, Wall MS, Markel MD (1998) Electrothermaly-assisted capsule shift (ETACS) procedure for shoulder instability. Oratec, Menlo Park, CA
[6] Habermayer P, Schweiberer L (1996) Schulterchirurgie. Urban & Schwarzenberger, Munich
[7] Hardy P, Thabit G III, Fanton GS, Blin JL, Lortat JA, Benoit J (1996) Arthroscopic management of recurrent anterior shoulder dislocation by combining a labrum suture with antero-inferior holmium:YAG laser capsular shrinkage. Orthopäde 25(1):91–93
[8] Hayashi K, Nieckarz JA, Thabit G III, Bogdanske JJ, Cooley AJ, Markel MD (1997) Effect of nonablative laser energy on the joint capsule: an in vivo rabbit study using a holmium:YAG laser. Lasers Surg Med 20(2):164–171
[9] Hayashi K, Thabit G III, Bogdanske JJ, Mascio LN, Markel MD (1996) The effect of nonablative laser energy on the ultrastructure of joint capsular collage. Arthroscopy 12(4):474–481
[10] Hayashi K, Thabit G III, Vailas AC, Bogdanske JJ, Cooley AJ, Markel MD (1996) The effect of nonablative laser energy on joint capsular properties. An in vitro histologic and biochemical study using a rabbit model. Am J Sports Med 24(5):640–646
[11] Imhoff A, Roscher E, König U (1998) Arthroskopische Schulterstabilisierung. Differenzierte Behandlungsstrategie mit Suretac, Fastak, Holmium:YAG Laser und Elektrochirurgie. Orthopäde 8:518–531
[12] Imhoff A, Ledermann T (1995) Arthroscopic subacromial decompression with and without the Holmium:YAG laser. A prospective comparative study. Arthroscopy 11(5):549–556
[13] Lane GJ, Mooar PA (1991) Holmium:YAG laser arthroscopic debridement. Lasers Surg Med Supp 3:53
[14] Markel MD, Hayashi K, Thabit G III, Thielke RJ (1996) Changes in articular capsular tissue using holmium:YAG laser at non-ablative energy densities. Potential application in non-ablative stabilization procedures. Orthopäde 25(1):37–41
[15] McGee P, Fanton GS, Shea K, Bradley JP (1998) Thermal shrinkage shows promise as less-invasive tool for shoulder instability. Orthopedics Today 18(7):10–16
[16] Obrzut SL, Hayashi K, Hecht P, Fanton K, Thabit GS, Markel MD (1998) The effect of radiofrequency energy on the length and temperature properties of the glenohumeral joint capsule. Athroscopy 14(4):395–400
[17] Saunier J, Indermühle F, Compère J (1993) Use of the holmium 2.1 laser in surgical arthroscopy. Rev Med Suisse Romande 113(2):129–132
[18] Schreiner C (1994) Laser in der Arthroskopie. Arthroskopie 7:148–153
[19] Sherk HH, Lane GJ, Black JD (1992) Laser arthroscopy. Orthop Rev 21(9):1077–1083
[20] Siebert WE (1992) Laseranwendung in der Orthopädie. Orthopäde 21:273–288
[21] Tibone JE, Shrader TA (1998) Glenohumeral joint translation after arthroscopic, nonablative, thermal capsuloplasty with a laser. Am J Sports Med 26(4):495–498
[22] Yoshida A, Ogawa K (1997) Extensive shoulder capsular tearing as a main course of recurrent anterior shoulder dislocation. J Shoulder Elbow Surg 6:1–5

IV Low-Level Laser

Preface to Low-Level Laser Therapy

Lasers with low energy levels have been used in the therapy of pain syndromes, rheumatoid arthritis, sports injuries and many other diseases for many years, often with surprisingly good success rates. The therapeutic effects especially in pain therapy have been striking. Sometimes combined with acupuncture and often used as a mere pain therapy, but always with energy levels much lower than those used during surgery, with wavelengths from red to near infrared, this type of therapy has spread widely all over the world. The World Association of Laser Therapy (WALT) deals with the application of low-level laser therapy in the different fields of medicine.

The section on low-level laser therapy in orthopedic medicine is composed of articles by two renowned experts, W. Glinkowski from Poland and S. Götte from Germany. They describe the history, the physics behind low-level laser application and the current state of medical application and experimental research including application modalities. Interested physicians, especially pain therapists and sports medicine doctors, will be intrigued by this very promising tool. The success rates are very good, especially for pain therapy of the musculoskeletal system, with hardly any side effects. More basic scientific research and clinical research are necessary to confirm these initial findings and the worth of this very promising field of laser application.

W. E. Siebert

Low-Level Energy Laser Therapy in the Musculoskeletal System

W. Glinkowski

Introduction

The curative effect of light was already described by the ancient Egyptians for treatment of some skin disorders. Later, the Greeks believed that sunlight brings strength and health to the organism. In the Middle Ages, sunlight was used to combat the plague. Physicians returned to light therapy by the late nineteenth century. Niels Finsen, the Nobel prize winner, utilized UV radiation to treat cutaneous tuberculosis. The concept of laser light application as light "medication" should therefore not be understood as new, having such antique roots. Low-energy lasers have been used in research and clinical applications for more than 30 years. Nevertheless, the mechanisms of the effects of low-energy lasers on living tissues, cells, and organisms are not as well understood and known as the high-power laser–tissue interactions, used as a method of physical therapy and rehabilitation. Basically, it is thought that laser irradiation alters cellular behavior in the absence of significant heating. First reports in Hungary and the Eastern Bloc countries in the mid-1960s showed an acceleration of wound healing and hair growth [57, 61, 74–76, 99]. Early investigators described the phenomenon as "laser biostimulation." Recently, low-intensity (low-level, low-power, or low-energy) laser therapy (LLLT) emphasizes the non-thermal, monochromatic, coherent light effect on living tissues. In Europe, Japan, South America, and the Middle East LLLT has wide indications and its popularity is increasing. In the United States, acceptance by the Food and Drug Administration (FDA) is minimal for any indication and low-energy lasers still await approval.

Discussion

In physical therapy hundreds of watts are delivered to the patient for heating therapy using radio-frequency diathermy and infrared (IR). Low-intensity lasers do not produce temperature elevations over 1.1 °C. The temperature changes are low and localized to the irradiated area only. They cannot produce significant physiological effects due to a rise in temperature.

Lasers utilized for LLLT emit light in the visible and IR spectrum. Recently, GaAs and GaA1As IR semiconductor laser diodes have become more available. HeNe devices are still widely used, but the majority of work is done with GaAs and GaA1As diodes with wavelengths between 635 nm and 980 nm. There is a growing belief that these latter devices are particularly effective. Ruby, Ar, and Kr lasers are no longer used for biostimulation.

Laser output powers did not exceed 1 mW initially, but improved technology has brought a power increase. Devices used therapeutically today have output powers from a few up to a few hundred milliwatts. New devices have allowed the treatment sessions to become shorter, but the total dose of energy usually delivered per session has remained at the same level over the last few years (1–4 J/cm^2). Only a few authors have described the effects of higher dosage application.

The mechanisms of action are still unclear, but interest has increased and expanded with new clinical and laboratory studies. Biochemical, biophysical, and physiological alterations have been described as the effects of low-energy laser irradiation. Cell process effects include the following: protein synthesis (collagen), cell growth and differentiation, cell motility, membrane potential and binding affinities, neurotransmitter release, phagocytosis, synthesis of ATP and prostaglandin, stabilization of cell membrane, increase of intracellular temperature, and release of endorphins [1, 2, 25, 43, 53–55, 57, 61, 62, 64, 71, 78, 84–86, 89, 91, 94, 118, 122]. Biophysical and physiological effects of LLLT include reflectance alterations, discovered recently, and neoangiogenesis. LLLT parameters include the following: typically, 632.8–980 nm (rarely, Nd:YAG or CO_2 defocused); average power: up to a few hundred milliwatts; mode continuous, pulsed, or modulated (1–10 000 Hz); dosage per single irradiated spot: 1–4 J/cm^2 (some authors suggest doses of 16 J/cm^2 or more), irradiated daily or on an alternate-days treatment regimen. Contact and noncontact techniques of irradia-

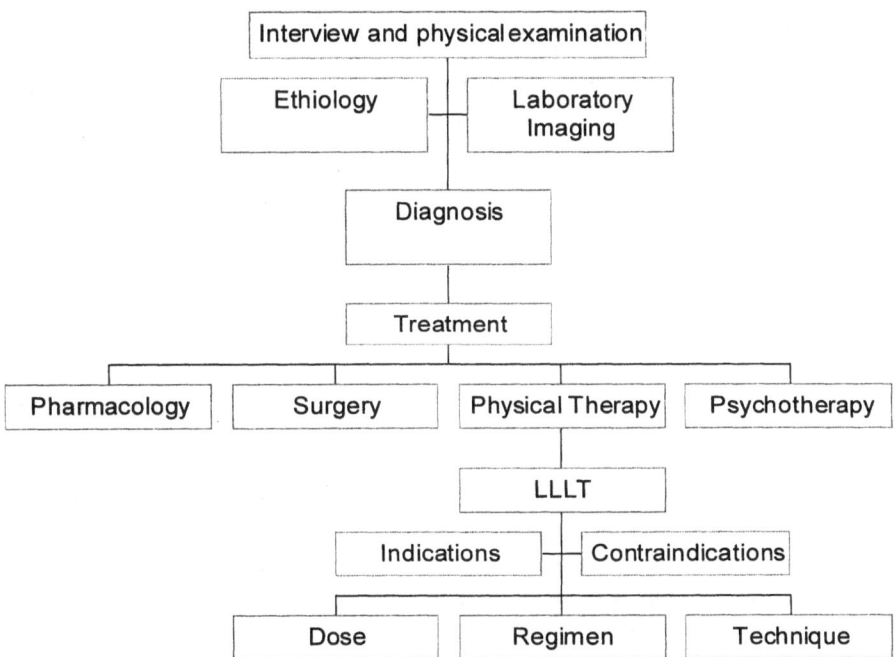

Fig. 1. Place of low-level laser therapy (LLLT) in relation to the overall structure of patient management

tion are used for the delivery of the laser beam. Non-contact techniques include hand-operated or automatic scanning. The contact techniques commonly used are the pressure, "sweep", and "woodpecker" techniques. Single or a combination of two wavelengths are used. Figure 1 shows the place of LLLT in relation to the patient management schedule as a whole. The therapist can irradiate sites over the lesion or painful area, around peripheral nerves innervating the area of interest, and over "trigger points" or acupuncture points. Irradiation of superficial sympathetic ganglia, intravascular, intraoperative, endoscopic, and in conjunction with photosensitizers can also be employed.

It is thought that human skin absorbs more than 80% of laser energy within a range of 3–4 mm. Rarely published experimental reports characterize the optical properties of tissues. The effective dose of laser energy at the level of the target tissue determines its therapeutic use. The depth of laser beam penetration depends on the optical characteristics of the particular tissue, the wavelength, and other optical phenomena. Laser beams can penetrate deeply enough into tissue to produce the reported effects. The different characteristics of penetration for different species, tissue types, and the most commonly used low-energy lasers have been studied extensively. Monochromaticity appears to be crucial for biological effects. Other laser beam features such as coherency and collimation may, due to scattering, lose their effect when passing through tissue [3].

Karu [53] showed that effects are present only within a narrow spectrum of stimulation. The wavelength emitted by a laser designed for laser therapy should not exceed the range of an "optical window" in the visible and IR portion of the tissue's spectrum, which extends from approximately 600 nm to 1300 nm. The specific absorption characteristics of a tissue's chromatophores are thought to play an important role in the effect of particular lasers (e.g., hemoglobin, 488–515 nm, for the Ar laser). While passing through the tissue, the laser beam is attenuated exponentially by the scattering and absorption. We can observe easily how the HeNe laser beam transilluminates a finger and creates a red light "ball" in the tissue. We can also assess laser energy at any given depth in the tissue with regard to light penetration and attenuation. The question of the effectiveness of low-energy laser at a deeply located target tissue still remains to be answered.

We have carried out an evaluation of tissue penetration [37]. Tissues were harvested from rats and humans at autopsy within 48 h post mortem. Several lasers typical for physical therapy were used as follows: continuous-wave, 830 nm, 40 mW; pulsed, 904 nm, 30 W; pulsed, 890 nm, 50 W; HeNe, continuous-wave, 25 mW; HeNe, continuous-wave, 12 mW. The harvested specimens completely covered the area of the photodetection window of a power meter. Tissue including skin, muscle, cartilage, and rib bone were excised and tested. We calculated an absorption coefficient for each particular tissue according to the Lambert–Beer equation. We found that the HeNe laser beam penetrates through muscle well, with less efficient penetration through cartilage and skin. The weakest penetration (highest absorption coefficient) was found through bone. No penetration was observed through plaster of Paris. The results of the penetration measurement are presented in Figs. 3 and 4. The expected high absorption coefficient values for HeNe laser penetration through tissues were not fully confirmed. The low-energy lasers' penetration results obtained in this experiment may suggest a nonlinear relationship between absorption and laser power.

Bone and skin have the highest absorption coefficients. Absorption coefficients differ among species. These findings may explain some of the lack of analogy between clinical and experimental applications and results. Biophysical changes after laser irradiation include changes in the reflectance of skin. We evaluated changes in the biophysical features of skin after low-energy IR laser irradiation. The system of multispectral image analysis for evaluation of media and surfaces of medical objects was used. Images of a patient's leg before and after irradiation (noncontact scanning diode, pulsed laser, 904 nm, 15 W peak power) were analyzed. Filters used for spectral analysis covered a range from 350 to 800 nm. Dissociation of reflectance values was observed (Figs. 5, 6). Differences in the near-IR region suggest better skin absorption after irradiation. The biophysical changes in skin features after irradiation may suggest a new hypothesis for the mechanism of LLLT. Our observations may also explain why some laser therapists prefer to begin low-power lasing by manual or automated scanning and then follow with local irradiation.

A description of laser therapy should include all laser parameters, site preparation details, technique, and the treatment regimen. For example, diode (GaAs) laser (890 nm or 904 nm, 3000 Hz, pulsed, 10–30 W/pulse) was employed most frequently in own studies. The treatment regimen usually involved the noncontact "sweep" technique, once daily, for 15 min.

Laser therapy can be applied as a monotherapy or, more usually, as one component of a complex therapy. The therapist should carefully interview patients to exclude those who are light-sensitive and to determine whether the patient's medication could interact with the particular laser irradiation.

LLLT has gained popularity in recent years as a treatment in the management of many localized painful musculoskeletal conditions. The clinical indications for laser therapy can be grouped into four main categories: wound healing [10, 26, 52, 60, 70, 92, 109], recent injuries, pain control, and arthritic joints. The evaluation of most trials and treatment outcomes is complicated. A review of controlled clinical trials of some investigated laser therapies sometimes shows benefits. Metaanalyses attempted by Beckerman et al. [14] and Gam et al. [27] surveyed and evaluated over 20 randomized studies of laser

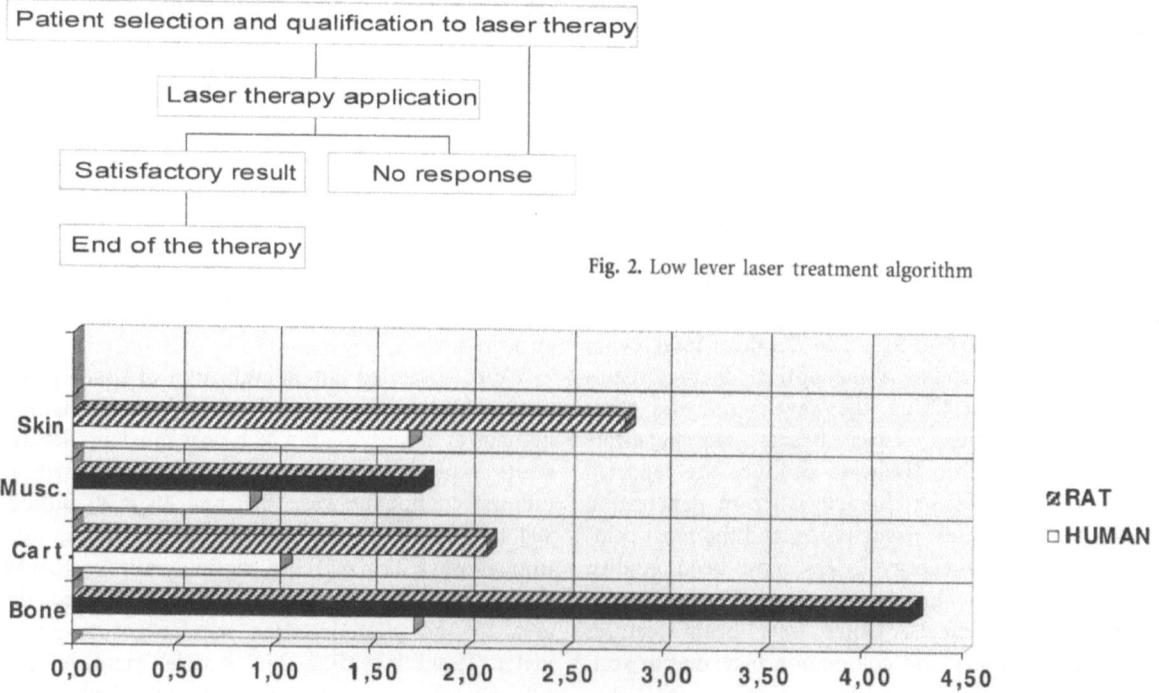

Fig. 2. Low lever laser treatment algorithm

Fig. 3. HeNe laser beam absorption in various tissues (1/mm)

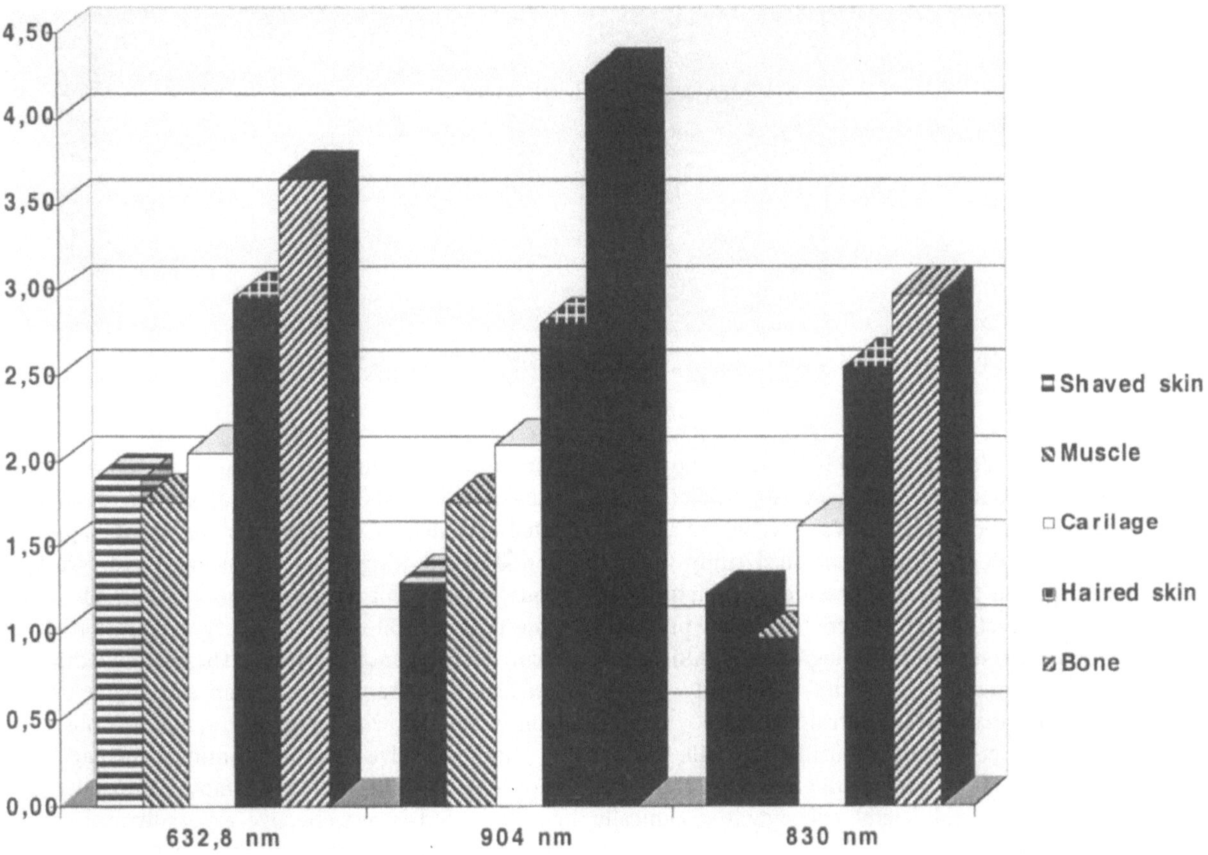

Fig. 4. Laser beam absorption of the different tissues at different wavelengths

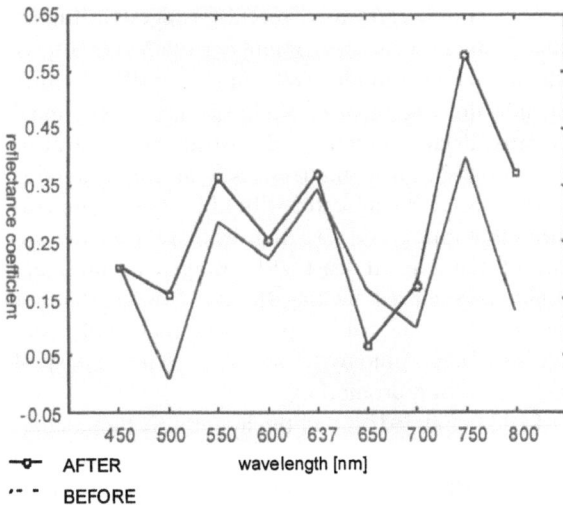

Fig. 5. Differences in reflectance coefficient of irradiated skin

therapy of musculoskeletal pain and skin disorders. The studies concluded that laser had only a tendency to be more effective than placebo treatment.

Several diseases and syndromes have been reported to be somehow effectively treated with laser therapy: arthritis (rheumatoid, ankylosing spondylitis), osteoarthritis (degenerative joint disease), periarthritis humeroscapularis, frozen shoulder, supraspinatus tendinitis, bicipital tendinitis, lateral epicondylitis (tennis elbow), medial epicondylitis, rotator cuff, Achilles tendinitis, entrapment syndromes (carpal tunnel syndrome), radiculopathy, acute and chronic musculoskeletal pain, low back pain, nerve repair, peripheral nerve repair, and various joint sprains [4, 6, 11, 12, 20, 21, 23, 28, 30, 38, 42, 47, 48, 63, 66, 69, 72, 73, 76, 88, 91, 97, 107, 111, 113]. Some of these diseases and syndromes have been selected more often for clinical trials than others.

Lateral epicondylitis (tennis elbow) is a well-known syndrome that typically presents in the form of lateral arm pain. Mechanical damage due to overuse is thought to be the most common etiological factor. Tennis elbow has a tendency to become chronic and recurrent, which makes treatment more difficult. The therapy is expected to control the inflammation, promote healing, improve pain-free range of movement, and reduce overload. Laser physiotherapy has been frequently proposed in recent years to treat this condition. Gartner [28] treated tennis elbow with laser (IR, 904 nm, 4–30 min, up to 22 sessions). In his opinion 87 % did not need any further therapy after the last laser session. Relapses were observed in only 20 % of this group after 5–15 months.

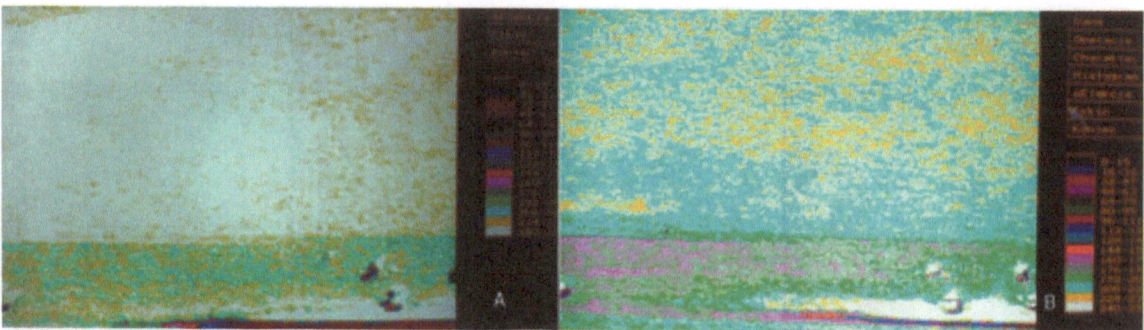

Fig. 6 A, B. Digital spectral analysis output images **A**, before and **B**, after irradiation (800-nm filter)

Haker and Lundeberg in 1990 [44] showed no benefit following acupuncture treatment with a pulsed GaAs IR device, power up to 12 mWs. Vasseljen et al. [113] performed a double-blind controlled study with an 18-mW pulsed 904-nm IR laser diode (eight 3.5 J/cm² local treatments). Laser treatment produced improvements in visual analog scale (VAS) scores and wrist extension strengths statistically significantly better than in the control group.

Simunovic et al. [101], considering LLLT to be a highly successful method for the treatment of modalities of medial and lateral epicondylitis, clinically studied IR diode laser (Ga AlAs, 830nm, continuous wave) treatment of trigger points (TPs), as well as HeNe (632.8 nm) combined with IR diode laser (904 nm, pulsed wave for scanner technique using TPs), and scanner application techniques, under placebo-controlled conditions. Total relief of the pain and, consequently, improved functional ability was achieved in 82% of acute and 66% of chronic cases, all of which were treated by a combination of TPs and scanner techniques. They also observed that under- and over-irradiation dosages can result in positive therapy effects being absent or even the opposite, negative (e. g., inhibitory) effects.

Haker and Lundeberg [45, 46] explored the pain-alleviating effect of low-energy laser (904 nm; average power output 12 mW; peak value 8.3 W; frequency 70 Hz; pulse, 8000 Hz) in lateral epicondylalgia. The laser (GaAs) was locally applied to six sites on and around the epicondyle. Each point was treated for 30 s, resulting in a dose of 0.36 J/point and an area of treatment of 0.2 mm². Patients were treated two to three times weekly, for a total of ten treatments. After the treatment period and at the three-month follow-up examination, some of the objective outcomes of the laser-treated group were significantly improved.

Melegati et al. [73] administered a protocol of treatment prescribing rest for two weeks, local cryotherapy, and iontophoresis of anti-inflammatory nonsteroidal agents. VAS and telethermography were used for evaluation. The laser therapy was conducted with a 50-W Nd:YAG apparatus, 1064 nm, fitted with defocusing lenses for therapeutic application. The following protocol was employed: two sessions per day for 12 days, power range 40–50 W, time per field 50 s, defocused spot diameter about 4 cm, energy about 150 J/cm². The therapy administered led to the rapid disappearance or attenuation of pain in patients with tennis elbow, and was observed as more effective than conventional management with iontophoresis and cryotherapy. The results suggest that LLLT is very effective, especially in the management of muscle and tendon exertion injuries in sportsmen. The effect of the Nd:YAG laser is immediately evident and persists over time. The increase in laser beam energies used recently suggests a higher effectiveness of therapy employing the Nd:YAG laser (defocused and diode; 980 nm, 200 mW). Studies include the treatment of ankle sprains, subacromial bursitis, delayed unions, and post-injury algodystrophy. Simple sports injuries such as ankle sprains recover faster when treated with LLLT. Local temperature after injury and swelling decrease after the 4th day of therapy. At least 75% range of movement could be achieved by the 9th to 11th day. Similar results were described by Beckerman [14] and Ohshiro [86]. Animal studies support the theory of tendon-healing promotion.

Reddy et al. [93] tested the hypothesis that a combination of laser phototherapy and mechanical load would further accelerate healing of experimentally tenotomized and repaired rabbit Achilles tendons. They found that the combination of laser photostimulation and early mechanical loading of tendons increased collagen production, with marginal biomechanical effects on repaired tendons. They also designed a study [94] to evaluate the influence of laser photostimulation on collagen production in experimentally tenotomized and repaired rabbit Achilles tendons. They treated animals daily for 14 days with a 632.8-nm HeNe laser at 1.0 J/cm². Biochemical analyses of the tendons revealed an increase in collagen concentration in the form of neutral salt-soluble collagen and insoluble collagen. They did not find statistically significant differences between treated and control tendons with regards to the concentrations of hydroxypyridinium cross-links and acid-soluble collagen.

Morselli et al. [82] reported on two years of experience with 25-W CO_2 automated scanning laser treatment of soft tissue sports injuries. Fast reduction of swelling and inflammation was described. Our own observations suggest that a combination of laser therapy with some other methods, for example, ultrasound, may bring synergistic effects. Synergy in the combination of laser and magnetic fields has also been reported.

Nissen et al. [83] applied low-energy laser therapy on shin splints (40 mW in 60 s per cm tender tibia edge) and found no significant differences between the groups regarding pain visual analog score and readiness to return to active duty after 14 days.

Minden et al. [80] observed a significant decrease of swelling and pain with GaA1As laser irradiation. Our own data show local improvement that was palpable and detectable by ultrasonic examination. Li [66] treated 60 cases of soft tissue injuries with laser (Ji4, CO_2, 10 600 nm, 15 W, and HeNe, 2–20 mW). Only 6.6% of the cases showed no effect from the laser treatment.

Conti [22] evaluated the efficacy of LLLT (830-nm GaA1As, 4 J) in patients with temporomandibular disorders with visual analog scale (VAS) and active range of motion (AROM). Laser treatment led to improvement in myogenous pain patients ($p \leq 0.02$) and active range of motion in arthrogenous pain patients.

Rotator cuff tendinitis, often resulting from repetitive trauma, is a common and painful soft tissue problem of the shoulders, usually affecting middle-aged and elderly athletes. Physical therapy and rehabilitation involve a wide range of options including heat, ice, rest, exercise, massage, nonsteroidal anti-inflammatory drugs, and corticosteroid injections. Shoulder tendinitis has often been reported as successfully treated with IR laser therapy [34–37, 39–41, 72, 88, 108]. Usage of 830-nm, 30-mW, continuous-wave laser was described by Vecchio et al. [114]. England et al. [24] and Glinkowski et al. [36] applied pulsed 904-nm lasers. The patients who received laser treatment improved significantly after treatment.

In spite of Longo and Clementi's [67] description that combined irradiation with CO_2 defocused and HeNe laser resorbs subacromial calcifications, we could not confirm this by ultrasonography and X-ray after diode laser therapy.

Patients with humeroscapular periarthritis were treated with pulsed 904-nm laser, using the noncontact "sweeping" technique, at a distance of 2 cm from the skin, 5 days a week, 8–11 sessions per therapy. Improvement after therapy was achieved in 90.9% of cases; more than 9% of the patients did not experience improvement at all. The range of shoulder joint movements rose in 63.4% of the cases. Siebert et al. [100] used HeNe and IR (904 nm) lasers to treat patients with tendinopathies, but no significant changes were found.

Low-energy lasers are often employed to treat rheumatoid arthritis [4, 15, 16, 29, 50, 51, 104, 111]. It is believed that laser therapy results in immune system modulation and depression of the inflammatory reaction. Biochemical benefits such as a decrease of immune complexes, C-reactive proteins (CRP), or sedimentation rates or increase in collagenase in the synovial fluid were reported. Clinical investigations have shown a decrease in pain, swelling, medication use, and morning stiffness following a variety of IR and visible laser treatments. Ankylosing spondylitis has been treated with HeNe and IR radiation with similar effects [31, 65].

The interaction of laser irradiation with nerve tissue is another area of intense research [9, 42, 68, 95, 96, 98, 112, 115–117, 119, 120]. Nerve growth and repair are important aspects of these studies. The important role of LLLT in pain relief and analgesia has been investigated extensively [4, 19, 20, 24, 44, 47, 58, 63, 81, 103, 115]. Analgesia may be produced by treating the injury itself, while successful treatment of neuropathic and radicular pain may indicate its influence by direct neurological effects.

Clinical and animal studies provide significant information about this interaction. Physiological studies usually show that laser irradiation can alter nerve conduction, repair, and evoked potentials. Walker et al. [117] reported that 1-mW HeNe laser irradiation diminishes pain, suppresses clonus, and triggers action potentials. Bork and Snyder-Mackler [17] found significant laser-mediated increases in superficial radial nerve distal latencies. Basford et al. [8] and Wu et al. [119] could not reproduce these findings with 1-mW HeNe lasers. Alterations of peripheral neurophysiological effects in the human median nerve with diode laser, 830 nm, were demonstrated as increases of antidromic nerve conduction [68].

Mohktar et al. [81] assessed the putative analgesic effect of combined monochromatic light/laser irradiation at low intensity (660–950 nm, 31.9 J/cm^2, pulsed at 16 or 73 Hz). Their results did not provide convincing evidence for the hypoalgesic potential of combined monochromatic light/laser irradiation.

The laser-treated group suffering from carpal tunnel syndrome demonstrated better outcomes than the control group. Some positive results were found by

Smith and Vangsness [102], who treated patients with carpal tunnel syndrome. One of the earliest low-power laser applications was stimulation of wound healing. The reports by Mester et al. [74–78] and other researchers from the late 1960s showed that 1–4 J/cm^2 of laser irradiation may induce healing of chronic ulcerations and wounds.

Laboratory experiments also provide some support for the use of low-intensity laser radiation in wound healing [10, 60, 71, 92, 105, 109]. It has found that visible and IR radiation stimulates capillary growth and granulation tissue formation and alters cytokine production, keratinocyte motility, and fibroblast movement. Improvements, particularly in the earlier phases of wound healing, have been reported following laser irradiation in many rabbit and rodent experiments. Well-controlled and blinded human wound healing studies are difficult to carry out, but applying these findings to humans may show some benefits, particularly in cases of delayed healing [26]. Lundeberg and Malm [70] treated patients with venous ulcers. One-half of the patients received HeNe laser irradiation twice a week for 12 weeks (4 J/cm^2, 6 mW) and the others were treated with a sham device. No significant differences in healing were demonstrated between the groups.

The diffuse nature of low back pain makes laser therapy useful for its treatment. Analysis by Klein and Eck [58] involved two groups of 20 subjects following a standard exercise program; one-half of the patients were irradiated three times a week for 4 weeks with 1.3 J/cm^2 from an array of pulsed 904-nm lasers. They found that low-energy laser stimulation plus exercise did not provide a significant advantage over exercise alone. Basford et al. [11] found 30-mW, 830-nm GaAlAs continuous-wave IR diode laser treatment three times a week for four weeks to be an ineffective but safe and well-tolerated treatment. Mika et al. [79] used IR laser (pulsed, 904 nm, 30 W per pulse, 2000 to 3000 Hz). They irradiated the area of pain by the "sweep" technique 6–8 min per area, and the trigger points 2 min each. The incident energy was 172–345 mJ/cm^2 during "sweeping" and 720–1080 mJ/cm^2 for point irradiation. Total pain relief after the fourth session was reported in 53 % of all cases. No effect was found in 5 % of the cases.

Patellofemoral disorders are classified into many clearly distinct diseases. Some of them can be treated with activity restriction, ice, vastus medialis strengthening, knee sleeves, and nonsteroidal anti-inflammatory medication. Therapists may find indications for laser therapy. Rogvi-Hansen et al. [97] described the results of 10-min treatments with either an active or a sham 1000-Hz pulsed 17-mW GaAs laser of arthroscopically documented chondromalacia patellae. At the end of the 5-week study no significant differences were found.

Laser trigger and acupuncture point irradiation are frequently reported [19, 44, 56, 87, 103], but this combination of methods is even more difficult to explain, because traditional Chinese medicine is not well understood and lacks scientific explanations.

Orthopedic surgeons have been searching for methods to accelerate fracture healing. The formation of the fracture callus may be modified by different physical stimuli: electric, magnetic and ultrasonic [13, 21, 40, 90, 121]. LLLT has been suggested as an effective adjuvant in the healing of bone fractures. However, there are still many unknown points regarding specific laser bioactivation mechanisms. In 1974, Shugharov and Voronkov [99] used HeNe laser along with an intramedullary rod to promote fracture healing. Since then other lasers have been employed for this purpose: He-Ne [110], CO_2 [21, 106], and 830-, 890- and 904-nm diodes [32–35, 39, 41, 109].

Bone healing involves complex physiological and biochemical processes, including collagen synthesis, deposition of inorganic salts, and osteogenesis, which could be affected by laser beam application. Active synthesis of collagen and other connective tissue components is necessary for optimal wound healing during the early period of repair [18]. An increase in collagen production may enhance inorganic metabolism of bone callus and speed up bone repair. Collagen synthesis enhancement with the use of low-intensity laser has been demonstrated by Mester, Kana, and Abergel et al. [1, 52, 77]. Chen and Zhou [21] demonstrated an increase in calcium, phosphorus, and hydroxyproline content after CO_2 laser bioactivation with an output of 2 W (wavelength 10 600 nm) and a power density of 255 mW/cm^2, every day, 10 min per session, for 7 consecutive days, using a model JG-6 CO_2 laser system, aiming the defocused beam at the region of the osteotomy from a distance of 10 cm. The calcium and phosphorus content in bone callus was demonstrated to be significantly increased by laser irradiation. The rise in the hydroxyproline content in the irradiated side within 28 days could indicate that LLLT stimulates bone collagen production. Promotion of mineralization by LLLT has been found experimentally and clinically. LLLT may influence fracture healing by stimulating vascular response directly or indirectly via prostaglandin E_2. Stimulation of the release of PGE_2, PDGF, FGF, TGF-β, and BMP activation are suspected to be possible mechanisms for the LLLT stimulation of bone remodeling. Other mechanisms confirmed in vitro, such as the promotion of fibroblast collagen synthesis, the stimulation of macrophages, neoangiogenesis, and the rise of capillary flow, may also play an important role in fracture healing. Regarding the influence of LLLT on osseous tissue, it has been reported in the literature that there is an affect of promoting fracture healing at the initial phase and an activity of accelerating osteogenesis. It is so far agreed that LLLT induces the healing-promoting effect by reducing edema in the initial phase of the inflammation process, due to the increased vascular drainage. During the period of bone healing, osteogenesis chiefly depends on blood circulation, which directly relates to the formation of bone matrix and its mineralization. The improved blood circulation and stimulated vessel growth may be the most important effects of LLLT on the healing process.

Most experiments in vivo provide only clues about the mechanism, but lack a standardized quantitative measurement of bone healing. The available statistical data are unreliable. It was therefore felt necessary to study the laser effect on bone healing with more convincing methods. Evaluation of X-rays by the naked eye could not differentiate slight changes in the callus. Therefore laser densitometry of radiographs, employing UltroScan XL (Pharmacia), was used to standardize and quantify the measurement of bone healing. It seems that laser densitometry employed to perform optical density evaluation of radiographs is a way of obtaining a numeric characterization of an X-ray view. In the near future new designs of ultrasonic bone defectoscopes may offer a more valuable method of fracture healing evaluation. One aim of the present author's previous studies was to evaluate the possibilities of low-energy laser stimulation of bone, muscle, and skin healing. Combined application of HeNe and HeCd lasers was demonstrated to stimulate fracture healing but their influence on bone was stronger when they were applied simultaneously. Two lasers were used simultaneously: 904 nm, 10 W pulsed, and HeNe, continuous wave 2 mW. Nine adult male WISTAR rats were used to investigate the influence of low-level HeNe and diode lasers (632.8 nm, 2 mW continuous wave and 904 nm, pulsed, peak power 10 W) irradiation on femoral defect healing. Reproducible defects were produced by drilling on the lateral side of the femoral shaft. Left femora were lased and right bones served as control. Tetracycline (20 mg/kg) was given intraperitoneally on the 8th and 15th days after surgery. Harvested femora were examined. The radiographs were evaluated using the UltroScan XL laser densitometer and the GelScan software; this examination was supplemented by analysis of digitized X-rays, using the RODIA System [59]. After 3 weeks of a daily regime of 0.2-J/cm^2 lasing, no significant difference was demonstrated either histologically or with a tetracycline test. Optical density changes around the defect on radiographs were not found. Only macroscopic enlargement of capillary vessels in subcutaneous tissue was observed in eight of nine cases. It was concluded that the neoangiogenesis observed in almost all cases suggests a positive response to LLLT, but the laser energy did not achieve therapeutic levels in the target tissue. Vascular effects were examined in our experiment on volunteers. Achilles tendons were irradiated and examined by Doppler ultrasonography [34]. Increased blood flow was observed after irradiation with either laser (830 nm, 30 mW continuous wave or pulsed 904 nm, 30 W/pulse). Another tibial fracture healing experiment was performed on mice. Eighteen BALB/C male mice, 4 months of age, were used. Three groups were irradiated with either 830-nm, continuous-wave, 30-mW, or 904-nm, pulsed, 30-W/pulse, or "sham" laser. Quantifiable and reproducible fractures were produced following the method of Borque et al. [18]. After 3 weeks of a daily regime of laser beam irradiation at 4.0 J/cm^2, it was demonstrated that the optical density on the radiographs of the irradiated calluses was significantly different ($p < 0.02$) from the control. Macroscopically, the calluses were found to be present on the last day of the experiment in all cases. The effect of the pulsed 904-nm laser was significantly greater than that of the 830-nm continuous-wave laser. Patients with delayed union of fractures in different long bones were stimulated with IR laser irradiation. From 1989 to 1995, 17 cooperative patients were treated with laser beam emitted from a diode (pulsed, 904 nm, 10–15 W peak power).

Patients in the irradiated group had previously either been treated conservatively or had been treated surgically but refused further surgery. Fractures with delayed union were most often located in the forearm or in the tibia. Treatment consisted of one or two series of laser irradiation every alternate day, 10 min, in contact mode, above the fracture gap, with a local frequency of 2.4–3 kHz. Each series of therapy consisted of 10 sessions. All patients finally achieved fracture consolidation, but only 13 experienced fracture consolidation just after therapy.

Four patients needed additional therapeutic series. One patient with pseudoarthrosis did not achieve fracture consolidation. The results suggest that LLLT may be expected to have a good therapeutic effect on cases of delayed union of superficially located fractured bones, where the laser beam has a thin layer of tissues to penetrate. No side effects or osteolysis was observed in the group of patients studied. The better fracture healing stimulation achieved with pulsed laser may be partially explained by a phenomenon known in acoustooptics: the laser beam generation of an ultrasonic wave in an anisotropic, porous medium, such as bone [5].

Conclusions

A clear and definitive consensus on LLLT has not yet emerged. Some laboratory studies support the concept that laser irradiation can modify cellular processes via a wavelength-dependent, nonthermal mechanism. To be effective on cells, laser energy should be delivered to the target tissues, with their optical properties taken into consideration.

In view of the present and other author's results, it can be postulated that LLLT possesses a potential for stimulating bone repair processes. In the author's own studies, not only continuous wave IR laser enhancement of bone healing was observed, but a more prominent influence of pulsed IR laser was also noted. The mechanisms of bone healing promotion after laser irradiation still need further study.

As mentioned by Basford [7], the basic problem in evaluating laser therapy remains the same: "similar but not identical" diagnoses, treatment, devices and methodologies produce different outcomes.

Although a definite trend of a therapeutic effect of LLLT has been seen, the manufacturers of low-level laser devices should be obliged to set up more double blind prospective trials to prove the clinical effects.

References

[1] Abergel RP, Meeker, CA, Dwyer RM, LeSavoy MA, Uitto J (1984) Nonthermal effects of ND:YAG laser on biological functions of human fibroblasts in culture. Lasers Surg Med 3:279–284
[2] Abergel RP, Meeker CA, Lam TS, Dwyer RM, Lesavoy MA, Uitto J (1984) Control of connective tissue metabolism by lasers: recent development and future prospective. J Am Acad Dermatol 11:1142–1150
[3] Anderson RR, Panish JA (1981) The optics of human skin. J Invest Dermatol 77:13–19
[4] Asada K, Yutani Y, Sakawa A, Shimazu A (1991) Clinical application of GaAlAs 830 diode laser in treatment of rheumatoid arthritis. Laser Ther 3:77–81
[5] Aussel A, le Brun JC, Baboux JC (1988) Generating acoustic waves by laser: theoretical and experimental study of the emission source. Ultrasonics 26:245–255
[6] Basford JR (1989) Low energy laser therapy: controversies and new findings. Lasers Surg Med 9:1–5
[7] Basford JR (1995) Low intensity laser therapy: still not an established clinical tool. Lasers Surg Med 16:331–342
[8] Basford JR, Daube JR, Hallman HO, Millard IL, Moyer SK (1990) Does low-intensity helium-neon laser irradiation alter sensory nerve action potentials or distal latencies? Lasers Surg Med 10:35–39
[9] Basford JR, Hallman HO, Matsumoto JY, Moyer SK, Buss JM, Baxter GD (1993) Effects of 830 nm continuous wave laser diode irradiation on median nerve function in normal subjects. Lasers Surg Med 13:597–604
[10] Basford JR, Hallman HO, Sheffield CG, Mackey GL (1986) Comparison of the effects of cold quartz ultraviolet, low energy laser, and occlusion on wound healing in a swine model. Arch Phys Med Rehab 67:151–154
[11] Basford JR, Malanga GA, Krause DA, Harmsen WS (1998) A randomized controlled evaluation of low-intensity laser therapy: plantar fasciitis. Arch Phys Med Rehabil 3:249–254

[12] Basfrord JR, Sheffield CG, Mair SD, Ilstrup DM (1987) Low-energy helium–neon laser treatment of thumb osteoarthritis. Arch Phys Med Rehab 68:794–797
[13] Basset C (1962) Current concepts of bone formation. J Bone Joint Surg 44A:1217–1244
[14] Beckerman H, de Bie RA, Bouter LM, de Cuyper HJ, Oostendorp RA (1992) The efficacy of laser therapy for musculoskeletal and skin disorders: a criteria-based meta-analysis of randomized clinical trials. Phys Ther 72:483–491
[15] Bendowski P, Lesiak A (1995) Laser biostimulation in rheumatology. In: Fiedor P, Kęcik T, Niechoda Z, Nowakowski, Nowicki M, Otto W, Pirożyński M, Stanowski E (eds) Outline of clinical laser applications. Ankar, Warsaw, pp 322–329 (in Polish)
[16] Bliddal H, Hellesen C, Ditlewsen P, Asselberghs J, Lyage L (1987) Soft-laser therapy of rheumatoid arthritis. Scand J Rheumatol 16:225–228
[17] Bork CE, Snyder-Mackler L (1988) Effect of helium-neon laser irradiation on peripheral sensory nerve latency. J Am Phys Ther Assoc 68:223
[18] Borque WT, Gross M, Hall BK (1992) A reproducible method for producing and quantifying the stages of fracture repair. Lab Animal Sci 42:369–374
[19] Brockhaus A, Elger CE (1990) Hypalgesic efficacy of acupuncture on experimental pain in man. Comparison of laser acupuncture and needle acupuncture. Pain 43:181–185
[20] Calderhead RG, Ohshiro T (1991) Progress in laser therapy. Wiley, Chichester
[21] Chen J, Zhou Y (1989) Effects of low level carbon dioxide laser radiation on biochemical metabolism of rabbit mandibular bone callus. Laser Ther 1:283–287
[22] Conti PC (1997) Low level laser therapy in the treatment of temporomandibular disorders (TMD): a double-blind pilot study. Cranio 15:2:144–149
[23] Emmanouilidis O, Diamantopoulos C (1986) CW IR low power laser application significantly accelerates chronic pain relief in rehabilitation of professional athletes. A double blind study. Laser Med Surg, Abstract no 175
[24] England S, Fanell AJ, Coppock JS, Struthers G, Bacon PA (1989) Low power laser therapy of shoulder tendonitis. Scand J Rheumatol 18:427–431
[25] Enwemeka CS (1992) Ultrastructural morphometry of membrane-bound intracytoplasmic collagen fibrils in tendon fibroblasts exposed to He:Ne laser beam. Tissue Cell 24:511–523
[26] Fiedor P, Glinkowski W, Kwiatkowski A, Rowiński W, Śladowski D (1993) Application of lasers generating near infrared irradiation for delayed wound healing. In: 7th national optoelectronic school, Zegrze, Poland, 27–29 April 1993, B54–69 (in Polish)
[27] Gam AN, Thorsen H, Lonnberg F (1993) The effect of low-level laser therapy on musculoskeletal pain: A meta-analysis. Pain 52:63–66
[28] Gartner C (1987) Laser treatment of therapy resistant tendinitis. Laser Med Surg, Abstract no 79
[29] Gartner C (1992) Low reactive level laser therapy (LLLT) in rheumatology: a review of the clinical experience in the author's laboratory. Laser Ther 4:107–115
[30] Gatev S (1989) Helium neon laser radiation in the rehabilitation of fracture patients. Voprosy Kurortologi i Lechebnoj Fiziczeskoj Kultury 2:28–30 (in Russian)
[31] Gembitskii EV, Ermolina LM, Serebrianskii IE (1989) Evaluation of the efficacy of laser irradiation in the combined treatment of patients with Bechterew's disease. Ter Arkh 61:83–87 (in Russian)
[32] Glinkowski W (1990) Delayed union healing with diode laser therapy (LLLT). Case report and review of literature. Laser Ther 2:107–109
[33] Glinkowski W, Gut G, Kornacki M (1998) Lack of effect of very low level laser irradiation on bone defect healing in rats. In: SPIE conference on three-dimensional and optical tomography, 21–22 Oct 1998, Warsaw

[34] Glinkowski W, Pokora L (1993) Lasers in therapy. Centrum Techniki Laserowej, Laserinstruments, Warsaw (in Polish)

[35] Glinkowski W, Szczypiorski P (1995) Laser biostimulation in traumatology, orthopedics and sports medicine. In: Fiedor P, Kęcik T, Niechoda Z, Nowakowski W, Nowicki M, Otto W, Pirożyński M, Stanowski E (eds) Outline of clinical laser applications. Ankar, Warsaw, pp 346–353 (in Polish)

[36] Glinkowski W, Szczypiorski P, Glinkowska B (1991) Laser therapy of shoulder tendinitis in sportsmen. Medycyna Sportowa 7(22):4–5 (in Polish)

[37] Glinkowski W, Szczypiorski P, Glinkowska B, Dąbrowska A, Gut G (1993) Application of low energy lasers in sports medicine. Basic and clinical study of rational laser therapy. Medycyna Sportowa 9(31):4–7 (in Polish)

[38] Glinkowski W, Szczypiorski P, Glinkowska B, Wasilewski L (1992) Influence of low-energy laser irradiation on sprained ankles healing. Chir Narz Ruchu Ortop Pol 57(Suppl 4):130–133

[39] Glinkowski W, Szczypiorski P, Serafin-Król M, Śladowski D, Fiedor P (1993) Low energy lasers in orthopedics and sports medicine. In: The 7th national optoelectronic school, Zegrze, Poland, 27–29 Apr 1995, B 70–101 (in Polish)

[40] Glinkowski W, Wasilewski L (1992) Nonunion and delayed union of fractures treatment with use of ultrasound therapy. The 3rd Conference of The International Society of Fracture Repair (ISFR-92), Brussels, (Book of Abstracts), p 154

[41] Glinkowski W, Wasilewski L (1994) Application of low power ultrasound and laser therapy to stimulate delayed union. Fizjoterapia 2(4):18–19 (in Polish)

[42] Greathouse DG, Cunier DP, Gilmore RL (1985) Effects of clinical infared laser on superficial radial nerve conduction. Phys Ther 65:1184

[43] Gum SL, Reddy GK, Stehno-Bittel L, Enwemeka CS (1997) Combined ultrasound, electrical stimulation, and laser promote collagen synthesis with moderate changes in tendon biomechanics. Am J Phys Med Rehabil 76:288–296

[44] Haker E, Lundeberg T (1990) Laser treatment applied to acupuncture points in lateral epicondylalgia. Pain 43: 243–247

[45] Haker E, Lundeberg T (1991) Is low-energy laser treatment effective in lateral epicondylalgia? J Pain Symptom Manage 6:241–246

[46] Haker EHK, Lundeberg TCM (1991) Lateral epicondylalgia: report of noneffective midlaser treatment. Arch Phys Med Rehabil 72:984

[47] Hansen HJ, Thoroe U (1990) Low power laser biostimulation of chronic orofacial pain: a double-blind placebo controlled cross-over study in 40 patients. Pain 43:169–179

[48] He JZ (1991) 154 cases of myogenic torticolis treated with low incident energy combination carbon dioxide and helium neon laser beam. Laser Ther 3:41–43

[49] Heckamn JD, Ryaby JP, McCabe J, Frey JJ, Kilcoyne RF (1994) Acceleration of tibial fracture healing by non-invasive, low-intensity pulsed ultrasound. J Bone Joint Surg 76A:26–34

[50] Hendrich C, Diddens H, Seara J, Siebert WE (1995) Photodynamic therapy for rheumatoid arthritis – a new therapeutic approach. Laser Surg Med; Suppl 7 (Abstact 149):32

[51] Iarema NZ, Nazar PS, Zoria LV (1987) Use of immunomodulating and laser therapy in rheumatoid arthritis patients. Vrach Delo 4:59–67 (in Russian)

[52] Kana JS, Hutschenreiner G, Haina D, Waidelich W (1981) Effect of low-power density laser radiation on healing of open skin wounds in rats. Arch Surg 116:293

[53] Karu T (1987) Photobiological fundamentals of low-power laser therapy. IEEE J Quant Elect 23:1703

[54] Karu TI (1988) Molecular mechanism of the therapeutic effect of low-intensity laser radiation. Lasers Life Sci 2:53–74

[55] Karu TI, Ryabykh TP, Fedoseyeva GE, Puchkova NI (1989) Helium–neon laser-induced respiratory burst of phagocytic cells. Lasers Surg Med 9:585–588

[56] King CE, Clelland JA, Knowles CJ, Jackson JR (1990) Effect of helium–neon laser auriculotherapy on experimental pain threshold. Phys Ther 70:24–30

[57] Kiss FA, Mester E, Krompecher ST, Tota JG, Kalabay L (1972) Laser-Strahlen und Vaskularisation. Radiobiol Radiother 13:123–132

[58] Klein RG, Eek BC (1990) Low-energy laser treatment and exercise for chronic low back pain: double-blind controlled trial. Arch Phys Med Rehab 71:34–37

[59] Kornacki M, Glinkowski W (1998) Relative optical density image analysis (RODIA) clinical application – preliminary report of FHM and IE subsystems usage. Med Sci Monit 4(Suppl 2):136–139

[60] Kovacs IB, Mester E, Gorog P (1974) Stimulation of wound healing with laser beam in the rat. Experientia 30:1275–1276

[61] Kriuk AS, Mostovnikov WA, Hohlov IV, Serdiuchenko NS (1986) Therapeutic effectiveness of low-intensity laser irradiation. Nauka i technika, Minsk (in Russian)

[62] Kubasova T, Kovacs L, Somosy Z, Unk P, Kokai A (1984) Biological effect of He-Ne laser investigations on functional and micromorphological alterations of cell membranes, in vitro. Lasers Surg Med 4:381

[63] Kuszelewski Z (1990) Infrared laser irradiation treatment of humeral epicondylalgia. Doctoral Thesis, Military Medical School, Warsaw

[64] Lam TS, Abergel RP, Meeker CA, Castael JC, Dwyer RM, Uitto J (1986) Laser stimulation of collagen synthesis in human skin fibroblast cultures. Lasers Life Sci 1:61–77

[65] Lerner LA (1988) Effectiveness of laser therapy in Bechterew's disease. Ter Arkh 60:134–136 (in Russian)

[66] Li XH (1990) Laser in the department of traumatology. Laser Ther 2:119–122

[67] Longo L, Clementi F (1992) CO_2 laser treatment of calcific metaplasias: In: Spinelli P, Dal Fante M, Marchesini R (eds) Photodynamic therapy and biomedical lasers. Excerpta Medica, Amsterdam, pp 186–190

[68] Lowe AS, Baxter GD, Walsh DM, Allen JM (1994) Effect of low intensity laser (830 nm) irradiation on skin temperature and antidromic conduction latencies in the human median nerve: relevance of radiant exposure: Lasers Med Surg 14:40–46

[69] Lundeberg T, Haker E, Thomas M (1987) Effects of laser versus placebo in tennis elbow. Scand J Rehabil Med 19:135–138

[70] Lundeberg T, Malm M (1991) Low-power HeNe laser treatment of venous leg ulcers. Ann Plastic Surg 27:537–539

[71] Lyons RF, Abergel RP, White RA, Dwyer RM, Castel JC, Uitto J (1987) Biostimulation of wound healing in vivo by a helium–neon laser. Ann Plast Surg 18:47

[72] Meier JL. Kerkour K (1988) Laser treatment of tendinitis. Med Hyg 46:907

[73] Melegati G, Miglio D, Respizzi S, Giani E, Volpi P, Roi GS (1994) Defocused Nd:YAG laser therapy in the treatment of humeral epicondylitis. J Sports Traumatol Relat Res 16(3):115–122

[74] Mester AF, Mester A (1986) Mester's method of laser biostimulation. In: Waidelich W, Kiefhaber P (eds) Laser opto-electronics in medicine. Springer, Berlin Heidelberg New York

[75] Mester E, Korenyi-Both A, Spiry T, Tisza S (1975) The effect of laser irradiation on the regeneration of muscle fibers. Z Exper Chir 8:258–262

[76] Mester E, Mester AF, Mester A (1985) The biomedical effects of laser application. Lasers Surg Med 5:31–39

[77] Mester E, Spiry T, Szende B, Tota JG (1971) Effect of laser rays on wound healing. Am J Surg 122:532

[78] Mester E, Toth N, Mester A (1982) The biostimulative effect of laser beam. Laser Basic Biomed Res 22:4

[79] Mika T, Orlow H, Kuszelewski Z (1990) Infrared laser irradiation treatment of low back pain. Wiad Lek 43:511–516 (in Polish)

[80] Minden A, Ipton C, Garvey M (1988) A pilot study to evaluate the efficacy of low power laser irradiation on the treatment of chronic Achilles tendonitis. Laser Med Surg 205 (Abstract)

[81] Mokhtar B, Baxter GD, Walsh DM, Bell AJ, Allen JM (1995) Double-blind, placebo-controlled investigation of the effect of combined phototherapy/low intensity laser therapy upon experimental ischaemic pain in humans. Lasers Surg Med 17:74–81

[82] Morselli M, Sorgani O, Anselmi C, Farinelli FF (1988) Very low energy density treatment by CO_2 laser in sports medicine. Laser Med Surg 205 (Abstract)

[83] Nissen LR, Astvad K, Madsen L (1994) Low-energy laser therapy in medial tibial stress syndrome. Ugeskr Laeger 156(49):7329–7331 (in Danish)

[84] Noble PB, Shields ED, Blecher PDM, Bentley KC (1992) Locomotory characteristics of fibroblasts within a three-dimensional collagen lattice: modulation by a helium/neon soft laser. Lasers Surg Med 12:669–674

[85] Ohshiro T (1991) Low reactive-level laser therapy. Practical application. Wiley, Chichester

[86] Ohshiro T, Calderhead RG (1988) Low level laser therapy. A pracitcal introduction. Wiley, Chichester

[87] Olavi A, Pekka R, Pertti K (1989) Effects of the infrared laser therapy at treated and non-treated trigger points. Acupunct Electrother Res Int J 14:9–14

[88] Pashniev C, Cherkasova G (1986) Laser therapy in diseases of the locomotor apparatus and skin at polyclinic. Voen Med Zh 3:42–44 (in Russian)

[89] Passarella S, Casamassima E, Quagliariello E, Caretto G, Jirillo E (1985) Quantitative analysis of lymphocyte–salmonella interaction and effect of lymphocyte irradiation by helium–neon laser. Biochem Biophys Res Comm 130:546

[90] Pilla AA, Mont MA, Nasser PR, Khan SA, Figueiredo M, Kaufman JJ, Siffert RS (1990) Non-invasive low-intensity pulsed ultrasound accelerates bone healing in the rabbit. J Orthop Trauma 4:246–253

[91] Poldi R, Beltrami GF, Montani G, Colana L (1982) Laser terapia nella traumatologia sportiva. Med Sport 35:15–20

[92] Rakocheev AP, Kiprienssky JB (1989) Experimental and clinical substantiation of laser therapy of wounds and trophic ulcers. Ortop Trawmatol Protez 66–70

[93] Reddy GK, Gum S, Stehno-Bittel L, Enwemeka CS (1998) Biochemistry and biomechanics of healing tendon. Part II. Effects of combined laser therapy and electrical stimulation. Med Sci Sports Exerc 6:794–800

[94] Reddy GK, Stehno-Bittel L, Enwemeka CS (1998) Laser photostimulation of collagen production in healing rabbit Achilles tendons. Lasers Surg Med 22(5):281–287

[95] Rochkind S, Alon M, Ouakine GE, Weiss S, Avram J, Rzon N, Doron A, Lubart R, Friedmann H (1991) Intraoperative clinical use of LLLT followup surgical treatment of the tethered spinal cord. Laser Ther 3:113–118

[96] Rochkind S, Barnea L, Razon N, Bartel A, Schwartz M (1987) Stimulatory effect of He-Ne low dose laser on injured sciatic nerves of rats. Neurosurgery 20:843

[97] Rogvi-Hansen B, Ellitsgaard N, Funch M, Dall-Jensen M, Prieske J (1991) Low level laser treatement of chondromalacia patellae. Int Orthop 15:359–361

[98] Schwartz M, Doron A, Erich M, Lavie V, Benbasat S, Belkin M, Rochkind S (1987) Effects of low-energy He-Ne laser irradiation of posttraumatic degeneration of adult rabbit optic nerve. Lasers Surg Med 7:51

[99] Shugharov NA, Voronkov DV (1974) Osseous tissues restoration treatment by intramedullary osteosynthesis combined with the influence of laser irradiation. In: 2nd thematic symposium of scientific practical papers on the problem of physical self regulation, pp 336–368

[100] Siebert W, Seichert N, Siebert B, Wirth CJ (1987) What is the efficacy of "soft" and "mild" lasers in therapy of tendinopathies? A double-blind study. Arch Orthop Trauma Surg 106:358–363

[101] Simunovic Z, Trobonjaca T, Trobonjaca Z (1998) Treatment of medial and lateral epicondylitis – tennis and golfer's elbow – with low level laser therapy: a multicenter double blind, placebo-controlled clinical study on 324 patients. J Clin Laser Med Surg 3:145–151

[102] Smith CF, Vangsness CT (1995) Treatment of repetitive carpal tunnel syndrome. Proc SPIE 2395:658–661

[103] Snyder-Mackler L, Barry AJ, Perkins AI, Soucek MD (1989) Effects of helium-neon laser irradiation on skin resistance and pain in patients with trigger points in the neck or back. Phys Ther 69:336–341

[104] Soroka WF (1989) The laser therapy of rheumatoid arthritis. Ter Arkh 61:124–127

[105] Surinchak JS, Alago ML, Bellamy RF, Stuck BE, Belkin M (1983) Effects of low-level energy lasers on the healing of full-thickness skin defects. Lasers Surg Med 2:267–274

[106] Tang XM, Chai BP (1986) Effect of CO_2 laser irradiation experimental fracture healing: a transmission electron microscopic study. Lasers Surg Med 6:346–352

[107] Ternowoi KS, Zhila I, Korolik IM (1987) Laser therapy in postraumatic arthrosis deformans. Ortop Travmatol Protez 44:30–32

[108] Thorsen H, Gam AN, Jensen H, Hojmark L, Wahlstrom L (1991) Lav-energi laserbehandling-effekt ved lokalisiert fibromyalgi i nakke og skylderregioner. Ugeskr Laegr 153:1801–1804

[109] Tkachenko SS, Rutskii g, Leskov NT, Tikhilov RR (1988) Possibilities of using computers in the optimization of the parameters of laser therapy in the treatment of bone and soft tissues wound. Ortop Travmatol Protez 11:6–10

[110] Trelles MA, Mayayo E (1987) Bone fracture consolidates faster with low-power laser. Lasers Surg Med 7:36–45

[111] Ushakow AA, Ermolina LM (1987) Laser therapy of rheumatoid arthritis and osteoarthrosis. Voen Med Zh 5:54–55

[112] Van Breugel H, Bar P (1993) He-Ne laser irradiation affects proliferation of cultured rat Schwann cells in a dose dependent manner. J Neurocytol 22:185–190

[113] Vasseljen O Jr, Hoeg N, Kjelödstad B, Johnsson A, Larsen S (1992) Low level laser versus placebo in the treatment of tennis elbow. Scand J Rehab Med 24:37–42

[114] Vecchio P, Cave M, Kind V, Adebajo AO, Smith M, Hazleman BL (1993) A double-blind study of the effectiveness of low level laser treatment of rotator cuff tendinitis. Br J Rheumatol 32:740–742

[115] Walker J (1983) Relief from chronic pain by low power laser irradiation. Neurosci Lett 43:339–344

[116] Walker JB (1985) Temporary suppression of clonus in humans by brief photostimulation. Brain Res 340:109

[117] Walker JB, Akhanjee LK (1985) Laser-induced somatosensory evoked potentials: evidence of photosensitivity in peripheral nerves. Brain Res 344:281

[118] Wollman Y, Rochkind S (1993) Muscle fiber formation in vitro is delayed by low power laser irradiation. J Photochem Photobiol B 17:287–290

[119] Wu W, Ponnudurai R, Katz J, Pott CB, Chilcoat R, Uncini A, Rapport S, Wade P, Mauro A (1987) Failure to confirm report of light-evoked response of peripheral nerve to low power helium–neon laser light stimulus. Brain Res 401:407

[120] Wylie L, Baxter GD, Walsh DM, Robinson J (1995) The hypoalgesic effects of low intensity infrared laser therapy upon mechanical pain threshold. Laser Med Surg suppl 7, abstract no 9

[121] Yasuda I, Nogychi K, Sata T (1955) Dynamic callus and electric callus. J Bone Joint Surg 37A:1292

[122] Young S, Bolton P, Dyson M, Harvey W, Diamantopoulos C (1989) Macrophage responsiveness to light therapy. Lasers Surg Med 9:497–505

Low-Level Laser Therapy

S. Götte

History

The development of all available medical laser systems is based on physical hypothesis and experiments. Already in 1917 Einstein hypothesized that accelerated electrons produce electromagnetic beams of a certain wavelength. In the following years, his theories were confirmed in experimental studies. Yet, not until 1960 did Maiman, a young American physicist, construct the first laser device, a ruby laser, which emitted visible light at a wavelength of 694.3 nm. In 1960 and 1961, Goldmann and Campbell used a ruby laser for dermatological and ophthalmologic treatment. However, it had taken many years until the laser became widely accepted for various medical applications. Alongside high-powered lasers that are used in surgery, low-level HeNe lasers and GaAs lasers have also been developed.

One of the pioneers of low-level laser medicine is the Hungarian surgeon Endre Mester, who first worked with the argon laser in 1964 and, later on, with the HeNe laser. He published many articles on his experience with low-level lasers and wound healing, his main research field. Low-level lasers are now accepted in a variety of medical disciplines. Their positive effect has been substantiated by approximately 2000 experimental and clinical publications.

Physics of Low-Level Lasers

The therapeutic effect of low-level lasers is based on the prinicple that light energy can be transformed into cell energy. The physical preconditions for a biological effect of low-level laser therapy is based on the quality of laser light and its following three characteristics:

- collimation
- coherence
- monochromaticity

These characteristics allow the laser to produce a specific spectrum of light with an intensity that is significantly higher than that of visible light. The pre-conceived opinion, that the effect of low-level laser energy is no greater than the effect of sunlight, can be disputed by the fact that the intensity of sunlight on the earth's northern hemisphere is on average 120 W/m^2 (12 mW/cm^2). This intensity is derived from all wavelengths ranging from 300 to 4000 nm. Half of the sun's intensity is produced by photons which, as in the laser, can penetrate tissue, thus resulting in an irradiation intensity of 6 mW/cm^2. If only the wavelengths of 630 nm and 900 nm (corresponding to the monochromatic HeNe and GaAs intensities of 0.13 mW/cm^2) and the water absorption of infrared light are taken into account, an intensity of 0.05 mW/cm^2 remains. In comparison, the more powerful HeNe laser has a peak energy intensity of 2 mW/cm^2, and that of the diode GaAs laser is 4 mW/cm^2.

Skin is particularly permeable for the wavelengths used in low-level lasers. This quality, the optical window of the skin, is biologically ideal for the effect of low-level lasers. The wavelengths 633 to 690, 780 to 850, and 904 nm are especially penetrative and have been shown to be most effective for biostimulative treatment. The red wavelengths, 633 to 690 nm, are more suitable for skin treatment, for example, for ulcers. The infrared range, 780–850 nm, is used for treatment of deeper-lying regions, for example, for muscular and ligamentous tissues. The pulsed infra-red wavelength 904 nm is also applied to deeper regions, but is being increasingly replaced by the 830-nm wavelength.

In the past years many hypotheses on the mechanisms of low-level lasers have been forwarded, the model by Warnke being the most reasonable and interesting. In the meantime his hypothesis has been confirmed in experimental studies.

Thus, the mechanism of low-level lasers is based on the absorption of laser-emitted photons by the flavin mononucleotide enzyme (FMN), which is found in mitochondria and is an activator of cellular respiration. Through this absorption, the synthesis of ATP from ADP is accelerated. ATP is the basic substance for metabolism activation. This process may be summarized as follows:

Respiratory chain enzymes
↓ ← Infrared laser
Accelerated ATP synthesis
↓
Metabolism is shifted from anaerobic to aerobic
↓ ↓ ↓
Pain reduction   Reduction of   Increased wound
inflammatory process   healing

The observed clinical changes allow us to summarize that, alongside increased cell activity, other processes are induced through low-level lasers, for example, nerve dipolarization or hormonal changes. However, this is only justifiable speculation and must be researched in further studies. The mechanisms behind laser light transfer also need further clarification, because, although the transfer of laser energy to deeper-lying tissues has been described, only a portion of the emitted energy reaches these tissues. In skin, the energy of HeNe light decreases by 50 % per 2 mm. Infrared light decreases by 50 % per 4 mm. Therefore, energy loss is reciprocally proportional to tissue depth. An increased emission rate causes deeper penetration, because more photons are produced and this increases the chance of deeper layers being reached. However, the energy density cannot be increased unlimitedly, because very high values will cause an inhibition of biological activity instead of an increase of biological activity. These effects have been observed and confirmed by many researchers, including Mester, and are the basis for low-level laser therapy. Accordingly, a biostimulative effect occurs between 1 and 4 J/cm^2. Below 1 J/cm^2 no measurable increase of cellular and/or tissue activity is observed. Above 4 J/cm^2 a gradual overloading effect is observed which leads to an inhibition of cellular metabolism. For safe and dosage-controlled low-level laser application, it is imperative that the correct energy density is determined.

The energy density, and its dosage, is given by the following formula:

$$D = \frac{P \times t}{A}$$

The dosage D, is measured in J/cm^2, P is the applied energy of the laser system in W. If energy is pulsed, then P is given as an average of the energy output; t is the application time and A is the treated region in cm^2. The values of GaAs laser energy densities (in J/cm^2) at three different energy output levels and different application times are given in Table 1.

The values of GaAs laser energy densities at an energy output level of 60 mW and over an area of 100 cm^2 are given in Table 2. The decrease of energy density over a larger area is conspicuous and necessitates a longer application time for biostimulative energy density levels to be reached. Therefore, alongside the value for energy dosage, the application time is also important and must be taken into account for the desired therapeutic effect to be reached. The application time (t, s) is given by the equation $t = (DA/P) (1 + d)$.

For example, if we plan to treat a certain area, e. g. an ulcus or a myotendopathic region, we must compute the application time according to the emitted energy of the used laser system. In case a certain dosage tissue layers is desired, the multiplicator $(1 + d)$ must be taken into account (d is 0–4 cm). The values 1–4 for d are valid for laser systems with deeper penetration such as GaAs lasers and GaAlAs lasers. In practice, the actual peak energy value of pulsed lasers corresponds to approximately one third of the theoretrical value. If a diode has a theoretical peak value of 30 W, then one third, 10 W in this case, should be used for computing the energy density.

Alongside energy density and energy output, the wavelength and frequency of the emitted laser light is important for determining the efficacy of a laser. Furthermore, whether the energy is continuous or pulsed is also of consequence. It has already been mentioned that GaAs and GaAlAs lasers have a

Table 1. GaAs laser energy density (D, J/cm^2) as a function of energy output (P, mW) and time (t)

	Application time, t					
	1 s	3 s	10 s	1 min	3 min	10 min
$P = 20$ mW	0.02	0.06	0.2	1.2	3.6	12
$P = 30$ mW	0.03	0.09	0.3	1.8	5.4	18
$P = 60$ mW	0.18	0.18	0.6	3.6	10.8	36

Table 2. GaAs laser density at an energy output level of 60 mW over an area of 100 cm^2 as a function of application time

Application time	30 s	1 min	3 min	10 min	30 min
Energy density, J/cm^2	0.02	0.04	0.1	0.4	1.1

deeper penetration in treated tissues. This is due to the fact that these lasers are always pulsed. The extremely intensive flashes of the GaAs lasers have a higher intensity in deeper tissues. There is not much published on the effect and application of pulse frequency in pulsed lasers. There is even less literature available on the question of which frequency is suitable for which treatment. However, experience has shown that inflammation and infections are responsive to high frequencies, whereas pain, neuralgia, edema, and soft tissue swelling should be treated within a lower frequency range, as summarized below:

- Pain, neuralgia: 10–100 Hz
- Edema and soft-tissue swelling: 1000 Hz
- General biostimulation: up to 250 Hz
- Inflammation: 5000 Hz
- Infections: 10,000 Hz

This list correlates with the above described observation that higher energy densities have an inhibiting effect on tissue metabolism.

The reflection properties of the area to be treated and the angle of incidence are further factors that must be taken into account for low-level lasers to be applied effectively. The laser beam should be applied at the correct angle to the treated area. A smaller angle will cause loss of energy density. Furthermore, the treated area should be free of reflecting materials such as hair or cream.

The most important and principal factor for effective and dose-dependent low-level laser treatment is the energy density and the calculation thereof.

According to clinical observation, the effect of low-level lasers on cell metabolism can be defined as follows:

1. Biostimulation
2. Analgesia
3. Muscle relaxation
4. Anti-edemic effect
5. Immunologic effect
6. Antibiotic effect

These effects conform with the results of many studies and observations.

Clinical Application

The effects of low-level lasers can be utilized for a variety of clinical applications. The biostimulative effect of low-level lasers is used to treat bradytrophic tissues. The analgesic effect can be exploited for treatment of a variety of pain symptoms, for example, musculoskeletal pain, all types of neuralgia (especially of cerebral nerves), pain following herpes zoster infections, and stump pain following amputation.

The effect of muscle relaxation is utilized for treatment of musculoskeletal overloading syndromes and acute injuries. Disorders of the musculoskeletal system can benefit from the anti-edemic effect which is also observed during treatment of skin lesions, varicose swelling and lymph edemas. An immunologic and antibiotic effect occurs in the treatment of herpes simplex infection, and was also found in experimental in vitro trials in which the bacterial growth was reduced especially after IR laser irradiation (904 nm). This effect has been observed in treatment of skin ulcers and odontological infections which healed faster.

Low-Level Laser Therapy in Orthopedic Medicine

Spine

Low-level laser therapy is potentially effective for treatment of spinal disorders that can be treated with conservative measures, especially muscle relaxation, analgesia, and antiphlogistica. Spinal disorders are characterized foremost by statically and degenerative myofascial pain in all of the spine. Low-level laser therapy will increase muscle relaxation and reduce pain and therefore augment physiotherapeutic treatment, which corrects the statics and reduces muscular dysbalance. Through the biostimulatory effect on tissue, bradytrophy is reduced or disappears; thus, a state ideal for regaining muscular balance is attained where training of insufficient and/or atrophic muscle groups is possible.

Furthermore, low-level laser therapy influences deeper-lying muscular and cartilaginous irritations, for example, advanced degenerative spondylosis deformans, osteochondrosis, spondylarthrosis, morbus baastrup, etc. The laser can alleviate severe muscle tension and muscular dysfunction, so that physiotherapy and/or manual therapy can be effectively applied, if it is still deemed necessary.

Low-level lasers can be used to treat acute injuries, for example, spinal distorsion, and can even be considered a feasible conservative alternative for therapy of nucleus prolapses. In these cases, the therapeutic effect is based on muscle-pain reduction and an anti-edemic effect, which influences swelling in the affected area, even reaching the arachnoidea space. To attain such an effect in deeper-lying soft tissues, the laser must be applied in the affected spinal section in such a manner that no energy is absorbed by bony tissues. Keeping spinal anatomy in mind, the patient should be in a kyphotic position, to increase the space between spinal processi. Inflammation of the spine such as spondylitis, for example, spondylitis ankylosans (morbus bechterew), can also be treated by low-level lasers. In these cases, an increased dosage must be applied to procure an inhibiting effect that will influence these proliferating diseases.

Extremities

For therapy of larger joints such as the hip and the shoulder joint, the low-level laser is mainly used for soft-tissue treatment. The shoulder joint responds very well to laser treatment: myotendopathia of the shoulder associated with spinal pain syndrome, insertion tendopathia, impingement syndrome, pain syndrome during rotator cuff rupture, arthrosis, periarthritis, and shoulder stiffness. The same observations have been made for hip-joint treatment. Symptoms of painful myotendopathia and limited movement are reduced after application of low-level laser, which has a muscle-relaxing and analgesic effect. It is more difficult to understand the effect of low-level laser on intraarticular structures, especially joint cartilage. An effect on the inflammatory mediators may play a role.

In smaller joints, such as the elbow, wrist, knee, and ankle, the low-level laser is used especially to treat tendopathia such as insertion tendinosis (e.g., epicondylitis, patella apex syndrome) and active chondropathia and arthrosis. As an example of the therapeutic efficacy of low-level lasers, the treatment of active gonarthrosis will be described later in this chapter. Low-level laser treatment of traumatic soft-tissue disorders of the extremities, e.g., muscle-fiber ruptures and acute tendopathia, offers very effective and fast-acting therapy that is often superior to physiotherapy and medication. Finally, it should be discussed whether low-level laser treatment is feasible for outlet syndromes (e.g., tarsal- and carpal-tunnel syndrome). Despite physical and anatomical predispositions, the occurrence of these disorders is often acute. Low-level laser therapy could be effective through reduction of pain and perineural swelling and inflammation.

The biostimulative effect of low-level lasers on bradytrophic tissues for the therapy of spinal disorders has already been described above. Of course, this effect can generally be used for treatment of the whole musculoskeletal system.

One point of discussion is the optimal type of low-level laser for orthopedic medicine. There are several different types of lasers available: laser scanners, laser cannons, and laser systems with point treatment.

As the name already suggests, the laser scanner allows treatment of an area with a more or less dispersed laser beam. Planar parts of the spine, torso, and extremities are ideal for this type of treatment. For therapy of very curved surfaces, for example, shoulder or hip joint, the treated area should be narrowed down to an area that is reached by the laser at a vertical angle. The area beyond the scope of the vertical laser beams will receive a reduced dosage due to the more slanted angle. The energy dosage must be determined with great care because of the curved surfaces and differing frequencies.

The laser cannon is the second main type of laser and treats a defined area of approx imately 5 cm² at a constant rate. These lasers are, of course, also used for treating the spine, but are mostly used for therapy of arm and leg joints. As results indicate, the optimal treatment of the shoulder joint consists of consecutively ventral, lateral, and dorsal application during one treatment session. Medial and lateral application is recommended for the knee.

Both above-mentioned laser types are often equipped with certain application instruments for trigger point treatment of very small areas, for example, for tendopathia. In cases where points of maximal pain within a whole painful area can be detected, it is helpful to specifically treat these points alongside the overall treatment. Furthermore, several reports describe the sole use of selective trigger point application for treatment of joint and spine disorders with satisfactory results. However, it is possible that the combination of both widespread treatment and trigger point treatment, that is, acupuncture, will be therapeutically more effective.

Clinical Studies

In my hospital, the therapy regime for low-level laser application is based on 12 single sittings within a four-week period. Immediate relief is not always observed, although some patients, especially patients suffering from pain, experience relief during the first or second sitting. Quite often, a positive effect is experienced after the whole treatment regime has been concluded. Resistant cervical syndrome and activated gonarthrosis often show an improvement only 2 weeks or more after low-level laser therapy has been concluded. This delayed effect may be due to a certain time span being necessary for affected areas in deeper tissue layers to be reached.

Results

So far, we have conducted three studies.

The first of these is a retrospective study on 560 patients after three years of treatment. The patients are asked to evaluate the success of laser therapy and also asked whether they would be willing to repeat laser treatment. The evaluation of results show very good success rates, especially when it is realized that most of the patients were suffering from a therapy-resistant disorder in which neither medication nor intensive physical therapy was effective. The results are shown in Figs. 1 and 2. The success rate correlates very well with the patients' readiness to repeat laser therapy. The patients were evaluated by means of the following follow-up questionnaire:

When did you receive laser treatment:

_____

Reason: _____

1. **Have your symptoms improved since receiving laser treatment?**
   yes/no

2. **When did your symptoms improve?**
   a) during therapy
   b) 3 weeks after the last therapy session
   c) 6 weeks after the last therapy session
   d) later than 6 weeks after
   e) no improvement

3. **When did your symptoms recur?**
   a) Less than ½ year after therapy
   b) ½ year to 1 year after therapy
   c) over 1 year after therapy
   d) symptoms have not recurred

4. **Would you receive laser treatment again?**
   yes/no

The second study is a randomized study comparing ibuprofen to low-level laser treatment for the therapy of shoulder disorders. Each group contained 20 patients. Ibuprofen (3–600 mg) was administered over the same period as low-level laser therapy. The success rate for low-level laser therapy was 75 % compared to 50 % for the ibuprofen group. In this study, low-level laser treatment is superior to analgesic treatment.

The third study is a randomized double-blind study, comparing parallel patient groups with activated gonarthrosis. One group with 20 patients was treated with low-level laser. The other group, also with 20 patients, received a placebo treatment. The success rate for low-level laser was 80 % and concurs with the results of the two studies described above and also with other published results. There is already a notable improvement after 12 days of laser therapy. The patients' opinion and the physician's opinion of the therapeutic result after 3, 5, and 7 weeks were also documented, and it was found that further improvement occurs during the 3rd and 5th week. These results correlate with other studies that describe a late post-therapeutic effect through low-level laser therapy.

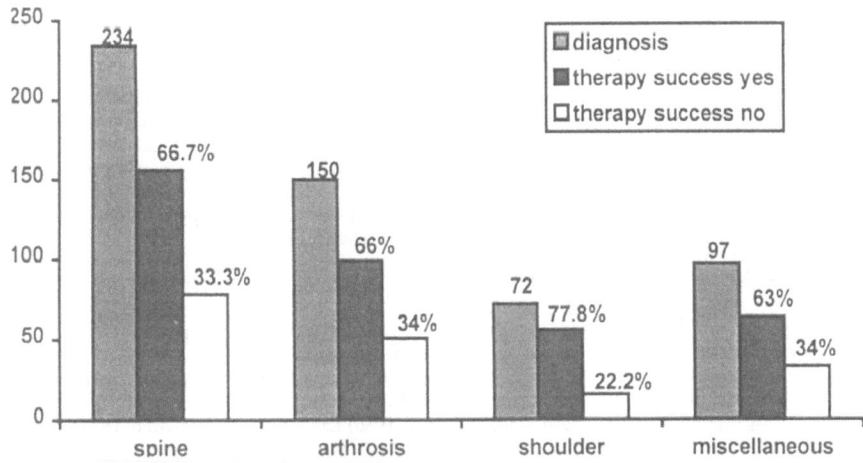

Fig. 1. Total number of patients diagnosed and therapy outcome

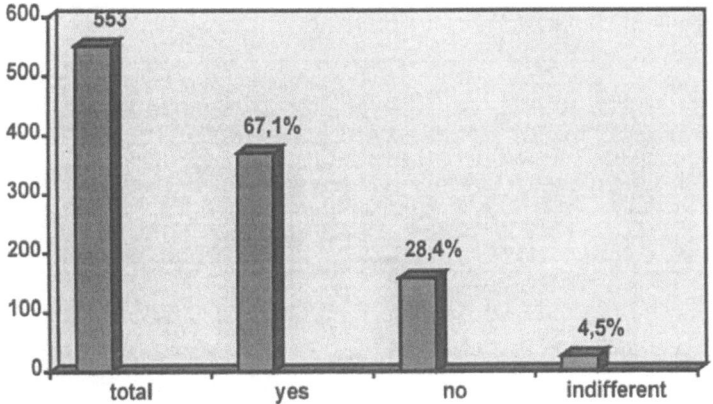

Fig. 2. The rate of patients' readiness to repeat laser treatment

Side Effects and Contraindications

Generally, direct laser light and also reflected laser light should not be pointed into or directed towards the eyes of the patient or the physician. All infrared-emitting, HeNe and class-3B collimated lasers can cause damage to the retina. Although this may be a potential risk, there have been no reports of retinal damage through low-level lasers. Nevertheless, protective goggles should be worn by the physician and the patient, especially during ventral applications near the head or in rooms with strongly reflecting objects and/or walls.

Potential skin burns can occur during treatment. On the other hand, the caloric effect is not notable under an energy density of 10 W cm². Energy densities of 100–150 W/cm² cause skin burns, for example; first-degree burns will occur if the laser is constantly focused on an area of 1 cm² with an energy density of 200 mW for 10 min. If low-level laser is used within the normal range of applications, such thermal damage is not possible.

Due to the biostimulative effect of low-level lasers, irradiation of the thyroid, ovaries, and testes should be avoided during laser treatment of orthopedic disorders. An increase in activity in these glands could occur. Due to the same biostimulative effect, irradiation of tumors and metastasis should also be avoided.

When children are treated, irradiation of the proliferative epiphysial disc should be strictly avoided.

References

[1] Bolton P (1991) Macrophage responsiveness to light therapy with varying power and energy densities. Las Ther 3:105–111

[2] Calderhaed G (1992) Meeting report: Proceedings of the 9th Congress of the International Society for Laser Surgery and Medicine, Anaheim, California, USA: 2–6 November 1991. Las Ther 4(1):43

[3] Dyson M (1991) Cellular and subcellular aspects of low-level laser therapy. In: Ohshiro T, Calderhead RG (eds) Progress in Laser Therapy. Wilew, Chichester, p 221

[4] Gärtner C (1989) Analgesy by low power laser (LPL): A controlled double blind study in ankylosing spondarthritis (SPA). Las Surg Med Suppl 1:30

[5] Götte S, Wirzbach E (1992) MID-Lasertherapie in der Orthopädie – Eine retrospektive Betrachtung der Therapieeffizienz. Jatros/Orthopädie/Traumatologie/Sportmedizin 7:5

[6] Götte S (1990) Lasertherapie – Reizwort mit magischer Wirkung. Jatros/Orthopädie/Traumatologie 5:8

[7] Götte S, Keyl W, Wirzbach E (1995) Doppelblindstudie zur Überprüfung der Wirksamkeit und Verträglichkeit einer niederenergetischen Lasertherapie bei Patienten mit aktivierter Gonarthrose. Quali Med 3:3

[8] Haimovici N et al (1988) Clinical use of antiinflammatory action of the laser in activated osteoarthritis of small peripheral joints. Laser. J Eur Med Laser Ass 1(2):4

[9] Karu T (1987) Photobiological fundamentals of low-power laser therapy. IEEE J Quantum Electronics 23(10):1703

[10] Karu T (1989) Photobiology of low-power laser effects. Health Physics 56(5):691–704

[11] Kubota J, Ohshiro T (1989) The effects of diode laser low reactive-level laser therapy (LOW LEVEL LASER) on flap survival in a rat model. Laser Ther 1(3):127

[12] Lievens P (1988) Effects of laser treatment on the lymphatic systems and wound healing. Laser. J Eur Med Laser Ass 1(2):12

[13] Lubart R, Wollman Y, Friedmann H, Rochkind S, Laulicht I (1992) Effects of visible and near-infrared lasers on cell cultures. J Photochem Photobiol B 12:305–310

[14] Mester E, Ludany G, Sellyei M, Szende B, Gyenes G, Tota GJ (1968) Studies on the inhibiting and activating effects of laser beams [in German]. Langenbecks Arch Chir 322:1022–1027

[15] Mester A, Mester A (1988) Scientific background of laser biostimulation. Laser. J Eur Med Laser Ass 1(1):23

[16] Mester E et al (1981) The biostimulating effect of laser beam. In: Proceedings of Laser-81, Opto-Elektronik, Munich, 1981

[17] Ohshiro T (1980) Treatment techniques to achieve superficial and intermediate LOW LEVEL LASER irradiation. Las Ther 3:153–155

[18] Rochkind S, Rousso M, Nissan M, Villarreal M, Barr Nea L, Rees DG (1989) Systemic effects of low-power laser irradiation on the peripheral and central nervous system, cutaneous wounds and burns. Las Surg Med 9:174

[19] Schindl L (1992) Effect of low-level laser irradiation on indolent ulcers caused by Bürger's disease. Las Ther 4(1):25

[20] Siebert W, Seichert B, Siebert B, Wirth CJ (1987) What is the efficacy of "soft" and "mild" lasers in therapy of tendinopathies? Arch Orthop Traum Surg 106:358–363

[21] Toya S et al. (1994) Report on a computer-randomized double blind clinical trial to determine the effectiveness of the GaAlAs (830 nm) diode laser for pain attenuation in selected pain. Las Ther 6:143

[22] Trelles M (1991) Infrared diode-laser in low reactive-level laser therapy (LOW LEVEL LASER) for knee osteoarthrosis. Las Ther 3(4):149

[23] Walker J (1983) Relief from chronic pain by low-power laser irradiation. Neurosc Lett 43:339

[24] Walker J et al (1987) Laser therapy for pain of rheumatoid arthritis. Clin J Pain 3(53):54

[25] Walker JB et al (1986) Laser therapy for pain of rheumatoid arthritis. Las Surg Med 6:171

V Spine

Preface

Laser techniques in spinal surgery evolved from key-hole methods of percutaneous manual discectomy as developed by Hijikata et al. (1975). Whilst Mainman developed the laser in 1960 upon the concepts by Albert Einstein in 1917, it was not until Ascher and Choy reported the application of laser energy to human disc tissue in 1987 that the era of lumbar laser-assisted spine surgery was born. With their concept of "laser disc decompression" with the Nd:YAG wavelength a wealth of efficacy studies followed. The technique was extrapolated to the cervical spine with success and found limited application in the thoracic spine. Subsequently, alternative wavelengths have been examined, including Ho:YAG, KTP 532 nm and 805 nm, but wavelengths with differing attributes such as those of CO_2 and erbium have been excluded because of the difficulty in conveying these wavelengths into the intradiscal space and spinal canal.

The development of improved rod lens systems and fibre-optic endoscopes together with side-firing laser probes has expanded the technical horizon and with it the evolution of laser-assisted endoscopic spinal surgery. This, in turn, has broadened, from an intradiscal appplication to an endoscopic exploration of the spinal canal and lumbar foramina combined with intradiscal procedures. Endoscopic surgery is being applied to cervical discs with removal of osteophytes and broad and narrow-based protrusions by the anterior approach.

Whilst these techniques hold the promise of improved outcome because of minimised tissue trauma, reduced destabilisation and loss of function, the major distinguishing feature is their use as an aware-state intervention. The feedback from the patient guides the surgeon to the source of the pain not only at the correct segmental level but directly to the causal and painful structure therein. This allows the surgeon to treat the pain source precisely and discretely, avoiding unnecessary tissue ablation and risk to adjacent tissues. All of this, conducted under the additional mantle of safety to neural structures, afforded by patient feedback, provides a promising pathway for future spinal surgery.

The absence of general anaesthetic allows these techniques to be conducted as day-case procedures, and makes possible their application to elderly and infirm patients, who would otherwise be condemned to continue with conservative measures and impaired lifestyle. The improved benefit/risk ratio of these techniques allows their wider use in patients outside the accepted inclusion criteria for conventional open procedures.

The emerging experience with such endoscopically guided techniques in the cervical, thoracic and lumbar spines heralds the employment of endoscopic surgery for the treatment of more advanced stages of disc degeneration and the promise of keyhole fusion, disc supplementation, vertebroplasty and endoscopic tumour surgery. At the same time these techniques are being increasingly supported with improved endoscopic instrumentation in the form of powered burrs, power osteotomes and electro-cautery and radio-frequency probes. Alternative radiation wavelengths are being explored, and although their use is still foiled by technical limitations at present, they, yet again, hold promise for the future. Their application will be linked to navigational planning and support and ultimately robotic assistance in the future.

This division was heavily oversubscribed and many contributions have had to be postponed with disappointment for all. I have selected papers to address surgical anatomy and the pathology of degeneration and laser effects on disc tissue. After the biomechanics of spinal function has been examined, the increasingly important area of economic outcome analysis of spinal surgery is addressed, to assist us in planning our future research to fulfill the needs of economic management in these days of fiscal constraint. Chapters follow on diagnosis, pain-source identification and patient selection. We then turn to prospective outcome studies of cervical and lumbar PLDD, endoscopic posterolateral and anterolateral lumbar surgery and finish with an analysis of complications related to the use of laser techniques.

In editing the manuscripts one cannot help but be impressed by the wealth of endeavour and innovation amongst all the authors who have submitted their research. Spinal surgery is still a young faculty of surgery and in many countries is not yet treated as a separate sphere. Whilst in its adolescence, it is being submitted to the inquisition of modern research concepts unlike other branches of surgery at similar stages in their evolution in the past. The Cochrane Collaboration has reported that spinal surgery has yet to prove itself to be better than conservative management or placebo effect. It is therefore paramount that spinal surgery as a whole and laser spinal surgery in particular incorporate the rigours of randomised controlled independent analysis using appropriate selection criteria and a meaningful battery of outcome measures. Efficacy studies often overestimate outcome by 20% and our own studies indicate a wide discrepancy between instruments such as the MacNab score and Oswestry disability index, both of which may be at variance with patient satisfaction scores and analogous pain scales. So the difficulties of setting up a randomised controlled clinical study are further compounded by the lack of ideal outcome instruments.

Reading the many submissions has highlighted the great dedication of the authors. It is hoped that the following publication will form a body of opinion and a platform from which we will launch truly idependently evaluated randomised controlled clinical trials (RCT) within the auspices of the International Musculoskeletal Laser Society. The congregation of expertise within the society should allow agreed RCTs to expand into becoming gold-standard multi-centred RCTs based upon targeted patient selection.

As the RCTs demonstrate the efficacy of laser-assisted techniques, it is hoped that they will then be used to assist the raft of patients currently denied conventional surgical treatment and who otherwise have to remain entirely reliant upon conservative measures and coping courses.

I hope that this section will promote a better understanding of the benefits of aware-state laser surgery and that it will assist aspiring spine surgeons to use these techniques. In the next edition we would expect to offer the evidence-based data required by governments and hospital managements worldwide to support the prescription of laser techniques on a wider basis.

Finally, I would like to thank Anukul Goswami, FRCS Orth., for his unstinting assistance during the extensive editing and revision of this section.

M. Knight

Anatomical Concepts in Applied Surgery of the Lumbar Spine: An Endoscopic View

A. Goswami · M. Knight

Introduction

The principal endeavour of the surgeon desiring to embark on minimally invasive spinal surgery is to avoid morbidity associated with open surgical techniques. There are two fundamental differences that make minimally invasive techniques unique. Firstly, they can be done in the aware state, allowing communication with the patient during surgery, thereby localising the source of pain. Secondly, when the portal of entry is postero-lateral, the intervertebral foramen and all foraminal, extraforaminal and discal pathology can be easily approached. Lateral recess stenosis and spinal pathology can be addressed to a lesser or greater extent depending on the accessibility of the site and the expertise of the surgeon. Therefore, for optimal use of the technique, good knowledge of the intevertebral foramen and its contents, and the pathological mechanisms that operate in the causation of back pain and radicular symptoms is required. This will greatly help when interpreting findings during endoscopic surgery. Needless to add, there is a steep learning curve. The purpose of this section is to highlight certain unique features of foraminal anatomy to facilitate that experience.

Foraminal Boundaries

The intervertebral foramen is tubular and must be visualised in three dimensions. From medial to lateral it has four zones: an osteum internum (lateral recess), the pedicle zone (mid zone), osteum externum (exit zone) and the far lateral zone [28]. Our experience indicates, more importantly, that it has three zones from its superior to inferior extent: the *superior notch*, from the superior pedicle to the apex of the ascending facet joint, the *inferior notch* from the inferior pedicle to the superior margin of the inferior vertebral body and, thirdly, the *subarticular zone* between the two notches, bounded mainly by disc and facet joint (Fig. 1). The shape and size of the intervertebral foramen is constantly changing with spinal movements and loading. An endoscopic surgeon who seeks to decompress the foramen and the lateral recesses must keep this in mind while performing the foraminoplasty. Success or failure to respond to the endoscopic procedures will depend on the effect dynamic activities have on the foraminal size and shape, and therefore on its contents.

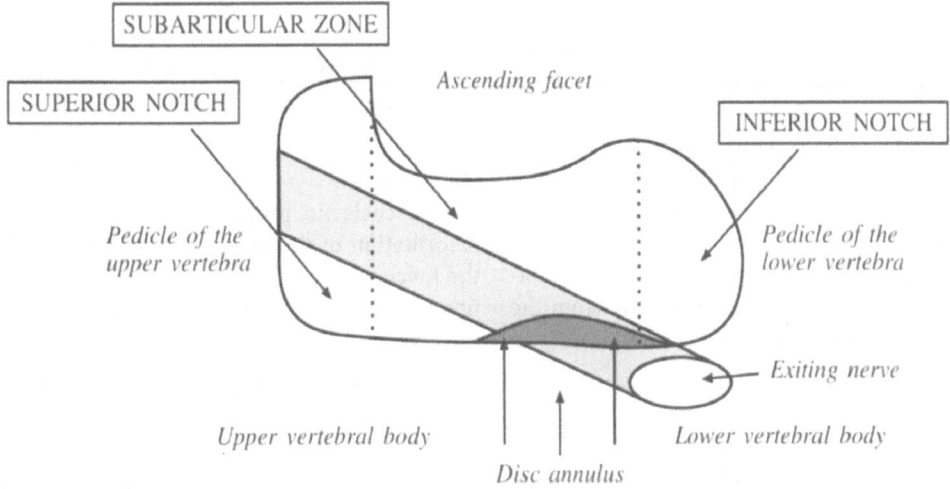

Fig. 1. Endoscopic zones of the intervertebral foramen

Bony Margins

The spinal foramen is the entry to the lateral aspect of the central spinal canal. It has an inverted pear-shaped appearance, broader in the cephalad direction and narrower caudally. It has a variable depth, the maximum being at L5–S1. Two adjacent vertebrae and the intervening disc participate in forming the boundaries. The specific components are the pedicles of the superior and inferior vertebrae, the posterior aspect of the adjacent vertebral bodies, ascending facet of the inferior vertebra and a portion of the descending facet of the superior vertebra.

The exiting nerve occupies between 7–33 % of the foraminal canal in an adult. The L5–S1 intervertebral foramen is the narrowest, and it has the thickest of the lumbar nerves. Thus, 33 % of the L5–S1 foramen is occupied by the nerve. At other levels, 7–22 % of the foramen is occupied by the nerve. In patients with severe degenerative spinal disease, the effective functioning of the neural structures depend on the interplay between the relative dimensions of nerve, the foramen and its contents. Thus, an alteration in the dimension of each component affects the ultimate dimension of the foramen. The morphological features of the pedicles, including height and width, facet morphology and orientation, vertebral body dimensions immediately below and above the pedicles, and the posterior height of the intervertebral disc need to be assessed radiologically.

Radiological assessment and CT findings can, however, easily overestimate the true dimensions of the foraminal canal, which undergoes alteration in shape and size dynamically with flexion and extension movements and with vertical compression [1]. We have found that weight-bearing analysis of spinal movements with the aid of dynamic x-rays during flexion and extension greatly assists interpretation.

We have found that the foramen is endoscopically divided into three zones (Fig. 1):

1. Superior notch: This is the space cephalad to an imaginary perpendicular line drawn from the junction of the proximal tip of the ascending facet to the posterior margin of the vertebral body of the superior vertebra.
2. Subarticular zone: This is between the superior and the inferior notch zones and is ventral to the facet joint.
3. Inferior notch: This is the space caudal to an imaginary vertical line projected posteriorly from the superior margin of the inferior vertebral body to the ascending articular process.

Articular Tropism

Facetal asymmetry include asymmetrical shape, size, surface area, inclination and abnormality of shape with degeneration. These, along with the asymmetry of the shape and size of pedicles, lamina and vertebral body, can significantly alter the shape of the neural canal [2]. Facetal tropism, whatever the origin (congenital, developmental, degenerative or pathological) can significantly alter the depth of the neural foraminal canal. The assessment of the facetal angle, the degree of its degeneration and olisthesis in the CT or MR scan prior to endoscopic procedure helps appropriate perception during surgery.

The foraminal depth of the interpedicular zone at L4–5 ranges from 8.2 to 10.2 mm while the corresponding figures of the L5–S1 foramen are 8.2 to 12.2 mm [26]. The average distance between the ligamentum flavum and the vertebral body is 7 mm. The radiographic measurements of the interpedicuar distance of L1–2 and L2–3 is 14–22 mm and of L3–4, L4–5 and L5–S1 is 12–20 mm.

Soft Tissues

The Intervertebral Disc

Desiccation and degeneration leads to progressive reduction in disc height. With the reduction of disc height, the "bulge" of the annulus increases, pushing the nerve dorsally; endoscopy reveals that this may be combined with superior and medial displacement. Adhesion of the nerve to the dorsal wall of the disc following inflammatory changes in the disc wall can restrict the mobility of the nerve.

The consequent vertical collapse of the functional spinal unit leads to a reduction in the foraminal dimensions, both anteriorly at the disc level and posteriorly at the facet joint. This is accompanied by proximal migration or overriding of the ascending facet of the inferior vertebral body. The normal height of the intervertebral foamen is 20–23 mm [3, 4, 5] with a cross-sectional area of 40–160 mm^2. With the reduction in the disc height, the foramen is further compromised by the lax posterior annulus of the disc. Discal prolapse or annular bulge at the lateral recess, foramen or in the far lateral zone compromise the foraminal dimension and may displace the exiting nerve toward the superior or inferior notch.

Spinal Ligaments

The viscoelastic properties of the ligaments allow deformation of the ligaments with loading. However, the mechanisms of failure of these ligaments depend upon the direction of loading and the intensity of the force vectors.

■ The Ligamentum Flavum.

The lateral extension of the ligamentum flavum forms the anterior capsule of the facet joint. The ligamentum flavum is seen in the superior notch extending in the cephalic direction, to be attached from the posterior inferior border of the superior pedicle and along the anterior margin of the descending facet. This attachment continues along the anterior medial aspect of the facet capsule and anterior aspect of the ascending facet along the medial border to the inferior pedicle. Endoscopically, the ligamentum flavum is thus seen to form the dorsal arch of the superior notch under which the nerve traverses. However, the distortion of this arch occurs with degenerative changes in the facet joint. Significant buckling of the ligamentum flavum occurs with reduction in disc height. This is often described as flaval hypertrophy. The infolding is seen to compress the nerve.

■ The Joint Capsule.

The ventral aspect of the facet joint capsule blends with the continuation of the ligamentum flavum. The capsular ligaments of the lumbar spine are thick and are the strongest of the spinal ligaments. However, with degenerative changes in the joint, the capsule develop tears and may allow sliding of the facet joints into the spinal canal [6].

A fibrofatty meniscus arising from the capsule has been described to occupy the deltoid space between the edges of the articular surfaces of the facet joints and the fibrous capsule [7]. Its role in the causation of spinal pain is unclear [30].

■ The Posterior Longitudinal Ligament.

The transverse fibres of the PLL (posterior longitudinal ligament) at the intervertebral region interdigitate with the fibres of the annulus fibrosus along the posterior surface of the intervertebral disc. The PLL is extensively innervated. Evidence of different types of nerve endings, which have been identified by immunohistochemical methods [8], has emerged. Parallel bundles of nerve fibres, which are arranged longitudinally, have been identified in the PLL. Studies in the rat have demonstrated that immunoreactive nerve fibres of similar nature supply the dura and the annulus in tandem with the PLL [9].

Contents of the Intervertebral Foramen

Intraspinal Neural Structures and their Attachments

Three groups of ligaments are known to contain neural structures linked to the PLL:

1. Midline Hofmann ligament which extends from the anterior dura to the PLL (Fig. 2)
2. Lateral Hofmann ligament which extends from the lateral aspect of the dura to the PLL (Fig. 2)
3. Lateral root ligament which arises from the dural extension around the nerve and the proximal root sleeve to the PLL and the periosteum of the pedicle (Fig. 3)

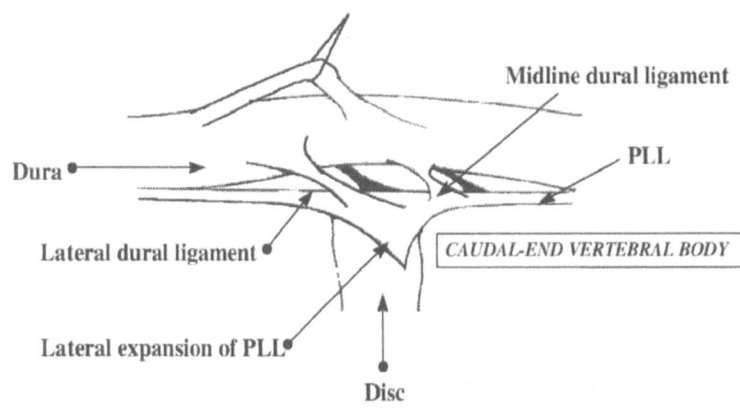

Fig. 2. Dural ligament complex of Hofmann. (Modified from Kirkaldy-Willis and Bernard Jr [15])

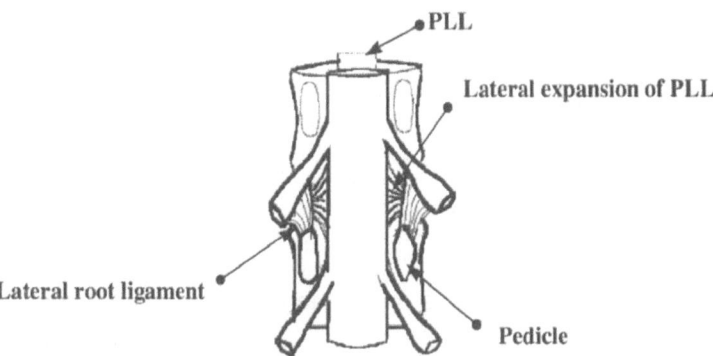

Fig. 3. The lateral root ligament. (Modified from Kirkaldy-Willis and Bernard Jr [15])

Transforaminal Ligaments and the Corporotransverse Ligaments

The transforaminal ligaments and the corporotransverse ligaments can reduce the supero-inferior foraminal dimensions by 31% [10]. The transforaminal ligament arises from the superior or the inferior articular processes or the articular joint capsule and is then ventrally inserted into one of three sites:

1. Above the disc: "superior type"
2. The posterolateral edge of the intervertebral disc: "intermedial type"
3. Distally: "inferior type"

The corporotransverse ligament is reported to arise from the posterolateral aspect of the disc and is attached to the transverse processes of the cranial or caudal vertebral, but is seldom recognised endoscopically.

Venous and Arterial Systems

The anterior intervertebral venous plexus (AIVVP) and the Batson's plexus form essential components of the anterior epidural space ventral to the PLL. The medial part of the AIVVP which receives the basivertebral veins is attached to the spinal canal through dense connective tissues, but is deficient over the dorsal aspect of the disc. The lateral component of the AIVVP lies longitudinally within the canal and is attached to adjacent structures by loose connective tissue.

The posterior internal vertebral venous plexus (PIVVP) occupies the epidural space between the ligamentum flavum and the laminae dorsally and the dura ventrally. These vessels are oriented longitudinally, traversing adjacent segments and have transverse anastomotic branches; these traverse anteriorly to the lateral longitudinal intervertebral venous plexus or reach out through the foramen into the external venous plexus [11].

The segmental artery which gains entry into the spinal canal through the spinal foramen supplies the anterior longitudinal arterial system on either side of the epidural space. The anterior arterial system which lies anterior to the PLL has longitudinal and transverse anastomotic components. Anterior and posterior radicular vessels are seen to follow the dorsal and ventral nerve roots within the foramina [12]. Branches from the anterior arterial system connect to the posterior longitudinal arterial systems, which supply the posterior intraspinal structures.

Microcirculation of the Intervertebral Nerves

A study reported by Corbin and further supported by Kobayashi [13] suggests that there are three types of artery supplying the spinal nerves:

1. Radiculomedullary arteries: These are the largest arteries, with an upward flow of blood, and supply very few branches to the nerve.
2. Radicular arteries: They run along nerve roots and receive communicating branches from the proximal (downward) and distal (upward) directions. A watershed area has been recognised in this arterial system where ramifying filaments of the nerve roots are bundled (Fig. 4).
3. T-shaped branches of the radicular artery: These are not affected by the direction of the blood flow in the radicular artery. Microangiograms have shown repeated T-branching in the system, which maintains intraradicular circulation even in the presence of nerve-root compression.

Kobayashi observes that the mechanism that can truly disturb the nerve root circulation is venous congestion from compression. The intraradicular oedema leads to the breakdown of the blood–nerve barrier, causing radicular pain and intermittent claudication.

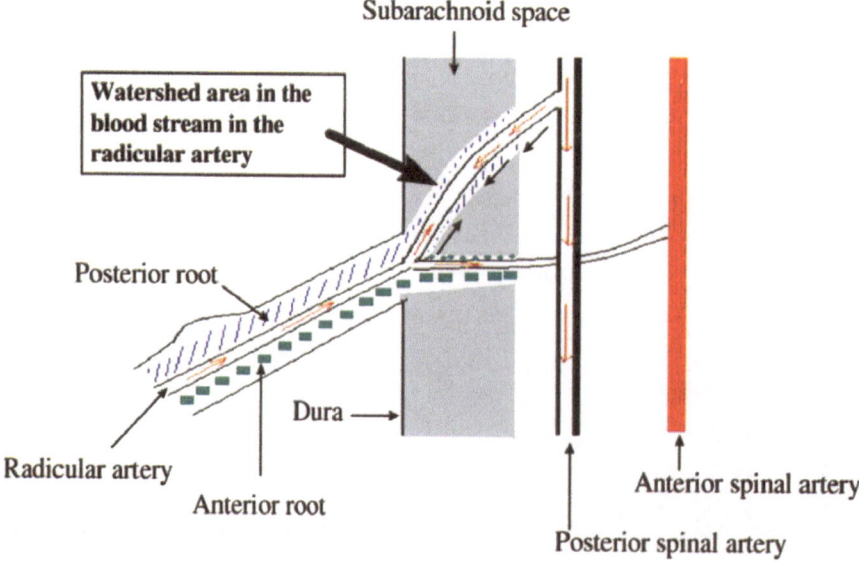

Fig. 4. The blood supply of the radicular artery and the watershed area. (Figure modified from Kobayashi et al. [13])

Neural Attachments

The nerve in the foramen has two mechanisms of attachment to the surrounding structures:
1. The lateral root ligament: This is the dural extension of the proximal root sleeve to the PLL and the periosteum of the inferior pedicle (Figs. 2–3).
2. Foraminal complex: These are multiple filaments or bands arising from the nerve sheath, and are attached centripetally within the bony boundary of the foramen in a spoke-like fashion [20]. Fibrous connections from the lateral aspect of the dorsal root ganglion are often seen as bands communicating with the joint capsule and to the circumference of the foramen [21].

Our endoscopic experience reveals that those bands noted to be filamentous in youth may be seen as thickened dense bands between the nerve and ascending facet joint in older patients with degenerative disc disease.

Nerve Distribution

Figures 5 and 6 show different views of the nerve supply to the lumbosacral spine. The sinuvertebral nerve arises from the primary ramus immediately distal to the bifurcation. These are usually two to four twigs of nerves, which obtain sympathetic fibres from the grey ramus communicans. These re-enter the spinal canal through the intervertebral foramen cephalad to the disc and ventral to the dorsal root ganglion. It gives out dorsal and ventral branches to supply the dorsal aspect of the dura, the ligamentum flavum and the periosteum. The ventral part of the sinuvertebral nerve has several branches that reach to adjacent levels. It supplies the periosteum, the PLL, the annulus of the disc, the ventral aspect of the dura and adjacent soft tissue.

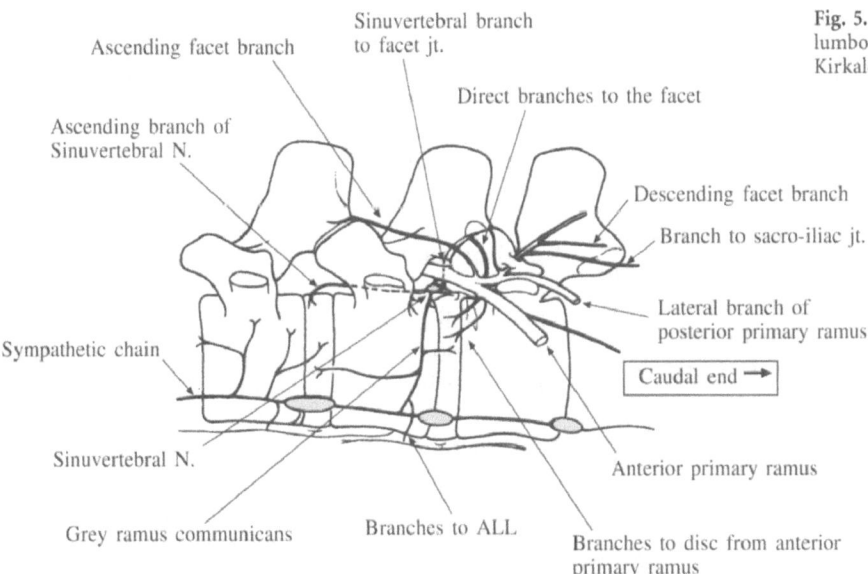

Fig. 5. Segmental nerve supply to the lumbo-sacral spine. (Modified from Kirkaldy-Willis and Bernard Jr [15])

Ascending facet branch

Sinuvertebral branch to facet jt.

Direct branches to the facet

Ascending branch of Sinuvertebral N.

Descending facet branch

Branch to sacro-iliac jt.

Lateral branch of posterior primary ramus

Caudal end →

Sympathetic chain

Sinuvertebral N.

Anterior primary ramus

Grey ramus communicans

Branches to ALL

Branches to disc from anterior primary ramus

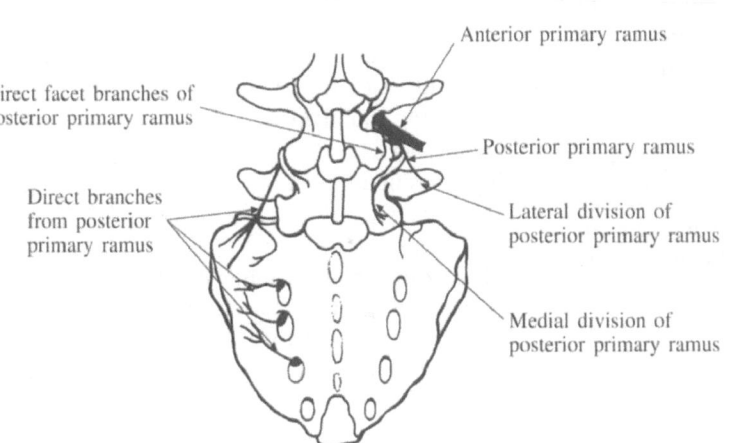

Fig. 6. Segmental nerve supply to the lumbo-sacral spine. (Modified from Kirkaldy-Willis and Bernard Jr [15])

Anterior primary ramus

Direct facet branches of posterior primary ramus

Posterior primary ramus

Direct branches from posterior primary ramus

Lateral division of posterior primary ramus

Medial division of posterior primary ramus

Autonomic Nervous System

The anterior and lateral aspects of the discs are well innervated by the sympathetic chain. That the sympathetic system innervates the outer intervertebral disc and the surrounding tissues has been proven histochemically [8]. Several mechanisms have been proposed to cause sympathetically induced back pain [22, 23]. Cunha et al. reduced cytokine-induced sympathetic pain by blocking interleukin-8 (IL-8) induced hyperalgesia after injecting propranolol locally [24].

Lumbar Dura

There is some evidence that the nerve-root sleeves and the lateral margins of the dura are innervated with fibres from the sympathetic system, which are recognised by the marker tyrosine hydroxylase (TH) [8]. These findings support the clinical study of El-Mehdi et al. that found the ventral dura and the nerve-root sleeve to be sources of pain [27].

Dorsal Root Ganglion

The dorsal root ganglion is implicated in the causation of back and leg pain symptoms in lumbar spinal pathology. It is usually located in the superior notch. Several pain-mediating neuropeptides, including substance P, are known to be produced and stored in the dorsal root ganglion. Mechanical stimulation or irritation of the ganglion can alter production and storage of the neuropeptides, causing pain and radicular symptoms. The L4 and L5 dorsal root ganglions are usually intraforaminal, while the first sacral dorsal root ganglion is intraspinal. The dorsal root ganglions of L1 to L3 also show considerable variation in their location but are usually intraspinal, but adjacent to the foramen in the lateral recess [25].

The root take-off angle (the angle that the nerve root subtends to the dura) usually remains constant at 40° from L1 to L5. However, this angle reduces to 22° at S1 and thereafter it continues to reduce to 4–5° at S4. The largest dorsal root ganglia are at L5 and S1 with an average width of 6 mm and length of 11 mm. There is progressive reduction in size of the dorsal root ganglion above and below L5 and S1 root levels.

The findings mentioned are confirmed endoscopically, but the ganglion may migrate distally and laterally in the presence of settlement and may be adherent to the superior foraminal ligament with aggravated irritation.

Spinal Contents

Several membranes have been identified in the epidural space. An epidural membrane has been reported to appear continuous with the PLL. A peridural membrane as a two-layered membrane has also been reported to line the spinal canal and to be attached to the deep layer of the PLL [26].

Internal Vertebral Nerve Supply

The recurrent meningeal nerve (sinuvertebral n.) supplies the structure of the spinal nerve (Fig. 5). The nerve consists of several filaments which arise from the anterior primary ramus and receive communicating branches from the sympathetic ganglion or the grey rami communicans. These communicating filaments along with the meningeal nerve return into the foramen, and ventral twigs lie immediately ventral to the dorsal root ganglion and supply the posterior longitudinal ligament, dura, periosteum and the outer wall of the annulus. The root sleeves are similarly supplied by the ventral branch. There is abundant anastomosis between nerves from one level to the other and from side to side. A few twigs from the meningeal nerve traverse immediately dorsal to the dorsal root ganglion and supply the ligamentum flavum, dorsal dura and the periosteum.

Sacroiliac Joints

The sacroiliac joints receive their nerve supply from the posterior primary ramus of L4, L5 and S1 with some contribution from S2 and S3.

Pathological Anatomy

Pathological bony changes: Degenerative and isthmic spondylolisthesis may significantly compromise the foraminal dimensions, allowing anterior translation of the cephalad vertebral body, causing compression of the exiting nerve. Bony outgrowths may occur as a result of several conditions affecting the spine [14]:
- Diffuse idiopathic skeletal hyperostosis (DISH)
- Paget's disease of the bone
- Ankylosing spondylosis
- Acromegaly
- Hyperparathyroidism
- Fluorosis
- Ocronosis
- X-linked hypophosphatemic osteomalacia

Foraminal and lateral recess stenosis may result from foraminal narrowing, which may be caused by [14]:
- Discal herniation (may be due to Paget's disease of vertebral body)

- Diffuse idiopathic skeletal hyperostosis (DISH): osteophytes involving the vertebral body or the articular processes
- Synovial cysts or tumours
- Spondylolisthesis

Subarticular of lateral recess stenosis, both of which produce bony hypertrophy around the facet joint, may be caused by [14]:

- DISH
- Paget's disease

Osteophytes

These may appear from any bony margins of the spinal foramen and the spinal canal. Endoscopically, the principal sites of clinically significant osteophytosis arise from the facet joints and the vertebral body margin dorsally, and the posterolateral corners of the vertebral bodies. The osteophytes arising from the posterolateral corners of the vertebral body along with displacements of the vertebrae (olisthesis or retrolisthesis) can significantly alter the shape and dimensions of the foramen (Fig. 7). The displacement, compression and especially the tethering of the exiting nerve appears endoscopically to generate irritation, inflammation and pain.

Dorsally, the vertebral end plate osteophytes may coalesce into a dorsal transverse bar (see Fig. 12). Very large osteophytes at these sites have been termed Heithoff–Dupuis spur (Fig. 7). In the endoscopic view of the foramen, however, a discrete osteophyte in the posterolateral corner of the superior vertebral body in line of the nerve and the ascending facet joint is seen. From its position, this prevalent bony projection has been termed the "shoulder osteophyte" (Figs. 8–9).

The shoulder osteophyte in the posterolateral corner of the vertebral body may displace the nerve either laterally or medially. When displaced laterally, the nerve exits from the superior notch. Conversely, when displaced medially, the nerve exits from the inferior notch. Of clinical significance is that the

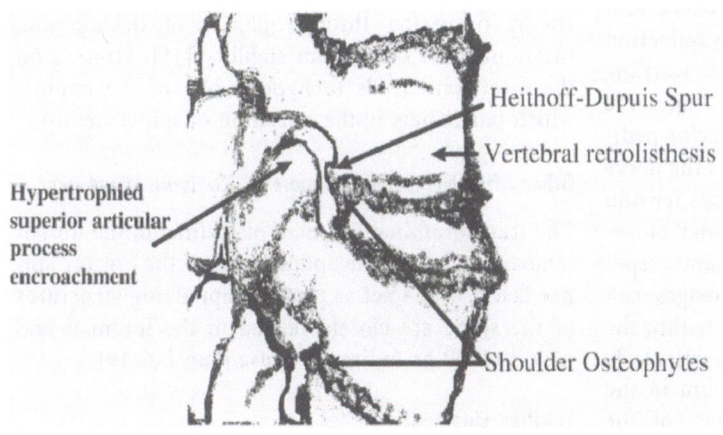

Hypertrophied superior articular process encroachment

Heithoff-Dupuis Spur

Vertebral retrolisthesis

Shoulder Osteophytes

Fig. 7. Hypertrophied facet joint, loss of disc height and associated retrolisthesis is shown here to significantly alter the foraminal dimensions. A large osteophyte from the lower end plate of the vertebral body (Heithoff-Dupuis spur) can cause foraminal and lateral recess stenosis affecting the exiting and the transiting nerve. Endoscopically, however, more commonly visualised osteophytes are small to fairly large, discrete and sharp osteophytes arising from the vertebral end plate, causing significant irritation and inflammation of the exiting nerve. These are the shoulder osteophytes. When fairly large, these osteophytes displace the nerve either medially or laterally

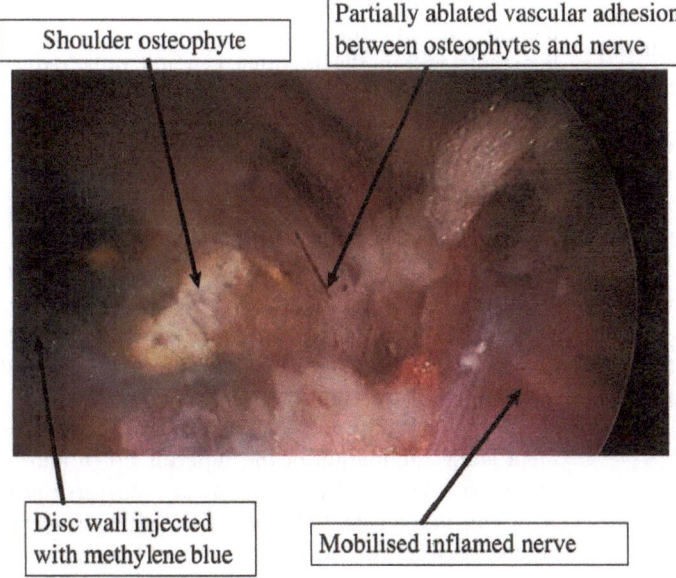

Shoulder osteophyte

Partially ablated vascular adhesions between osteophytes and nerve

Disc wall injected with methylene blue

Mobilised inflamed nerve

Fig. 8. An endoscopic view of the left L4–5 foraminal "floor" in a prone patient as seen through the posterolateral approach. The head end of the patient is towards the bottom of the picture and the left side of the picture is towards the midline. The disc injected with methylene blue after discography is identified by its blue colour. The osteophyte is seen projecting lateral to the disc. The exiting nerve has been mobilised laterally (right side of the picture) to visualise the osteophyte. The nerve is seen grossly inflamed and tender and has been mobilised with the guard tube (cannula). Grossly tender, hypervascular tissue is seen binding the nerve to the osteophyte, which is seen partially ablated with laser. In patients with narrow foramen these "shoulder osteophytes" cause significant irritation of the exiting nerve

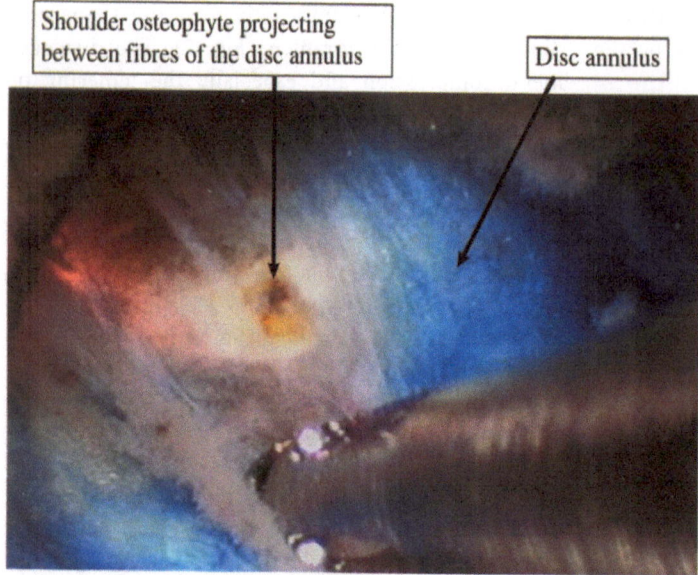

Shoulder osteophyte projecting between fibres of the disc annulus

Disc annulus

Fig. 9. An endoscopic view of the right L5–S1 foraminal "floor". Left side of the picture is towards the lateral aspect of the vertebral body. A large shoulder osteophyte is seen arising from the end plate splitting the fibres of the disc annulus. The nerve has been mobilised laterally (to the left of the picture) and is protected by the guard tube during lasing

nerve is often found adherent to the osteophyte. With adhesion or where the osteophyte is found in the angle between the dura and the exiting nerve root at the apex of the safe working zones, gross reduction in the neural mobility is observed. The safe working zone is the triangular space between the exiting nerve root, the transiting nerve root and the inferior pedicle. The reduction in neural mobility makes the nerve vulnerable to deformation or irritation from tension or compression at different stages of spinal movement. Osteophytes arising from the facet joints, especially those with significant arthritic changes can incite local irritation of the exiting nerve within the foramen and the lateral recess. These are particularly noticeable hidden in the ligamentum flavum in the superior notch or in relation to the apex of the ascending facet.

If the degenerative changes of the facet are extensive, with osteophytes and facet hypertrophy encroaching into the foramen dorsally, then, in conjunction with the vertebral body osteophytes and displacements from the ventral aspect, the pear-shaped foramen becomes constricted in the middle (Fig. 7). This almost splits the foramen into an oval opening at the cephalad end and a narrow oblong opening in the caudad end. The resultant effect on the exiting nerve root is its displacement either supero-laterally and towards the cephalad end (superior subpedicular region) or infero-medially towards the narrower caudad region of the foramen. The medical displacement of the nerve may compromise non-endoscopic laser disc decompression as the nerve may block the access to the approach to the disc.

Facet and Laminar Hypertrophy

Kirkaldy–Willis described the progressive facet hypertrophy occurring through phases of dysfunction, instability and subsequent stability [15]. Stresses on the facet joint leads to hypertrophy of the lamina, which participate in the causation of spinal stenosis.

Other Often-Neglected or Ignored Soft-Tissue Structures

The transforaminal ligament of Hofmann, the dorsolumbar fascia and the aponeurosis of the erector spinae fascia which act as passive supporting structures of the spine are closely related to the foramen and may directly or indirectly cause pain [16–19].

Calcified Ligaments

The transforaminal ligaments, corporotransverse ligaments, Hofmann ligaments, the PLL and the ligamentum flavum may show calcification. Calcified ligaments within the foramen can not only reduce the dimensions of the foramen, but can also compress the nerve during spinal movements.

The "Superior Foraminal Ligament"

The effect of the impact of a ligament in the superolateral aspect of the foramen has been observed to compromise neural function (M. T. N. Knight, unpublished data). This ligament, termed the "superior foraminal ligament" (Fig. 10), arises from the lateral aspect of the descending facet and the apex of the ascending facet and continues anteriorly to its attachment along the margin of the superior notch and to the inferior aspect of the base of the transverse process. This is a substantial structure, readily visualised endoscopically. The superior foraminal ligament may

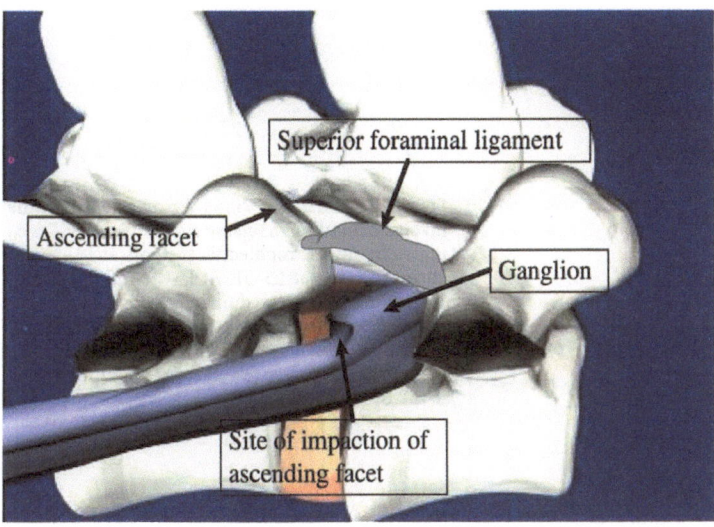

Fig. 10. The location of the superior foraminal ligament

be observed to be partially or completely calcified, and division of this ligament leads to considerable decompression and widening of the foramen. The nerve may be seen endoscopically to be discretely hyperaemic and adherent at the region and margin of the superior foraminal ligament.

The anatomic variables are classified as follows [28]:
1. Ligaments:
   a. Ligamentum flavum: hypertrophy, calcification, ossification
   b. PLL calcification
2. Disc:
   a. Bulging annulus
   b. Severe loss of disc height
   c. Protrusion
3. Facet joint: synovitis with synovial hypertrophy and effusion
4. Bone:
   a. Articular process: osteophyte formation, uncommon shape or orientation
   b. Vertebral body: osteophyte formation posteriorly or laterally
   c. Lamina: hypertrophy, spondylolysis with granulation tissue

Vertebral Displacement

Anterior olisthesis and retrolisthesis: The importance of lateral views of the lumbosacral spine in flexion and extension, obtained as weight-bearing x-rays of the sitting and standing patient can give an advance warning of the vertebral displacement which occurs during motion of intervetebral segments. These abnormal movements have a direct effect on the reduction of the foraminal dimensions, leading to compression of the neural structures and the dorsal root ganglion at the lateral recess and the foramen.

Sudden mechanical irritation of these structures may present as "mechanical instability" with the "catch", or present as symptoms of dynamic stenosis.

Neural Anomalies

Anomalous nerve origins, most of which present as conjoined nerves, are found in 14% of patients. The nerves may arise high or low. Complex combinations, anastomosis or a double set of nerves may occupy more space than normal, and cause symptoms arising from entrapment [26].

Claudication

Claudicant symptoms of spinal stenosis cannot be purely from bony compression. Several soft tissue structures within and adjacent to the foramen can encroach into the spinal canal and cause compression of the nerve. This compression on the nerve may be severe and sufficient to prevent appropriate conduction of neural signals. Symptoms may arise from relative minor compression, by reduction of the vascular supply of the nerve from compression of the arterial or venous microvasculature of the nerve. Extensive scarring can similarly affect the microvasculature, causing persistent neurological symptoms [13]. The altered microcirculation in conjunction with the physiologic changes from tissue hypoxaemia can alter neural transmission in the presence of abnormal micromovements aggravated by malposture.

Neural function can be markedly altered when the nerve is partially under compression at two levels (Figs. 11–13). This affects the site of compression as well as the intermediate segment [29]. It may be further accentuated by "instability" in the segment. These findings have been supported by the studies of Olmarker and Rydevik [30] and Takahashi et al [29].

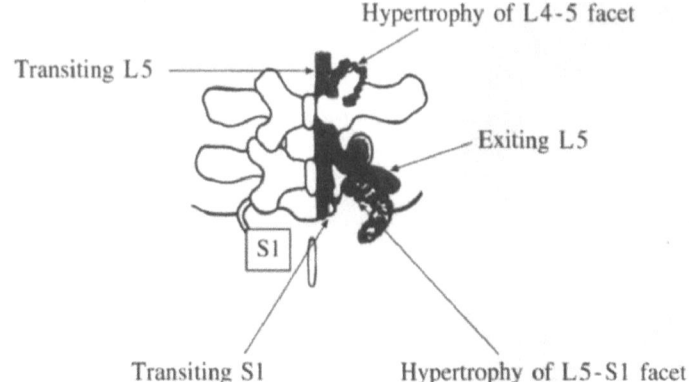

Transiting L5

Hypertrophy of L4-5 facet

Exiting L5

S1

Transiting S1

Hypertrophy of L5-S1 facet

Fig. 11. This diagram shows the mechanism of the involvement of the L5 nerve root at two levels, i. e., under the hypertrophied facet joints at L4–5, and at the foramen at L5–S1. At L5–S1 the transiting S1 nerve is compressed under the hypertrophied L5–S1 facet joint. Thus, a single nerve may be involved at two sites, or a single site may cause symptoms involving two nerves. (Modified from Kirkaldy-Willis and Bernard Jr. [15])

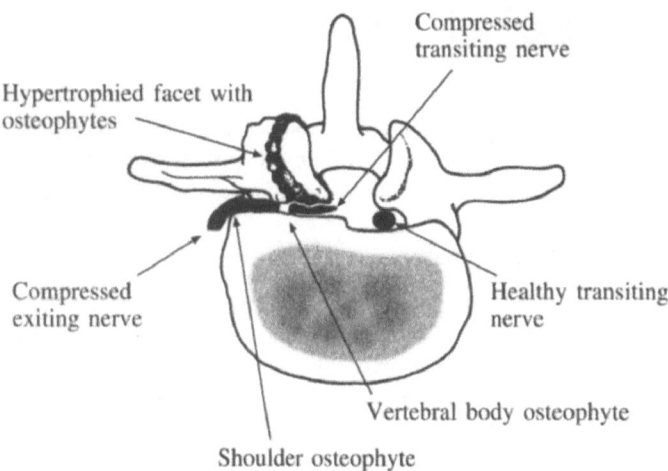

Hypertrophied facet with osteophytes

Compressed transiting nerve

Compressed exiting nerve

Healthy transiting nerve

Vertebral body osteophyte

Shoulder osteophyte

Fig. 12. Facet hypertrophy and osteophytes arising from the vertebral end plate and facet is shown narrowing the foramen and causing lateral recess and foraminal stenosis. (Modified from Kirkaldy-Willis and Bernard Jr. [15])

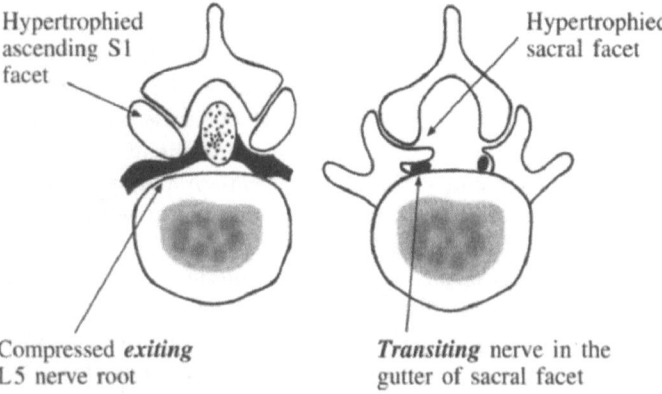

Hypertrophied ascending S1 facet

Hypertrophied sacral facet

Compressed *exiting* L5 nerve root

Transiting nerve in the gutter of sacral facet

Fig. 13. Facet joint hypertrophy affecting the exiting and the transiting nerve at one level. (Modified from Kirkaldy-Willis and Bernard Jr. [15])

Summary and Conclusions

The outcome of the minimalist endoscopic intervention depends largely on a careful analysis of all the factors that may be implicated in the causation of pain, and focuses one's attention on those factors that are newly accessible by endoscopy. The available literature broadly classifies the causation of pain and sciatica into three interrelated groups (Fig. 14). These are:
1. Mechanical and physical factors

2. Tissue changes: neovascularisation, neoneuralisation
3. Biochemical factors: cytokines, pain mediators, alteration in pH, ionic changes, etc.

In the performance of the endoscopic or minimally invasive spinal procedures, the surgeon needs to consider the effect of alteration of the effect of alteration of the foraminal anatomy on its contents. This alteration is seen with the rotation of vertebrae, scoliosis, previous trauma, previous surgery, inter-transverse

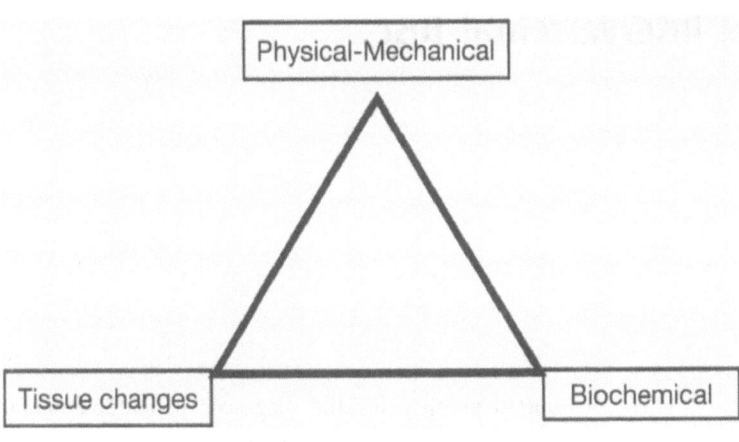

Fig. 14. The three interrelated groups of causes of pain and sciatica

grafting, incorrectly placed pedicular screw, instability arising from degeneration or decompression surgery, spondylolisthesis, and anatomical variations arising from the displacement of tissues secondary to settlement or olisthesis. Their effect upon tissues in and around the foramen cannot be overemphasised.

References

[1] Schönström N, Lindahl S, Willën J, Hansson T (1987) Dynamic changes in the dimensions in the lumbar spinal canal: an experimental study in vitro. J Orthopaed Res 7:115–121
[2] Panjabi M, Goel V, Oxland T, Takata K, Duranceau J, Krag M, Price M (1992) Human lumbar vertebrae, quantitative three-dimensional anatomy. Spine 17:299–306
[3] Hasegawa T, Mekawa Y, Watnabe R, An H (1996) Morphometric analysis of lumbosacral nerve roots and dorsal nerve root ganglia by magnetic resonance imaging. Spine 21:1005–1009
[4] Hasegawa T, An H, Haughton V, Nowicki B (1995) Lumbar foraminal stenosis: critical heights of the intervertebral discs and the foramen. J Bone Joint Surg [Am] 77:32–38
[5] Stephens M, Evens J, O'Brien J (1991) Lumbar intervertebral foramens: An in vitro study of their shape in relation to intervertebral disc pathology. Spine 16:525–529
[6] Andersson GBJ (1999) Biomechanics of lumbar spine. In: Kirkaldy-Willis WH, Bernard TA Jr (eds) Management of low back pain, 4th edn. Churchill Livingstone, Philadelphia, Pennylvania
[7] Bogduk N, Engel R (1984) The menisci of the lumbar zygoepiphyseal joint: A review of their anatomy and clinical significance. Spine 9:454
[8] Kallakuri S, Cacanaugh JM, Blagoev DC (1998) An immunohistochemical study of human lumbar spinal dura and longitudinal ligament. Spine 23(4):403
[9] Imai S, Konttinen YT, Tokunaga Y, Maeda T, Hukud S, Santavarta S (1997) An ultrastructural study of calcitonin generelated peptide immunoreactive fibres innervating the rat posterior longitudinal ligament. Spine 22(17):1941
[10] Bakkum BW, Mestand M (1994) The effects of trans-foraminal ligaments on the sizes of T11 to L5 human intervertebral foramina. J Manipulative Physiol Ther 17:517–522
[11] Roy PV, Barbiax E, Clarijs JP (1999) Anatomy of the lumbar canal, foramen and ligaments, with references to recent insights. In: Gunzburg R, Szpalski M (eds) Lumbar spinal stenosis. Lippincott Williams and Wilkins, Philadelphia, PA
[12] Dupuis PR (1999) Anatomy of the lumbosacral spine. In: Kirkaldy-Willis WH, Thomas A, Bernard TA Jr (eds) Management of low back pain, 4th ed. Churchill Livingstone, Philadelphia, PA
[13] Kobayashi S, Yoshizawa H, Nakai S (2000) Experimental study on the dynamics of the lumbosacral nerve root circulation. Spine: 25(3):298–305
[14] Devogelaer J, Maldague B (1999) Lumbar spinal stenosis in metabolic bone disease. In: Gunzburg R, Szpalski M (eds) Lumbar spinal stenosis. Lippincott Williams and Wilkins, Philadelphia, PA
[15] Kirkaldy-Willis WH (1999) Pathology and pathogenesis of low back pain. In: Kirkaldy-Willis WH, Bernard TA (eds) 4th edn. Churchill Livingstone, Philadelphia, PA
[16] Golub BS, Silverman B (1969) Transforaminal ligament of the lumbar spine. J Bone Joint Surg 51A:947–956
[17] Bogduk N, Macintosh JE (1984) The applied anatomy of the thoracolumbar fascia. Spine 9:164–170
[18] Bogduk NA (1980) A reappraisal of the anatomy of the human lumbar erector spinae. J Anat 131:525–540
[19] Tencer AF, Allen BL Jr, Ferguson RL (1985) A biomechanical study of the thoracolumbar spine fractures with bone in the canal: Part III. Mechanical properties of the dura and its tethering ligament. Spine 10:741–747
[20] Sunderland S (1974) Meningeal–neural relations in the intervertebral foramen. J Neurosurg 40:756
[21] Spencer DL, Irwin GL, Miller JAA (1983) Anatomy and significance of fixation of lumbosacral nerve roots in sciatica. Spine 8:672
[22] Roberts WJ (1986) A hypothesis on the physiological basis for causalgia and related pains. Pain 24:297
[23] Gillette RG, Kramis RC, Roberts WJ (1994) Sympathetic activation of cat spinal neurons responsive to noxious stimulation of deep tissues in low back. Pain 56:31
[24] Cunha FQ, Lorenzetti BB, Poole S, Ferreira SH (1991) Interleukin-8 as a mediator of sympathetic pain. Br J Pharmacol 104:765
[25] Jenis LG, An HS (2000) Spine update: Lumbar foraminal stenosis. Spine 25(3):389–394
[26] Roy PV, Barbiax E, Clarijs JP (1999) Anatomy of the lumbar canal, foramen and ligaments, with references to recent insights. In: Robert Gunzburg R, Supalski M (eds) Lumbar spinal stenosis. Lippincott Williams and Wilkins, Philadelphia, PA
[27] El-Mehdi MA, Latif FYA, Kanko M (1981) The spinal nerve root innervation, a new concept of clinicopathological innervations in back pain and sciatica. Neurochirurgia 24(4):137
[28] Akkerveeken PF (1994) A taxonomy of lumbar stenosis with emphasis on clinical applicability. Eur Spine J 3:130–136
[29] Takahashi K, Olmarker H, Holm S, Porter RW, Rydevik B (1993) Double level cauda equina compression: an experimental study with continuous monitoring of internal blood flow in porcine cauda equina. J Orthop Res 11:104–109
[30] Eisenstein SM, Parry CR (1987) The lumbar facet arthrosis syndrome–clinical presentation and articular surface changes. J Bone Joint Surg 69B:3–7
[31] Cohen MS, Wall EJ, Brown RB, Rydevik B, Grafin SK (1990) Cauda equina anatomy. Part II: Extrathecal nerve roots and dorsal ganglia. Spine 15:1248–1251

The Pathobiology of the Intervertebral Disc

A. J. FREEMONT

Introduction

The normal intervertebral disc consists of an outer fibrous tissue component known as the annulus fibrosus and an internal cartilaginous component called the nucleus pulposus. The annulus fibrosus is attached to the rims of the adjacent vertebrae at entheses and the nucleus pulposus is separated from the underlying vertebral bone by a thin zone of cartilage known as the cartilaginous end plate, which consists of hyaline cartilage in many respects similar to the articular cartilage of synovial joints. The intervertebral disc is, with the exception of the outer third of the annulus fibrosis, both avascular and aneural.

It has long been recognised that, with age and following trauma, there are profound changes to the intervertebral disc [1, 2, 3, 4, 5] and some have been associated with back pain. There is, however, an increasing body of evidence showing that many of these changes are seen in asymptomatic individuals [6]. There have been no large systematic studies comparing the discal pathology of patients with and without back pain.

In this chapter, I will describe novel data from this laboratory which have given new insights into the understanding of spinal disease and back pain. We have performed four studies, two in cadavers and two from operative specimens, that shed more light on the aetiopathogenesis of these disorders.

Cadaveric Studies

Cadaveric Study 1

The first of these was a cadaveric study performed on 50 individuals. Twenty of these were symptomatic with longstanding low-back pain of more than 3 years duration. This was well documented, but in every case had been managed conservatively, the only invasive procedure being myelography which had been performed in 14 cases. All 20 had died of conditions unrelated to the back pain. The other 30 individuals were a sequential group of patients com-

ing to autopsy for the diagnosis of sudden death. Most had died of myocardial infarction, pulmonary embolism or acute intracranial haemorrhage. Criteria for inclusion in the "control" group of the study were that the patient should have had no history of venous hypertension, endocrine disease, spinal instrumentation or any documented history of back pain sufficient to have necessitated seeing their general medical practitioner or a hospital specialist.

The lumbosacral spine was removed in every case and fixed in neutral buffered formalin. After fixation, it was cut longitudinally, and tissue blocks incorporating the intervertebral root canal (IVRC) and the hemisected spinal canal were taken from alternate sides from L1/L2 to L5/S1. The blocks were decalcified and serially sectioned. Histological analyses were performed and the area of the intervertebral root canal occupied by the nerve complex and veins was calculated histomorphometrically. The proportion of the nerve root occupied by fibrous tissue and by neural tissue was also calculated.

Subjectively, there was little difference between the changes seen in symptomatic patients or controls. Discal bulging, or frank sequestration, was seen in a high proportion of the specimens examined (41% of levels in the control group and 59% in the symptomatic group). The protruding disc impinged on vascular structures and fat within the intervertebral root canals and spinal canal, but only in the most severe sequestrations, usually associated with massive osteophyte formation, was direct nerve-root compression seen. Vascular compression and oedema in the lower part of the intervertebral root canal was always associated with prominent dilatation of the vessels of the venous plexus proximally in the intervertebral root canal (Fig. 1).

A common finding was the presence of fibrin deposition within the dilated vascular channels of the intervertebral root canal. In places, this amounted to occlusive thrombus formation showing organisation, absolute evidence for the thrombus having formed prior to death (Fig. 2). Fibrosis was present around and within nerve roots and spinal nerves.

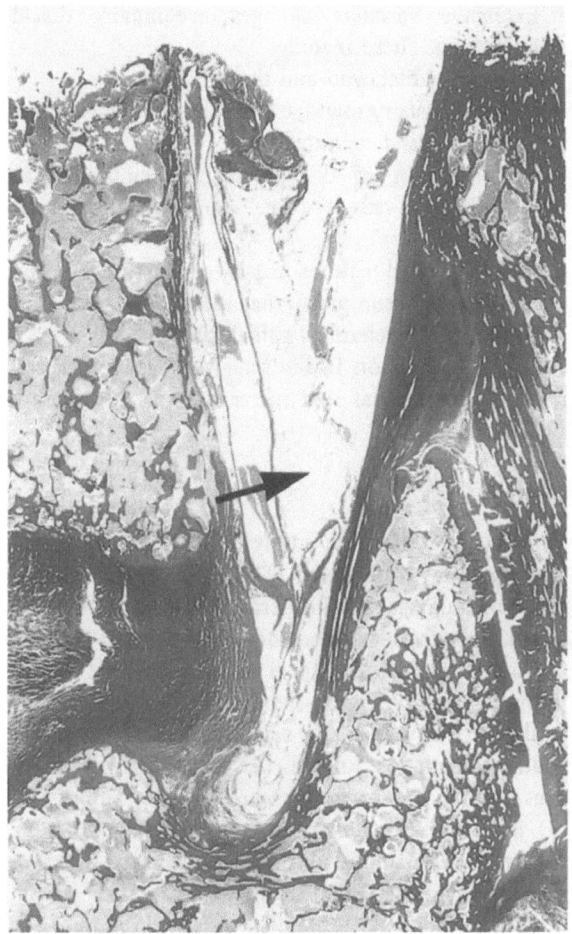

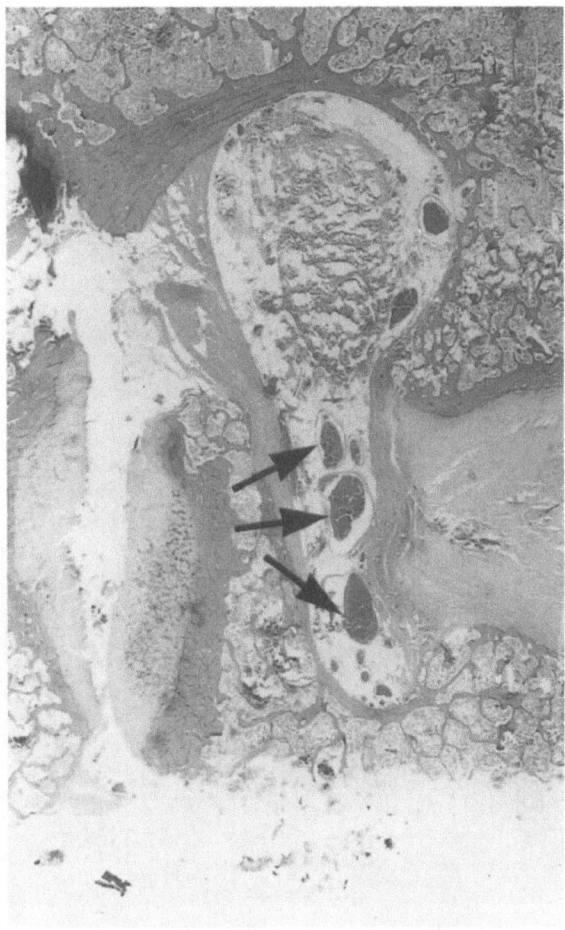

Fig. 1. A bulging disc is compressing the vascular channels at the inferior pole of the IVRC. The more caudal vessels are dilated (*arrowed*) (H & E, × 4)

Fig. 2. The dilated vessels of the IVRC contain thrombus (*arrowed*) (H & E, ×4)

The area of the intervertebral root canal occupied by veins was directly related to the proportion of the adjacent nerve-root complex occupied by perineural and intraneural fibrous tissue (Fig. 3).

Further changes were seen in the soft tissues around the nerve. Frequently, the fat cells that occupy the majority of the intervertebral root canal showed the histological changes associated with early fat necrosis. The microvessels around the nerve root were characterised by extensive thickening of their basement membranes and, where the meninges still covered the nerve roots, there was arachnoid cell proliferation and psammoma body formation. In other tissues these changes are considered evidence of tissue ischaemia.

In all cases of discal bulging and sequestration there were degenerate changes within the disc. Typically these changes included chondrocyte proliferation and myxoid change in the matrix. In addition, the disc frequently contained propagated intradiscal fissures. These were cracks or splits running through the disc, usually entering into and through the fibres

of the posterior annulus where they turned caudally to end at the vertebral end plate adjacent to the vertebral rim. In these cases there was usually damage to the vertebral end plate or rim, manifest as defects in the bone and cartilage of the vertebral end plate or bone of the rim. Through these defects, new vascular channels extended into the disc and propagated along the edges of the fissures.

In purely subjective terms, the type or extent of the pathological changes in specimens of the symptomatic and asymptomatic individuals showed no obvious differences. However, when the changes described above were analysed over all five levels from each spine, differences appeared.

When spines from symptomatic and asymptomatic patients were compared, discal pathology (disc protrusion or sequestration) was seen in the former in 95 % of cases compared to 23 % of the latter; venous dilatation in 95 % compared to 47 %; multiple level venous dilatation in 45 % compared to 6 %; periradicular fibrosis in 100 % as compared to 32 %; intradicular fibrosis in 85 % versus 12 %; and organising

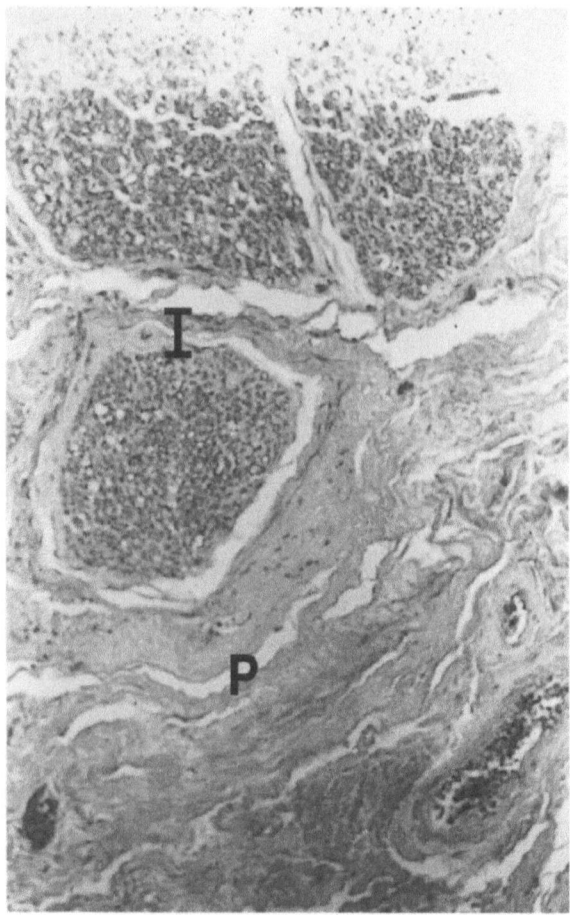

Fig. 3. Intra (*I*) and peridural (*P*) fibrosis (H & E, × 25)

3. Extensive vascular changes accompany discal pathology. These include:
   a) Venous dilatation and thrombosis
   b) Extensive ingrowth of vessels into dense connective tissues, notably the IV disc
   c) Thickening of the basement membranes of exchange vessels (e. g. capillaries and venules)
4. Morphological features usually suggestive of tissue ischaemia accompany the discal and vascular changes in mechanical spinal disease.
5. Venous dilatation in the intervertebral root canal and periradicular and intraradicular fibrosis are linked.

Cadaveric Study 2

The second cadaveric study examined the discal pathology in more detail. The study material consisted of cadaveric lumbosacral spinal tissue removed at necropsy from selected individuals.

The general selection procedures were very similar to the first study. Eighty-five spines were selected for study. In every case the selection criteria were (1) sudden death of known (or autopsy-established) cause, (2) no history of severe spinal trauma, and (3) no evidence of cardiac failure, metabolic bone disease or abnormality of thyroid or adrenal function prior to or at the time of autopsy.

Of the 75 spines sutdied, 50 were from individuals who, on subsequent examination of case notes held by the FHSA, were discovered never to have visited their family doctor complaining of lumbosacral back pain (no-pain group). The other 25 had complained of low-back pain of sufficient severity to have warranted their being seen in hospital (back-pain group), although none had been treated surgically. Treatment of the back-pain group had included analgesics, nonsteroidal anti-inflammatory drugs, corsetry, physiotherapy and, in 11 cases, epidural injections of lignocaine and/or steroids.

The age of the patients in the non-pain group was 61.3 years (range = 19–85) and in the back-pain group 57.7 (range = 31–79). The male to female ratio for the non-pain group was 29:21 and for the pain group was 11:14.

In each case, the lumboscral spine was removed by cutting through the T12/L1 vertebral body with a knife and through the alae of the sacrum with a saw. The spine was sectioned longitudinally in the sagittal plane, and blocks of tissue consisting of the halved intervertebral disc, small amount of adjacent vertebral body, the inververtebral root canal, and zygapophyseal joints were taken from the L1/2 IV disc to the L5/S1 disc, making five specimens from

thrombus in 15 % of symptomatic patients but only 5 % of asymptomatic patients. All these differences were significant at the $p = < 0.01$ level.

Histomorphometric analyses also disclosed two aspects of the pathology in which statistically defined differences could be identified between the symptomatic and asymptomatic groups. Taken overall, the proportion of the area of the intervertebral root canal occupied by dilated veins was 28.8 % ± 5.9 % in symptomatic patients and 10.6 ± 3.8 % in asymptomatic patients ($p = < 0.001$). The proportion of the nerve root occupied by fibrous tissue was 35.1 % ± 7.2 % in symptomatic patients and 18.4 ± 6.6 % in asymptomatic patients ($p = < 0.005$).

Conclusions from Cadaveric Study 1

There are a number of conclusions that can be drawn from this study:

1. The presence of discal and associated pathologies is not necessarily associated with significant back pain.
2. The greater the number of spinal levels affected, the greater the likelihood that an individual will develop back pain.

each spine. Histological preparations were examined with conventional stains.

In all, 375 discs were examined. Five individuals in the no-pain group were below the age of 30. Because of their age, lack of pain, and the similarity of their discal morphology to that of previous descriptions of normal IV discs, we called these the "normal" controls. The other members of the no-pain group are known as the "older non-pain group" (45 cases).

As in the first study, the spectrum of changes was very similar in both groups, only the extent of the changes within each spine differed between groups. The discal changes are best described in terms of anatomical structure. As a general rule, the deviation from the appearances of the 25 "control" discs (see below) was greatest in the L4/5 and L5/S1 discs. In the normal discs, the fibres of the annulus were almost vertical. When assessed relative to a line drawn between the original bony corners of adjacent vertebral bodies, the disc bulged both anteriorly and posteriorly, but in none of the 25 discs was the bulge more than 3 mm.

Of the 225 discs from the older no-pain patients, 103 appeared to have the similar general shape of those in the control group. In the rest, the intervertebral distance was decreased. In 84 of these, the disc bulged more than those of the control group, with a mean bulge of 6.1 mm. In 49 there was sequestration of discal tissue through the fibres of the annulus. Twenty-one of the 84 bulged discs and 22 of the 38 sequested discs were associated with osteophytes.

In the pain group, 36 discs appeared similar to those in the control group. Increased bulge was seen in 44 and in the remaining 45 there was sequestration. Twenty of the 44 bulged discs and 24 of the 45 sequestered discs were associated with osteophytes.

Annulus Fibrosus

In all of the normal discs, the annulus fibrosus was clearly demarcated from the nucleus pulposus. It consisted of well-organised and orientated collagen fibres at right angles to the surfaces of the vertebral body. The insertions of the annulus into the vertebral rims were uniform, there being no disruption of the fibres of the annulus or the bone of the end plate.

In 145 (64%) of the discs in the older no-pain group, the annular entheses were similar to those in the younger patients, in the remainder they were disrupted. The pattern of disruption varied. It included tearing of annular fibres from the vertebral rim (often associated with damage to the bone of the rim), interposition of cartilage between the annular fibres and the bone of the rim, and separation of the fibres by blood vessels growing into the annulus from the rim. These changes were seen most commonly at the posterior inferior aspect of the disc.

Similar changes were seen in 60 discs (57%) in the pain group. In 187 (83%) of the discs of the older patients in the no-pain group, and 103 (84%) of the discs of the pain groups, the fibres of the annulus distant from the rims were separated, either by vessels growing in from the outer surface of the annulus or from the rim, or by aggregates of fibro-chondroid material resembling that seen in the nucleus. In all these 290 discs (187 from the older no-pain patients and 103 from the pain patients), the annulus appeared broader than in the control group. In the latter, the anterior and posterior parts of the annulus occupied approximately 25% of the sagittal diameter of the disc, whereas in the 290 discs, tissue resembling annulus occupied approximately 40%.

Nucleus Pulposus

In the control patients, all of the nuclei pulposi consisted of hypocellular myxochondroid matrix. When viewed in polarised light, there was very few fibrillar arrays within the disc.

In 270 (77%) of the other discs, there were one or more of the following features:

(a) Fibrosis, recognised by the presence of polarisable fibres within the annulus (64%). The presence of fibrosis was defined as polarisable fibrous collagen within the disc. The area of the nucleus pulposus consisting of polarisable fibrous tissue was measured in each case. The mean area of fibrosis was greater in the discs from the pain patients, but this failed to reach statistical significance, largely bcause of the great range of results in each group.

(b) Longitudinal splits in the nucleus were seen in 182 discs (52%). In about 60% of these discs, the splits propagated anteriorly or posteriorly into the annulus, the latter being about twice as frequent as the former. Although there was no statistically significant differnce between the frequency of the longitudinal slits, the proportion in which they extended into the annulus was significantly greater in the pain group.

(c) Areas of hypocellularity (64%). The normal, relatively even distribution of chondrocytes was disturbed in many cases. This was due either to a focal but obvious local paucity in the number of chondrocytes to form clusters or clones. None of these parameters differed significantly between the pain and non-pain groups.

(d) "Microcysts" containing acellular myxoid or chondroid material (38%).

(e) Chondrocyte cluster (clone) formation (24%).

(f) Foci of "necrotic" matrix (28%).

(g) Vascularisation – One prominent feature of these IV discs was the presence of blood vessels within the discal material; they could all be followed to either the bone marrow of the rim (most commonly) or to the extra-discal connective tissues. There was a marked difference between the frequency of vascularisation within the disc of the pain and non-pain groups. The vessels most commonly followed the splits in the nucleus. They consisted of thin-walled capillaries and venules (20 %).

Vertebral Rim

Frequently, damage to the annular enthesis was associated with changes in the vertebral rim. In the normal group, the vertebral rim (that area of the superior or inferior surface of the vertebra between its junction with the horizontal cortex and the hyaline cartilage of the end plate) consisted of bone with inserting fibres of the annulus on the discal side and haemopoietic marrow on the other. In the other discs the abnormalities included avulsion of annular fibres, fracture of the cortex (30 %), with disruption of continuity of the bone (16 %) and fracture callus formation (19 %). These changes were usually associated with a zone of loss of haemopoiesis from the adjacent marrow, and ingrowth of vessels from the marrow into the disc (Fig. 4). The incidence was no different in the pain and non-pain groups.

In 87 discs (25 %), areas of marginal osteophyte formation were seen. They were more frequently seen in the back-pain patient group.

End Plate

The end plate in the normal group consisted of a sheet of hyaline cartilage (the cartilaginous end plate) overlying a thin bony end plate of cortical bone. Of the 350 discs in the older no-pain and pain groups, 77 (22 %) showed damage to the end plate. This consisted of fracture and disruption of the normal architecture of the central portions of the end plate (13 %) or erosion and disruption at the periphery, invariably associated with a vertebral rim lesion, (17 %). The end-plate damage, of all types, was greater in the back-pain group than in the no-pain group.

In 37 % there was bowing of the end plate into the vertebral body; this was not usually associated with fracture of the end plate.

Vertical Vertebral Body Cortex

Although not strictly part of the disc, damage to the disc (particularly the annulus) was associated with "traction spur" formation in the adjacent vertebral cortex in 3 % of cases. This was unrelated to the presence of back pain.

Differences Between the Pain and No-Pain Group

All the features described were seen to varying extents in the older no-pain and pain groups. The extent of the change and the number of vertebrae

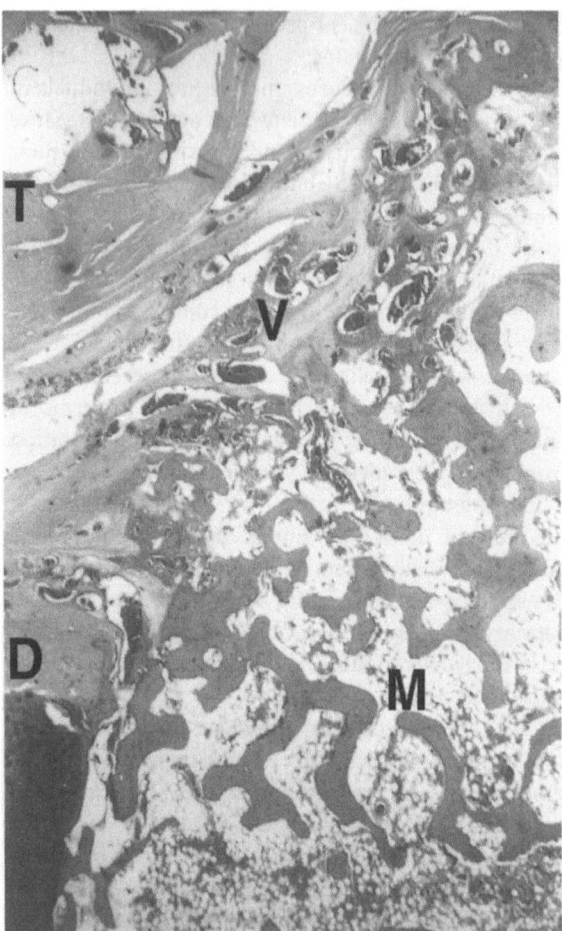

Fig. 4. A defect in the vertebral rim (*D*). Vessels (*V*) pass from the marrow devoid of haemopoietic cells (*M*) into the discal tissue (*T*) (H & E, × 50)

affected in each case varied in the two groups. Only those parameters for which there was a statistically significant difference in the number of affected discs per spine or whose subjective assessment appeared markedly different will be described.

(a) Although the two groups had very similar proportions of discs exhibiting splits, the number of discs with splits propagated through the fibres of the annulus to the vertebral rim was much greater ($p = 0.001$) in the pain group, where they were found, on average, in 2.6 discs per spine, compared with 0.86 discs per spine in the no-pain group.

(b) Vascularisation. The incidence of vascularisation of the discs was 19 % in the pain group and 4 % in the no-pain group. This was significant at $p = 0.001$. There was no difference between the number of discs per spine showing vascularisation.

(c) Vertebral rim damage. Because the process of vascularisation most commonly extended from the vertebra into the discs through defects in the rim, the trend of erosion and fracture of the rim, as expeded, matched that of vascular ingrowth, and was greater in the pain group than in the no-pain group ($p = 0.02$). However, the incidence of rim damage was much greater than that of vascularisation, and so this was not a constant relationship.

(d) Fracture of the end plate. True fracture of the end plate was uncommon in the non-pain group, but much less so in the pain group ($p = 0.01$).

(e) Osteophytes. Osteophytes usually arose at sites of rim damage and followed the incidence of rim lesions.

Conclusions from Cadaveric Study 2

The conclusions from this study are that if the young, no-pain patients discs are regarded as "normal", then many of the lumbar discs examined in this study show abnormalities. They can be divided into three main categories on pathological principles; they are mixed in their number, type, and distribution, in any one spine:

(a) Degeneration – alteration in the discal matrix with blurring of the distribution of annular and nuclear matrix, necrosis of matrix and clustering of chondrocytes.

(b) Traumatic – avulsion of annular fibres, and fracture of the rim and end plate.

(c) Reactive – osteophyte formation, neovascularisation and displacement of haemapoetic marrow. It is interesting to note that a classic cellular inflammatory infiltrate was never encountered within the disc.

The pathology is best interpreted as being that of (i) trauma and repair and (ii) degeneration and attempted stabilisation. These two sets of processes can be combined to formulate a hypothesis for how the observed changes occurred.

Hypothesis Based on Data from the Cadaveric Studies

An alteration in the matrix of the intervertebral discs leads to a decrease in hydration and loss of height of the disc. This process affects the nucleus pulposis predominantly. The fibres of the annulus do not reduce in length, and the potential for increased movement between the vertebrae and within the nucleus increases, rendering the disc at greater risk for traumatic damage. Alteration in matrix constituents and increased motion lead to split formation and instability, causing increased load on the annular enthesis and increased risk of inducing a traumatic enthesopathy and fracture of the vertebral rim. The local trauma induces neovascularisation as a repair process and perhaps loss of haemopoietic marrow, perhaps mediated by similar changes in the chemical environment.

Ingrowth of vessels (angiogenesis) in other tissues is associated with production of matrix-degrading enzymes. In the disc, production of these enzymes could further weaken the structure of the disc and thus initiate a spiral of increasing discal injury. The other aspect of neovascularisation is repair or scarring, which would be manifest as a further change in the matrix.

This hypothesis would explain the presence of osteophytes, on the basis of a stabilising response to increased discal motion.

Clearly, any hypothesis would need to take into account more major changes to the disc, such as end plate fracture, that are so severe and require such loading that they are unlikely to be caused just by the increased discal mobility associated with the processes described above. Thus, some of the changes at the vertebral rim and traction spurs could be explained by true "exogenous" trauma such as excessive loading.

We have shown no absolute association between any specific discal lesion and chronic back pain, but have demonstrated an association betweeen increased extent and multi-level disease with pain.

Biopsy Studies

There have been two biopsy studies. One relates to perivascular tissues, and enlarges upon observations made on the vascular pathology in the IVRC and its relationship to fibrosis; the other relates to neovascularisation of the IV disc.

In both studies, we have employed two techniques, immunohistochemistry (IHC) and in situ hybridisation (ISH), to obtain a better concept of the cell and molecular biology of the spinal tissues.

Immunohistochemistry [7, 8] is used to establish the presence of detectable final gene product. Labelled antibodies are applied to the tissue and the site of their binding is detected by a coloured reaction [9].

In situ hybridisation [10] employs radiolabelled riboprobes (specially designed strings of RNA bases with a complementary sequence to the messenger RNA being studied). It allows gene transcription to be studied [11, 12, 13]. Hybridisation is detected autoradiographically.

Both techniques were used together to obtain the greatest amount of information from the tissue. It is important to combine the techniques. For instance, where one is looking for a rapidly secreted molecule, loss of gene product from the cell precludes an accurate IHC assessment of the extent of product being synthesised, but changes in product production are often mediated by altered gene transcription, in which case the increased mRNA for the molecule under study is more stable evidence of upregulation. Where both techniques are applicable to a single molecule, a comparison of the relative changes in mRNA and protein can allow more detail to be derived about the level (transcriptional or translational) at which the alterations in regulation occur.

Biopsy Study 1

This study involved histological and in situ cell and molecular biology observations on biopsies taken from periradicular structures at the time of primary spinal surgery for mechanical spinal disease. These biopsies incorporated vascular fibrous and adipose tissue. When compared with normal periradicular tissue excised from "fresh" cadavers (within 4 h of death) and similar specimens excised from one organ donor at the time of organ donation, very extensive changes were seen in the fibrous tissue and in the vessels.

At the morphological level, the surgical specimens showed tissue fibrosis, fibrin deposition in thin-walled vascular channels, endothelial vacuolation (Fig. 5) and neovascularisation of a type not seen in controls.

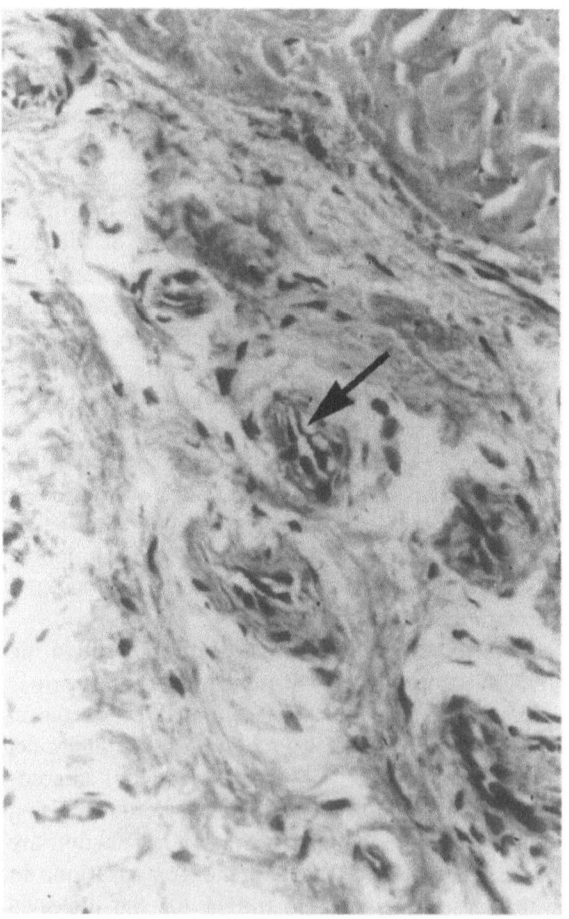

Fig. 5. Vacuolated endothelial cells in periradicular blood vessels (*arrowed*) (H & E, × 100)

ISH and IHC studies of von Willebrand factor (vWF), a product of endothelial cells whose release is associated with platelet aggregation and thrombus formation, showed loss of immunostainable vWF but increase in its mRNA in endothelial cells of the operative group. vWF is normally stored in endothelial cell cytoplasm within organelles called Wiebel–Palade bodies. When the endothelial cell is stimulated, the vWF is discharged and is no longer immunodetectable. If stimulation continues, vWF mRNA is upregulated; this increases the detectable in situ hybridisation signal, but because the gene product is continuously secreted, not enough is available under these circumstances to be detected immunohistochemically within the cell. It follows, therefore, that in symptomatic patients with mechanical spinal disease, venous channels around nerve roots are subject to endothelial stimulation leading to release of vWF which causes, in turn, platelet aggregation and thrombosis. In our study, upregulation of vWF mRNA was associated with an increase in intravascular accumulation of platelets detected by the presence of platelet glycoprotein IIa.

These studies also revealed other changes in endothelial function in the operated group of patients. These included endothelial cell expression of the fibrogenic cytokines IL-1 and TGF-B1. Fibroblasts within the fibrous tissue surrounding these vessels showed a marked increase in mRNA for type I collagen. Although it is not possible to quantify the absolute amount of protein or mRNA from the density of the immunohistochemical or in situ hybridisation reaction products, the relative densities of staining suggested that the increase in type I collagen mRNA was directly related to the level of cytokine expression.

Both morphological studies and histochemical probing of the tissue with antibodies directed towards cell-surface antigens expressed only on B lymphocytes, T lymphocyte subsets, macrophages and mast cells failed to reveal an inflammatory cell infiltrate in any specimen.

Conclusions from Biopsy Study 1

The conclusions from this study are that blood vessels within diseased spines exhibit disturbed endothelial function, initiating thrombosis and perivascular fibrosis.

Biopsy Study 2

The second study was used to examine neovascularisation and associated events in the intervertebral disc. Because slits can be mistaken for vessels, a marker of blood-vessel endothelial cells (CD31) was used to prove that vessels had penetrated into the disc beyond the outer third of the annulus fibrosus (the normal extent of vascular ingrowth into the IV disc). It is recognised that nerve fibre ingrowth is associated with angiogenesis to support vasoregulation. Therefere, the distribution of nerve fibres into the IV disc was also examined with neural markers. These markers included the nerve-specific molecule PGP9.5, the neurotransmitter substance P and the marker of active neural growth GAP 43.

IV discs were taken from patients undergoing anterior spinal fusion. Wedge-shaped sections of two or three discs, including the disc at the symptomatic level and a disc above and/or below were taken at the time of surgery and processed routinely.

These studies confirmed the cadaveric findings that blood vessels, as determined by the possession of CD31 on their lining cells, can penetrate deep into the IV disc. Thirty-two discs from 13 spines were examined. Of these, 15 showed vascularisation of otherwise avascular tissue. Many discs contained more vessels than predicted on the basis of morphology alone, probably because vessels can be difficult to identify morphologically in a collapsed state. Nerves were shown to grow into the discal tissue of 11 discs,

along the course taken by ingrowing blood vessels. These nerves expressed PGP9.5. In addition and unexpectedly, nerve twigs were seen growing into the disc away from blood vessels (Fig. 6). These nerves consisted of fine single nerve fibres and reacted for the neurotransmitter, substance P, which is nociceptive. Many were also positive for GAP43, evidence of active growth at the time of biopsy. In the vicinity of the ingrowing blood vessels, discal chondrocytes expressed the matrix-degrading enzymes MMP-1, 3 and 9 (Fig. 7); this suggests a role for chondrocytic chondrolysis in vascular ingrowth.

Of the 15 discs showing vascularisation, 10 were at the identified "pain level". Similarly, of the 11 showing neural ingrowth, 9 were from the "pain level" disc.

Conclusions from Biopsy Study 2

Vascularisation (66 %) and neural ingrowth (82 %) are features of discs at the level of pain symptoms; this suggests a relationship between pain levels and these features.

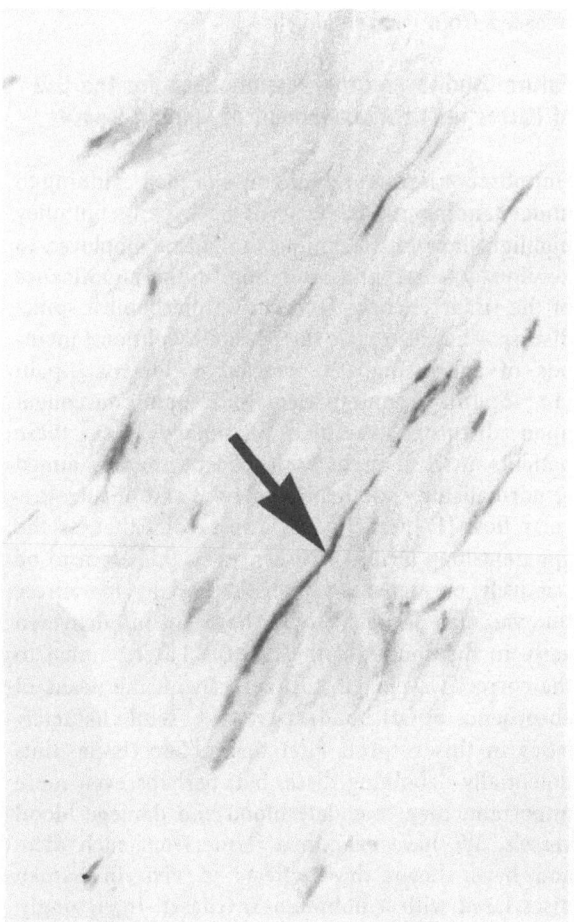

Fig. 6. A nerve twig (*arrowed*) in the annulus fibrosus reactive for PgP 9.5 (Immunoperoxidase, × 200)

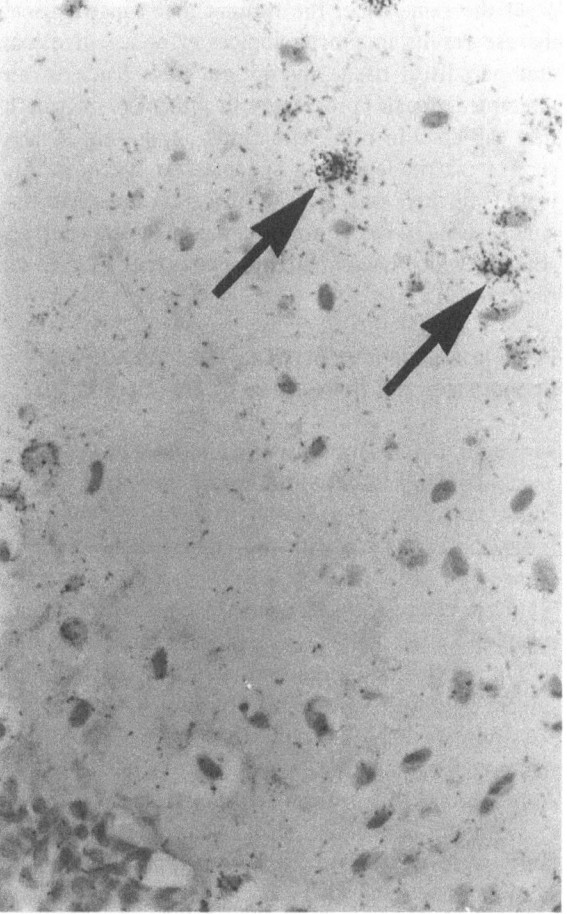

Fig. 7. Discal chondrocytes containing MMP-9 mRNA (*arrowed*) (ISH, × 150) (autoradiograph)

A Unifying Hypothesis Derived from Cadaveric and Biopsy Study Data to Explain Some of the Tissue Changes Seen

Although our studies have shown associations between various types of pathological change within the spines of patients with mechanical spinal disease, the only causal links that could even be inferred from these studies relate vascular changes to radicular fibrosis and ingrowth of vessels and nerves into the discs. Piecing these data together indicates that discal disease leads to venous compression in the lower part of the intervertebral root canal and disturbed blood flow. In multi-level disease, particularly significant impairment of venous outflow from the spinal cord occurs as a consequence of discal disease, to lead to venous hypertension in the cord. This is manifest as venous dilatation. The poor blood flow causes tissue ischaemia, endothelial dysfunction and thrombus formation within the vessels of the intervertebral root canal. Simultaneously, changes in endothelial function lead to the synthesis of fibrogenic cytokines. The contribution of new cytokine synthesis and tissue ischaemia results in increased collagen synthesis by local fibroblasts.

At the same time, the trauma that caused discal disease results in morphological evidence of discal and paradiscal tissue disruption. This leads to an attempted repair process with vascular ingrowth into the disc. In other situations, ingrowing vessels secrete matrix-degrading enzymes. In the disc, this would further weaken the discal connective tissues. These vessels are accompanied by nerves, some of which have nociceptive branches into discal tisue.

Possible Associations Between the Pathological Appearances and the Genesis of Low-Back Pain

Although there is circumstantial evidence to indicate a relationship between fibrosis and pain, our studies could only hint at potential mechanisms for pain induction associated with mechanical disease of the spine.

It has been proposed that direct nerve-root compression causes pain. There is substantial evidence to support this in patients with acute discal prolapse, but we have been unable to show any significant association between chronic back pain and direct nerve-root compression.

Inflammation has also been implicated in the genesis of pain, but in neither our cadaveric nor biopsy study were we able to identify, morphologically or immunohistochemically, any conventional inflammatory cell infiltrate within the soft tissues inside the spinal and nerve-root canals. Furthermore, our studies would suggest that the redness often noted at surgery in the peridural tissues and annulus, and reported as inflammation, is not a manifestation of inflammation as such, but rather a consequence of vascular dilatation and/or increased local vascularity.

In addition to nerves penetrating the disc that could be prone to physical stimulation under load, our investigations indicate another potential mechanism by which nerves might be stimulated in spinal disease. Dense aggregates of nerves are distributed around periradicular veins and are associated with vessels in traumatised and degenerate discs. These vessels show evidence of platelet aggregation and thrombus formation and the adjacent tissues exhibit features usually associated with ischaemia. Nociceptive nerve endings can be stimulated by a variety of chemical mediators, including the kinins, 5-hydroxytryptamine, prostanoids, lactic acid and potassium ions. In the context of our observations on blood vessels and the distribution of nerve endings, it is interesting to note that kinins are formed during coagulation, 5-hydroxytryptamine is released from activated, aggregated platelets and prostanoids, lactic acid and potassium ions are released from ischaemic cells.

Future Studies and the Possible Basis for the Use of Lasers in the Management of Spinal Disease

Our observations represent only a crude beginning to understanding mechanisms of back pain, but they highlight how our techniques might be employed to develop a better understanding of the significance of the tissue changes recorded in mechanical spinal disease. They also raise the possibility of novel methods of addressing the problem of low back-pain [14, 15, 16]. If some patients have pain consequent upon disturbed vascular physiology, then these patients at least might be helped by therapy aimed at normalising endothelial function, and/or intravascular flow [17]. One would also predict that, as the apparent long-term consequences of this seem to be relatively permanent, a realistic strategy to redress the vascular lesions would have to be delivered early in the course of the disease. Lasers, tuned to the correct wavelength to interact with the peaks of absorbance of OH bonds, have two useful characteristics in this respect. First they ablate tissue, thus potentially debulking discs, but, perhaps even more important, they coagulate blood and damage blood vessels. We have examined tissue from such discs and have shown these effects in vivo in human discs lased with a holmium-YAG laser. Intriguingly, it appears that the laser energy can also stimulate regrowth of connective tissue cells [18]. Perhaps highly selected lasers such as the erbium-YAG laser with a peak of absorbance at 294 nm [19, 20] could be the future evidence-based treatment strategy for mechanical disc disease.

References

[1] Goldie I (1958) Granulation tissue in the ruptured intervertebral disc. Acta Pathol Scand 42:300–304

[2] Hanson HJ (1952) A pathologic–anatomical study on disc degeneration in dogs. Acta Orthop Scand Suppl 11:1–117

[3] Hirsch C (1959) Studies on the pathology of low back pain. J Bone Joint Surg 41B:237–243

[4] Hoyland JA, Freemont AJ, Jayson MIV (1989) Intervertebral foramen venous obstruction. A cause of periradicular fibrosis. Apine 14:558–568

[5] Hoyland JA, Freemont AJ (1991) The incidence and significance of psammoma bodies within nerve roots of lumbar spines. Neuro-Orthopaedics 11:83–89

[6] Buirski G, Silberstein M (1993) The symptomatic lumbar disc in patients with low back pain. Magnetic resonance imaging appearances in both asymptomatic and control population. Spine 18:1808–1811

[7] Fitzmaurice RJ, Pitalia A, Freemont AJ (1992) Effects of prolonged processing in standard and isotonic trichloroacetic acid (TCA) on cellular preservation in bone marrow trephines. J Clin Pathol 45:631–632

[8] Pitalia AK, Liu-Yin JA, Freemont AJ, Morris DJ, Fitzmaurice RJ (1993) Immunohistological detection of human herpes virus 6 in formalin-fixed, paraffin-embedded lung tissue. J Med Virol 41:103–107

[9] Braidman IP, Davenport LK, Carter DH, Selby PL, Mawer EB, Freemont AJ (1995) Preliminary in situ identification of estrogen target cells in bone. J Bone Min Res 10:74–80

[10] Andrew JG, Hoyland JA, Freemont AJ, Marsh D (1993) Insulinlike growth factor gene expression in human fracture callus. Calcif Tissue Int 53:97–102

[11] Marles PJ, Hoyland JA, Parkinson R, Freemont AJ (1991) Demonstration of variation in chondrocyte activity in different zones of articular cartilage – an assessment of the value of in situ hybridisation. Int J Exp Pathol 72:171–182

[12] Hoyland JA, Thomas JT, Donn R, Marriott A, Ayad S, Boot-Handford RP, Grant ME, Freemont AJ (1991) Distribution of type X collagen in normal and osteoarthritic human cartilage. Bone and Mineral 15:151–164

[13] Andrew JG, Hoyland JA, Andrew SM, Marsh D, Freemont AJ (1993) Demonstration of TGF-B1 in normally healing fracture callus by in-situ hybridisation. Calcified Tissue International 52:74–78

[14] Innes D, Sevitt S (1964) Coagulation and fibrinolysis in injured patients. J Clin Pathol 17:1–13

[15] Klimiuk PS, Pountain GD, Keegan AL, Jayson MIV (1987) Serial measurements of fibrinolytic activity in acute low back pain and sciatica. Spine 12:925–928

[16] Mitchell WS, Illingworth KJ, Jayson MIV (1988) Fibrinolytic enhancement therapy in the treatment of severe chronic low back pain. Br J Rheumatol A2:12

[17] Pountain GD, Keegan AL, Jayson MIV (1987) Impaired fibrinolytic activity in defined chronic back pain syndromes. Spine 12:83–86

[18] Freemont AJ, Charlton A, King T (1992) Post-operative healing of erbium-YAG laser incisions. Lasers in Medical Science 7:449–453

[19] Charlton A, Dickinson MR, King TA, Freemont AJ (1991) Homium-YAG and erbium-YAG laser interaction with hard and soft tissue. SPIE 1427:189–197

[20] Herdman RCD, Charlton A, Hinton AE, Freemont AJ (1993) An in-vitro comparison of the erbius:YAG laser and the carbon dioxide laser in laryngeal surgery. J Laryng Otol 107:908–911

Open Lumbar Discectomy After Percutaneous Laser Disc Decompression (PLDD): Clinical and Histological Results

K. Mahlfeld · R. Kayser · K. Radig · U. Mahlfeld · J.-U. Greinert · H. Grasshoff

Introduction

Neodynium:YAG (Nd:YAG) PLDD was first introduced by Ascher in 1986 and has become an accepted minimally invasive procedure for prolapsed disc protrusions, subject to strict inclusion criteria (Ascher and Choy 1986). Since then, many clinical results have been published (Ascher 1991; Choy et al. 1992; Siebert et al. 1996). The reported early success rate is between 70–80 % and it therefore lies within the same range as other minimally invasive disc-treating procedures (e.g., Choy 1991; Davis et al. 1994; Hellinger 1994; Siebert 1996). In 7–20 % of PLDD-treated cases, open discectomy is required (Choy 1991; Leu et al. 1994; Siebert et al. 1996).

The degenerative disc has often been examined histologically (e.g., Scott et al. 1994). Alongside the common H & E stain, many other specialized stains (Elastica, Alzian-PAS, Berlin blue, Mowry, etc.) are used for histological identification of disc degeneration (cell number, fiber quality, pathological markers). Through histochemistry, the progression of disc degeneration has been described (Holm 1993).

The aim of our study was to evaluate the clinical outcome of patients who had undergone discectomy following Nd:YAG PLDD and to analyze the histological progression of disc tissue changes after PLDD.

Materials and Methods

From February 1, 1992 to September 1, 1996, 403 patients suffering from symptomatic lumbar disc disorders were treated in our hospital with the Nd:YAG laser, wavelength 1320 nm.

The patients were selected according to the indication criteria of Choy and Siebert (Choy 1991; Siebert et al. 1996). Average applied laser energy was 2500 J. Due to persisting symptoms, 53 patients needed subsequent open microsurgical discectomy of the PLDD-treated segment on the same side. The extracted disc tissue was examined histologically.

All 53 patients were included in the study. Average follow-up time was 40 months after open surgery following PLDD and 43.5 months after primary open discectomy. Follow-up included clinical examination, subjective assessment of back and leg pain, pain-free walking distance, medication, as well as performance at work and during recreational activities. Distribution of age, gender and follow-up period was homogeneous.

The results were then compared to those of another group of patients who had undergone only primary open discectomy (Table 1).

Results

The patients consisted of 38 men and 15 women, with an average age of 38.2 years, who were treated with discectomy after PLDD. This was performed at the L3–4 level in one patient, L4–5 in 23 patients and L5–S1 in 29 patients. The operations were on the right side for 19 patients and on the left side for 34 patients. Intraoperative findings are given in Table 2. If PLDD failed to relieve symptoms, open surgery

Table 1. Distribution of age, gender, operated levels and follow-up period

		Open discectomy after PLDD	Primary discectomy only
Number		53	352
Age		38.2 years	40.6 years
Gender, %	Male	71	67
	Female	29	33
Operated levels, %	L3/4	1.8	3.2
	L4/5	43.5	44.8
	L5/S1	54.7	48.7
	Other	0	3.1
Follow-up time		40 months	43.5 months

Table 2. Intraoperative findings during open discectomy after PLDD ($n = 53$)

Diagnosis	Rate in %
Free sequester	45
Prolapse	32
Protrusion	18
Narrow spinal canal	5

was performed after an average period of 104 days (6 to 450 days).

At the time of follow-up, the clinical examination showed that the back pain of more than 80 % of the patients of both groups was completely relieved, markedly improved (63 % of patients with open discectomy following PLDD and 63 % of patients with open discectomy only) or improved (21 % vs. 19 %, respectively). Details are given in Table 3. Nearly 80 % had complete disappearance of leg pain or were markedly improved. Details are given in Table 4. More than 80 % of the patients of both groups took either no analgesics (61 % vs. 61 %) or occasional analgesics (21 % vs. 31 %) (Table 5). Of the patients, 59 % vs. 47 % were able to walk a distance of 5 km or more without pain (Table 6).

Table 3. Relief of back pain

	Open discectomy after PLDD, %	Primary discectomy only, %
Very satisfied	22	23
Markedly improved	39	40
Improved	21	19
The same	13	13
Worse	5	5

Table 4. Relief of leg pain

	Open discectomy after PLDD, %	Primary discectomy only, %
Very satisfied	53	41
Markedly improved	29	27
Improved	8	18
The same	5	11
Worse	5	3

Table 5. Use of analgesics

Table 6. Ability to walk pain-free

	Open discectomy after PLDD, %	Primary discectomy only, %
No restriction	59	47
1–5 km	22	29
0.5–1 km	15	17
< 500 m	9	7

Table 7. Subjective satisfaction

	Open discectomy after PLDD, %	Primary discectomy only, %
Very satisfied	36	34
Markedly improved	28	29
Improved	25	24
The same	8	10
Worse	3	3

On the visual analogue pain scale of 0–10, the preoperative value was 7.1 in those patients who had undergone open surgery after PLDD and 7.3 in the group of primary open surgery. The value was reduced after operation to 3.6 vs. 3.3.

The ability to work and undertake recreational activities was notably improved in 85 % of the patients of both groups. Of the patients, 58 % with discectomy following PLDD and 59 % with only open discectomy were either without any restrictions or had negligible restrictions.

Altogether, 89 % of patients who had PLDD before open discectomy and 87 % of the patients who had received subsequent open surgery were satisfied with the results. Of the patients, 64 % vs 63 % were completely cured or markedly improved (Table 7).

The histological examination of the disc samples extracted after ND:YAG lager PLDD showed moderate to severe degeneration (fibrillated cartilage, pseudocysts, necrosis, separation of intercellular substance, fiber exposure, cell rarefaction, encapsulation) (Fig. 1). While the histological changes in the disc demonstrated classical changes of the disc degeneration in both the groups, patients who had previous laser disc intervention demonstrated fibrolymphocytic infiltrations and foreign-body reactions (Figs. 2, 3).

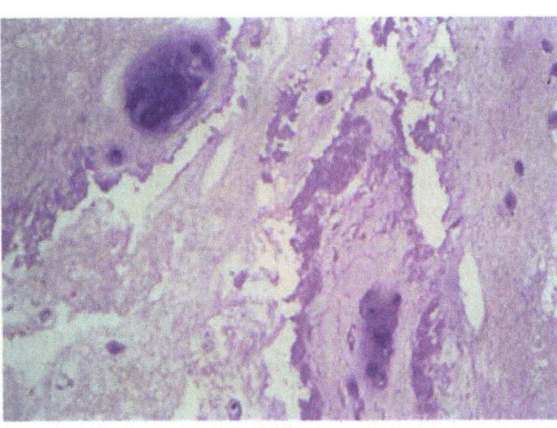

Fig. 1. Severe degenerative discopathia with typical degeneration; 50 days after PLDD. H & E stain, 1:500

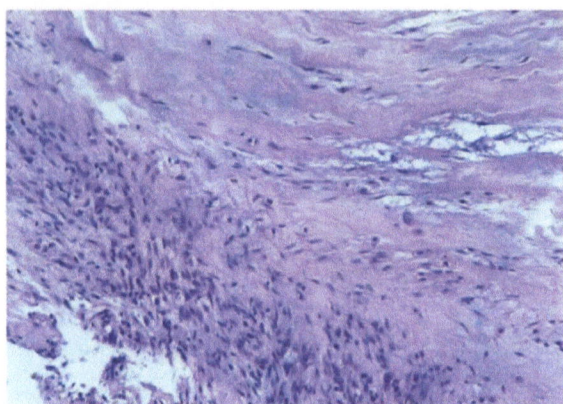

Fig. 2. Fibrohistiocytic infiltration after laser induction. Degenerative discopathia; 16 days after PLDD. H & E stain, 1:500

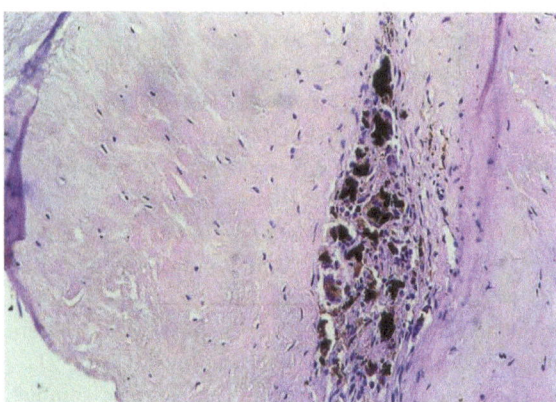

Fig. 3. Foreign-body reaction with giant vells. Degenerative discopathia; 450 days after PLDD. H & E stain, 1:500

Discussion

The reported success rates of 70–80 % following PLDD encompass a surgical revision re-surgery rate of 7 to 20 %. Our reoperation rate after PLDD was 13.1 %, twice as high as the rate given by Siebert et al. (1996). Choy reports a reoperation rate of 21.6 % (Choy et al. 1992).

The analysis of our intraoperative results show (Table 1) a free sequestrated disc in 45 % of the patients. This finding suggests that in the presence of a sequestrated disc, minimally invasive PLDD is contraindicated. In the presence of an extrusion or sequestration, a microsurgical procedure may be expected to achieve a higher success rate than a PLDD. However, revision surgery has been necessary after primary open discectomy in 3–15 % of the cases (e. g., Davis et al. 1994). Furthermore, open surgery carries the risk of instability at the treated segment and postoperative scarring of the spinal canal and perineural fibrosis, leading to long-term morbidity which is difficult to treat.

The results of our follow-up examinations of reoperated patients are the same as those of patients who had primary open discectomy. It may therefore be concluded that poor outcome in some patients following PLDD is not a complication but is the result of inadequate decompression.

One of the first reports on histological changes after conventional nucleotomy was published by Haas in 1949. Recently, more attention has been paid to the histological analysis of disc tissue (e. g., Scott 1994). Histological signs of disc tissue degeneration have been found in samples extracted during PLDD. In addition, several studies describe histological changes after laser treatment (Buchelt et al. 1992; Choy et al. 1992; Gropper et al. 1984). This has been verified in animal experiments (Yonezawa et al. 1990; Qi et al. 1994; Turgut et al. 1996). The histological changes are divided into two periods: an early period of fibrocytic and cartilagenic activity in the defect area and a later period of fibrocartilagenic proliferation in the defect area (Yonezawa et al. 1990; Qi et al. 1994; Turgut et al. 1996). We also observed fibrolymphocytic infiltration and foreign-body reactions, which we surmise to be a vital tissue reaction against laser-induced necrosis. Thus, the evident chronological course of tissue reaction to laser application becomes comprehensible. As vital tissue reactions need a certain time span before occurring, tissue changes will not be visible in patients who are reperated soon after PLDD. We believe this time span commences after 8 to 14 days. An exception, which we observed in a few cases, were nonreactive foreign bodies. In our study, the histological tissue changes were not consistent. In order to histologically classify tissue changes after PLDD, further studies need to be conducted.

If due care is taken to adhere to the indications, PLDD would be the first choice for disc decompression. Aggressive open surgical procedures may be reserved for patients who fail to respond to the minimally invasive PLDD.

References

[1] Ascher DW, Holzer P, Sutter B, Tritthart H (1991) Nucleus-pulposus Denaturierung bei Bandscheibenprotrusionen. In: Siebert WE, Wirth CJ (eds) Laser in der Orthopädie. Thieme, Stuttgart pp 169–172

[2] Bonati AO (1991) Arthroscopic lumbar laser discectomy. In: Abstracts of the 1st international symposium on lasers in orthopaedic surgery, San Francisco pp 4–5

[3] Buchelt M, Kitschera HP, Katterschafka T, Kiss H, Schneider R, Ullrich R (1992) Erb:YAG and Hol:YAG laser ablation of meniscus and intervertebral disc. Lasers Surg Med 12: 375–381

[4] Choy DSJ, Case RB, Ascher P (1987) Percutaneous laser ablation of lumbar discs. In: 33rd anual meeting of the orthopaedic research society 1:19

[5] Choy DSJ, Ascher PW, Saddekui S, Alkaitis D, Liebler W, Hughes J, Diwan S, Altmann P (1992) Percutaneous laser disc decompression. Spine 12:949–956

[6] Choy DSJ, Michelsen J, Getrajdman G, Diwan S. (1992) Percutaneous laser disc decompression. An update – Spring 1992. J Clin Laser Med Surg 177–184

[7] Choy DSJ (1991) Percutaneous laser disc decompression (PLDD). In: Abstracts of the 1st international sympsium on lasers in orthopaedic surgery. San Francisco pp 24

[8] Davis JK (1994) Laser-assisted percutaneus lumbar discectomy. Laserscope, San Jose

[9] Gropper GR, Robertson JH, McClellan G (1984) Comparative histological and radiographic effects of CO_2 laser versus standard surgical anterior cervical discectomy in the dog. Neurosurgery 14:42–47

[10] Leu HJ, Imhoff A, Schrieber A (1994) Perkutane Nukleotomie mit Diskoskopie. Erste Erfahrungen mit der Excimer-Photoablation. In: Siebert WE, Wirth CJ (eds) Laser in der Orthopädie. Thieme, Stuttgart pp 163–167

[11] Hellinger J (1994) Nonendoscopic percutaneous 1064 – Nd:YAH laser decompression: mechanism, technique and experience. In: Abstracts of the 3rd symposium on laser-assisted endoscopic intervention in orthopaedics, Orthopaedic University Clinic Balgrist, Zürich, 1

[12] Qi Q, Dang GD, Cai QL (1994) Laser ablation of intervertebral disc: animal experiment. Chung Hua Wai Ka Chin. 32:187–189

[13] Scott JE, Boswoth TR, Cribb AM (1994) The chemical morphology of age-related changes in human intervetebral disc glycosaminoglycans from cervical thoracal and lumbar nucleus pulposus and annulus fibrosus. J Anat 184:73–82

[14] Siebert WE, Ksinsik B, Wirth CJ (1991) In-vitro-Untersuchungen zur thermischen Belastung der Bandscheibe bei der Laserablation. In: Siebert WE, Wirth J (eds) Laser in der Orthopädie. Thieme, Stuttgart, pp 150–153

[15] Siebert WE, Berendsen BT, Tollgard J (1996) Die perkutane Laserdiskusdekompression (PLDD). Orthopäde 25:42–48

[16] Turgut M, Ozcan OE, Sungur A, Sargin H (1996) Effect of Nd:YAG laser on experimental disc degeneration. Acta Neurochir 138:1355–1361

[17] Yonezawa T, Onomura T, Kosaka R (1990) The system and procedures of percutaneous intradiscal laser nucleotomy. Spine 15:1175–1185

Quantitative Analysis of the Ablation Effects of Holmium:YAG and Neodymium:YAG Laser in Human Spinal Disc Tissue

J. Krott · R. Sroka · W. Stummer · H.-J. Reulen

Introduction

For several years lasers have been used routinely in percutaneous nucleotomy. However, there still is very little standardized data on the effect of specific laser parameters on the ablation rate of spinal disc tissue. The aim of our study was to quantify the effects of the Ho:YAG and Nd:YAG lasers on disc tissue ablation, by systematically changing specific energy parameters, to determine the optimal parameter combination for tissue ablation.

Materials and Methods

The experiments were conducted on spinal disc tissue samples from fresh cadavers, within 12 h after removal, to avoid desiccation or autolysis. A Ho:YAG laser ($\lambda = 2130$ nm) and a Nd:YAG laser ($\lambda = 1064$ nm), BLM 800, Basel-Medizintechnik/Starnberg, were used. The single pulse energy level was changed stepwise from 0.5 to 5 J. The repetition rate was altered stepwise from 1 to 8 Hz. The maximal performance of the laser systems was limited to 15 W. The maximum total energy applied was 150 J. The experiments were conducted in both contact mode (laser fiber touching the disc surface) and in noncontact mode (constant distance of 1 mm kept between laser fiber and disc surface). The volume of the ablated craters was calculated by measuring the depths, calculating the diameters microscopically, and using the cylinder formula.

Results

Results with the Ho:YAG Laser

In both contact and noncontact mode, the volume of ablated disc tissue increased as total energy increased (Fig. 1). Although the total volume of ablated tissue was the same in the contact and noncontact mode, the depth and diameter were different. The depths of the lesions produced in contact mode were significantly larger than those produced in noncontact mode (Fig. 2). On the other hand, the diameters of

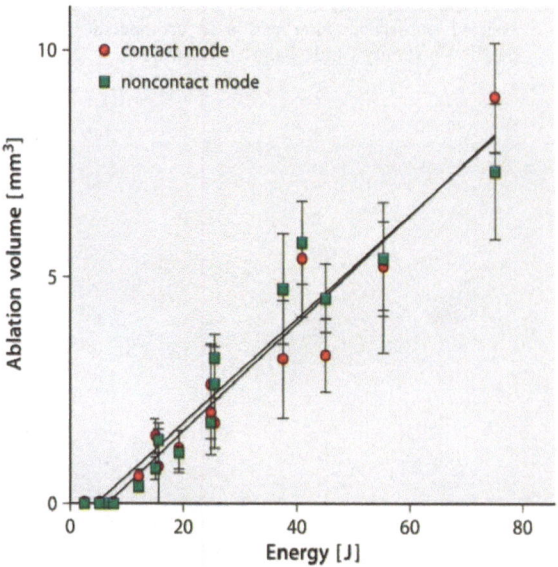

Fig. 1. Ablation volume in contact and noncontact mode when the Ho:YAG laser is used

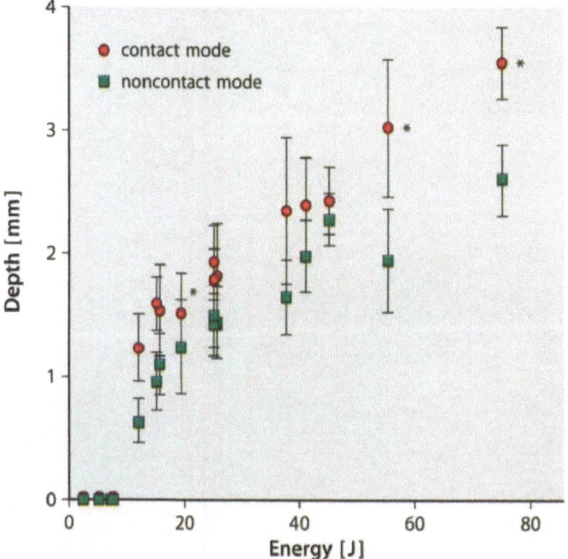

Fig. 2. Depth of the ablation lesions in contact and noncontact mode when the Ho:YAG laser is used (* $p < 0.05$ vs. noncontact mode)

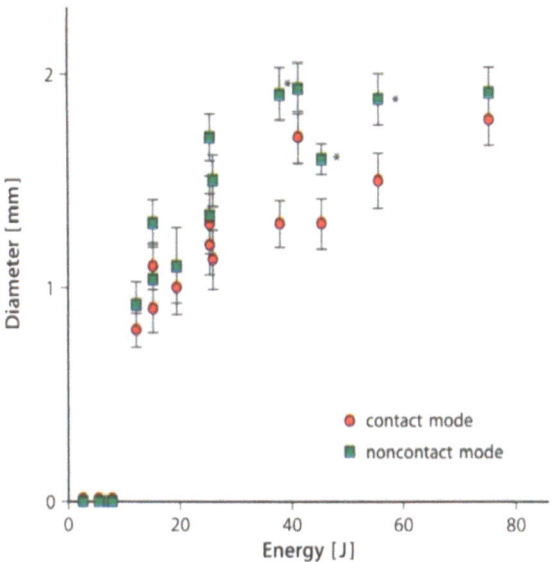

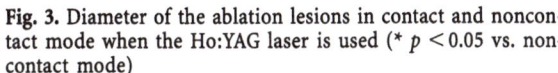

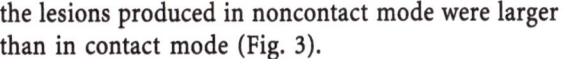

Fig. 3. Diameter of the ablation lesions in contact and noncontact mode when the Ho:YAG laser is used (* $p < 0.05$ vs. noncontact mode)

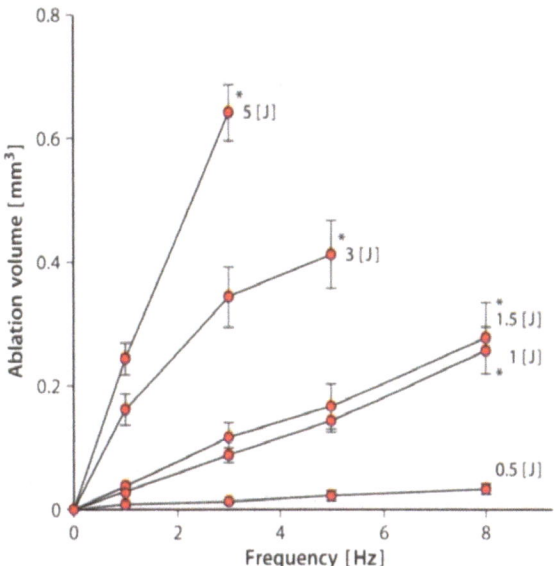

Fig. 4. Ablation volumes in contact mode per single impulse level when the Ho:YAG laser is used (* $p < 0.05$ vs. noncontact mode)

the lesions produced in noncontact mode were larger than in contact mode (Fig. 3).

The total energy is the product of the single energy pulses and the repetition rate. To separately analyze the effect of each single parameter on the disc tissue, the energy of a single impulse was increased stepwise from 0.5 to 5 J in each experiment, whereas the total energy and the repetition rate remained constant. The same experiments were then conducted with stepwise increased repetition rates (1 to 8 Hz); the single impulse and total energy values were constant.

At a constant total energy level, each increase of single impulse energy led to a significant enlargement of the ablation crater, except at the 0.5-J level. The increase of the repetition rate from 1 to 8 Hz at constant single impulse energy and total energy levels also caused an increase in ablation volumes. The largest ablation volume per single laser impulse was caused at the following combination of parameters: single impulse energy, 5 J, repetition rate, 3 Hz (Fig. 4).

Results with the Nd:YAG Laser

The ablation volumes were significantly smaller in all experiments with the Nd:YAG laser in comparison to the Ho:YAG laser. The Nd:YAG laser caused a measurable lesion only in contact mode; in noncontact mode no ablation effect could be found (Fig. 5).

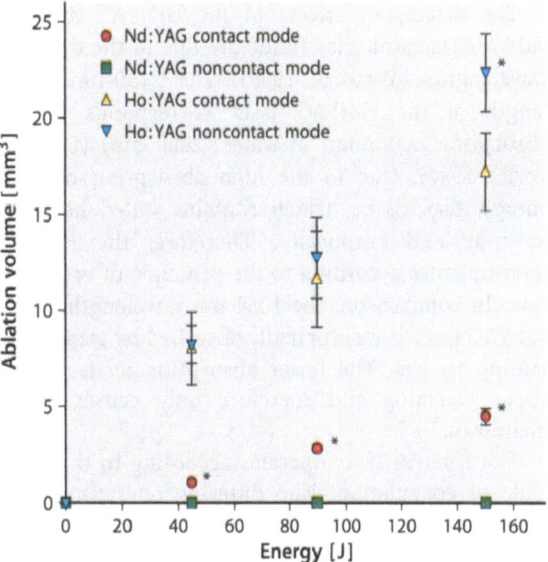

Fig. 5. Ablation volumes of the Ho:YAG and Nd:YAG lasers in contact and noncontact mode (* $p < 0.05$ vs. noncontact mode)

Discussion

Since 1987, the laser has been used in percutaneous nucleotomy procedures, as introduced by Hijikata (Hijikata 1975; Choy 1987). Although application has been clinically successful (Ohnmeiss 1994; Caspar 1996), there is no universally calid information indicating which laser and which parameters are most suited for spinal disc tissue ablation (Quigley 1994).

Our experiments with the Ho:YAG laser show that the ablation volume is not only dependent on the total energy applied, but also depends on the single impulse energy, the repetition rate, and the distance between the laser fiber and the disc surface. The side effects of the energy of a single impulse and the repetition rate are ablation and tissue carbonization. This is undesirable because carbonization absorbs laser energy and hinders further tissue ablation (Helfmann 1989).

In contact mode, the laser beam penetrates disc tissue vertically. In noncontact mode, the laser beam penetrates the tissue at a larger exit angle according to the distance between the laser fiber and disc surface and the numerical settings of the laser fiber. Compared to contact mode, a larger area is irradiated in noncontact mode, with less intensity per irradiated area. This explains why noncontact mode causes ablation craters with wider diameters and why contact mode causes deeper craters. A similar effect occurs during tissue carbonization. In comparison to contact mode. The beam intensity in noncontact mode is lower than in contact mode, and therefore produces less carbonization.

The discrepant effects of the HO:YAG and the Nd:YAG lasers on disc tissue are due to the different wavelengths (Vorwerk 1989). The 2130-nm wavelength of the Ho:YAG laser corresponds to the absorption maximum of water (2000 nm) (Domankevitz 1996). Due to the high absorption of laser energy, disc tissue, which contains water, heats up abruptly and evaporates. Therefore, the Ho:YAG laser operates according to the principle of vaporization. In comparison, the 1064-nm wavelength of the Nd:YAG laser is insufficiently absorbed by water-containing tissues. The lower absorption leads to less tissue warming and therefore only causes tissue meltdown.

The Nd:YAG laser operates according to the principle of coagulation. The differing operating principles lead to different ablation rates, with the Ho:YAG laser ablating faster than the Nd:YAG laser.

When ablation and carbonization are compared, our experiments show that the Ho:YAG laser, which was first used in 1991 (Quigley 1991), is the most suitable for disc tissue ablation, at energy parameters

of 5-J single impulse and a 3-Hz repetition rate in noncontact mode. These good results were confirmed by Siebert (Siebert 1993). Because the laser can remove smaller amounts of disc tissue precisely, and there is no uncontrolled temperature spread to adjacent tissues (Buchelt 1995), it is feasible to use laser for treatment of sequesters or discs near sensitive tissues such as nerve roots. First results on the success of minimally invasive therapy of sequestered prolapsed discs by percutaneous laser sequestrectomy have already been published (Seibel 1997).

References

[1] Buchelt M, Schlangmann B, Schmolke S, Siebert W (1995) High power Ho:YAG laser ablation of intervertebral discs: effects on ablation rates and temperature profile. Laser Surg Med 16(2):179–183
[2] Caspar GD, Hartman VL, Mullins LL (1996) Results of a clinical trial of the Holmium:YAG laser in disc decompression utilizing a side-firing fiber. Laser Surg Med 19(2): 90–96
[3] Choy DSJ, Case RB, Fielding W (1987) Percutaneous laser nucleolysis of lumbar discs. N Engl J Med 317:771–772
[4] Domankevitz Y, McMillan K, Nishioka NS (1996) Characterization of tissue ablation with a continuous wave holmium laser. Laser Surg Med 19(1):97–102
[5] Helfmann J, Brodzinski T (1989) Thermische Wirkungen. In: Berlien H-P, Müller G (eds) Angewandte Lasermedizin, 1st edn. economed, Landsberg, pp 1–8
[6] Hijikata S, Yamagushi M, Nakayama T, Oomari K (1975) Percutaneous nucleotomy – A new treatment method for lumbar disc herniation. J Tode Hosp 5:39–42
[7] Ohnmeiss DD, Guyer RD, Hochschuler SH (1994) Laser disc decompression. The importance of proper patient selection. Spine 19(8):2054–2058
[8] Quigley MR, Shih T, Elfrifai A, Loesch DV, Maroon JC (1991) Laser discectomy: comparison of Hol:YAG and Nd:YAG systems. Surg Forum 42:507–509
[9] Quigley MR, Shih T, Elrifai A, Maroon JC, Lesiecki ML (1994) Laser discectomy: a review. Spine 19(1):53–56
[10] Seibel RMM (1997) Mikroendoskopische minimal-invasive Therapie von sequestrierten Bandscheibenvorfällen. Medizin und Bild 1:51–57
[11] Siebert W (1993) Percutaneous laser disc decompression: the European experience. Spine: State of the Art Reviews 7(1):103–133
[12] Vorwerk D, Husemann T, Blazek V, Zolotas G, Guenther R (1989) Laserablation des Nucleus pulposus: Optische Eigenschaften von degeneriertem Bandscheibengewebe im Wellenlängenbereich von 200–2200 nm. Fortschr Röntgenstr 151:725–728

Biomechanics of the Spine: The Engineer's View

D. W. L. Hukins · J. R. Meakin · J. C. Leahy

Introduction

The spine is a series of rigid vertebrae connected by joints to form a flexible column. Spinal flexibility enables the body to twist and bend to adopt a wide range of postures [16].

The behaviour of a "motion segment" is often used to describe the mechanics of the spine. A motion segment consists of two adjacent vertebrae and the flexible joints between them. Each motion segment contains two zygapophyseal joints (diarthrodial-synovial joints) and the intervertebral joint (whose major component is the intervertebral disc). Movement of a motion segment arises from flexion–extension in the sagittal plane, lateral bending in the coronal plane and rotation in the axial plane of the spine. Spinal movement is then the sum of the movements of the individual motion segments.

The spine is also subjected to axial compression. This compression arises from the weight of the body and any external loads being supported. Measurement of pressure within the disc indicates that most of the compression arises from muscular activity [29]. Movement of the spine is initiated by contraction of muscles; models also indicate the importance of the musculature for the control of spinal motion [26]. These muscles include the oblique muscles of the abdomen (which initiate rotation) as well as the muscles of the back. Because of their directions, the forces generated by these muscles have components which tend to compress the spine. The ability of the intervertebral joint to withstand compression should not be confused with shock absorption (the ability to filter out transient axial compression), which is achieved by the intact spine and its muscles [33]. The next three sections consider the mechanics of a motion segment, the effect of removing the nucleus from its disc and how it can be stabilised, when necessary.

Mechanics of a Motion Segment

The flexible tissues of the intervertebral joint are reinforced by collagen fibres. These fibres prevent the tissue being damaged by the forces acting on the joint. They also provide the stiffness that prevents excessive stretching of tissues. However, collagen can only perform these functions if its fibres are oriented in the direction in which the tissue will be stretched by joint movement.

Flexion stretches the posterior longitudinal ligament, the ligamenta flava and the posterior annulus fibrosus, which then resist excessive motion. Flexion will also cause the zygapophyseal joint space to open, stretching the joint capsule. Although the supraspinous and interspinous ligaments are extended in flexion, the arrangement of their collagen fibres is such that they are unlikely to resist this motion [18]. In extension, the anterior longitudinal ligament and the anterior annulus fibrosus are stretched. On further extension, the tips of the inferior anterior processes of the upper vertebra impact on the lamina of the vertebra below. Extreme extension may also cause the spinous processes to impact [1]. During flexion and extension, the nucleus pulposus moves within the disc – posteriorly during flexion, and anteriorly during extension [8]. Lateral bending is resisted by the lateral parts of the annulus fibrosus with little contribution by the posterior elements [22, 32].

The first few degrees of rotation will be resisted by the collagen fibres in the annulus fibrosus. The alternating angle of orientation in subsequent layers of the annulus means that only the fibres oriented in the direction of rotation will be stretched by the movement [15]. At approximately $3°$ of rotation, the movement will be resisted by the impaction of the facets of one of the zygapophyseal joints. This protects the annulus which risks failure at this point [7]. Rotation is unlikely to strain the ligaments [18].

Axial compression of a motion segment is resisted by the intervertebral disc. The incompressibility of the nucleus (a feature of its high water content) means that height loss must be accompanied by radial expansion. This exerts a pressure on the annulus, causing it to bulge outwards (Fig. 1a) and therefore places the collagen fibres in tension. A pressure is also transmitted to the end-plates of the disc.

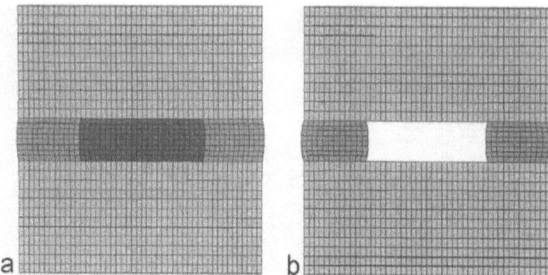

Fig. 1. A simple computer model, developed with the finite element method, of an intervertebral disc subject to an axial compression (Meakin and Hukins, unpublished). In **a** the nucleus (*dark shading*) is present and the walls of the annulus are pushed outwards; in **b** the nucleus has been totally removed and now the inner walls bulge inwards. In this model, the vertebrae (*pale shading*) are assumed to be rigid

They will tend to bulge into the vertebral body [14] and be supported by the cancellous bone. The tension in the annulus and end-plates thus enables them to contain the pressurised nucleus. Maintaining axial compression causes water from the nucleus to be lost gradually. This is responsible for the creep (change in height over time for a fixed load) and stress relaxation (change in stress over time for a fixed displacement) effects seen in an intervertebral disc. Extreme compression may also result in the tips of the inferior articular processes of the upper vertebrae impacting on the lamina below [4].

Removal of Nucleus Pulposus

Several procedures, including laser ablation, reduce the volume of the nucleus pulposus with the intention of decompressing the intervertebral disc to relieve sciatic pain. A number of changes can subsequently be observed, which have immediate effects on the mechanics of the motion segment and may have further repercussions.

The changes most easily observed are those of reduced disc height and increased bulging of the external margins of the annulus [5, 23, 31]. This height loss may compromise the alignment of the zygapophyseal joints in such a way that they are then subject to higher pressures, possibly causing pain [6]. It has also been found that experimental removal of nucleus pulposus reduces intradiscal pressure [5, 20, 31] and stiffness [23] while the rate of creep and stress relaxation is increased [23].

Internal changes to the disc can also be observed, particularly in the inner margins of the annulus. Investigation of decompressed sheep lumbar discs showed that the inner layers of the annulus had folded inwards towards the centre of the disc [13]. Experiments and computer models to investigate the behaviour of the annulus during axial compres-

sion, before and after total nucleotomy, also demonstrate that while the outer layers of the annulus bulge outwards, the inner walls move outwards before nucleotomy (Fig. 1a), and inwards after nucleotomy (Fig. 1b). Where the inner and outer margins of the disc move in opposite directions, the successive layers of the annulus may be pulled apart and lead to delamination and disc degeneration [11]. To counter this phenomenon, due consideration may need to be given to the proposal that the nucleus pulposus be replaced with some biologically inert, synthetic material, to allow restoration of near-normal discal mechanics.

Stabilisation of a Motion Segment

Decompression of the intervertebral disc is one factor which can sometimes lead to spinal instability. The spine can be stabilised by fusion of the affected level. The increasing variety of implants being developed has led to much research into the biomechanics of spinal fixation.

Spinal implants are currently evaluated before implantation in two ways: computer modelling with the finite element technique and mechanical testing. Finite element modelling [24] can provide useful information on the stresses induced in an implant, or one of its components, under defined loading conditions (Fig. 2). Modelling is important at the development stage to avoid excessive prototyping. However, any information obtained from a finite element analysis is only as good as the information put into the model. Finite element analysis is a useful tool only if applied sensibly to the design process.

The use of different test methods and test protocols has led to difficulties in comparing the mechanical characteristics of different implant. However, the American Society for Testing and Materials' standard

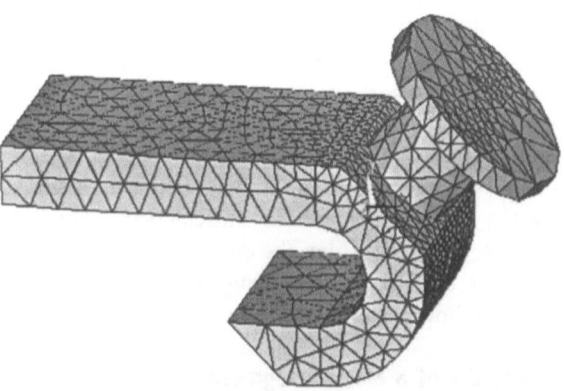

Fig. 2. A finite element model of a hook designed for attachment to the lamina of a vertebra. In this model, the hook is broken down into small three-dimensional elements. The stress in each element was calculated to determine the stress distribution in the hook

on the testing of spinal implants, by a corpectomy model [3], contains guidelines on test configurations and protocols for all cervical, thoracic and lumbar spinal implants. It is now standard practice to perform a number of static axial compression, static compression bending, static tension bending and static torsion tests on implants. However, problems can occur during torsional testing of some implant designs [21]. A compression bending fatigue test is also recommended to obtain information on the performance of a construct over time. Both finite element analysis and mechanical testing are essential for assessing spinal implant in vitro. However, these techniques cannot provide information on implant performance in vivo. This can only be assessed clinically or radiologically.

The primary goal of spinal instrumentation is to stabilise a motion segment in order to allow solid bony fusion to take place. Fusion is encouraged by preventing excessive load transfer and intervertebral movement at the index level. However, the implant must allow sufficient mechanical load transfer across the fusion site to enhance bone growth and prevent bone resorption through stress shielding. It is impossible to predict the exact effect of a stabilisation system on the fused level and those adjacent to it. In a canine model, bone mineral content was reduced in the vertebra adjacent to the implant [34]. This is consistent with the results of McAfee et al. [25], who found that rigid internal fixation leads to stress-shielding of the vertebral bodies within the stabilised segments. An increase in spinal stenosis/spondyloysis, both above and below the fusion level, has also been noted [10]. Concerns about these effects of rigid stabilisation have led to the development of both semi-rigid and, more recently, flexible devices.

Flexible devices such as the Global System (SEM, Montrouge, France) are used to stabilise the spine without fusion. By locking the zygapophyseal joints with a force of 50 N [30], it has been found that these flexible devices can stabilise the spine while allowing a limited amount of motion [35]. Early results of flexible fixation have been very promising [12]. Fixation by flexible stabilisation is quicker, less invasive than conventional stabilisation methods, and is used without bone grafting [9]. These reasons alone indicate that flexible fixation may be the stabilisation technique of choice for some patients.

Whole Spine

Although the behaviour of a motion segment does provide certain useful information for the understanding of the biomechnics of the spine, it fails to provide comprehensive information on the functioning of the whole spine. The observation that fusion of a vertebral level may affect the behaviour of the motion segments at adjacent levels necessitates consideration of the mechanics of the whole spine.

For many purposes, muscles need to be considered as part of the spine. The forces generated by the muscles are not only meant to initiate spinal movement but are also needed to maintain spinal equilibrium [36]. Furthermore, muscular actions must control spinal movements, bring about sudden acceleration and deceleration of the moving body and cause the moving body to stop or maintain it in a desired position [17, 26]. The distinction between the forces generated by connective tissues, such as ligaments, and the forces generated by muscles is that the former are passive whereas the latter are active. Passive components can only exert a force because they tend to recoil to their original dimensions when they have been deformed by an applied force. Active components produce a force without the need for an external force being applied to them; thus muscles generate a force by converting chemical energy (from the hydrolysis of ATP) into mechanical energy. In addition, spinal flexibility and the musculature are essential for shock absorption [33]. Thus the spine requires its active muscular components, as well as its passive ligamentous components, for static equilibrium and control of movement.

Spinal curvature is an obvious structural feature which is expected to have biomechanical consequences. Biomechanical factors in the aetiology of idiopathic scoliosis provide an example [28]. The importance of curvature and flexibility for the function of the spine have been described recently; this description demonstrates that an increase in abdominal pressure and tension in the thoraco–lumbar fascia provides mechanical support to the spine [2]. This description is one of several models for the biomechanics of the intact spine [27].

It may be concluded that the understanding of spinal biomechanics requires a comprehensive understanding of the function of the entire spinal column and its supporting structures. This not only involves a detailed analysis of the structure and function of the individual components of the spine, but also the entire musculo–skeletal system that may have direct or indirect bearing on spinal mechanics in static and dynamic states.

■ Acknowledgments.

We thank the Biotechnology & Biological Sciences Research Council, Smith & Nephew Group Research Centre and Surgicraft Ltd for supporting this research.

References

[1] Adams MA, Dolan P, Hutton WC (1988) The lumbar spine in backward bending. Spine 13:1019–1026

[2] Aspden RM (1995) The curved, flexible spine and the functions of ligaments and muscles. In: Aspden RM, Porter RW (eds) Lumbar Spine Disorders: Current Concepts. World Scientific, Singapore, pp 1–14

[3] ASTM (American Society for Testing and Materials) (1996) Standard test methods for static and fatigue for spinal implant constants in a corpectomy model. F1717/ASTM

[4] Bogduk N, Twomey LT (1991) Clinical Anatomy of the Lumbar Spine, 3nd edn. Churchill Livingstone, Melbourne

[5] Brinckmann, P, Grootenboer H (1991) Change of disc height, radial disc bulge, and intradiscal pressure from discectomy. An in vitro investigation on human lumbar discs. Spine 16:641–646

[6] Dunlop RB, Adams MA, Hutton WC (1984) Disc space narrowing and the lumbar facet joints. Journal of Bone and Joint Surgery B66:706–710

[7] Farfan HF, Cossette JW, Robertson GH, Wells RV, Kraus H (1970) The effects of torsion on the lumbar intervertebral joints: the role of torsion in the production of disc degeneration. Journal of Bone and Joint Surgery 52A:468–497

[8] Fennell AJ, Jones AP, Hukins DWL (1996) Migration of the nucleus pulposus within the intervertebral disc during flexion and extension of the spine. Spine 21:2753–3757

[9] Gardner ADH (1995) Lumbo-sacral and spondylo-pelvic arthrodesis. In: Aspden RM, Porter RW (eds) Lumbar Spined Disorder: Current Concepts. World Scientific, Singapore, pp 185–208

[10] Goel VK, Lim T-H, Gwon J, Chen J-Y, Winterbottom JM, Park JB, Weinstein JN, Ahn J-Y (1991) Effects of rigidity of an internal fixation device. A comprehensive biomechanical investigation. Spine 16:s155–s161

[11] Goel VK, Monroe BT, Gilbertson LG, Brinchmann P (1995) Interlaminar shear stresses and laminae separation in a disc: finite element analysis of the L3–L4 motion segment subjected to axial compressive loads. Spine 20:689–698

[12] Grevitt MP, Gardner ADH, Spilsbury J, Shackleford IM, Baskerville R, Pursell LM, Hassaan A, Mulholland RC (1995) The Graf stabilisation system: early results in 50 patients. European Spine Journal 4:169–175

[13] Gunzburg R, Fraser RD, Moore R, Vernon-Roberts B (1993) An experimental study comparing percutaneous discectomy with chemonucleolysis. Spine 18:218–226

[14] Holmes AD, Hukins DWL, Freemont AJ (1993) End-plate displacement during compression of lumbar vertebra-disc-vertebra segments and the mechanism of failure. Spine 18:128–135

[15] Hukins DWL (1988) Disc structure and function. In: Ghosh P (ed) The Biology of the Intervertebral Disc. CRC-Press, Boca Raton, vol 1, pp 1–39

[16] Hukins DWL (1994) Biomechanics of the spine, In: Klippel JH, Dieppe PA (eds) Rheumatology. Gower Medical, London, pp 5.3.1–5.3.8

[17] Hukins DWL (1995) What is lumbar instability? In: Aspden RM, Porter RW (eds) Lumbar Spine Disorders: Current Concepts. World Scientific, Singapore, pp 26–37

[18] Hukins DWL, Kirby MC, Sikiryn TA, Aspden RM, Cox AJ (1990) Comparison of structure, mechanical properties, and functions of lumbar spinal ligaments. Spine 15:787–795

[19] Jacob RP, Mack CA, Fessler RG (1994) Pedicle screws: biomechanics, uses, and current assessment of outcomes. Neurosurgery Quarterly 4:39–50

[20] Leonard D (1995) The effect of arthroscopic microdiscectomy (AMD) on the response to loading of lumbar motion segments. PhD thesis, University of Manchester

[21] Leahy JC, Anthony ME (unpublished work) Experience of testing spinal constructs to the ASTM standard in torsion

[22] Markolf KL (1972) Deformation of the thoracolumbar intervertebral joints in response to external loads: a biomechanical study using autopsy material. Journal of Bone and Joint Surgery 54A:511–533

[23] Markolf KL, Morris JM (1974) The structural components of the intervertebral disc. A study of their contributions to the ability of the disc to withstand compressive forces. Journal of Bone and Joint Surgery 56A:675–587

[24] Mathias KJ, Meakin JR, Heaton A, Brian MW, Mierendorff S, Aspden RM, Leahy JC, Hukins DWL (1997) Orthopaedic applications of finite element analysis. Proceedings of the NAFEMS World Conference 97. NAFEMS, Glasgow, pp 752–762

[25] McAfee PC, Farey ID, Sutterlin CE, Gurr KR, Warden KE, Cunningham BW (1989) Device-related osteoporosis with spinal instrumentation. Spine 14:919–926

[26] Meakin JR, Hukins DWL, Aspden RM (1996) Euler buckling as a model for the curvature and flexion of the human lumbar spine. Proceedings of the Royal Society B263:1383–1387

[27] Meakin JR, Aspden RM, Hukins DWL (1998) Biomechanical models of the human lumbar spine. Comments on Theoretical Biology 5:49–68

[28] Millner PA, Dickson RA (1996) Idiopathic scoliosis: biomechanics and biology. European Spine Journal 5:362–373

[29] Nachemson A (1987) Lumbar intradiscal pressure. In: Jayson MIV (ed) The Lumbar Spine and Back Pain, 3rd ed. Churchill Livingstone, Edinburgh, pp 191–203

[30] Papp T, Porter RW, Aspden RM, Sheppard JAN (1997) An in vitro study of the biomechanical effects of flexible stabilization on the lumbar spine. Spine 22:151–155

[31] Shea M, Takeuchi TY, Wittenberg RH, White AA III, Hayes WC (1994) A comparison of the effects of automated percutaneous discectomy and conventional discectomy on intradiscal pressure, disc geometry, and stiffness. Journal of Spinal Disorders 7:317–325

[32] Schultz AB, Warwick DN, Berkson MH, Nachemson AL (1979) Mechanical properties of human lumbar spine motion segments. Part 1: Responses in flexion, extension, lateral bending, and torsion. Journal of Biomechanical Engineering 101:46–52

[33] Smeathers JE (1994) Shocking news about discs. Current Orthopaedics 8:45–48

[34] Smith KR, Hunt TR, Asher MA, Anderson HC, Carson WL, Robinson RG (1991) The effect of a stiff spinal implant on the bone-mineral content of the lumbar spine in dogs. Journal of Bone & Joint Surgery 73A:115–123

[35] Strauss PJ, Novotny JE, Wilder DG, Grobler LJ, Pope MH (1994) Multidirectional stability of the Graf system. Spine 19:965–972

[36] Yettram AL, Jackman MJ (1980) Equilibrium analysis for the forces in the human spinal column and its musculature. Spine 5:402–411

Clinical Instability of the Lumbar Spine After Microdiscectomy

E. KOTILAINEN

Introduction

According to various reports, the postoperative results after microdiscectomy have been good or excellent in 75% to 96% of the patients [1, 6, 11, 13, 19, 29, 39, 50]. Yet, the occurrence of subsequent low back pain has been quite common in many series. Up to 38% of the patients who have undergone lumbar discectomy have an unsatisfactory outcome [1, 6, 10, 11, 15, 21, 33]. Recurrent disc herniation, central or lateral stenosis, epidural fibrosis and scarring are regarded as the most common causes of the failed back surgery syndrome [3, 5, 22, 30, 38]. Segmental instability of the lumbar spine is another potential source of unsatisfactory results after lumbar disc surgery [2, 3, 14, 27, 34, 40].

Segmental Instability of the Lumbar Spine

Segmental instability of the lumbar spine is defined as abnormal motion between two or more vertebrae [17, 27, 44]. When extensive, the movement may cause mechanical deformation of the intraspinal nerve tissue and, thereby, induce pain and/or neurologic deficits. The clinical history associated with this condition may include recurrent episodes of low back pain, sometimes associated with scoliosis [25, 41, 45]. Frequently, the patient has pain in the leg and signs of nerve root tension. The pain episodes are thought to become more frequent and severe as the condition progresses [48]. Although segmental instability of the lumbar spine is frequently cited as a potential cause of the low back pain, the clinical importance of this entity has so far not been definitely proven [4, 8, 37, 48]. Correlation between radiological findings and clinical findings has been poor [16, 37, 45]. Equally, radiological evidence of instability does not always correlate with the clinical presentation of a patient [4, 8, 12, 16, 18, 45, 46, 48].

Methods to Detect Instability

Radiological and clinical methods are used to determine segmental instability of the spine. The radiographic signs of this condition include traction spurs, disc-space narrowing, asymmetric collapse of the disc flexion–extension movements, malalignment of the vertebrae in the sagittal plane and abnormal translation and/or retrolisthesis during flexion and extension [26, 31].

Radiological Instability

According to Selby [47] and Frymoyer and Selby [17], lumbar-spine instability can be radiologically divided into five different types:
- *Instability associated with disc herniation or disc degeneration* is the most common form of instability. Approximately 17% to 35% of all patients with low back pain and disc herniation have findings indicative of lumbar instability [17, 35, 42, 49]. In addition, isolated disc resorption may lead to instability and intractable back pain [7]. The patient often has a specific history of significant trauma although there are no radiographic signs of skeletal injury. The only diagnostic clue may be the reproduction of the pain during discography.
- *Rotational instability* occurs most often at the L4–L5 or L5–S1 levels. This type of instability is due to the horizontal alignment of the facet joints. X-rays may show traction spurs [31]. Forward subluxation may be demonstrated on flexion–extension radiology.
- *Translational instability* is the classic form of instability. It may be verified radiographically in flexion–extension views as a forward translation and increased angulation at the disc space [26]. There is a particular increase in the back pain, frequently accompanied by ratcheting, as the patient rises from a bent to an erect position.
- *Retrolisthesis* is a backward subluxation of a vertebra commonly found at the L5–S1 level. The condition is more common in males than in females.

Retrolisthesis with increased angulation can be demonstrated radiographically on flexion–extension films and may be a variant of rotational instability.

- *Postsurgical instability* may develop after extensive laminectomies. Removal of 30 % to 50 % of the facets may be sufficient to produce postoperative instability [17, 43].

Clinical Instability

The three most important criteria of clinical instability have been described [25, 27, 36, 37, 41, 45]. The criteria include (1) the "instability catch", (2) the "painful catch" and (3) "apprehension".

When the "instability catch" is examined for, the patient is asked to bend the body forward as far as possible and then return to an erect position. The test result is abnormal if the return from the bent position fails because of a sudden attack of low back pain. The "painful catch" is studied by asking the patient to lift up a straight leg and then let it slowly return to the examination table. The test result is abnormal if the leg frops suddenly because of sharp pain in the lower back. Finally, if the patient feels anxiety because of a sensation of collapse of the low back due to sudden onset of back pain when moving, the "apprehension" symptom is present.

Occurrence of Clinical Instability After Discectomy

So far, little is known about the development and progression of spinal instability after lumbar-disc surgery. It is, however, clear that extensive laminectomy, when used to treat spinal stenosis, may accelerate lumbar instability [9, 23, 24]. Lumbar-disc surgery (i. e., laminectomy or radical curettage of the disc material) may increase the risk of instability [20]. Taken together, it seems prudent to reason that in patients with instability, sparing operative methods might be preferable to standard disc surgery. In this regard, the theoretical benefits afforded by microinvasive discectomy are to be preferred. This technique permits decompression and evacuation of the bulge of the disc herniation without damaging the facets and articular processes, thus leaving the structures important to segmental stability uncompromised [34].

Kotilainen et al. [27] found that the clinical signs and symptoms of lumbar instability as defined by "instability catch", "painful catch" and "apprehension" occurred in 22 % of 190 patients who had previously undergone microdiscectomy. Correlation between spinal instability and an unsatisfactory outcome was strong. Clinically, instability was significantly associated with a loss of working capacity,

the occurrence of low back pain and disability in daily activities. The symptom of "apprehension" was present in 81 % of the patients. By logistic regression analysis, the "apprehension" symptom was the most strongly associated with an unsatisfactory postoperative outcome as indicated by the occurrence of low back pain, poor working capacity and disability in daily activities. Moreover, of the three instability criteria, only "apprehension" was significantly associated with postoperative sciatic pain. These findings suggest that patients presenting with sciatica and low back pain should be examined for the "apprehension" symptom in order to identify those who may have instability.

In a subsequent study [28], clinical instability of the lumbar spine was detected preoperatively in 24 % of 45 patients who underwent percutaenous nucleotomy. In these patients, clinical instability was significantly associated with an unsatisfactory postoperative outcome: patients with instability again lost their working capacity and suffered from low back pain and sciatica significantly more often than those without instability did.

Conclusion

All patients submitted to lumbar surgery should be carefully examined for the presence of clinical instability. Only a careful examination can aid in selecting the most appropriate operative method for each individual patient. The indications for surgery must be seriously considered in patients with clinical and radiological signs of instability, since their postoperative recovery may be poor. The poor outcome in patients with instability indicates that there is a need to seek alternative therapeutic approaches for the treatment of this specific patient group. Further studies are also needed to evaluate the development and progression of lumbar instability in patients treated by different surgical methods for lumbar disc herniation.

References

[1] Andrews DW, Lavyne MH (1990) Retrospective analysis of microsurgical and standard lumbar discectomy. Spine 15:329–335
[2] Barr JS (1951) Protruded disc and painful backs. J Bone Joint Surg 33-B:3–4
[3] Bernhard TN Jr. (1993) Repeat lumbar spine surgery. Factors influencing outcome. Spine 18:2196–2200
[4] Boden SD, Wiesel SW (1990) Lumbosacral segmental motion in normal individuals. Have we been measuring instability properly? Spine 15:571–576
[5] Burton CV, Kirkaldy-Willis WH, Yong-Hing K, Heithoff KB (1981) Causes of failure of surgery on the lumbar spine. Clin Orthop 157:191–199
[6] Caspar W, Campbell B, Barbier DD, Kretschmer R, Gottfried Y (1991) The Caspar microsurgical discectomy and comparison with a conventional standard lumbar disc procedure. Neurosurgery 28:78–87

[7] Crock HV (1986) Internal disc disruption. A challenge to disc prolapse fifty years on. Spine 11:650–653

[8] Dvorak J, Panjabi MM, Novotny JE, Chang DG, Grob D (1991) Clinical validation of functional flexion–extension roentgenograms of the lumbar spine. Spine 16:943–950

[9] Ebara S, Harada T, Hosono N, Inoue M, Tanaka M, Morimoto Y, Ono K (1992) Intraoperative measurement of lumbar spinal instability. Spine 17(3S):S44–S50

[10] Ebeling U, Kalbaryck H, Reulen HJ (1989) Microsurgical reoperation following lumbar disc surgery. Timing, surgical findings, and outcome in 92 patients. J Neurosurg 70:397–404

[11] Ebeling U, Reichenberg W, Reulen H-J (1986) Results of microsurgical lumbar discectomy. Review of 485 patients. Acta Neurochir (Wien) 81:45–52

[12] Feffer HL, Wiesel SW, Cuckler JM, Rothman RH (1985) Degenerative spondylolisthesis: To fuse or not to fuse. Spine 10:287–289

[13] Frizzell RT, Hadley MN (1993) Lumbar microdiscectomy with medial facetectomy. Techniques and analysis of results. Neurosurg Clin N Am 4:109–115

[14] Frymoyer JW (1981) The role of spine fusion. Question 3. Spine 6:284–290

[15] Frymoyer JW, Hanley E, Howe J, Kuhlmann D, Matteri R (1978) Disc excision and spine fusion in the management of lumbar disc disease. A minimum ten-year follow up. Spine 3:1–6

[16] Frymoyer JW, Hanley EN, Howe J, Kohlmann D, Matteri RE (1979) A comparison of radiographic findings in fusion and in nonfusion patients ten or more years following lumbar disc surgery. Spine 4:435–440

[17] Frymoyer JW, Selby DR (1985) Segmental instability. Rationale for treatment. Spine 10:280–286

[18] Gertzbein SD, Seligman J, Holtby R, Chan KH, Kapasouri A, Tile M, Cruicskhank B (1985) Centrode patterns and segmental instability in degenerative disc disease. Spine 10:257–261

[19] Goald HJ (1981) Microlumbar discectomy: follow-up of 477 patients. J Microsurg 2:95–100

[20] Goel VK, Nishiyama K, Weinstein JN, Liu YK (1986) Mechanical properties of lumbar spinal motion segments as affected by partial disc removal. Spine 11:1008–1012

[21] Gurdjian ES, Ostrowski AZ, Hardy WG, Lindner DW, Thomas LM (1961) Results of operative treatment of protruded and ruptured lumbar discs. J Neurosurg 18:783–791

[22] Hirabayashi S, Kumano K, Ogawa Y, Aota Y, Maehiro S (1993) Microdiscectomy and second operation for lumbar disc herniation. Spine 18: 2206–2211

[23] Iida Y, Kataoka O, Sho T, Sumi M, Hirose T, Bessho Y, Kobayashi D (1990) Postoperative lumbar spinal instability occurring or progressing secondary to laminectomy. Spine 15:1186–1189

[24] Johnsson K-E, Redlund-Johnell I, Uden A, Willner S (1989) Preoperative and postoperative instability in lumbar spinal stenosis. Spine 14:591–593

[25] Kirkaldy-Willis WH, Farfan HF (1982) Instability of the lumbar spine. Clin Orthop 165:110–123

[26] Knutsson F (1944) The instability associated with disc degeneration in the lumbar spine. Acta Radiol 25:593–609

[27] Kotilainen E, Valtonen S (1993) Clinical instability of the lumbar spine after microdiscectomy. Acta Neurochir (Wien) 125:120–126

[28] Kotilainen E, Valtonen S (1994) Percutaneous nucleotomy in the treatment of lumbar disc herniation; results after a mean follow-up of 2 years. Acta Neurochir (Wien) 128:47–52

[29] Kotilainen E, Valtonen S, Carlson C-A (1993) Microsurgical treatment of lumbar disc herniation: Follow-up of 237 patients. Acta Neurochir (Wien) 120:143–149

[30] La Rocca H, MacNab I (1974) The laminectomy membrane. J Bone joint Surg 56B: 545–550

[31] MacNab I (1971) The traction spur: An indicator of segmental instability. J Bone Joint Surg 53A:663–670

[32] Markwalder T-M, Battaglia M (1993) Failed back surgery syndrome. Part 1: Analysis of the clinical presentation and results of testing procedures for instability of the lumbar spine in 171 patients. Acta Neurochir (Wien) 123:46–51

[33] Maroon J, Abla A (1985) Microdiscectomy versus chemonucleolysis. Neurosurgery 16:644–649

[34] Maroon JC, Onik G, Vidovich DV (1993) Percutaneous discectomy for lumbar disc herniation. Neurosurg Clin N Am 4:125–134

[35] Morgan FP, King T (1957) Primary instability of lumbar vertebrae as a common cause of low back pain. J Bone Joint Surg 39B:6–22

[36] Nachemson A (1985) Lumbar spine instability: A critical update and symposium summary. Spine 10:290–291

[37] Nachemson AL (1991) Instability of the lumbar spine. Pathology, treatment, and clinical evaluation. Neurosurg Clin North Am 2:785–790

[38] Naylor A (1974) The late results of laminectomy for lumbar disc prolapse. A review after ten to twenty-five years. J Bone Joint Surg 56B:17–29

[39] Nystrom B (1987) Experience of microsurgical compared with conventional technique in lumbar disc operations. Acta Neurol Scand 76:129–141

[40] O'Brien JP, Dawson MHO, Heard CW, Momberger G, Speck G, Weatherly CR (1986) Simultaneous combined anterior and posterior fusion. A surgical solution for failed spinal surgery with a brief review of the first 150 patients. Clin Orthop 203:191–195

[41] Paris SV (1985) Physical signs of instability. Spine 10: 277–279

[42] Pope MH, Panjabi M (1985) Biomechanical definitions of spinal instability. Spine 10:255–256

[43] Robertson PA, Grobler LH, Novotny JE, Katz JN (1993) Postoperative spondylolisthesis at L4–5. The role of facet joint morphology. Spine 18:1483–1490

[44] Rydevik BL (1992) Pathophysiology of the neural elements in the lumbar spine. J Spinal Disord 5:139–140

[45] Sano S, Yokokura S, Nagata Y, Young SZ (1990) Unstable lumbar spine without hypermobility in post laminectomy cases. Mechanism of symptoms and effect of spinal fusion with and without spinal instrumentation. Spine 15: 1190–1197

[46] Sato H, Kikuchi S (1993) The natural history of radiographic instability of the lumbar spine. Spine 18:2075–2079

[47] Selby DK (1983) When to operate and what to operate upon. Orthop Clin N Am 14:577–588

[48] Stokes IA, Frymoyer JW (1987) Segmental motion and instability. Spine 12:688–691

[49] Weiler PJ, Eng P, King GJ, Gertzbein SD (1990) Analysis of sagittal plane instability of the lumbar spine in vivo. Spine 15:1300–1306

[50] Williarns RW (1993) Lumbar disc disease. Microdiscectomy. Neurosurg Clin N Am 4:101–108

Optical Properties of the Human Lumbar Intervertebral Disc

W. Glinkowski · E. Łukowiak · M. Brzozowska

Introduction

Laser surgery is investigated as a recent alternative approach to arthroscopic and spinal endoscopic surgery. In this field, Nd:YAG (1064 nm, 1320 nm, 1440 nm), Ho:YAG (2100 nm) and Excimer (308 nm) lasers are commonly used [8,10]. Recent reports on the application of different laser systems for ablation and other orthopaedic procedures have been encouraging [1, 3, 8, 9, 10]. The effect of irradiation on a given tissue depends on the laser type, conditions of irradiation and optical properties of the particular tissue. The optimal wavelength and energy output for surgical ablation of connective tissues have not yet been clearly determined. The rationale for using a particular laser type was the assumption that the surgical laser should optimally operate at the same wavelength at which the given tissue has its absorption maximum. Vangsness et al. [12] determined the absorption spectrum for the human meniscus in the 300 to 2500 nm wavelength range. They observed increased absorption at the infrared end of the spectrum; this suggests that the meniscus could also have an absorption peak around 2000 nm, the wavelength of the Ho:YAG laser beam. An aim of the studies was to determine the absorption characteristics of human lumbar intervertebral discs and to find the most efficient wavelength for its laser ablation.

Materials and Methods

Tissue samples of intervertebral discs L4–L5 and L5–S1 were obtained from cadavers at the Department of Legal Medicine. Sampling occurred within 48 h post mortem; the individuals were aged 25 to 50, and their deaths resulted from severe accidents. Specimens were stored in 0.9 % NaCl solution at 4 °C before examination. Spectroscopic measurements were performed within 48 h of sampling. Specimens were classified as healthy tissue on the basis of macroscopic evaluation. Fibrocartilage of the annulus fibrosus and nucleus pulposus were excised and examined separately. The approximate size of each sample was 0.2 mm × 5 mm × 10 mm. Square sections of tissue were prepared at room temperature. For transmission spectroscopy, a Cary Varian 2300 spectrophotometer was employed. The spectral range investigated extended from 221 nm (ultraviolet) to 2800 nm (infrared). Absorption range differences were compared for different tissue samples. Average absorption versus wavelength graphs were plotted for meniscal and intervertebral discs. Baseline glass and water transmission measurements were also made.

Results

Digitized and averaged results of the absorption spectra of the examined tissue are presented in Figs. 1 and 2. Absorption peaks were found in the ranges 236 to 269 nm (max.: 236 nm), 1390 to 1495 nm (max.: 1443 nm), 1875 to 2039 nm (max.: 1908–1921 nm), and 2407 to 2597 nm (max.: 2538 nm) for the nucleus pulposus (Fig. 2). The annulus fibrosus absorption maxima were found in the ranges 223 to 393 nm, 1397 to 1475 nm, 1875 to 2052 nm, and 2439 to 2600 nm. Absorption peaks were consistently found for all specimen sections at 236 nm and 1902–1921 nm, with a smaller peak at 1436 nm (Fig. 1).

The glass absorption curve (Fig. 3) may interfere with the results in a narrow range of ultraviolet and at the end of the examined infrared spectrum. As with the water absorption curve, absorption increases with increased wavelength in the infrared spectrum.

Discussion

The wavelength-dependent transmission properties of fibrocartilage and other musculo-skeletal tissues may be the basis for laser–tissue interaction, hence optimal ablation or coagulation would require a suitable wavelength. This may contribute to the selection or construction of appropriate laser systems for articular and spinal surgery.

Optical properties of biological tissues, as demonstrated by spectroscopic analysis, may underlie the

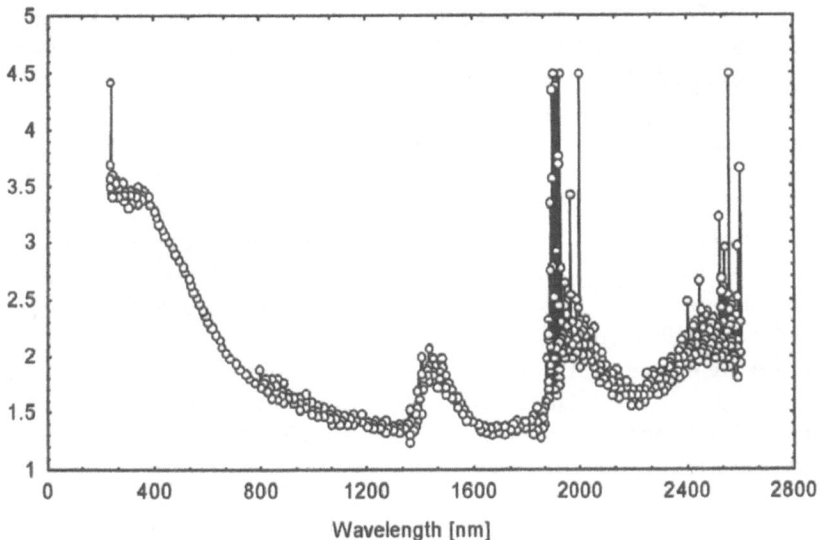

Fig. 1. Average absorption curve for horizontal sections from the annulus fibrosus of the intervertebral discs

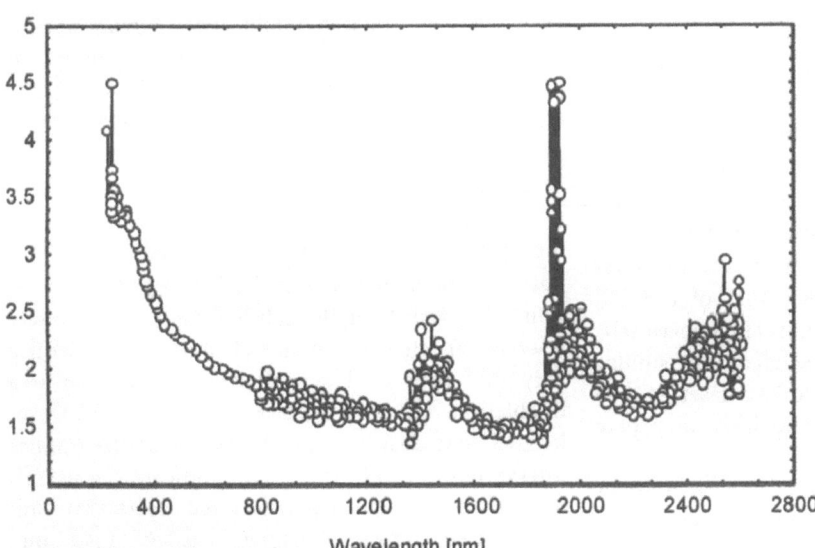

Fig. 2. Average absorption curve for horizontal sections from the nucleus pulposus of the intervertebral discs

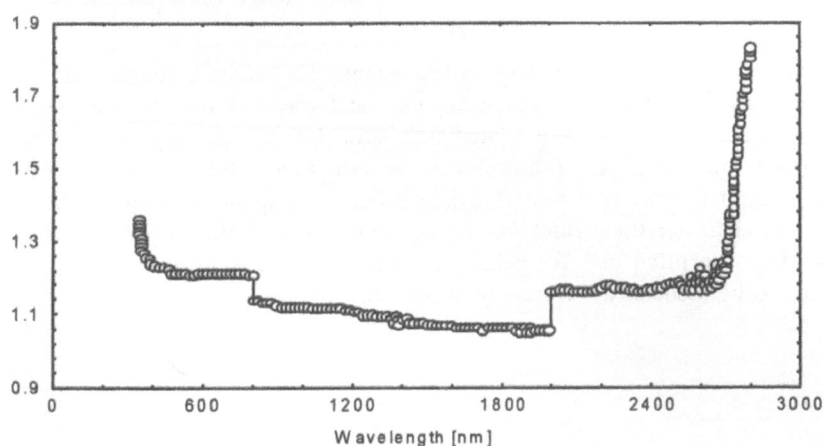

Fig. 3. Absorption curve for glass

mechanisms of laser–tissue interaction [2, 5, 11]. Such an analysis may also predict thermal energy deposition in tissue; from this its consecutive ablation may be determined. Some papers report large differences between in vivo measurements and previous in vitro measurements [4]. More accurate values for the optical properties could be obtained by pulse photothermal radiometry and time-resolved reflectance spectroscopy [2, 4, 6]. These techniques can be used in noninvasive in vivo measurements. Optical properties measured in vitro are still used as estimates for in vivo values, which are diffcult to measure.

It is thought that the efficacy of laser energy-tissue coupling increases with light absorption. The wider spectrophotometer range allowed evaluation of wavelengths from the electromagnetic spectrum ranging from 221 to 2800 nm. It is expected that the CO_2 laser (10600 nm) may have greater absorption, but strict measurements have not been performed.

High absorption peaks appear around 1900 nm, below 350 nm, and above 2500 nm. The results indicate the usefulness of the excimer laser, and the potential usefulness of the Er:YAG laser in this field. Spectrophotometry has not provided an explanation for the clinical observation that the Ho:YAG laser beam perfectly ablates the meniscus. The level of absorption at 2100 nm equals that of a small peak of absorption around 1400 nm. The intervertebral disc absorption could be considered to be similar for the Ho:YAG laser and the Nd:YAG laser – 1440 nm. Other features of the Ho:YAG laser may play an important role.

Vangsness et al. noted that tissue from different zones and tissue planes of different tissue thicknesses and of different ages have similar absorption curves [12]. The observed similarities also apply for intervertebral discs, but this needs to be confirmed by another study.

There were no significant differences between the optical properties of the nucleus pulposus and the annulus fibrosus.

The similarities between the absorption curves of water and the intervertebral disc suggest that water content mainly influences absorption characteristics in the infrared region. The increasing absorption in the UV range has been considered to be associated with the presence of collagen proteins [12]. Chromophores of fibrocartilage (water and collagen proteins) are considered to be key factors for the absorption peaks of the spectrophotometer curves.

The temperature increase within the tissue was suggested [7] to be an important factor influencing irreversibility of changes in optical properties after laser irradiation. This phenomenon seems to be less important when normal saline or Ringer solution is used to clean the superficial coagulated or charred layer of the tissue.

If tissue-specific absorption characteristics related to spectral analysis are taken into consideration, the problem of selective tissue ablation may be finally solved.

Conclusions

Selective laser ablation would allow a reduction in iatrogenic damage, if it is applied toward the optical properties of normal pathological joint tissue. Spectrophotometer evaluation of musculo-skeletal tissue predicts the laser type that could be successfully used for spinal endoscopic surgery. Thermal laser-tissue interaction brings about some alterations in the optical properties of the irradiated tissue. This observed phenomenon may lead to a reduced ablation effectiveness of the selected laser. An accurate laser is expected to produce ablation craters with a very thin layer of damaged tissue around the area of ablation. The results presented indicate the wavelengths best absorbed by the tissue of the lumbar intervertebral discs. The results indicate the usefulness of the ultraviolet and infrared lasers that emit in selected ranges (excimer, Nd:YAG–1440 nm, Ho:YAG and potentially Tu:YAG and Er:YAG laser), to obtain the optimal ablative effect on the intervertebral disc.

■ **Acknowledgements.** The authors thank Prof. A. Dubrzyński, head and Chair of the Department of Legal Medicine, and Mr. T. Jędral, ASC, for his technical help in obtaining tissue specimens. The authors acknowledge the support of Prof. W. Stręk and Dr. G. Dominiak-Dzik, PhD, Institute of Low Temperatures and Structural Research, Polish Academy of Sciences, Wroclaw.

References

[1] Buchelt M, Kutschera H-P, Katterschafka, T, Kiss H, Schneider B, Ullrich R (1992) Erb:YAG and Ho:YAG laser ablation of meniscus and intervertebral discs. Lasers in Surgery and Medicine 12:375–381

[2] Cheong WF, Prahl SA, Welch AJ (1990) A review of the optical properties of biological tissues. III J Quantum Electron 26(12):2166–2185

[3] Glinkowski W, Brzozowska M, Ciszek B, Rowiński J, Stręk W (1996) Effects of Er:YAG laser irradiation on human cartilage. Proc SPIE 2781:184–187

[4] Graaff R, Dassel ACM, Koelink MH, de Mul FFM, Aarnoudse JG, Zijlstra WG (1993) Optical properties of human dermis in vitro and in vivo. Appl Opt 32(4):435–447

[5] Izatt JA, Albagli D, Britton M, Jubas JM, Itzkan I, Feld MS (1991) Wave length dependence of pulsed laser ablation of calcified tissue. Lasers in Surgery and Medicine 11:238–249

[6] Prahl SA, Vitkin IA, Bruggemann U, Wilson BC, Anderson RR (1992) Determination of optical properties of turbid media using pulse photothermal radiometry. Phys Med Biol 37(6):1203–1217

[7] Raunest J, Scharzmaier H-J (1995) Optical properties of human articular tissue as implication for a selective laser application in arthroscopic surgery. Lasers in Surgery and Medicine 16:253–261

[8] Sherk HH (1993) The use of lasers in orthopaedic procedures. J Bone Joint Surg [Am] 75:768–776

[9] Sherk HH, Black JD, Prodoehl JA, Diven J (1995) The effects of lasers and electrosurgical devices on human meniscal tissue. Clin Orthop Rel Res 310:14–20

[10] Siebert W (1993) Percutaneous laser disc decompression (PLDD); the European experience. Spine 7:103–132

[11] Torres JH, Welch AJ, Cilesiz I, Motamedi M (1996) Tissue optical property measurements: overestimation of absorption coefficient with spectrophotometric techniques. Lasers in Surgery and Medicine 14:249–257

[12] Vangsness CT, Huang J, Smith CF (1995) A spectrophotometer analysis of light absorption in the human meniscus. Clin Orthop Rel Res 310:27–29

Clinical Results of Percutaneous Laser Disc Decompression and Targeted Literature Review

S. Schmolke · F. Gossé · O. Rühmann

Introduction

Introduced in 1986, percutaneous laser disc decompression (PLDD) has become one of the most frequently performed routine procedures in the management of herniated lumbar intervertebral discs. Due to its minimally invasive character, this procedure is often recognized as the last "conservative" treatment possibility [2, 4, 9, 22]. The principal points of criticism are its highly selective indication and occasionally the short-term effect [4]. Over the past few years, PLDD has been a controversial subject, necessitating a review of the indications and application of this procedure [5, 16, 23, 27].

The aim of this retrospective study was to investigate the medium-term results of PLDD. Pain and specifically back pain present in different ways in patients. Depending on the degree of activity and the subjective pain sensitivity, back pain can restrict day-to-day life in several different ways [11, 14, 18, 20, 21]. For our investigation, we used the clinical questionnaires compiled by Roland and Morris in 1983 for the assessment of back pain [20, 21]. The score system was expanded with a visual analog chart for pain and another visual analog chart for patients to enter their own assessment of the result of the operation. Since almost one-third of all patients undergoing PLDD lived further than 250 km away, a questionnaire was used to gather the information without these patients being required to turn up for clinical examination. The preoperative and postoperative results were analyzed with regard to age and sex.

Materials and Methods

The questionnaires were filled out by 150 of 180 patients. Two patients died during the course of this study and 28 patients moved and failed to leave a forwarding address. Final follow-up cohort integrity was therefore 84%. The patients were placed into five groups; each group representing one of five periods of follow-up between one and five years postoperatively.

The Roland–Morris score (RMS) served to form the subjective assessment of back pain. The score system is based on the restrictions faced by the patients in their day-to-day life and estimates the degree of activity of the individual. The maximum score of 24 points corresponds to the most severe case of restriction of day-to-day activity. Lower scores indicate less severe restriction within the social environment [20, 21]. The Roland–Morris score (RMS) was supplemented with a visual analog chart for pain with values between 0 to 10 points. A further analog chart with points between 0 to 10 was presented to each patient from which he/she could make an individual assessment of the operation result. The highest level of pain is indicated by 10 points on the pain chart and 0 points indicate that the patient is completely pain-free (Fig. 1). Between 1990 and 1996, 180 patients were treated with PLDD at the Orthopedic Clinic, Hannover Medical School, mostly presenting with complaints in the region of L4/L5 and L5/S1. These criteria for selection and exclusion of patients are given in Tables 1 and 2 [5, 9, 12, 16, 18].

Inclusion Criteria

In each case, the level treated was restricted to radiologically proven nonsequestered herniated intervertebral discs. All patients demonstrated a clear correlation between the clinical symptoms and the radiological findings [4, 18, 16, 22].

A Nd:YAG laser was used for 31 patients and a Ho:YAG laser was used for 149 patients. Several studies have already shown that the choice of the laser system for the lumbar spine region has no significant influence on the success of the treatment (Table 3). A decisive factor is the amount of energy transmitted to the target discal volume and the changes in the biochemical milieu in the intervertebral disc tissue [1, 6, 8, 10, 17, 24, 26, 27].

Statistics

The statistical evaluations for comparison of average differences between the recorded preoperative and postoperative scores were carried out using the

Medizinische Hochschule Hannover

Orthopedic Department

Name: _____

Date: _____

- ☐ I stay at home most of the time because of my back
- ☐ I change position frequently to try and get my back comfortable
- ☐ I walk more slowly than usual because of my back
- ☐ Because of my back I am not doing any of the jobs that I usually do around the house
- ☐ Because of my back, I use a handrail to get upstairs
- ☐ Because of my back, I lie down to rest more often
- ☐ Because of my back, I have to hold on to something to get out of an easy chair
- ☐ Because of my back, I try to get other people to do things for me
- ☐ I get dressed more slowly than usual because of my back
- ☐ I only stand up for short periods of time because of my back
- ☐ Because of my back, I try not to bend or kneel down
- ☐ I find it difficult to get out of a chair because of my back
- ☐ My back is painful almost all the time
- ☐ I find it difficult to turn over in bed because of my back
- ☐ My appetite is not very good because of my back
- ☐ I have trouble putting on my socks (or stockings) because of the pain in my back
- ☐ I only walk short distances because of my back
- ☐ I sleep less well because of my back
- ☐ Because of my back pain, I get dressed with help from someone else
- ☐ I sit down for most of the day because of my back
- ☐ I avoid heavy jobs around the house because of my back
- ☐ Because of my back, I am more irritable and bad tempered with people than usual
- ☐ Because of my back, I go upstairs slower than usual
- ☐ I stay in bed most of the time because of my back

Pain Scale

no pain |⌐ 0 1 2 3 4 5 6 7 8 9 10 ⌐| intolerable pain

With the operation, I'm

very satisfied |⌐ 0 1 2 3 4 5 6 7 8 9 10 ⌐| not satisfied

no change

- ☐ repeat intervertebral disc operation on .... due to persistent complaints

- ☐ administration of pain killers
  - ☐ regularly   ☐ from time to time

Fig. 1. Patient questionnaire

Table 1. Indications for PLDD

Clinical	Morphological
Unsuccessful conservative therapy (3-months outpatient, 2-weeks inpatient therapy)	Protrusion
Radicular symptoms	Subligamentous prolapse (contained herniation)
Clinical symptoms with correlating radiological findings (CT/MRI)	

Table 2. Contraindications for PLDD

Clinical	Morphological
Cauda syndrome	Free sequestered disc herniation
Failed back surgery syndrome	Osseous nerve-root compression
General contraindications, e.g., instable angina pectoris, coagulation defects	Severe instability of the mobile segment
Suspended compensation procedure	
	Recurrence following PLDD of the same intervertebral disc

Table 3. Comparison of success rates (PLDD)

Author	Success rate	Criteria	Laser system	Follow-up	Reference
Casper 1995	84%	McNab criteria	Ho:YAG	1 year	[3]
Choy 1995	75%	McNab criteria	Ho:YAG Nd:YAG	5 years	[5]
Liebler 1995	75%	McNab criteria	KTP	1 year	[14]
Liebler 1995	70%	McNab criteria	Nd:YAG	1 year	[14]
Ohnmeiss 1994	71%	dependent on patient selection	KTP/532	1 year	[18]
Siebert 1996	78%	psychological assessment, "pain-drawings"	Ho:YAG	4 years	[26]

t-test for dependent random samples. To identify the impact of each of the factors under study in the five groups of patients, analysis of variance (ANOVA) was used with a 95% confidence interval. For evaluation of validity of the final results given by the Roland–Morris score and the pain chart, the correlation between the corresponding preoperative and postoperative pairs of values was recorded. For interval-scaled variables which were not "normal", the Spearman rank correlation tests were performed.

Percutaneous Laser Disc Decompression – Indication and Technique

The mildly sedated and anesthetized patients were placed in a prone or side position with the affected side facing up. The patient would have to be in a cooperative state during the procedure. After infiltration of the skin with 5 ml of 1% lidocaine, a stab incision was made and infiltration of the subcutaneous tissue and musculature continued along the puncture channel to the intervertebral space. The intervertebral disc itself was punctured with a discography needle under image intensifier control. Entering through a corridor 9–12 cm lateral to the midline, the needle was pushed to an angle of 45° in a horizontal direction to the intervertebral disc. A final discography pattern under image intensifier control was documented in two planes and the correct position was confirmed. Should a so-called memory pain be induced, then radicular irritation in the corresponding intervertebral disc was inferred. Memory pain was not triggered in all patients. This has been documented by other authors as well [1, 3, 26]. An important factor is that no contrast medium should flow out of the intervertebral space. Outflow of contrast medium though a damaged annulus would be seen as a contraindication for PLDD. The discography needle was then changed for a gold-covered laser cannula over a guide wire. After careful preparation, and after particular attention had been paid to the correct length of fiber, the laser fiber was finally inserted into the intervertebral disc. The projection of the fiber tip was maintained at approximately 3–4 mm beyond the cannula tip. Laser energy was then applied to the disc with continual neurological observation. The position of the needle was confirmed regularly under image intensifier control. A few seconds break was given when each energy aliquot of 50 J had been reached [24]. A drainage device connected to the laser cannula served to drain off any water vapor and products of tissue combustion. This helped to reduce intradiscal pressure and to speed up the cooling process. In the intervertebral disc L4/L5, 1600 J was applied; at the L5/S1 level, 1200 J was applied, independent of the type of laser system used. The operation was completed by the application of a sterile bandage and a final neurological check-up. The position of the laser cannula would usually be shifted around 1 cm after one-half of the required amount of energy had been delivered.

Results

A total of 67 women and 83 men took part in this study. The mean follow-up time was 39 months. The average age of the patients was 46 years with a median of 46 years. The youngest patient was 19 years old, the oldest was 87 years old. Altogether 8 % of patients were younger than 30 years, 56 % were between 31 and 50 years and 36 % were over 50 years.

A further operation within the study period was necessary for 23 patients, (average age 46 years), almost half of which were done in other clinics.

All five groups of patients showed no significant difference with regard to their ages and sex distribution ($p = < 0.001$). There was no difference between the preoperative score of the groups under study. The demographics of the five groups were similar.

The average preoperative Roland–Morris score was 17. The average postoperative Roland–Morris pain score was 8.5. The Roland–Morris score thus showed a decrease of 9 units following laser treatment. This was independent of the follow-up period (Fig. 2).

Sensitivity to pain was reduced on average by 4 units to 4.5 points. The subjective assessment of results came to a value of 3 points on the 0-to-10 scale.

The postoperative scores are those following percutaneous laser disc decompression and are not the scores following revision surgery.

The score results included all the patients who had to undergo repeat surgery showed no statistical difference between the preoperative scores of the whole group (Fig. 3). All groups were classified into three age groups to determine any correlation between age and operation outcome. But here there was no significant difference between the scores of the individual groups either (Fig. 4). A high correlation (0.82) (ONEWAY analysis of variance and the multiple-range test–student–Newman–Keuls procedure) was found between the postoperative scores obtained by using different scales, namely the postoperative evaluation of the Roland–Morris score and the pain scale, and the Roland–Morris score and the self-assessment result.

The main outcome of this study is that there is a significant decrease in the Roland–Morris score and pain after percutaneous laser disc decompression. This significant reduction of scores is independent of the interval between PLDD and follow-up within the 5-year postoperative period.

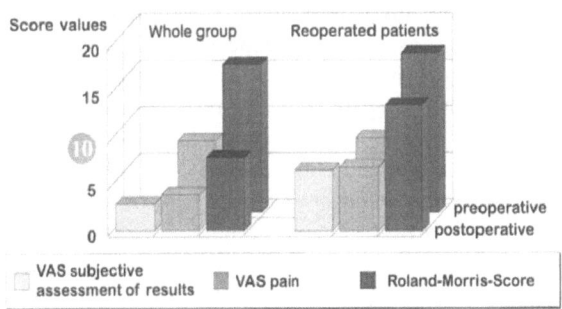

Fig. 3. Results after PLDD – reoperated patients

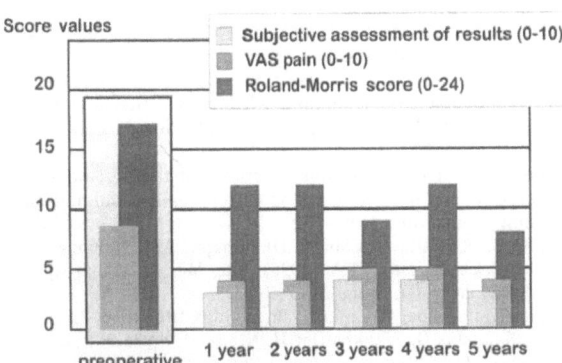

Fig. 2. Results after PLDD

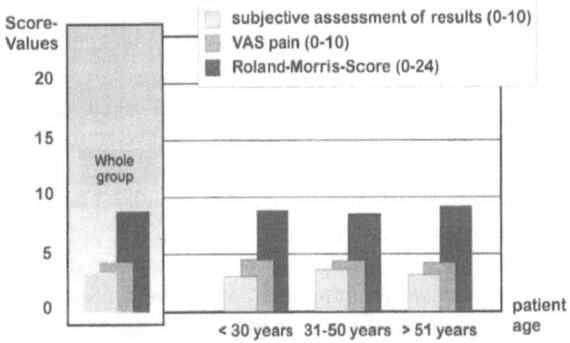

Fig. 4. Results after PLDD – according to age of patients

Discussion

This study looked at PLDD as an intradiscal procedure for the treatment of herniated lumbar intervertebral discs, and reports on the medium-term results following therapy. The outcome is not dependent on the age of the patient or the degree of preoperative activity. The improvement in the pain level after laser treatment and the degree of activity as determined by RMS does not give any evidence of medium-term deterioration over the following 5 years.

In 78 % of the cases, PLDD resulted in an improvement in the RMS; in 55 % of cases, the reduction was more than 10 points. The symptoms of 19 % of the patients did not improve. The scores showed deterioration in 4.3 % of the patients. On the pain scale, 79 % of the treated patients showed a decrease in pain, with 55 % demonstrating more than 3.5 points reduction in the pain scale. However, only a few cases were found to be completely free of pain.

In older patients, the herniated intervertebral disc is not always the sole reason for back pain. Our patients had radiological evidence of degenerative changes (spondylarthrosis, osteochondrosis). Laser treatment was helpful in reducing the intradiscal pressure and the pressure on the afflicted nerve roots. Apart from this, there was definitely a simultaneous change in the biochemical milieu of the intervertebral disc, with liberation of inflammatory substances and stimulation of nociceptors [8, 15, 17, 27]. The sustained improvement suggests that the subsequent liberation was interrupted by this technique.

The study assessed the impact of surgery on the painful disc and the disabilities of the afflicted patients, that is, pain and the restrictions in their day-to-day lives. An assessment with more complex methods of follow-up evaluation to determine the success of the operation, such as pain-drawings for planimetric quantification of pain assessment can only be carried out on a restricted basis. This study shows that the outcome of the treatment is positive for patients. Follow-up studies using the McNab criteria reveal a success rate of between 72 % and 84 % [3, 4, 5, 10, 22, 25, 26]. For several years, the Roland–Morris score has been recognized and has been a widely used scoring system for the subjective assessment of back pain.

Failures have also been reported for PLDD treatment. Unsuccessfully treated patients have retrospectively been found to have moderate spondylarthrosis as an additional cause of persistent complaint besides the unavoidable recurrent intervertebral disc problem.

The fear that post-lasing carbonization particles could cause an inflammatory foreign body reaction, and thus cause increased pain, is not supported by this study.

Conclusion

When indicated, PLDD is a useful and effective method of treatment in a staged treatment plan for patients with symptomatic herniated lumbar intervertebral disc. The intraoperative risks and postoperative complications are insignificant compared to other surgical procedures. The use of the technique outside of strict selection criteria must be considered most critically. Taking into account the possible complications arising from PLDD (discitis, vascular and nerve injury), this minimally invasive procedure must be performed with care. PLDD, like other minimally invasive procedures, requires only a short treatment period.

Recent experimental investigations have revealed that the effectiveness of PLDD is mainly based on the ablation of the nociceptors and the changes in the biochemical milieu [8, 10, 24, 26]. Only around 5 % of the nucleus pulposus tissue can be removed [24]. This indicates that the effect of PLDD is mainly symptomatic rather than effecting major anatomical changes in the disc. It appears to offer a minimally ablative therapeutic procedure.

References

[1] Black PW, Rhodes A, Lane GJ, Uppal GS, Sherk HH (1993) The chronic effects of anterior cervical and percutaneous lumbar discectomy using the Holmium;YAG laser – an animal model. In: Sherk HH (ed) Spine – laser discectomy; vol 7 no 1. Hanley and Belfus, Philadelphia, pp 31–35

[2] Black WA (1995) A neurosurgical perspective on PLDD. J Clin Laser Med Surg 13:167–171

[3] Casper GD, Hartman VL, Mullins LL (1995) Percutaneous laser disc decompression with the Holmium:YAG laser. J Clin Laser Med Surg 13:195–204

[4] Choy DS, Botsford J, Black WA (1995) Patient selection: Indications and contraindications. J Clin Laser Med Surg 13:157–160

[5] Choy DS (1995) Clinical experience and results with 389 PLDD procedures with the Nd:YAG laser, 1986 to 1995. J Clin Laser Med Surg 13:209–214

[6] Choy DS, Altman PA, Case RB, Trokel SL (1991): Laser radiation at various wavelengths for decompression of intervertebral disc. Clin Orthop 267:245–250

[7] Dauch WA, Fasse A, Brücher K, Bauer BL (1994) Prädiktoren des Behandlungserfolges nach mikrochirurgischer Operation lumbaler Bandscheibenvorfälle. Zentralabl Neurochir 55:144–155

[8] Franscon RC, Saal JS, Saal JA (1992) Human disc phospholipase A2 is inflammatory. Spine 17 Suppl:129–132

[9] Gottlob C, Kopchok G, Peng S-H, Tabbara M, Cavaye D, White RA (1992) Holmium:YAG laser ablation of human intervertebral disc: Preliminary evaluation. Lasers Surg Med 12:86–91

[10] Hellinger J (1999) Technical aspects of the percutaneous cervical and lumbar laser disc decompression and nucleotomy. Neurol Res 21:99–102

[11] Keller RB, Atlas SJ, Singer DE, Chapin AM, Mooney NA, Patrick DL, Deyo RA (1996) The Maine lumbar spine study, PartI-III. Spine 21:1769–1795

[12] Larequi-Lauber T, Vader JP, Burnand B, Brook RB, Kosecoff J, Sloutskis D, Frankhauser H, Nerney J, de Tribot N, Paccaud F (1997) Appropriateness of indications for surgery of lumbar disc hernia and spinal stenosis. Spine 22:203–209

[13] Leu H, Schreiber A (1992) Endoskopie der Wirbelsäule: minimal-invasive Therapie. Orthopäde 21:267–272

[14] Liebler WA (1995) Percutaneous laser disc nucleotomy. Clin Orthop 310:58–66

[15] Min K, Leu H, Zweifel K (1996) Quantitative determination of ablation in weight of lumbar intervertebral disc with Holmium:YAG laser. Lasers Surg Med 18:187–790

[16] North RB Campell JN, James CS, Conover-Walker MK, Wang H, Piantadosi S, Rybock JD, Long DM (1991) Failed back surgery syndrome: 5-year follow-up in 102 patients undergoing repeated operation. Neurosurgery 28:685–691

[17] O'Donnell JL, O'Donell AL (1996) Prostaglandin E2 content in herniated lumbar disc disease. Spine 21:1653–1656

[18] Ohnmeiss DD, Guyer RD, Hochschuler SH (1994) Laser disc decompression. The importance of proper patient selection. Spine 19:2054–2058, diskussion 1059

[19] Robertson JT, Huffmon GV, Thomas LB, Leffler CW, Gunter BC, White RP (1996) Prostaglandin production after experimental discectomy. Spine 21:1731–1736

[20] Roland M, Morris R (1983) A study of natural history of back pain. Part I: Development of a reliable and sensitive measure of disability in low-back pain. Spine 8:141–144

[21] Roland M, Morris R (1983) A study of natural history of back pain. Part II: Development of guidelines for trials of treatment in primary care. Spine 8:145–150

[22] Rudolph H, Studtmann V (1996) Der Lasereinsatz in der perkutanen Therapie lumbaler Bandscheibenvorfälle. In: Berlien HP, Müller G (eds) Angewandte Lasermedizin, III-3.11.2. Ecomed, Landsberg

[23] Scale D, Zichner L (1994) Spontanverlauf beim lumbalen Bandscheibenvorfall. Orthopäde 23:236–242

[24] Schlangmann B, Schmolke S, Siebert WE (1996) Temperatur- und Ablationsmessungen bei der Laserbehandlung von Bandscheiben gewebe. Orthopäde 25:3–9

[25] Sheppard J (1992) 50 percutaneous intradiscal decompressions comparing necleotomy and posterior discectomy. J Bone Joint Surg [Br] 74–70

[26] Siebert WE, Berendsen BT, Tollgard J (1996) Die perkutane Laserdiskusdekompression (PLDD). Erfahrungen seit 1989. Orthopäde 25:42–48

[27] Zweifel K, Panoussopoulos A (1996) Laser und Bandscheibenchirurgie – Balfrist Erfahrungen. In: Berlien HP, Müller G (eds) Angewandte Lasermedizin, III-3.11.3. Ecomed, Landsberg

Economic Measurement in Spinal Surgery – The Contribution of Quality-Adjusted Life Years

M. James

Introduction

It is no longer sufficient to establish the efficacy of health care interventions – in an environment with increasing and competing demands on health care resources, it is important to establish efficiency, that is, the benefit per unit of cost, of a health care intervention. In spinal surgery, the comparison may be between surgical techniques, or between surgery and conservative management of back pain. It is therefore impossible to talk about outcomes, in health economics, without relating them to costs. Importantly, choices are always being made both in life and in the surgical specialty of spinal surgery. These choices may be between physical therapy or surgical treatment for back pain, or between a health authority funding either an extra spinal discectomy or an extra hernia repair.

Technical Definitions

Economics has, as one of its main tenets, the concept of efficiency in health care. Economics has as one of its primary objectives the maximisation of efficiency.

Efficiency is the maximisation of benefit per unit of cost (or resource), or, conversely, the minimisation of cost per unit of benefit. That is, in the production of any health care intervention, the aim is not to pursue the cheapest alternative, but to undertake that intervention that will produce the most benefit for a single unit of resource spent. Failure to pursue this objective will result in lost opportunities, not only to the individual, but to society.

Efficiency can be defined in the single product, or across goods and service.

Technical efficiency seeks to maximise benefit per unit of resource in the single product. If, for example, the choice is between two surgical techniques for the treatment of lateral recess stenosis, economics will choose the treatment that maximises the benefit per unit of resource.

Allocative efficiency seeks to maximise the benefits per unit of resource across a range of goods and services. This requires spinal surgery to demonstrate its relative position against other competing health interventions. It further requires measurement of both costs and benefits that enable such comparison. It is with this in mind that this chapter will focus upon the use of utility measurements in spinal surgery and, in particular, the use of the Quality-Adjusted Life Year (QALY), the use of cost utility analysis and league tables as they may apply to spinal surgery. Cost utility league tables allow the comparison of efficiency for a range of goods and services in terms of cost per unit of benefit generated from a health care intervention, where the outcome of the intevention is expressed in terms of cost per quality-adjusted life year.

A *Quality-Adjusted Life Year (QALY)* is a function of the quantity and the quality of life. It recognises that not only is the length of life or the length of a health care intervention important, but that the quality of that life is equally important. It is, importantly, a measure of the *change* following an intervention. Hence, it represents the difference between the quality of life before and after an intervention, or that with and without treatment. It is a measure of change, not a measure of final or absolute outcome.

Opportunity cost is the value of the good in its next-best alternative. Essentially, money spent in general surgery is money no longer available to be spent in spinal surgery. If resources are to be removed from discectomy, where could they be better spent? Could they, for example, be used to fund additional laser surgery? Essentially, quantifying opportunity cost or lost opportunities again requires systematic measurement of benefits and costs in spinal surgery.

Cost: A central element in the production of economic efficiency is cost. It should, however, not be taken to be synonymous with financial valuation; it is, instead, concerned with real resources. The real resources of a health care intervention are those of staff, capital and consumables required to produce that health care intevention. The monetary price is the attempt to attach a financial valuation to such resources.

The choice of benefit measure: To achieve efficiency, that is to maximise the benefit per unit of cost, it must be possible to measure the surgical *outcome* in an objective and comparative fashion.

Three scenarios are possible in the measurement of outcome: clinical methods, disease-specific measures, and generic measures. Although clinical outcomes have dominated in the past, increasing emphasis is being placed on patient-focused and functional outcomes of care.

This is not to dismiss the clinical and disease-specific measures which have an important role in the evaluation in spinal surgery, and provide the measure of benefit required by such economic tools as cost-effectiveness analysis. Clinical indicators are a useful measure of benefit where the desired outcome is a change in the clinically significant indicator. Where clinical indicators fall short is in capturing all the significant outcomes following a health care intervention. To this end, disease-specific scales have been developed across a range of specialties. Disease-specific scales have the advantage of both brevity and sensitivity in small but clinically significant changes in health status (Bowling 1995). Disease-specific scales in back pain include the Roland–Morris (Roland and Morris 1982) and Oswestry disability scales (Fairbank et al. 1980) and measures such as the Million pain index in back pain (Million et al. 1982).

Domain-specific scales, however, may not capture the broad nature of quality of life and are not appropriate for making comparisons of disease outcomes across differing diseases or conditions. The alternative is therefore to use a generic measure of health status. Such measures can be separated into two types of indices and profiles. Profiles measure a range of differing dimensions in health status but do not make any attempt to weigh the various dimensions or to collapse them into a single figure to indicate health status. This presents the decision-maker with the dilemma of rating the relative importance of each dimension. They are often intended not so much as a measure of outcome or change but, instead, as a point-in-time measurement of health status. The index measure seeks to measure change in a number of different dimensions of health status, such as usual activities and pain, but then to collapse such measurements into a holistic and all-encompassing indicator for health status, in the form of a single number. An index measures the change in health status before and after, or with and without, an intervention. The production of a single number, however, can restrict the number, range, and sensitivity of items that can be included in the instrument, and hence may not capture all the clinically significant factors of

the change in health status following a health care intervention.

The remainder of this book will illustrate the choices of disease-specific and clinical measures that are used in the measurement of outcome in spinal surgery. This chapter will focus on the still relatively new concept of a generic index tool in spinal surgery, and the use of the Quality Adjusted Life Year.

Measurement Viewpoint and the Concept of Need

Back pain affects 40 % of the adult population during a year. In the population of back-pain sufferers, 40 % will consult their GP, and 13 % of the population aged 16 to 64 cited back pain as preventing them from taking paid employment (Croft 1996). This evidence indicates that back pain is a crucial issue not only to the health service, but also to the individual and to society.

The perspective or viewpoint adopted is important for measuring the costs and benefits in an economic evaluation.

Possible viewpoints for a study would include:
- the patient
- the patient's family or other carers
- one health care provider (e.g. an acute hospital)
- the broader NHS (adding the primary and community sectors to the above)
- wider governmental services (such as social services
- voluntary services
- society as a whole

In back pain and, hence, spinal surgery, the establishment of the viewpoint will determine the study design and the enumeration of the associated costs and benefits. Back pain is one of the major causes of time lost from employment (Underwood 1998) and, as such, the burden, not only on the patients and their relatives, but on society, in terms of lost production, is considerable. Back pain is, furthermore, a major factor that results in a primary care consultation; hence, any secondary care intervention will have considerable implications for primary and rehabilitative services such as physiotherapy.

It is important to distinguish among the various perspectives, and to clarify the relationship between the concepts of need, health, inequality, and outcome (James 1999).

First, need can be defined as an instrumental concept, that is, the need for something. This is most commonly expressed as the need for a desirable end state (e.g. health or happiness; Lightfoot 1995). The demand for an intermediate state, for example, a health care intervention, is in economics a product of derived demand, as it reflects the desire to attain the end state. People, for example, demand freedom from back pain to enjoy the utility that this brings and because it enables them to pursue their usual activities, such as work or leisure. The direct link between need and outcome is explicitly made here, and Culyer (Culyer 1976) argues that a focus on the need for health is central. However, the definition of health as a desirable end state is fraught with difficulties.

Second, need can be defined by professionals using expert standards. The clearest example is what Bradshaw (Bradshaw 1972, 1994) calls normative need. Another important aspect of understanding need as socially constructed is the voice of the citizens (or users of health/social services). Within the field of social policy, reference is often made to Bradshaw's taxonomy of need (Bradshaw 1972), which defines four different types of need: normative (expert), felt (individually experienced), expressed (demand), and comparative (against a reference group). The problem is then to balance needs against limited resources both within back pain and across other areas of medical care.

Economists have expressed concern about the concept of need (Culyer 1976) and prefer to focus upon understanding the end state required, that is, the outcome and as such the known ability or capacity to benefit from health care. In essence, the key distinction between the economists' definition of need, the capacity to benefit, and need as defined by Doyal and Gough (1993), Soper (1993) and Bradshaw (1972, 1994) is that the latter deal with the "absolute" pre-intervention state, whereas economics examines change in the state once an intervention has been initiated. Hence, economics is concerned with the marginal benefits yielded by competing interventions and with the most efficient ways of meeting needs.

The Concept of Outcome

The concern with using resources efficiently has made the measurement of health outcomes an accepted part of decision-making. Health outcomes can be defined as the changes in health status (of groups or individuals) brought about by an intervention, for example, spinal surgery. Wilkin et al. (1992) state that measuring outcome intends to establish a causal relationship between antecedent and subsequent conditions or events, which in the area of health tends to be seen in terms of achievement or failure to achieve desired goals.

Outcome in the world of health care has, however, until relatively recently focused upon mortality and life expectancy. This represents a rather limited definition of outcome. The crucial issue in outcome assessment is the before and after (or the with and without) measurement of the patient's health state. Calculating the difference in the patient's health state in order to yield a meaningful measure of health gain is the central objective. Therefore, emphasis is placed upon the additional benefit (or the marginal benefit) yielded as a consequence of explicit intervention(s), rather than the final health state being valued for its intrinsic worth per se. This can then be compared to the marginal cost of achieving the health state.

Outcome in health is, however, a function of both quality of life and quantity of life. This implies that, when measuring an individual's (or group's) health status, the question of judging the relative importance of the different dimensions of health cannot be avoided. We move from assessing the intrinsic health state (or outcome) to the contextual valuation of a health state. Or to put it more concretely, what is a desired outcome for the individual or group within the specific societal and cultural context?

The implications of a health care intervention in back pain or, more specifically, spinal surgery are far-reaching and cannot be confined to the measurement of pain alone. The effects or spinal surgery will affect the whole range of an individual's ability regarding mobility, participation in their usual activities, and, indeed, their ability to take care of themselves. Measurement of outcome of benefit in spinal surgery lends itself not only to clinical or disease-specific measures of health care benefit, but to more generic or holistic approaches such as Quality-Adjusted Life Years.

Prioritisation is the hierarchical ranking of competing claims upon health care resources, so that need is minimised or outcome is maximised; such choices in economics must always be made with recourse to limited resources. The allocation of health care resources can thus be pursued either with efficacy or efficiency. Under efficacy, resources are allocated lexicographically, dependent upon "greatest" need or capacity to benefit until all resources are exhausted. To pursue efficiency, resources need to be allocated where maximum benefit is yielded per unit of resource.

Economic Tools

The type of outcome tool affects the economic analysis possible. There are four main methods of economic analysis: cost minimisation, cost benefit, cost effectiveness and cost utility (Drummond et al. 1998). All the methods seek to quantify the resources involved in an intervention in financial terms. Where each method differs is in their measurement of outcome.

Cost minimisation does not attempt to address outcome, but assumes it is equivalent across interventions. Cost-benefit analysis seeks to evaluate all benefits in purely financial terms, and seeks to place a financial figure on mortality and morbidity. Cost-effectiveness analysis seeks to determine the cost per unit of effect, where a single measure of effect is used to determine the outcome, for example the radiological result or a disease-based approach, as in, for example, the Roland–Morris assessment of back pain (Roland and Morris 1982).

Cost utility takes a more holistic view of the patient outcome, across a number of spectra. Utility is expressed in terms of a single composite measure of health effect. It is the combination of the morbidity indicator with the duration of the health state that determines the Quality-Adjusted Life Year (Williams 1987). The measure of utility is then combined with the cost of the intervention to yield a cost per Quality-Adjusted Life Year (C/QALY). It is on the measurement of utility and, as such, cost utility that the remainder of this chapter will focus.

Cost per QALY calculations performed in a number of different specialties and interventions can be used to construct cost per QALY league tables to compare the relative cost and effects of such interventions. If the objective is to maximise efficiency, then interventions that produce a QALY at the least cost (see Drummond et al. 1993) will be ranked as the first choice interventions in a league table. If, for example, a neurosurgical intervention for head injury costs £240 to produce a single unit of QALY benefit, and a hip replacement was £1180 per QALY, then neurosurgical intervention would rank above the hip replacement. Ultimately, if a strict efficiency rule is followed, all interventions at the top of a priority list or cost utility league table would be chosen first, and the process would continue until all available resources for health care had been allocated as in the Oregon experiment (Hadorn 1991; Dixon and Welch 1991). The final section of this chapter will present the results of a cost-utility league table for spinal surgery.

Measures of Quality-Adjusted Life Year

The QALY measures the quality and the quantity of life. Hence, the QALY is calculated by multiplying the quality indicator (index value) by the quantity indicator (years of life).

The benefit measured by the QALY is expressed in terms of a composite numerical index commonly between zero and one, where one is equivalent to 1 year in perfect health and zero indicates death or unconsciousness. The QALY, or index measures in particular, can combine many different aspects of quality of life, for example, pain and mobility, into a common index. Cost-utility analysis expresses the benefits and cost of the procedures studied, in terms of cost per QALY gained from each of the procedures.

The following is an illustration for calculating QALYs. Health gain (q) is the difference between the final outcome and the initial outcome, that is:

$$q = \Sigma OF - \Sigma QI$$

where q = Quality of life or benefit in terms of QALYs
  QI = Initial QALY score
  QF = Final QALY score
  y = Duration of the health care intervention

The average QALY or index number is then the sum of the individual stream of benefits over time. This must be adjusted by factors such as life span (duration of benefits), the possible need for revisions or retreatment, and the potential decay rate of benefits.

For example, before spinal surgery, the patient may have a quality of life of 0.3, which, following surgery, rises to 0.8, a gain of 0.5. This benefit may accrue for 10 years.

Hence, $q = 0.8 - 0.3 = 0.5$; $y = 10$. The QALY gain is 0.5×10, or 5 QALYs.

There are a number of tools for measuring QALYs. In British and European studies, the Rosser classification of illness states (Kind et al. 1982) and EuroQol (EuroQol Group 1990) are commonly used. The Rosser classification of illness states provides pairwise groupings of four distress and eight disability states, which are experienced by the patient, and which can be converted into a composite numerical index. Gudex and Kind (1987) described the use of this index in detail.

EuroQol is a classification system that includes additional aspects of health. There are five dimensions of health, each with a one (best health) to three (worst health) rating scale. The dimensions are mobility, self care, usual activities, pain/discomfort and anxiety/depression. The five states convert into a composite numerical index.

A Case Study in Spinal Surgery – The Use of Quality-Adjusted Life Years

If Quality-Adjusted Life Year measurements are to play a role in measuring the quality of life with back pain or after spinal surgery, they must be responsive to change in the single intervention, and must allow meaningful comparison of the cost per Quality-Adjusted Life Year gained by spinal surgery with that gained by competing health care interventions.

The study took place in West Lancashire Health Authority in the Northwest of England, from 1990 to 1992 (James et al. 1996). It developed the application of cost-utility analysis into a range of orthopaedic procedures and, importantly, spinal discectomy. Currently, the literature on outcome assessment in orthopaedics is heavily clinically dominated and contains little on the patients' functional and psychological assessments of outcome (Wilcock 1981; Wroblewski 1985; Walter et al. 1986; Eftekhar 1987; Dallenbach et al. 1990; Casper et al. 1996; Timm 1994).

Orthopaedic surgery was chosen as the speciality, because it has a set of discrete procedures, each with relatively clear indications for their use and each leading to potential benefits that could be assessed after a relatively short time. Elective orthopaedics, of which spinal surgery is a part, had notoriously long waiting times (Yates 1987) and is believed to be one of the major elective areas where substantial health gains may be made.

The study used two index measures to determine health status or benefit following surgery: the Rosser classification of illness states and the EuroQol. The EuroQol tariff used was from Frome, Somerset.

Method

The study population comprised all patients under the care of each of the participating orthopaedic surgeons at a single speciality orthopaedic hospital, between May and August 1991, for one of the nine procedures shown in Fig. 1. The patients were assessed pre-operatively and 6 months post-discharge.

The nine procedures were those that constituted the greatest proportion of the orthopaedic waiting list, and, furthermore, the greatest proportion of the activity within the speciality. The patients' conditions were chronic, with little change in health status expected without surgical intervention. The procedures undertaken affect quality of life, rather than life expectancy, and were well established as technically successful. The patients completed Rosser and EuroQol self-reported health states before and after surgery.

Costs were attached to all the procedures in the analysis. These were calculated as patient-based individually derived costs, obtained by detailed data extraction from the casenotes. They comprised detailed ingredient costs for each procedure, including information on drug usage, pathology/haematology tests, X rays, aids and appliances, length of stay, outpatient appointments and readmissions.

Costs and benefits do not remain constant over time, and it is the stream of costs and benefits over time that are important for cost-utility analysis and cost per QALY calculations. In this analysis, factors taken into consideration were the patients' life span and, where appropriate, length of life of the prosthesis; the probability of complications (derived from the consultants' own data and the literature), probability of failure (included in the calculations by percentage that benefit), decay point, that is, the point in time from which the prosthesis starts to decay and decay rate of benefit over time were also taken into account. The net gain in quality of life is therefore calculated by subtracting the initial health state valuation from the final one, multiplied by the years of remaining life, and subject to the adjustments factors detailed above (see Appendix).

Results

The Rosser and the EuroQol classification systems successfully differentiated between the pre-operative and post-operative states in the cohort of elective orthopaedics and spinal discectomy, that is, the measures detected a positive change in the patients'

The Sample

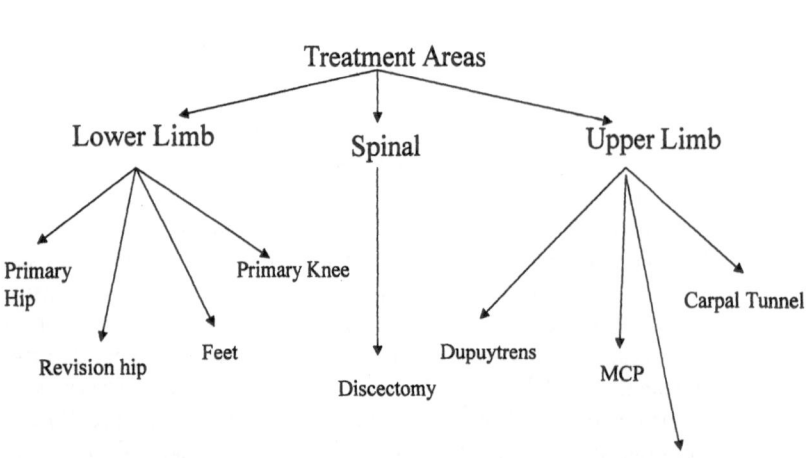

Fig. 1. The orthopaedic procedures that were studied

Table 1. Net health gain determined by using the Rosser index with patient valuation, patient-based costs and cost-utility ratios in British pounds

Operation	Net health gain, patient valuations	Cost (£)[b]	Cost per QALY (£)
Spinal discectomy	4.841	2044	422
Revision hip	1.762	5078	2881
Primary hip, age ≥ 40[a]	1.496	3112	2080
Metacarpophalangeal	0.799	2910	3644
Primary hip, age < 40[a]	0.783	3546	4528
Flexor Tenosynovectomy	0.666	2032	3049
Primary knee	0.647	4134	6392
Carpal tunnel	0.457	132	290
Dupuytren's	0.132	708	5350
Feet general	−0.172	1679	−9761

[a] Primary hips, < 40 and ≥ 40 are those patients aged under 40 and 40 or above, respectively.
[b] Revision × % of expected revisions are discounted by 5 years.

Table 2. Net health gain determined by using the EuroQol index with patient valuations, patients-based costs and cost-utility ratios in British pounds

Operation	Net health gain, patient valuations	Cost (£)[b]	Cost per QALY (£)
Spinal discectomy	6.830	2044	299
Primary hip ≥ 40[a]	6.270	3112	496
Primary hip, < 40[a]	6.108	3546	580
Primary knee	2.955	4134	1399
Revision hip	1.651	5078	3074
Carpal tunnel	1.309	132	101
Dupuytren's	1.263	708	561
Flexor tenosynovectomy	0.190	2032	10672
Metacarpophalangeal	−0.133	2910	−21864
Feet general	−1.377	1679	−1220

[a] Primary hips, < 40 and ≥ 40 are those patients aged under 40 and 40 or above, respectively.
[b] Revisions × % of expected revisions are discounted by 5 years

health states after an intervention. For all the procedures, the final health status valuation was statistically significantly different ($p < 0.001$, Wilcoxon matched pairs) from the original health status measure, hence both quality of life measures were sensitive to changes in the patients' quality of life.

Tables 1 and 2, respectively, show the Rosser QALY and EuroQol net gains in quality of life [final – initial health state valuation, by life span (adjusted)], alongside costs and costs per QALY. The first column shows the health state valuation obtained from the patients' assessment of their health status; the second column shows the cost of the procedure. The final column represents cost divided by QALY. This makes costs and QALYs comparable and shows, for each procedure, how much must be spent to gain an additional QALY per person. Hence, the smaller the figure in this final column the more cost-effective is the procedure. To illustrate this from Table 2, spinal surgery is the most efficacious procedure, producing 6.830 QALYs per patient, hence is ranked in top position with respect to efficacy. In terms of QALYs it costs £299 to generate an additional QALY when a

spinal discectomy is performed, and it costs £101 per QALY for a carpal tunnel. Hence a carpal tunnel operation generates more QALYs per unit of cost than a spinal discectomy does and spinal discectomy drops to second place in the ranking. However, this demonstrates that spinal discectomy is not only an efficacious procedure, but also that it is an efficient procedure.

Table 3 presents a summary of the results ranked in order of greatest benefit and also ranked in ascending order of cost per QALY.

Discussion

This study indicates that the cost-utility analysis (CUA) approach appears to be feasible in providing a framework that will assist purchasers in making health care decisions and for valuing interventions in spinal surgery relative to other orthopaedic interventions.

The measure of outcome or benefit used in the study should depend on the objectives of the study. To compare a large number of disparate treatments

Table 3. Summary of the Rosser and EuroQol health gain and cost-utility rankings. Ranked according to greatest health gain and least cost per QALY

Rank	Health gain – Rosser	Health gain – EuroQol	Cost-utility ratio – Rosser	Cost-utility ratio – EuroQol
1	Discectomy	Discectomy	Carpal tunnel	Carpal tunnel
2	Revision hip	Primary hip, $\geq$ 40	Discectomy	Discectomy
3	Primary hip, $\geq$ 40	Primary hip, < 40	Primary hip, $\geq$ 40	Primary hip, $\geq$ 40
4	Mcp	Primary knee	Revision hip	Dupuytren's
5	Primary hip, < 40	Revision hip	Flexor	Primary hip, < 40
6	Flexor	Carpal tunnel	Mcp	Primary knee
7	Primary knee	Dupuytren's	Primary hip, < 40	Revision hip
8	Carpal tunnel	Flexor	Dupuytren's	Flexor
9	Dupuytren's	Mcp	Primary knee	Feet general
10	Feet general	Feet general	Feet general	Mcp

and conditions requires a common simple and comparable unit of benefit. Index measures permit the comparison of differing dimensions of health by converting the dimensions into a single health state valuation, hence allowing treatments to be ranked within and between specialities.

Quality-of-life measurements showed that patients for spinal surgery who underwent discectomy obtained the most health care benefits of all the elective procedures studied, and the change in outcome, measured by QALY, was hown to be statistically significant. Equally, in terms of absolute QALYs gained by performing spinal surgery, both the Rosser QALY and the EuroQol methods showed that the gain in Quality-Adjusted Life Year from surgery was high.

The most important application of index measures is to provide cost-utility ratios and hence to rank treatments. Cosideration of some of the general rankings of procedures within this study raises interesting points. The high-cost, high-publicity operations such as hip and knee replacements, do not necessarily rank highest in the list, either in terms of their cost-utility ratios or in terms of benefit alone, and are out-ranked by the procedure of spinal discectomy in terms of both efficacy and efficiency. Although out-ranked by the carpal-tunnel operation, spinal surgery still ranked second by both QALY instruments. Spinal discectomy was a highly cost-effective procedure, with cost per QALY rated as £422 and £299, respectively, by the Rosser and EuroQol instruments.

Measuring quality of life in spinal surgery is important and goes beyond the realm of the purely clinical or disease-specific measures. Studies in spinal surgery must increasingly be prepared to evaluate the broader functional dimensions of health as they affect the patient. Equally, purchasers of multiple health care interventions must be able to utilise tools that enable them to assess the relative worth of interventions. The challenge for spinal surgeons will be to effectively utilise and develop a suite of tools for systematically evaluating surgical interventions in spinal surgery.

Appendix

Derivation of Costs and Benefits Over Time

Costs

The baseline cost is derived from the extra-contractual referral (ECR) price or the patient-based costs adjusted by follow-up visits.

Where revision of a prosthetic replacement occurs as a genuine complication of the host hospital, (rather than failure of a joint replaced at another hospital or long-term wear and tear) it is assumed that a revision occurs on average approximately 5 years after the initial joint was replaced.

The final-cost figure for each procedure is therefore:

Baseline cost + (cost of revision × probability of revision) discounted by 5 years (assuming a 6% test discount rate) + (cost of complication × probability of complications) + (cost of readmissions × probability of readmissions).

or

$$C = C_b + (C_r \times P_r) \, 1/(1 + 0.06)^5 + (C_c \times P_c) + (C_{ra} \times P_{ra})$$

Where

C = Total cost

C_b = Baseline cost

C_r = Revision cost

C_c = Complication cost (excluding hospital admissions)

C_{ra} = Cost of readmission (excluding readmission as a consequence of revision)

P_r = Probability of revision

P_c = Probability of complication

P_{ra} = Probability of readmission

Benefits Over Time

Benefit calculations are derived separately for the Rosser QALY and the EuroQol.

The baseline benefit is the difference between the sum of the final outcome and the sum of the initial outcome (by procedure):

$QL = \Sigma QF - \Sigma QI$

QL = Quality of life or benefit in terms of QALYs

QI = Initial QALY score

QF = Final QALY score

QL is presented as an average for each procedure, hence the QALY score by procedure (QT) is:

$QT = \Sigma QL/n$

Where n = Sample size.

Life expectancy to death (LYD) for each procedure = average years life until death males $\times$ % males in the sample + average years life left until death females $\times$ % of females in the sample

Total prosthesis life (TPL):

$TPL = PL_{ND} + PL_D$

PL_{ND} = Prosthesis life before any substantial decay occurs in the prosthesis

PL_D = Additional years of prosthesis life after the prosthesis has started to decay

$1/D$ = Decay rate of the prosthesis

m = Mortality rate for the individual hospital

R = Reoccurrence rate

LYD_R = Lost years of benefit from point of reoccurence

When the total benefit in QALY calculations is determined, the percentage that benefit would normally need to be built into the QALY calculation; however, in this sample, the average benefit figure already takes into account the percentage that benefit for each procedure.

Total benefit over life:

$QT_{TOTAL} = QT (PL_{ND} + PL_D \, 1/D(LYD - PL_{ND}))$
$- \% \, m(QI) - \%R(\Sigma LYD_R(QL))$,

where $LYD > PL_{ND}$

If $LYD < PL_{ND}$, or no prosthesis is involved:

$QT_{TOTAL} = QT (LYD) - \% \, m(QI)$
$- \% \, R\Sigma((LYD_R(QT))$

References

[1] Bowling A (1995) Measuring disease – A review of disease-specific quality of life measurement scale. Open University Press, Buckingham, Philadelphia
[2] Bradshaw J (1972) A taxonomy of social need. In: MacLachlan G (ed) Problems and progress in medical care, 7th series. Oxford University Press, Oxford
[3] Bradshaw J (1994) The contextualisation and measurement of need: a social policy perspective. In: Popay J, Williams G (eds) Researching the people's health. Routledge, London
[4] Casper DG, Hartman VL, Mullins LL (1996) Results of a clinical trial of the holmium:YAG laser in disc decompression utilising a side-firing fiber: a two-year follow-up. Lasers in Surgery and medicine 19:90–96
[5] Croft P (1996) Health care needs assessment: Low back pain. Radcliffe, Abingdon
[6] Culyer AJ (1976) Need and the national health service. Martin Robertson, Oxford
[7] Dallenbach HG, Gillespie WJ, Daellenbach US (1990) Economic appraisal of new technology in the absence of survival data – the case of total hip replacement. Social Science and Medicine 31(12):1287–1293
[8] Dixon J, Welch HG (1991) Priority setting: Lessons from Oregon. Lancet 337:891–894
[9] Doyal L, Gough I (1993) A theory of human need. Macmillan, London
[10] Drummond MF, O'Brien B, Stoddart GL, TZorrance GW (1998) Methods for the economic evaluation of health care programme, 2nd ed. Oxford University Press, Oxford
[11] Drummond MF, Maynard A, Wells N (1993) Purchasing and providing cost-effective health care. Churchill Livingstone, Edinburgh
[12] Eftekhar NS (1987) Long-term results of cemented total hip arthroplasty. Clin Orthop Relat Res 225:207–217
[13] EuroQol Group (1990) EuroQol – a new facility for the measurement of health-related quality of life. Health Policy 16:199–208
[14] Fairbank JCT, Davies J, Couper J, O'Brien J (1980) The Oswestry disability questionnaire. Physiotherapy 66:271–273
[15] Gudex C, Kind P (1987) The QALY toolkit discussion, paper 76, Centre for Health Economics. University of York, York
[16] Hadorn DC (1991) Setting health care priorities in Oregon. Cost effectiveness meets the rule of rescue. J Am Med Assoc 265(17):2218–2225
[17] James M, St Leger S, Rowsell K (1996) Prioritising elective care: a cost utility analysis of orthopaedics in the north west of England. J Epidemiology Community Health 50:182–189
[18] James M (1999) Towards an integrated needs and outcome framework. Health Policy 46:165–177
[19] Kind P, Rosser R, Williams A (1982) Valuation of quality of life: some psychometric evidence. In: Jones-Lee MW (ed) The value of life and safety. North Holland, Holland
[20] Lightfoot J (1995) Identifying needs and setting health care priorities: Issues of theory policy and practice. Health and Social Care 3:105–114
[21] Million R, Hall W, Haacick-Nilsen K, Baker RD, Jayson MIV (1982) Assessment of the progress of the back pain patient. Spine 7:204–212
[22] Roland M, Morris R (1982) A study of the natural history of back pain. Spine 8(2):141–144
[23] Soper K (1993) Review: A theory of human need. New Literature Review 197:113–128
[24] Timm KE (1994) A randomized-control study of active and passive treatments for chronic low back pain following L5 laminectomy. J Orthop Sport Phys Ther 20(6):276–286
[25] Underwood MR (1998) Crisis: what crisis? Eur Spine J 7(1):2–5
[26] Walker SJ, Sharma P, Parr N, Cavendish ME (1986) The long-term results of the Liverpool mark II knee prosthesis. J Bone Joint Surg 68:111–116
[27] Wilcock GK (1981) A comparison of total hip replacement in patients aged 69 years or less and 70 years or over. Gerontology 27:85–88
[28] Wilkin D, Hallam L, Doggett MA (1992) Measures of need and outcome for primary health care. Oxford University Press, Oxford
[29] Williams A (1987) Measuring quality of life: a comment. Sociology 21(4):565–566
[30] Wrobleski BM (1985) Charnley low friction arthroplasty in patients under the age of 40 years. In: Sevastik J, Goldie I (eds) The young patient with degenerative hip disease. Almqvist & Wiksell International, Stockholm
[31] Yates J (1987) Why are we waiting? Oxford University Press, Oxford

MRI Scans of the Lumbosacral Spine Under Compression

D. S. J. CHOY

Introduction

Nachemson [1] in 1964 studied in vivo intradiscal pressures in human lumbar spines in sitting, standing, and supine positions, and in flexion. Sitting pressure averaged 150–200 kPa, while standing pressures were in the neighborhood of 50 kPa. Expressed differently, these are 1125 to 1500 mmHg and 375 mmHg, or almost 2 atm versus 0.5 atm, or roughly 30 and 7.5 psi, respectively. The common observation that patients with herniated lumbar disc disease are more comfortable in the supine, and least comfortable in the sitting positions, may at least be partially due to these pressure differences.

At the 1995 Laser Association of Neurosurgeons International (LANSI) meeting in Salzburg, this author highlighted the lack of association between the MRI findings in herniated lumbar disc disease and the severity of clinical symptoms. Dr. Ferenc Jolecz, in support of the author's argument, presented three slides (Figs. 1–3) showing MR images of L5–S1 disc protrusion that noticeably increased when the patient sat upright.

At the time of writing this paper, there were only two MRI machines (one at Harvard and the other at Zurich) that allow MR imaging both in the supine and the sitting positions. In order to circumvent the relative lack of access to MR imaging of the spine in a loaded mode, the author designed a wooden frame, which is both inexpensive and easy to use.

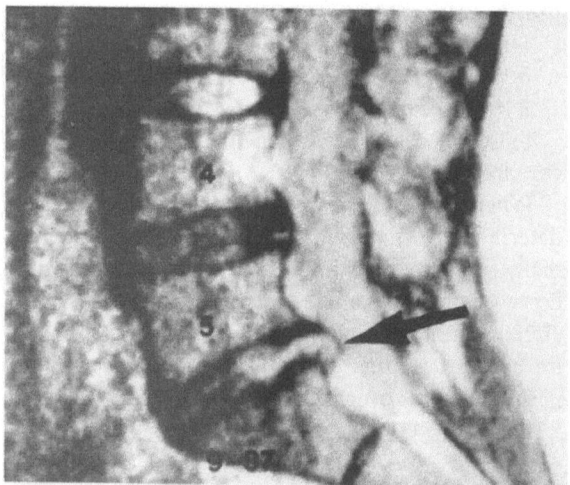

Fig. 2. The same disc imaged with the patient sitting

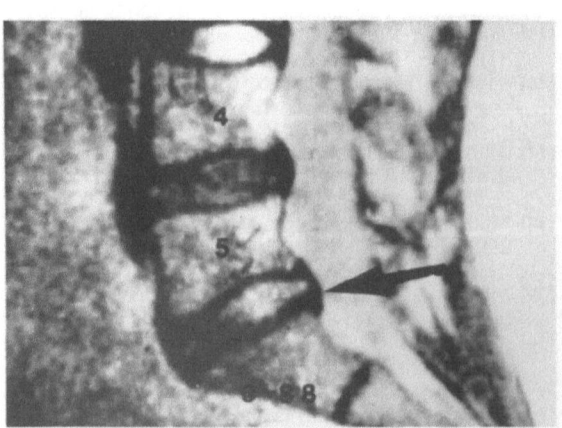

Fig. 1. L5–S1 disc imaged in the supine position

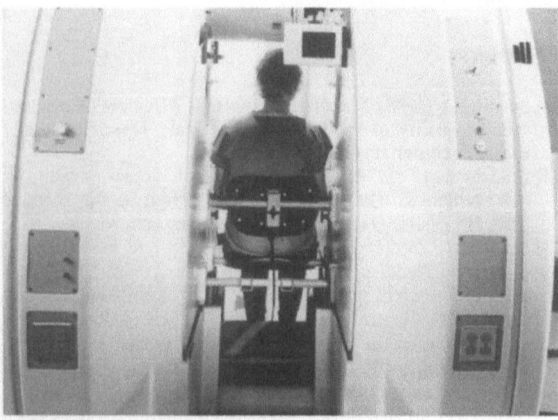

Fig. 3. The patient sitting in the special MRI machine at Harvard

Method

Frame: The frame consists of a ¾ inch × 16 inch × 7 foot plywood base. At one end there are two fixed padded shoulder restraints. At the other end, an adjustable foot board is attached to the base with hardwood dowels which are 0.5 inch in diameter and pass through the base of the foot board into 0.5-inch holes drilled into the base at 0.5-inch intervals (Fig. 4). Thus the foot board can be moved on the base board by 0.5 inch at a time. The length of the patient from the shoulders to the soles of the feet is measured (L1).

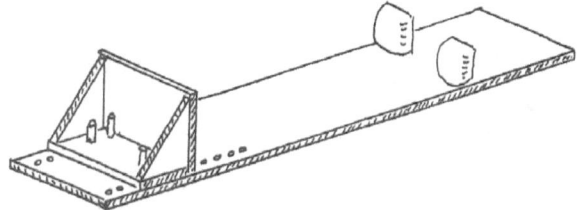

Fig. 4. An all-wood frame with fixed shoulder restraints and a movable foot board fixed with hard-wood 0.5-in. dowels

The first scan is performed. The distance between the shoulder restraints and the foot board is adjusted to a distance that corresponds to the length of the patient from the shoulder to the sole of the feet (L1) minus 3 inches (L2). The patient is then placed in the frame with his/her knees slightly bent to accommodate the shorter distance. Once placed in the MR tube, the patient is asked to fully extend both knees, thereby exerting a compressive load on the lumbosacral spine. The second scan is then performed.

Results

Seven patients with suspected herniated lumbar disc disease were studied. MR imaging was performed both in the standard supine position with a GE 1.5-Tesla scanner and repeated with the lumbosacral spine under compression. In four patients, lumbosacral compression augmented disc protrusion significantly (Figs. 5 and 6). This was associated with increased pain in all of these patients. Similar tests carried out on three asymptomatic subjects, who served as a control group, lying in the jig with and without compression produced no disc protrusion.

Discussion

The physiologic rationale for bed rest in conservative treatment of herniated disc disease as well as the various decompressive therapeutic modalities (microdiscectomy, percutaneous laser disc decompression)

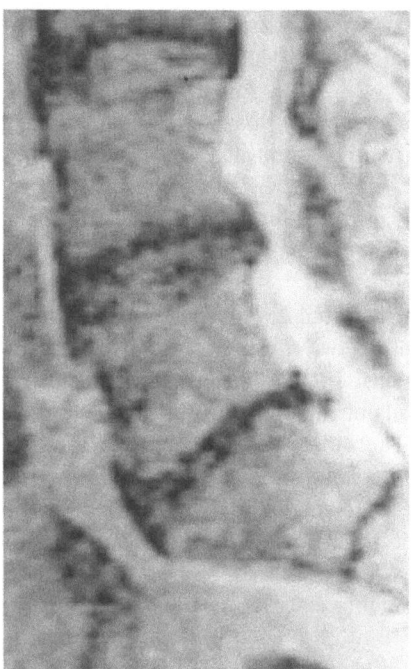

Fig. 5. L5–S1 disc imaged with the patient supine, with no L/S compression

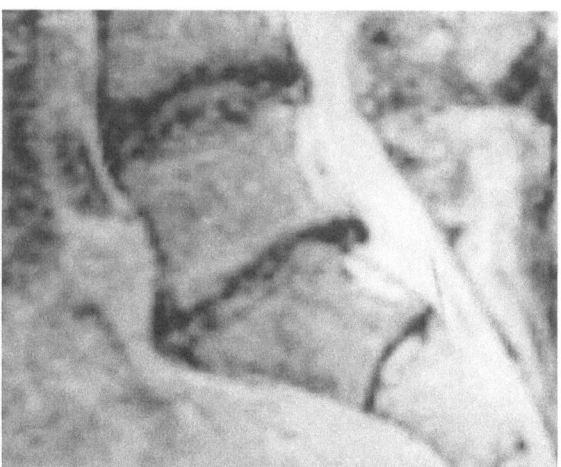

Fig. 6. The same disc imaged with the patient lying in the compressive frame, with knees extended. Note the pronounced disc protrusion

is based on Nachemson's work on intradiscal pressures. Ramos and Martin [3] described linear fall of intradiscal pressure in five patients subjected to axial stretching. This report describes MRI changes with axial compression.

In patients with severe sciatic syndrome, in the absence of supporting MRI evidence, decisions on therapeutic intervention can be facilitated by MR imaging of the lumbosacral spine appropriately loaded and under compression, which could demonstrate herniated disc with greater clarity. Some laser spine surgeons [2] routinely perform discography to:
1. Rule out the presence of free disc fragments

2. Induce sciatic pain to identity the painful discal level, especially in patients with multiple disc involvement

The author believes that this step is unnecessary because discography is an invasive procedure with a possibility of increased morbidity. With the availability of MR imaging of the lumbosacral spine in loading, identification of the responsible symptomatic disc is simplified.

Only one-third of the day is spent in the supine position; the other two-thirds are in the sitting or standing positions. In the erect position, approximately two thirds of the body weight presses on the lumbar discs. The more "physiological" orientation of the body is therefore the sitting or standing positions. MR scans of the highest diagnostic value in the management of back pain are best obtained with patients' lumbosacral spine appropriately loaded to simulate the standing erect spinal position.

With only two "sitting" MRI machines available at the present time, the author proposes the wider-spread use of this "poor-man's sitting MRI" simulation frame where the only investment is US$75 for a wood compressive frame. This will be useful to the spinal surgeons of both types–the "scalpel users" and the "laser users".

References

[1] Nachemson A, Morris J (1964) In vivo measurements of intradiscal pressure. Discometry, a method for the determination of pressure in the lower lumbar discs. J Bone Joint Surg 46A(5):1077–1092
[2] Botsford JA (1993) Radiological considerations: percutaneous laser disc decompression, J Clin Laser Med and Surg 11(5):223–231
[3] Ramos G, Martin W (1994) Effects of vertebral axial decompression on intradiscal pressure. J Neurosurg 81:350–353

Patient Selection for Percutaneous Laser Discectomy

J. A. BOTSFORD

Introduction

Percutaneous laser discectomy (PLD) is a safe and effective alternative treatment for the lumbar herniated nucleus pulposis (HNP) that is contained by an intact annulus/posterior longitudinal ligament (PLL) complex and connected to the parent disc of origin. When rigid patient selection criteria are applied, published success rates meet or exceed those of traditional open surgery. In addition to plain film radiography, multiple other radiological examinations including myelography, computed tomography (CT), magnetic resonance imaging (MRI), and CT-discography (CT-D) (Table 1) have been used alone or in combination to preoperatively identify those patients with an HNP that will benefit from percutaneous intradiscal therapy. Each of the available imaging modalities has a different sensitivity and specificity in diagnosing the contained lumbar disc herniation. Therefore, even when abnormal, they may not be equally useful for the prospective selection of patients for PLD.

Table 1. Radiological examination techniques

Plain radiography – non-weight-bearing   – weight-bearing
Myelography
Unenhanced computed tomography (CT)
Iodinated contrast-enhanced CT
CT myelography
Unenhanced magnetic resonance imaging (MRI)
Gadolinium contrast-enhanced MRI
Discography
CT-discography

Patient Selection

All physicians involved in the selection and treatment of patients by laser discectomy must be familiar with the radiologic concepts appropriate to this procedure to optimise patient selection, thereby improving results and decreasing complications. The lumbar discovertebral unit has been likened to a closed hydraulic space subject to a pressure and volume relationship [1, 2, 3]. Other investigators [4, 5] have shown that a small reduction in central intradiscal volume by mechanical removal, chemical dissolution or laser ablation results in a reduction of pressure within the enclosed space. This pressure reduction will be transmitted through the posteriorly projecting nuclear material, provided it remains in continuity with the parent disc of origin and the annulus and posterior longitudinal ligament (PLL) complex is still intact. Contiguous but non-contained herniations that have ruptured through the annulus and PLL complex (extrusions) as well as herniations that have broken free into the epidural space (sequestrations) violate the closed-space principle and are not suitable for PLD.

In addition, any surgical therapy directed at the abnormal nucleus including PLD may produce suboptimal results unless there is pretreatment confirmation that altered intradiscal pressure is related to the patient's typical pain. The importance of these factors in the selection of patients for PLD cannot be overstated. Incorrect preoperative classification of a herniation as contained and/or symptomatic will lead to inappropriate application of the technique and a less than optimal success rate. The radiographic study that most reliably provides both these pieces of information will be the best at predicting a successful outcome [6].

Plain film radiographs and contrast myelography are of limited use in the evaluation of the unoperated patient with clinical symptoms consistent with a lumbar herniated nucleus pulposis (HNP) [7]. Both computed tomography (CT) and magnetic resonance imaging (MRI) can accurately diagnose a generic "herniated disc" [7–14]. However, neither of these cross-sectional imaging modalities consistently characterizes the herniation as contained (protruded or focally herniated) or non-contained (extruded or sequestered) [7]. Moreover, not all patients with abnormal lumbar disc morphology on MR imaging are symptomatic and the mere presence of a contained HNP does not prove causality of clinical symptoms [15, 16]. Thin-needle non-ionic water-soluble discography followed by thin-section CT of the injected disc (CT-discography or CT-D) is the most specific test prior to intradiscal therapy [17, 18]. It correctly predicts the type of disc herniation as contained or non-contained (extruded or sequestered) in the highest percentage of any radiologic study [19]. CT-D is the only diagnostic examination that combines anatomic information with a physiologic pain provocation challenge to the lumbar disc [20, 21]. It should only be considered positive when there is both anatomic abnormality and familiar pain reproduction during injection [22].

Although it has proven valuable in the PLD candidate [6, 18], CT-D should *not* be used as the primary method of diagnosing the lumbar HNP. CT or MRI are unquestionably superior in the initial evaluation of a suspected lumbar radiculopathy [9, 23]. Instead, CT-D should only be performed to confirm containment and causality where the cross-sectional imaging study has suggested an appropriate disc herniation and treatment by PLD is being considered.

Conclusion

Recent work has confirmed that the symptomatic patient who has both a contained HNP on preoperative cross-sectional imaging and a positive CT discogram will have a much higher chance of a successful PLD outcome than one who has only an abnormal CT or MRI exam [6]. These principles have been integrated into a diagnostic imaging algorithm for the evaluation of the PLD candidate (Fig. 1).

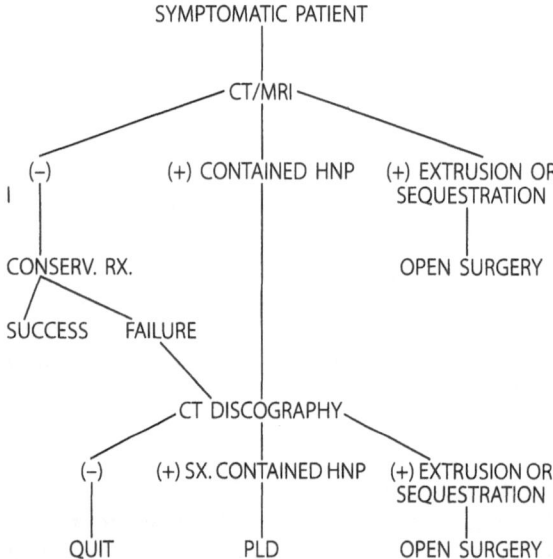

Fig. 1. Diagnostic evaluation scheme

References

[1] Adams MA, Hutton WC (1989) Mechanics of the intervertebral disc. In: Ghosh P (ed) The biology of the inververtebral disc. CRC Press, Boca Raton
[2] Nachemson A (1981) Disc pressure measurement. Springer 6:93–97
[3] Choy DSJ (1993) Intervertebral disc pressure as a function of fluid volume infused. Spine: State of the art reviews 7(1):11–15
[4] Brock M, Gorge H, Curio G (1984) Intradiscal pressure volume response: A methodological contribution to chemonucleolysis. J Neurosurg 60:1029–1032
[5] Choy DSJ, Altman P (1993) Fall of intradiscal pressure with laser ablation. Spine: State of the art reviews 7(1):23–29
[6] Botsford JA (1994) Radiological considerations: patient selection for percutaneous laser disc decompression. J Clin Laser Med & Surg 12(5):255–259
[7] Thornbury JR, Fryback DG, Turski PA, Javid MJ, McDonald IV, Beinlich BR, Gentry LR, Sackett JF, Dasbach EJ, Martin PA (1993) Disc-caused nerve compression in patients with acute low back pain. Diagnosis with MR, CT myelography, and plain CT. Radiology 186:731–738
[8] Firooznia H, Nebjamin V, Kricheff II, Mahvash R, Golimbu C (1984) CT of the lumbar spine disc herniation: correlation with surgical findings. AJR 142:587–592
[9] Modic MT, Masaryk TJ, Boumphrey F, Goormastic M, Bell G (1986) Lumbar herniated disc disease and canal stenosis: prospective evaluation by surface coil MR, CT, and myelography. AJR 147:757–765
[10] Thornbury JR, Fryback DG, Lawrence WF, Turski PA, Javid MJ, McDonald JV, Beinlich BR, Gentry LR, Sackett JF, Dasbach EJ, Martin PA (1994) Reply: diagnostic accuracy, patient outcome, and economic factors in lumbar radiculopathy. Radiology 190:21–30
[11] Haughton VM (1988) MR imaging of the spine. Radiology 166:297–301
[12] Modic MT, Masaryk TJ, Ross JS, Carter JS (1988) Imaging of degenerative disc disease. Radiology 168:177–186
[13] Ross JS, Tkach J, VanDyke C, Modic MT (1991) Clinical MR imaging of degenerative spinal disease: pulse sequences, gradient-echo techniques, and contrast agents. JMRI 1:29
[14] Ross JS, Modic MT (1992) Current assessment of spinal degenerative disease with magnetic resonance imaging. Clin Orth Rel Res 279:68–81
[15] Modic MT, Ross JS (1990) Morphology, symptoms and causality. Radiology 175:619–620
[16] Bozzao A, Gallucci M, Masciocchi C, Aprile I, Barile A, Pasariello R (1992) Lumbar disc herniation: MR imaging assessment of the natural history in patients treated without surgery. Radiology 185:135–141
[17] Edwards WC, Orme TJ, Orr-Edwards G (1987) CT discography: prognostic value in the selection of patients for chemonucleolysis. Spine 12:792–795
[18] Botsford JA (1994) CT discography: Prognostic value in patient selection for percutaneous laser disc decompression (PLDD). Abstract no 265. In: 94th annual meeting of the American Roentgen Ray Sciety (ARRS), New Orleans, LA, 24–20. April 1994
[19] Bernard TN (1990) Lumbar discography followed by computed tomography. Spine 15:690–707
[20] Milette PC, Melanson D (1987) Lumbar discography. Radiology 163:828–829
[21] Vanharanta H, Sachs BL, Spivey MA, Huyer RD, Hochschuler SH, Rashbaum RF, Johnson RA, Ohnmiess D, Mooney V (1987) The relationship of pain provocation to lumbar disc deterioration seen by CT discography. Spine 12:295–298
[22] Walsh TR, Weinstein JN, Spratt KF, Lehman TR, Aprill C, Saure H (1990) Lumbar discography in normal subjects. J Bone and Joint Surg 72-A(7):1081–1088
[23] Seidenwurm D, Russel EJ, Hambly M (1994) Diagnostic accuracy, patient outcome, and economic factors in lumbar radiculopathy. Radiology 190:21–30

Endoscopically Determined Pain Sources in the Lumbar Spine

M. T. N. KNIGHT

Background

Since 1990, we have used aware-state surgery to treat spinal disorders as part of the process of viviprudence. Viviprudence is the evaluation cascade of in-depth questionnaires, postural analysis, extended clinical examination and weight-bearing X-rays which underpin initial examination. This is followed by extended postural restabilisation and motor reprogramming physiotherapy for 6–12 weeks, after which persistent debilitating symptoms merit MRI scanning. This is followed by spinal probing and discography wherein spinal probing is the most valuable entity. Multiple-point probing serves to pinpoint pain sites at the facet margin, neural margins, annulus and in the safe working zone (SWZ). The safe working zone is a triangular region bounded by the dura or traversing nerve medially, the medial border of the exiting nerve laterally, and the superior endplate margin of the inferior-bounding vertebra. Discography reproduces pain in only 27 % of patients with non-compressive radiculopathy but is valuable in defining the disposition of degeneration within the disc and the integrity of the annulus. Discography defines most leaks and the direction of emission from them. The acceptance volume of radio-opaque dye defines the degree of degeneration present.

For those cases where pain is either incompletely reproduced or where there is overlap in the symptoms reproduced, differential discography is particularly valuable. Differential discography uses the intradiscal instillation of methylprednisolone acetate (Depo Medrone Upjohn), iohexol (Omnipaque 240 Nycomed Amersham), or bupivacaine hydrochloride (Marcaine 0.5 % Astra) to produce amelioration of symptoms for 6–10 days, 12–18 h, or 5–8 h respectively, to determine the contribution to a symptom complex from each specific segment.

Our experience with aware-state surgery commenced in 1990 when we performed percutaneous discectomies. The 12.5 % annual recurrence rate led us to explore laser disc decompression as a minimal alternative to treating compressive and non-compressive radiculopathy. In 1992 we developed biportal

endoscopic intradiscal discectomy, but found that whilst this technique could address more significant lesions such as disc extrusion and large focal protrusions, it was extremely susceptible to lateral recess stenosis. This led us to develop a method of foraminal decompression termed endoscopic laser foraminoplasty (ELF) which provides the means to explore the epidural, foraminal and extraforaminal zones as well as effect intradiscal discectomy, all by the posterolateral route and in the aware state. Clinical implementation of uniportal endoscopic laser foraminoplasty started in 1994.

The system of viviprudence and aware-state endoscopic examination has been used to address lateral recess stenosis, epidural scarring, osteophytosis, settlement, listhesis, disc extrusion, spondylolytic spondylolisthesis, "instability", sequestration, "failed back syndrome" and "failed back surgery syndrome" in over 775 patients. This experience has demonstrated numerous unsuspected causes of pain arising in degenerative disc disease. This will be discussed in more detail in the section "Anatomy and Pathology" of this chapter.

Surgical Protocol

The patients underwent a staged procedure consisting of:
- Spinal probing and discography at suspected levels, approached on the side of maximal symptoms.
- Endoscopic laser foraminoplasty consisting of exploration of extraforaminal, foraminal and epidural zones with flexible endoscopic intradiscal discectomy, neurolysis, undercutting of facets and osteophytectomy as required. However, the final decision for this second stage (endoscopic laser foraminoplasty) was made only after spinal probing and discography had reproduced a description of the type, intensity and distribution of pain that agreed with that normally experienced by the patient.
- Where symptom reproduction was imperfect, a differential discogram was performed with the

instillation of 2 ml of methylprednisolone acetate at the presumed level. If postoperative observation revealed a reduction of symptoms for 5–10 days, then those affected symptoms could be expected to be modified by endoscopic laser foraminoplasty at the said level.

Spinal probing differs from discography in that it relies upon specific probing of the anterior margin of the facet joint, perineural structures and the disc wall at several points. The essential and distinctive step in "viviprudence" is therefore spinal probing and differential discography. Discography defines the distribution of degeneration within the disc and the acceptance volume and the presence of annular leaks. If discography on a contained disc produces radicular pain then this further endorses that that disc is the index level for the compressive pain. Similarly, if a leak reproduces the patient's compressive or non-compressive pain, this then identifies the targeted disc as a contributor to that evoked pain. Where probing evokes pain, the subsequent endoscopic aware-state examination then confirms these structures to be sources of pain. Endoscopy demonstrates the contribution to the pain arising from inflamed disc, disc pad and foraminal structures.

Operative Technique

Neuroleptanalgesia (aware-state analgesia) was performed using 0.03 mg/kg midazolam (Hypnovel, Roche) bolus at the onset of the operation, 2–5 µg/kg fentanyl and 30–70 µg/kg droperidol. Patient feedback is essential in cases where the presence of perineural scarring is often unexpectedly dense and masks the neural structures. A bolus dose of 1.5 g cefuroxime was given at the onset of operation. The skin and subcutis were infiltrated with the local anaesthetic anhydrous lignocaine hydrochloride (Xylocaine 0.25 % (0.75–1.5 mg/kg), Astra) with 1:200 000 adrenaline.

Push-Up Test

The push-up test consisted of the patient extending the arms, hyperextending the lumbar spine whilst the abdomen is allowed to sag in the prone position on the operating table, prior to surgery. If this manoeuvre evoked the patient's leg or back pain prior to surgery then the absence of the same pain at the end of the procedure indicated that sufficient clearance of the cause of the pain had been achieved and the manoeuvre constituted a "positive push-up test".

Lasing Technique

The probe is replaced with a guide wire and under biplanar X-ray control a 4.6-mm dilator tube is railroaded to the exit-root foramen. During the entire

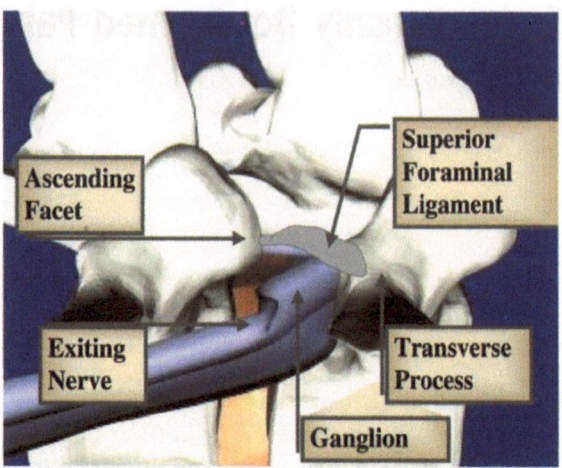

Fig. 1. Foraminal anatomy; the superior foraminal ligament and the impacting ascending facet joint margin deforming the nerve and ganglion

procedure an image intensifier is used at intervals to ensure the correct position of the endoscope and the laser probe. The trocar is removed and a Richard Wolf endoscope with an eccentrically placed 2.5-mm working channel and two irrigation channels are inserted. A side-firing 2.1-mm diameter laser probe with internal irrigation is inserted through the endoscope. The extraforaminal zone and margin of the foramen are cleared (Fig. 1). The ascending and descending facet joint surfaces are then excavated and undercut to allow admission of the endoscope beyond the isthmus of the foramen into the epidural space. Vertebral body and facet joint osteophytes, ligamentum flavum and superior foraminal ligament, perineural and epidural scarring are ablated and the facet joint undercut until the annulus and epidural space are displayed.

The exiting and transiting nerve roots are mobilised and decompressed medially and laterally until the functional axilla of the root at the apex of the safe working zone are displayed. The nerve is cleared of perineural fibrosis. The bone margin of the superior notch and the superior foraminal ligament are then addressed. Osteophytes along the ascending facet joint and in the superior notch, dorsum of the vertebral margin and the vertebral shoulder (shoulder osteophytes) are ablated under endoscopic vision. In the presence of a disc protrusion in the epidural or foraminal zone, disc degeneration, annular collection or leaks, the disc is entered and cleared by laser ablation and manual punches.

Anatomy and Pathology

Experience of over 1200 endoscopic laser foraminoplasties and 173 flexible endoscopic intradiscal discectomies has taught us that new pathological enti-

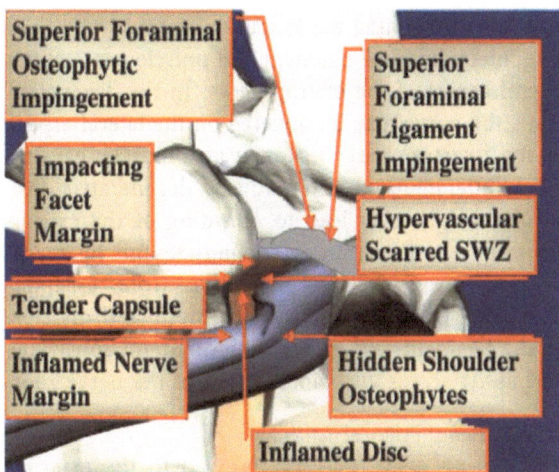

Fig. 2. Some of the new foraminal pathologies demonstrated by endoscopic aware-state evaluation of the foramen by the posterolateral approach

ties lie in the foramen and extraforaminal regions (Fig. 2). These include:

- Superior foraminal ligament impingement
- Superior notch osteophytosis
- Dorsal and shoulder osteophytes
- Facet joint impaction
- Facet joint cysts
- Pars interarticularis tethering
- Safe working zone and notch engorgement
- Ligamentum flavum infolding
- Disc pad
- Posterior longitudinal ligament irritation
- Intertransverse ligament and muscle entrapment
- Inferior external pedicular tethering
- Annulus
- Annular tears
- Shoulder osteophytes
- Lateral osteophytosis
- Paravertebral bone graft tethering
- Post-fusion discitis
- Instrumentation neural tethering
- Perineural and neural tethering and irritation

Superior Foraminal Ligament Impingement

The superior foraminal ligament passes from the ascending facet to the base of the transverse process. As settlement occurs, so this ligament bears down on the exiting nerve, and the exiting nerve may become tethered, causing local hyperaemia and irritation of the nerve at that point. This irritation is further aggravated by calcification of the ligament. The ligament is often found adherent to the nerve and the nerve is then inflamed and tender at that point. While normal radicular symptoms may be elicited from quiescent sections of the same nerve, the inflamed nerve may produce atypical dysaesthesiae.

Superior Notch Osteophytosis

When the superior foraminal ligament is resected, superior notch osteophytes may be displayed in the superior notch adherent to the exiting nerve, resulting in local inflammation. These osteophytes arise from the superior facet joint margin.

Dorsal and Shoulder Osteophytes

Osteophytes are covered by a soft tissue cap which increases their compressive effect on adjacent tissues. This effect is worsened by tethering between the osteophyte fibrous cap and the nerve, posterior longitudinal ligament or dura. Shoulder osteophytes can be found as a peripheral extension of dorsal osteophytes or as individual entities. Usually the dorsal osteophyte arises from the upper vertebral body margin and produces midline or medial foraminal tethering and inflammation and displacement of the nerve pathway. This tethering or displacement is especially noticeable during flexion. Shoulder osteophytes may also occur on the superior or inferior vertebral margin in the foramen or lateral foramen lying anterior to the nerve and tethering same. These are often hidden from view unless an active search is made on the medial or anterior (deep) surface of the nerve. These appear to lie in the pathway of the abutting impacting ascending facet joint and may indeed arise as a consequence of such impaction. The endoscopy cannula can be used to mobilise and retract the nerve whilst the nerve is separated from the fibrous cap of the osteophyte and whilst it is subsequently ablated.

Facet Joint Impaction

Facet joint impaction arises from the ascending facet joint impacting upon the exiting nerve root or the tissues in the safe working zone. The consistent presence of tissues tethering the nerve to the facet margin increases the effect of the impaction when disc degeneration leads to overriding of the facet joints during settlement and displacement. The effect is worsened as retrolisthesis and anterior listhesis occurs. Tethering between the facet joint needs to be resected and the facet joint needs to be undercut to remove the dynamic impaction. Such dynamic impaction may be the mechanism underlying many instances of so-called instability.

Facet Joint Cysts

Facet joint cysts can cause compression on exiting and traversing nerves; they can increase in size during activity and can be marsupialised after the foraminal isthmus has been enlarged and traversed.

Pars Interarticularis Tethering

Pars interarticularis defects cause tethering to traversing and exiting nerve roots. The tethering to the fibrous defect and to the bone of the anterior pars fracture site can be resected and the nerve root mobilised and decompressed. In the presence of anterior displacement, the disc wall is deformed and causes dorsal displacement of the traversing nerve roots and often, in addition, a knuckle of disc wall is displaced into the foramen, further compromising the exiting nerve root. Each of these elements can be resected under vision, with amelioration of symptoms without fusion.

Safe Working Zone and Notch Engorgement

Hypervascular tissue consisting of scarring hypervascular veins and arterioles can be found in the superior and inferior notch and in the safe working zone. This can become engorged, producing stenotic and claudicant symptoms and may itself be directly tender when inflamed.

Ligamentum Flavum Infolding

The ligamentum flavum infolds as disc height is reduced. The infolding crowds the exiting nerve root in the superior notch and in the inferior notch if the nerve is displaced. On occasion, the ligamentum flavum may be found to blend with the posterior disc pad and posterior longitudinal ligament. Resection of the ligamentum flavum at these sites serves to decompress the exiting and traversing nerve roots and to mobilise these nerve roots from local tethering. The procedure should be combined with anterior mobilisation of the nerve at the index level to achieve full mobilisation.

The ligamentum flavum may blend with the posterior foraminal ligament that passes from the superior notch, blends with the capsule and extends to the inferior notch, but of itself does not appear to cause compression.

Disc Pad

On the posterior aspect of the disc, a pad of tissue may be found which is thick and contains inflammatory blood vessels and nerves which may be locally tender in contradistinction to the annulus itself which, if not injected, is often pain-free to probing. Removal may produce immediate relief of local back pain. This may occur in the absence of a posterior collection of dye in the annulus or a leak, but it is more common to find this in association with the collection of dye.

Posterior Longitudinal Ligament Irritation (PLL)

The posterior longitudinal ligament may be inflamed and locally tender but is usually found in this state when adjacent tissues such as the disc are inflamed. Local neurolysis and ablation of adjacent tissues can resolve the inflammation. Probing of the inflamed PLL will produce pain arising in territories normally expected to be subtended by both the index and adjacent levels.

Intertransverse Ligament and Muscle Entrapment

The intertransverse ligament and muscle pass on the lateral aspect of the exiting nerve. In the degenerate state, the nerve may be tethered on the lateral aspect of the intertransverse ligament and muscle, causing local inflammation. Alternatively, degenerative loss of disc height may lead to crowding of the exiting nerve by the intertransversus muscle and ligament, so preventing the exiting nerve from escaping ascending facet. Endoscopic neurolysis and division of the ligament and muscle relieve lateral constraint and assist access and mobilisation of the nerve root.

Inferior External Pedicular Tethering

The exiting nerve may be tethered to the external surface of the inferior pedicle, especially following previous surgery and prior posterolateral bone grafted fusion. Local endoscopic neurolysis is valuable in mobilising the nerve root from the pedicle and when combined with resection of dorsally placed hypertrophic tethering bone graft.

Annulus

The annulus may be extruded or may protrude into the foramen, lateral foraminal zone or epidural posterolateral or central zones. Discectomy or resection of the central or posterolateral bulging disc may be appropriate and concur with expected clinical findings. However, protrusions in the lateral foramen may impact upon the exiting nerve and produce unexpected clinical signs, especially where this is tethered to the nerve. The disc protrusion in this area may be surprisingly small and yet produce a significant impact upon the nerve, especially where the nerve is tethered to the disc wall. Under these circumstances the disc protrusion may be imperceptible on the MRI scan. In situations of degenerate disc height loss, the wall of the disc may play only a limited role in the pathogenesis of symptoms, and under these circumstances the wall of the disc may be shrunk thermoplastically with the laser rather than be removed, further damaging the degenerate remnants of the disc. In 68 % of cases, intradiscal clearance may be performed without pain. This indicates that in these cases the inosculation of blood vessels and nerves into the annulus had either not contributed to the symptom complex or was not extensive.

Annular Tears

The annulus may be the site of intradiscal tears which may breach the annulus either under the posterior longitudinal ligament (PLL) (subligamentous) or through the PLL (transligamentous), occasioning symptoms according to the point of liberation of breakdown products. The most symptomatic are those ejecting breakdown products directly onto the nerve in the foramen. Their effect is amplified where the nerve is tethered adjacent to the exit portal of the tear. The reaction to the leakage may be formation of perineural scarring, causing adherence of the nerve to the disc, thus impeding movement of the nerve away from the point of leakage during flexion or rotation. The fibrous response may cause encapsulation of the leakage, resulting in containment and concentration of the breakdown products around the nerve. These effects worsen the symptoms and are found in patients with long-term preoperative symptom durations.

Clearance of the perineural scarring and mobilisation of the nerve should be complemented by opening of the radial tear orifice and removal of debris often holding the tear open. The course of the tear is often serpiginous, so the route of the tear can not be fully explored. It is recommended that the nucleus be explored and that degenerate material be removed manually and by laser ablation. The wall of the disc is then treated by thermoplastic annealing.

Lateral Osteophytosis
Lateral osteophytes displace the exiting nerve root dorsally and into the inferior notch, amplifying compression by the redundant annulus at that point. In addition, the lateral osteophytes cause displacement of the nerve into the middle section of the foramen, thus placing it in the path of the impacting facet joint. Partial resection of the osteophytes where they displace the nerve is valuable as part of general undercutting and enlargement of the foramen.

Paravertebral Bone Graft Tethering
Following instrumented and non-instrumented fusion, paravertebral bone graft causes anterior tethering to exiting nerve roots, with profound entrapment, often in the presence of a secure and technically correct fusion. Wide neurolysis on the anterior surface of the graft results in nerve-root mobilisation and resolution of symptoms resulting from tethering caused by such extraforaminal entrapment.

Post-fusion and Aseptic Discitis
Post-fusion discitis and aseptic discitis are manifested by a highly inflamed and tender annulus which can be relieved by manual and laser discectomy under endoscopic control. If clinical evidence of infection exists, then a fine cannula can be placed intradiscally to insert antibiotics until intravenous conversion is appropriate. However, in cases of aseptic discitis, removal of the inflamed disc contents serves to significantly reduce the back pain with subsequent resolution over a short ensuing period.

Instrumentation and Neural Tethering
Pedicle screw instrumentation can produce neural tethering either by direct impingement of the metal work or by tethering of the nerve to misplaced metalwork or microfractures of adjacent pedicles. The former, when identified, should be treated by endoscopic mobilisation of the nerve and removal of the metalwork. The latter should be treated by mobilisation of the nerve only.

Perineural Tethering and Nerve Irritation
Perineural tethering may arise as a consequence of direct irritation from a disc protrusion or facet joint impaction or the release of breakdown products. The nerve may be reddened because it is entrapped by an impacting facet joint, osteophytes and inflamed engorged hypervascular tissues in the notch. The inflammation may be aggravated by displacement of the nerve by scarring, lateral small knuckles of disc protrusion and shoulder osteophytes. The nerve may be found adjacent to annular tears adjacent to annular tears which by direct release of intradiscal breakdown products on to the nerve cause inflammation.

The exiting or traversing nerve root will produce normal radicular signs with compression. However, the irritated reddened nerve will often produce dysaesthesiae of unexpected distribution. Interestingly, adjacent sections of the nerve not irritated produce symptoms in expected territories. This may explain the cause of persistent symptoms after conventional surgery using conventional guidelines rather than the results of aware-state feedback, which may indicate that the nerve is being irritated at an adjacent and unexpected level.

Endoscopic Laser Foraminoplasty Outcome
The results of endoscopic laser foraminoplasty [1] indicate that this technique provides a minimal means of exploring the extraforaminal zone, the foramen and the epidural space and of performing discectomy, osteophytectomy and perineural neurolysis with encouraging results. It incorporates the prophylactic advantage of foraminal undercutting and provides a promising means of identifying and treating the pain of "failed back surgery" and back pain and sciatica of indeterminate origin and patients with "instability". Done in the aware state, it serves to identify and localise the source of pain generation at the time of surgery and the relevance of these findings. Endoscopic laser foraminoplasty avoids the morbidity associated with open spinal surgery and serves as a useful means of effecting "keyhole" neurolysis without extensive exploration and fusion. Current improvements in equipment promise wider application and more encouraging results in the future.

Discussion

Instability is not a diagnosis but merely a mechanism, the treatment of which requires an understanding of the effects that such abnormal micro-movements may be having upon adjacent tissues and structures. These micro-movements become, in effect, micro-trauma and as such produces inflammation and irritation in the adjacent structures, with consequent symptoms.

The posterolateral approach conducted in the aware state with the additional benefit of endoscopic evaluation has confirmed that the foramen and extra-foraminal zone is the source of hitherto unknown causes of pain, parasthesiae and neurological deficits. In the foramen, the facet joint is consistently found to be tethered to the nerve and may be tethered to the disc. When there is partial settlement or listhesis, micro-movements graduate to quite extensive ones which result in abnormal movements and cause particular impaction between the facet joint, the nerve or bulging disc. Repetition stimulates irritation and sensitisation of nerve receptors and evokes pain. This nerve compromise arises at the foramen as the nerve leaves the spinal canal; the distribution matches that normally attributed to segmental disease at the level above. This leads to maldiagnosis and incorrect indications for surgery.

Other features of the foraminal construct provide unfamiliar causes of symptoms. The superior foraminal ligament may contain small osteophytes. Either individually or in combination, the superior foraminal ligament or the contained osteophytes may impinge upon the exiting nerve root. This is often seen as reddening at the point of impact. Again, the guillotining action of these structures is aggravated by settlement or short pedicles. The nerve may be tethered directly to the disc, which, if inflamed or focally weak at the point to tethering, will distort and irritate, causing pain in the exiting or occasionally the transiting nerve. Again, this would be attributed to the superior adjacent disc level, especially as the MRI scan will not demonstrate small areas of focal annular weakness nor tethering to the disc. After prior surgery or trauma or in the case of settlement or facet joint hypertrophy, the nerve may be displaced medially or occasionally be displaced superiorly and laterally. The displacement is then held by perineural scarring. Under these circumstances, the nerve cannot deploy normally into the superior or inferior notches during flexion, extension and rotation, and is vulnerable to impact from the facet joint, the focally distorted or broad-based bulging disc, or a combination of these.

Shoulder osteophytes on the shoulder of the vertebral rim lie anterior to the exiting nerve and usually arise from the superior vertebral margin in the plane of the impacting facet. They result in tethering of the exiting nerve and local irritation and marked sensitivity. Their presence prior to a successful fusion or conventional decompression may account for persistent symptoms following technically satisfactory surgery and contribute to the "failed back-surgery" syndrome.

Conventional discectomy, decompression or fusion and height restoration fail to treat, for instance, the nerve tethered to the disc wall or the superior notch and superior foraminal ligament tethering and may, indeed, aggravate them. Endoscopy would determine the presence of such pathology and, specifically, treat it without the need for extensive surgery such as a fusion.

Tears and leaks are a common source of elusive pain. The distribution of pain depends on the direction of the leak and the containment of irritative breakdown products around the exiting or transiting nerve or dispersal along and around the posterior longitudinal ligament. Lumbar leakage may produce global dysaesthesia, urinary irritation, partial weakness, partial numbness, disproportionate back buttock or leg pain, individually or in any combination. Endoscopic aware-state examination indicates that, in cases of non-compressive radiculopathy or mild compressive radiculopathy, the text book guidelines to the source of the pain may be seriously misleading. Elusive back pain and referred pain may arise from a variety of sources which may be difficult to determine from clinical examination, X-rays and scans alone.

Spinal probing and endoscopy, however, do provide a reliable method of identifying pain sources and treating these specifically, accurately and discretely.

The conventional diagnostician favours an axial diagnosis or a facet-joint arthropathy but ignores the adjacent level foramen and may therefore be misled into addressing the wrong level. In our experience, facet-joint injections may be misleading because the steroid injection, rather than affecting the joint itself, is in fact influencing the pathology in the foramen on the anterior aspect of the joint.

The failures of conventional treatment may often arise because the pathology is not in or around the epidural space but is, surprisingly commonly, associated with the same nerve as it exits the subjacent foramen. We pay lip service to the fact that conventional surgery may fail because the incorrect level has been addressed. In fact, it may not just be the wrong level, but the wrong structure that has been addressed.

Acknowledging the prerequisite to address the correct level, surgeons seem peculiarly reluctant to define the pain site accurately before proceeding to intervention. Aware-state surgery and endoscopy provide an ideal solution to identifying the level and the aetiopathology.

The inexplicable severity or persistence of symptoms should not be classed as "illness behaviour" but rather should spark a quest to further identify the remaining pain source and treat this specifically. After all, effective hip or knee replacement in patients with long-term pain means that surgeons do not need to resort to concepts of "memory pain", "centrally perpetuated pain", "coping courses", or "psychiatric support", because the source of the pain has been eradicated effectively.

Aware-state surgery offers us the opportunity to learn more about the mechanisms of pain arising in the back and neck as well as referred pain, and to address these by consevative rehabilitation or minimal surgical intervention. It has already shown us that there are many extremely sensitive pain sources hitherto unappreciated in and about the foramen.

I belive that aware-state endoscopic surgery allows us to step forward from diagnostic "guesstimating" to precise definition of pain sources and allows us to devise specific discrete, conservative or minimal treatment thereof.

References

[1] Knight MTN, Goswami AKD, Patko J (1999) Endoscopic laser foraminoplasty and aware-state surgery: a treatment concept and outcome analysis. Die Arthroskopie 2:1–12

Laser Disc Decompression – A Treatment Algorithm

J. R. Tatay Manzanares

Introduction

According to Wisneski and Rothman [1], the success of an orthopaedic surgeon treating patients with lumbar pain at reaching the preset objectives does not depend so much on the surgeon's technical capability, but depends rather on the precision with which one chooses the correct therapeutic measures.

The following treatment algorithm seeks to achieve the following treatment targets for laser disc surgery:
- To recover functional performance.
- To re-establish normal spine function.
- To reduce costs for patients and society.
- To optimise the selection of available effective treatments.

Critical Evaluation of Conservative and Surgical Treatment

Hakelius [2] reported follow-up results of 583 patients with L5–S1 radiculopathy, comparing surgically and nonsurgically treated patients. Two months after treatment, 81 % of operated patients and 52 % of conservatively treated patients reported improvement. At six months there was no significant difference between the two groups. At final follow-up, 48 % of the operated patients had back pain, whereas this was present in 71 % of the conservatively treated patients. This data indicates that short-term results are similar, but surgery gives better long-term results.

It is accepted that a progressive neurological crisis requires emergency surgery.

But in cases of enduring symptoms, persisting after three months of conservative treatment without any significant and demonstrable improvement, surgical treatment should also be considered.

Background

In 1934 Mixter and Barr [3] published their observations on the role of nucleus pulposus herniation in causing lumbar pain. Laminectomy, introduced later, served to relieve lumbar and radicular pain. With the introduction of the microscope, surgical morbidity has been reduced considerably.

Indirect approaches to the lumbar spine to minimise morbidity started with Craig (1956) [4], who carried out a percutaneous posterolateral vetebral biopsy. The concept of using an indirect approach to decompress the herniated lumbar disc was first described by Smith [5] in 1963. He used chymopapain, an enzyme, to digest the proteoglycans of the nucleus pulposus. This enzyme was injected into the centre of the disc to digest the nucleus and to relieve intradiscal pressure and sciatica due to disc protrusion.

Indirect mechanical decompression of the lumbar disc was first performed in Philadelphia in 1973 (Philadelphia Medicine). Hijikata et al (1975) [6] described the technique of percutaneous discectomy through the posterolateral approach. Using specially designed instrumentation, enough disc material could be removed through a 6-mm incision to relieve radicular pain in 75 % of the patients. Kambin [7, 8] developed his own instrumentation and highlighted the fact that with dorsolateral opening of the annulus there is a rapid drop in the intradiscal pressure resulting in the easing of sciatic pain. Suezawa et al. [9, 10] used Hijikata's instrumentation in association with an optic fibre. Onik et al. (1984) [11, 12] introduced automated percutaneous lumbar discectomy. Mayer and Brock [13] designed nondisposable instruments that allowed the aspiration of the nucleus.

On the basis of Einstein's theory of 1917, Mainman introduced the first functional laser device in 1960. Ascher and Choy (1986) [14, 15] carried out the first laser discectomies with a Nd:YAG laser. Their results were published in 1987. Johnstone [16] made a comparative study of discectomy with laser and other techniques in the treatment of lumbar disc herniation.

Choy [17, 18, 19] and Yonezawa [20, 21] researched the effects of laser on the discs of experimental animals and proposed that the application of 1000 J of Nd:YAG laser energy to the nucleus pulposis will reduce intradiscal pressure by 50 %. Other chapters in this book disclose the results of different laser wavelengths used as percutaneous laser disc decompression (PLDD) and endoscopic laser assisted surgery (ELAS), but this paper focuses on a functional algorithm for their use.

Treatment Algorithm

Preoperative Stage

Criteria for Patient Selection

The selection of patients for surgery depends on precise diagnosis of the herniation by analysis of clinical presentation, appropriate clinical tests, assessment of psychosocial behaviour and non-invasive investigations.

The important features of clinical presentation are:
- Sudden onset or recurrence of lumbago.
- Intensity and distribution of the sciatica.
- Predominance of sciatica over lumbago.
- Radicular pain, increasing with coughing or straining and decreasing with rest.
- Presence of paraesthesiae, muscle weakness, coldness in the limbs.
  Clinical examination pinpoints:
- Abnormalities of posture.
- Abnormalities of gait, walking on tiptoe and on heels.
- Loss of intersegmental mobility.
- Control of rocking onto tiptoes or heels.
- Sciatic nerve-root stretching manoeuvres.
- Neurological deficit (sensitive and/or motor).
- Deficiencies of osteotendinous reflexes.
  Non-invasive investigations:
- Plain x-rays (AP and lateral weight-bearing).
- MRI scan of the affected area. Correlation of clinical and MR scan results is essential.

The contraindications to percutaneous techniques may be divided into absolute and relative contraindications.
  Absolute contraindications:
- Malignant spine tumour, either primary or metastasis.
- Noncontained and migrated herniations.
- Vertebral fractures.

- Central-spinal bone stenosis.
- Bleeding disorders.
- Uncontrolled diabetes.
- Multiple myeloma.
- Pregnancy.
  Relative contraindications:
- Congenital spinal deformities that do not allow access to a determined area.
- Patients with excessively high iliac crests.
- Patients with reduced intervertebral spaces and retrolisthesis or olisthesis.
- Anxious patients who may need deep sedation impairing their responses to questions during surgery.
- Spinal infections.

Operative Stage

Prior to surgery, the surgeon plans an appropriate technique to address the pathology; the choice of technique is based on the fulfilment of the clinical criteria and presentation and Bonatti's MRI classification of disc herniation. The Bonatti classification is as follows:
- Type I: 1-mm bulge, normal disc hydration, no clinical findings.
- Type II: 1–3 mm bulge, constant radiculopathy that disappears with rest.
- Type III: 3–4 mm bulge, constant radiculopathy unrelieved by conservative treatment.
- Type IV: 5 mm bulge, constant pain needing continuous medical treatment.

At surgery, discography will be used to define the technique to be used, for example, PLDD or endoscopic techniques, according to the discographic classification of Adams et al. [22] (Fig. 1, see next page). The surgical techniques employed, based on this classification system, are:
- Type I and II: PLDD, at 800–1200 J for the lumbar, and 400–600 J for the cervical region.
- Type III, IV, V: Endoscopic techniques.
- Typ VI: Microsurgery and laser ablation.

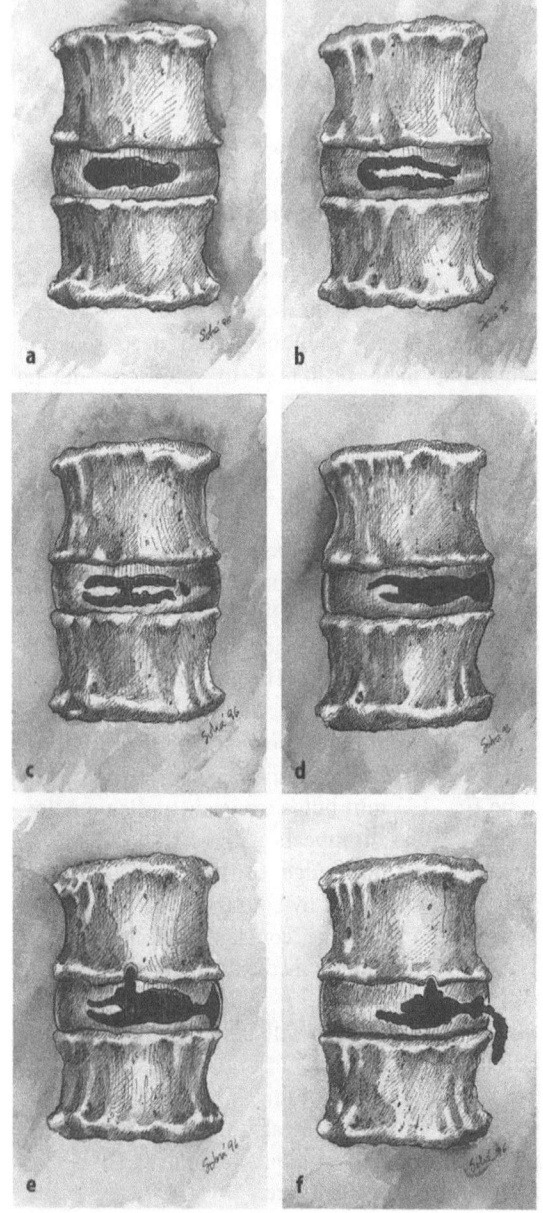

Fig. 1a–f. Discographic classification according to Adams et al. [22] into Types I to VI (*a* to *f*) (Reproduced by permission of ...)

References

[1] Wisneski RJ, Rothman RH (1985) The pennsylvania Plan II. an algorithm for the management of lumbar degenerative disc disease. Instr Course Lect 34:17–36

[2] Hakelius A (1970) Prognosis in sciatica. A clinical follow-up of surgical and non-surgical treatment. Acta Orthop Scand Suppl 129:1–76

[3] Mixer WJ, Barr JS (1934) Rupture of the intervertebral disc involvement of the spinal canal. N Eng J Med 2A:210–215

[4] Craig FS (1956) Vertebral body biopsy. J Bone Joint Surg 38A:93–102

[5] Smith L (1964) Enzyme dissolution of the nucleus pulposus in humans. JAMA 187(2):137–140

[6] Hijikata H, Yamagishi M, Nakayama T (1975) Percutaneous discectomy: a new treatment method for lumbar disc herniation. J Todenhops 5:5–13

[7] Kambin P, Casey K, O'Brien E, Zhou L (1996) Transforaminal arthroscopic decompression of lateral recess stenosis. J Neurosurg 84(3):462–467

[8] Kambin P, Zhou L (1996) History and current status of percutaneous arthroscopic disc surgery. Spine 21(24 Suppl):57S–61S

[9] Suezawa Y, Ruttimann B (1983) Indications, methods and results in percutaneous nucleotomy in lumbar disk hernia (in German). Z Orthop Ihre Grenzgeb 121(1):25–29

[10] Suezawa Y, Jacob HA, Schreiber A (1987) Percutaneous nucleotomy. An alternative to spinal surgery for lumbar disc herniation. Acta Orthop Belg 53(2):293–299

[11] Onik G, Helms CA, Ginsberg L, Hoaglund FT, Morris J (1985) Percutaneous lumbar discectomy using a new aspiration probe: porcine and cadaver model. Radiology 155(1):251–252

[12] Onik G, Maroon J, Day A, Helms C (1988) Automated percutaneous discectomy: preliminary experience. Acta Neurochir Suppl (Wien) 43:58–61

[13] Mayer HM, Brock M (1989) Differential therapy of lumbar intervertebral disc protrusion (in German). Zentralabl Chir 114(8):489–502

[14] Choy DS, Case RB, Fielding W, Hughes J, Liebler W, Ascher P (1987) Percutaneous laser nucleolysis of lumbar discs. N Engl J Med 317(12):771–772 (letter)

[15] Choy DS, Ascher PW, Ranu HS, Saddekni S, Alkaitis D, Liebler W, Hughes J, Diwan S, Altman P (1992) Percutaneous laser disc decompression. A new therapeutic modality. Spine 17(8):949–956: Erratum (1993) Spine 18(7):939

[16] Johnstone B (1987) Structure and biosynthesis of human intervertebral disc proteoglycans. Ph. D. thesis, London University

[17] Choy DS, Altman P, Trokel SL (1995) Efficiency of disc ablation with lasers of various wavelengths. J Clin Laser Med Surg 13(3):153–156

[18] Choy DS, Altman P (1995) Fall of intradiscal pressure with laser ablation. J Clin Laser Med Surg 13(3):149–151

[19] Case RB, Choy DS, Altman P (1995) Change of intradisc pressure versus volume change. J Clin Laser Med Surg 13(3):143–147

[20] Xonezawa T, Onbomura T, Kosaka R, Miyaji Y, Tanaka S, Watanabe H, Abe Y, Imachi K, Atumi K, Chinzei T et al (1990) The system and procedures of percutaneous intradiscal laser nucleotomy. Spine 15(11):1175–1185

[21] Sato K, Kikuchi S, Yonezawa T (1999) In vivo intradiscal pressure measurement in healthy individuals and in patients with ongoing back problems. Spine 24(23):2468–2474

[22] Adams M, Dolan P, Hutton W (1986) The stages of disc degeneration as revealed by discograms. J Bone Joint Surg 68B:36–41

An X-ray Jig to Facilitate
the Percutaneous Posterolateral Approach to the Lumbar Spine

M. T. N. KNIGHT

Background

Received wisdom suggests that the ideal percutaneous approach to the lumbar spine is parallel to the endplates in the lateral projection (sagittal orientation) and at 45° to the sagittal axis in the coronal plane for intradiscal surgery. This angle is too acute for the more challenging endoscopic procedures where the ideal approach is 30–35°. This allows the dilator tube and endoscope to enter the foramen and so facilitate undercutting and exploration. More shallow approaches of less than 30° tend to become blockaded by the nerve, obscuring vision. Pelvic anteversion and hyperextension inconvenience conventional "eyeball" alignment even for the experienced surgeon. Lateral intradiscal tilting can impede access dramatically and cause serious misplacement of probes and devices within the disc space. The transverse process in patients with grossly settled discs impedes access and sometimes requires to be trimmed if comprehensive access to the L5/S1 foramen safe working zone is to be effected. This is particularly the case in males with a genetically narrow pelvis. Whilst other approaches such as the transiliac approaches have been devised to gain access to L5/S1, the use of this jig has so far rendered alternatives unnecessary.

Description

The jig (Figs. 1, 2) consists of a flat beam with a longitudinal slot. A slide is affixed to the slot and attached to a side arm which can be swung out from the line of the main beam and locked at any angle. The apex of the angle can be varied by adjusting the side before locking the side arm.

The longitudinal borders of the beam are tubular to receive the pendular arms. These tubes have locking screws to hold the pendulae at any desired angle. The pendulae can be extended beyond the extent of the beam to accommodate broad patients. Each pendulum arm has an adjustable bob which can be moved along the pendulum to any desired position but easily slotting into circular slots spaced at 0.5-

cm intervals. The bob friction can be adjusted by a friction grub screw. The main beam has mm and cm measurements marked from the midline outwards and reaching to the longitudinal borders. The use of the jig takes the idiosyncrasies of skeletal structure into account and optimises the approach.

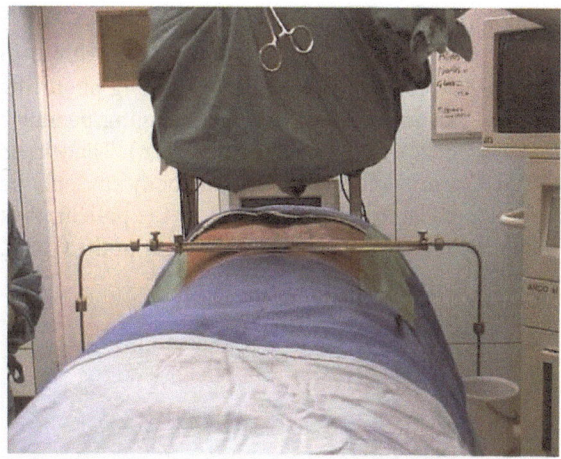

Fig. 1. The caudally directed view of the jig positioned across the patient at L4/5 with pendulae hanging free

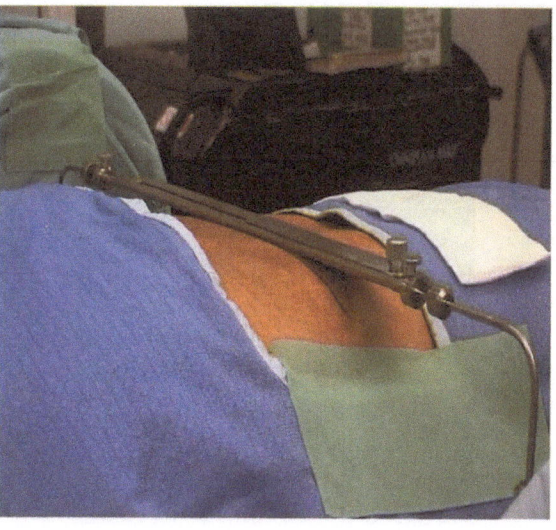

Fig. 2. Cephalically directed view of the jig aligned on the L4/5 disc

The Standard Approach to L3/4 and L4/5

The approach to levels L3/4 and L4/5 uses the standard technique. The point of skin entry should be at right angles to the point of entry into the disc in the lateral plane. Entry into any lumbar disc is ideally effected at the midpedicular line in the anteroposterior (AP) projection and on the posterior annulus. Ideal alignment may be confounded by intradiscal tilting, asymmetrical vertebrae or scoliosis. The use of the jig will assist in minimising these distorting effects, when the C arm is set parallel to the endplates in the AP projection and the dorsal spines are equidistant between the pedicles and overlap of the endplate margin in the AP plane is avoided at the outset.

The lower margin of the jig is then aligned with the midpoint of the disc space in the AP projection and a line is drawn on the skin along the lower border of the jig (Fig. 3). This line is drawn out to the flank and represents the "transverse line" (A).

The C arm is rotated into the lateral position. In the lateral projection the C arm is swung about the vertical axis until the vertical free-hanging pendulae overlap and are therefore parallel (Fig. 4). The wheels of the C arm are locked so that the body can only be moved parallel to the sagittal axis of the patient, thus retaining the ideal transverse alignment of the C arm.

The pendulum "bob" on the emitter side is then raised or lowered until it overlies the "midpoint" of the disc for a 45° approach to the disc and foramen. However, we would recommend that the bob is set for length to the "anterior" margin of the disc to produce an angle of approach of approximately 35° to the foramen. These chosen angles are used for specific but separate applications. The midpoint marker approximates a 45° approach to the disc and allows access to the safe working zone (SWZ) for small (2 mm) diameter instrumentation in procedures such as laser disc decompression. For endoscopic approaches this angle will cause the dilator tube to impinge on the lateral aspect of the facet and cause pressure on the exiting nerve root. This vertically may force the surgeon to excessively displace the exiting nerve or mistakenly to operate lateral to the nerve. This will preclude access through the foramen, especially in cases where there is disc settlement or facet joint hypertrophy. The anterior border of the disc is preferred as the marker for endoscopic laser foraminoplasty as it facilitates an approach medial and posterior to the exiting nerve root and facilitates the exploration of the epidural space and the SWZ. The selected length is measured as the bob length (B). This length (B) is marked from the midline along the transverse line (A) and marks the entry portal for the desired procedure.

The L5/S1 Approach

When addressing the L5/S1 level, the surgeon should make every effort to choose the optimal skin incision, for the L5/S1 approach is more awkward than that at L3/4 or L4/5. However, the portal can often be used to approach both L5/S1 and L4/5 levels.

For the L5/S1 approach, the jig is set up and aligned as described above on L4/L5 in the AP and lateral planes (Fig. 5). The overlapping pendulae and L4 vertebra are positioned at the junction of the cephalad/middle third of the x-ray frame (Fig. 6). The L5/S1 disc space should lie at or just above the

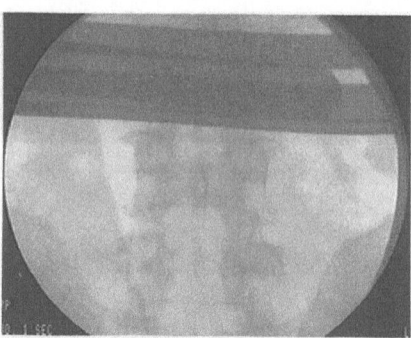

Fig. 3. AP view of jig aligned to tilted L3/4

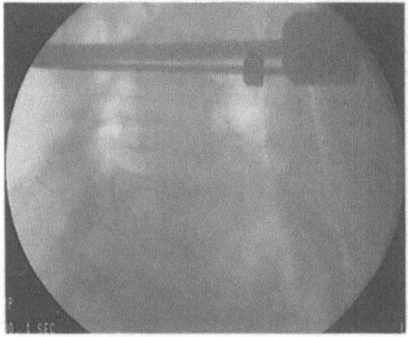

Fig. 4. Pendulae almost aligned in the lateral plane on L3/4

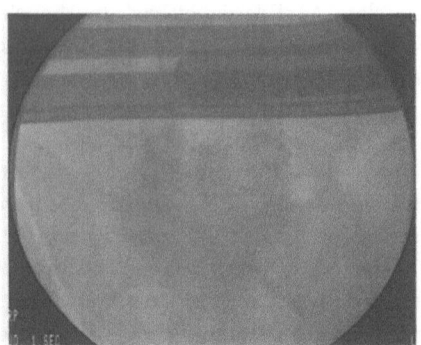

Fig. 5. AP x-ray view of lower margin of jig aligned on the lower border of L4

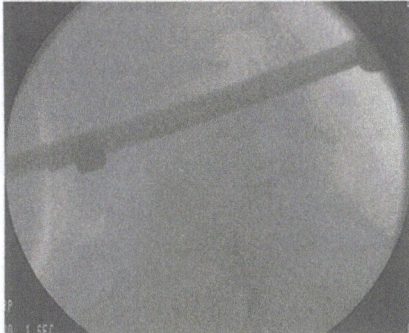

Fig. 6. Lateral x-ray view of pendulae overlapping over the L4/5 disc with pendulae mid- to upper screen

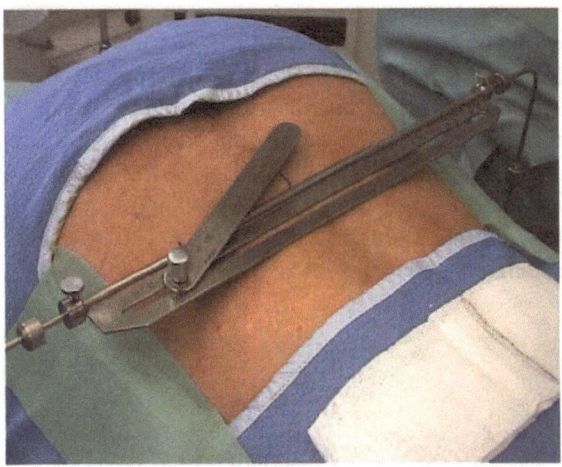

Fig. 7. The bob length is marked from the midline along the lower margin of the jig. The side arm is rotated caudally, crossing the jig margin at this mark

caudal third junction of the screen. Thereafter the pendular arms are flexed to lie in the midlateral plane of the L5/S1 disc space and are locked in position parallel to the endplate of L5. The pendulae may lie above or below the S1 endplate in this preliminary position because they do not overlap. The body of the C arm is then moved caudally but parallel to the sagittal axis of the patient until the pendulae overlap once again. The position of the jig should be adjusted superiorly or inferiorly until the pendulae clear the lower margin of the transverse process of L5. Adjustment must be associated with alteration in the position of the body of the C arm to maintain the overlap of the pendulae and retention of parallel alignment with the lower margin of the L5 endplate.

The transverse line (A) is redrawn along the lower border of the jig in the new position. The midpoint marker approximates a 45° aopproach to the disc and allows access to the SWZ for small (2 mm) diameter instrumentation in procedures such as laser disc decompression. For endoscopic approaches this angle will cause the dilator tube to impinge on the lateral aspect of the facet and cause pressure on the exiting nerve root.

This verticality may force the surgeon to excessively displace the exiting nerve or mistakenly to operate lateral to the nerve. This will preclude access through the foramen, especially in cases where there is disc settlement or facet joint hypertrophy.

The anterior border of the disc is preferred as the marker for endoscopic laser foraminoplasty as it facilitates an approach medial and posterior to the exiting nerve root and facilitates the exploration of the epidural space and the SWZ.

The selected length is measured as the bob length (b) (Fig. 7). This length is measured *along* the pendulum rather than vertically. This distance is marked from the midline elong the transverse line (A) and marks the distance from the midline for the entry portal for the desired procedure, but does not

account for the idiosyncratic obliquity or the approach enforced by the iliac crests.

The C arm is restored to the AP projection and the vertical angle is adjusted to match the angle of the pendulae locked on the L5 endplates (Fig. 8).

The L5/S1 level approach is compromised by factors including the obstructive presence of the iliac crests, higher in males, the narrowness of the android pelvis, the presence of L5 vertebral retroversion, disc settlement, posterior and lateral osteophytes, hypertrophic facet joints and pelvic anteversion, large transverse processes and pseudarthroses. The jig seeks to optimise the approach by addressing these problems by the use of the side arm line (S). The side arm is swung out from the lower border of the jig until the lower free margin of the side arm ruler passes below the pedicle of L5 and marks the midpedicular point on the L5/S1 annulus. The C arm is moved mediolaterally until the hinge lies at the midpoint of the outer third of the screen. The axial hinge of the side arm is moved mediolaterally

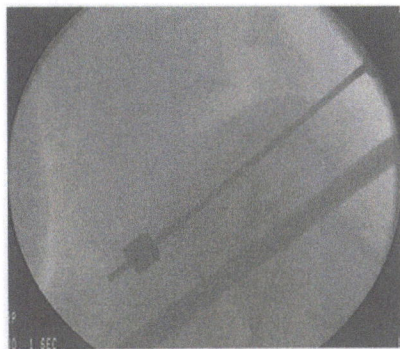

Fig. 8. Lateral x-ray with pendulae rotated until parallel with lower border of L5

until the lower margin of the ruler abuts the outline of the iliac crest on the AP x-ray. The medial alignment must be maintained below the pedicle of L5. The C arm should be adjusted so that the hinge of the side arm lies between the midpoint of the screen and the lateral third junction (Figs. 9–12). The lower border of the side arm is marked as the side arm line (S). The entry protal is defined as the point of coincidence between the lower border of the side arm

ruler where this crosses the transverse line (A). Where this crossing point is short of the length established as the bob length (B), then the entry point is arrived at by migrating along the side arm line (S) until the bob length (B) is obtained, but measured parallel to the transverse line (A) (Figs. 13, 14).

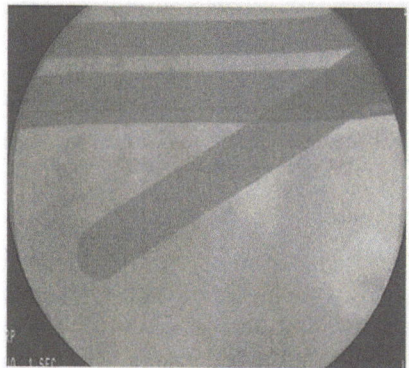

Fig. 12. The side arm is adjusted until it passes midway between the ipsilateral pedicles and abuts the free border of the iliac margin

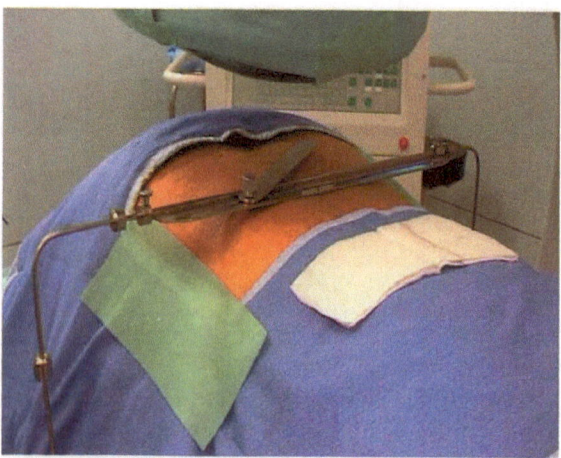

Fig. 9. The sidearm is adjusted under x-ray control until it passes midway between the ipsilateral pedicles and abuts the free border of the iliac margin

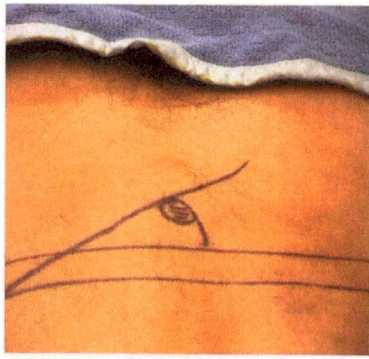

Fig. 13. A line is drawn along the inferior boder of the side arm and is projected until it coincides with the distance from the midline established by the bob length

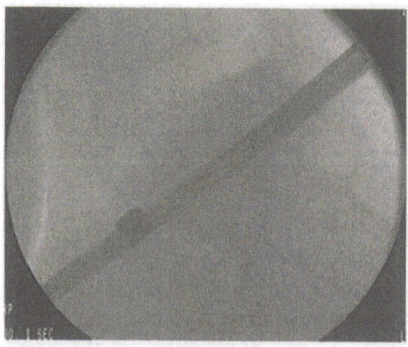

Fig. 10. Lateral x-ray with pendulae rendered parallel by moving C-arm base

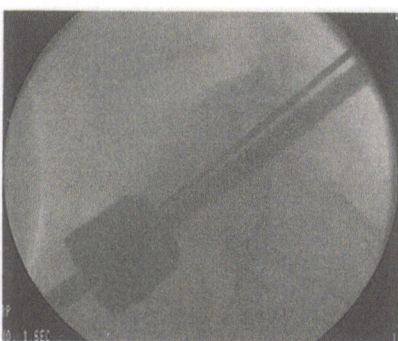

Fig. 11. The large "bob" is adjusted until the upper margin is flush with the anterior border of L5

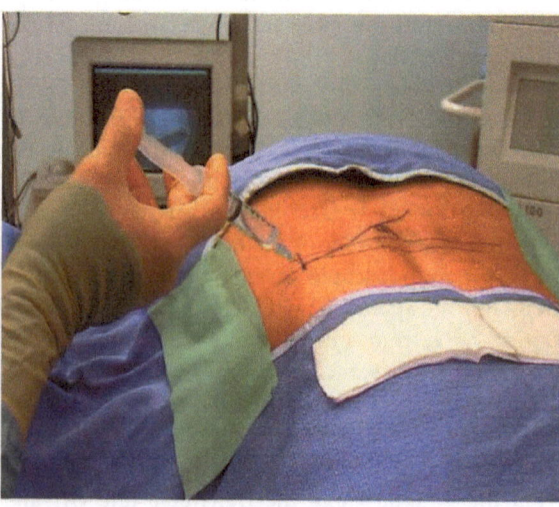

Fig. 14. Local anaesthetic is inserted of the defined coincidence point

This technique should allow the approach to pass close to the iliac crest and bring the approach probe to the annulus avoiding impediment from the transverse process of L5 and allow direct approach to the L4/L5 disc under normal circumstances, thus limiting the number of incisions (Figs. 15, 16). It may result in proximal migration of the entry point but maintains obliquity at approximately 35° to the foramen, avoids the L5 transverse process, and accommodates for the iliac crest.

Whereas others have advocated a skin portal measured 12 cm from the midline, this rigid concept does not accommodate for postural variation and height and weight variation. The above technique has facilitated this approach in males and females of widely varying frames and also accommodates variation in obesity. This technique was reproducible in 50 cases redrawn by a second operator to arrive at an identical entry point in 46 cases and within 2 mm in the remainder. It is therefore valuable for those in training as well as for the experienced practitioner.

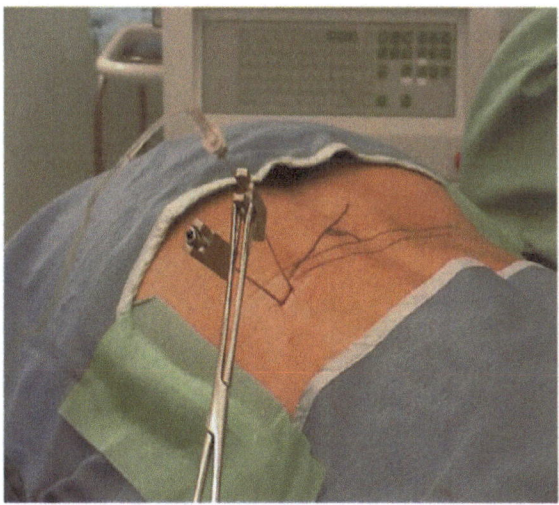

Fig. 15. Separate incisions are used for L5/S1 and L4/5, but they can be combined

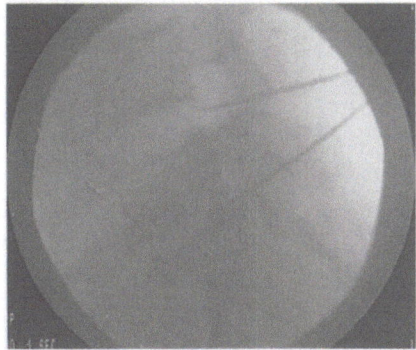

Fig. 16. Probes inserted from a single portal

The L1/2 and L2/3 Approach

Access to L1/2 and L2/3 is forced by the lower rib margin to be oblique. The procedure starts as that described for the L3/L4 level and is modified inversely as with the L5/S1 approach. The C arm is set in the AP projection and adjusted until the end plates are parallel and free from overlap at the target disc. The jig is placed upon the patient in the "inverted" postion with the pendulae cephalad. The jig is applied and aligned to the midpoint of the disc and parallel to the L2/3 end plates in the AP projection. The C arm is rotated into the lateral plane and aligned about the vertical until both pendulae overlap. The transverse line (A) is marked along the superior margin of the jig. The pendulae are rotated to lie parallel to the superior margin of the inferior vertebra abutting the target disc. With the C arm locked about the vertical axis it is moved en masse cephalad until the pendulae overlap again. In the case of the L1/2 disc, the jig may need to be moved cephalad until the pendulae clear the transverse process of L1 and the C arm moved cephalad or caudally until the penduale overlap.

The midpoint marker approximates a 45° approach to the disc and allows access to the SWZ for small (2 mm) diameter instrumentation in procedures such as laser disc decompression. For endoscopic approaches this angle will cause the dilator tube to impinge on the lateral aspect of the facet and cause pressure on the exiting nerve root. This verticality may force the surgeon to excessively displace the exiting nerve or mistakenly to operate lateral to the nerve. This will preclude access through the foramen, especially in cases where there is disc settlement or facet joint hypertrophy.

The anterior border of the disc is preferred as the marker for endoscopic laser foraminoplasty as it facilitates an approach medial and posterior to the exiting nerve root and facilitates the exploration of the epidural space and the SWZ. The selected length is the bob length (B). This length is measured *along* the pendulum rather than vertically. This distance is marked from the midline along the transverse line (A) and marks the distance from the midline for the entry portal for the desired procedure but does not account for the idiosyncratic obliquity of the approach enforced by the rib margin and the need to circumvent the visceral space and kidneys.

The C arm is restored to the AP projection and the vertical angle is adjusted to match the angle of the pendulae locked on the L1 or L2 end plates. The jig seeks to optimise the approach by the use of the side arm line (S). The side arm is swung out from the upper border of the jig until the superior free margin of the side arm ruler passes above the pedicle of L2 or L3 and marks the midpedicular point on the target annulus. The C arm is moved mediolaterally until the hinge lies at the midpoint of the outer third of the screen. The axial hinge of the side arm is moved mediolaterally until the upper margin of the ruler abuts the outline of the lowest rib on the AP x-ray. The medial alignment must be maintained above the selected pedicle. The C arm should be adjusted to the hinge of the side arm that lies between the midpoint of the screen and the lateral third junction.

The upper border of the side arm is marked as the side arm line (S). The entry portal is defined as the point of coincidence between the upper border of the side arm ruler where this crosses the transverse line (A). Where this crossing point is short of the length established as the bob length (B), the entry point is arrived at by migrating along the side arm line (S) until the bob length (B) is obtained but measured parallel to the transverse line (A). This technique should allow the approach to pass close to the lowest rib and bring the approach probe to the annulus, avoiding impediment from the transverse process of L2 and allowing direct approach to the L1/L2 or L2/L3 disc under normal circumstances, thus limiting the number of incisions.

The approach to L1/2 and L2/3 levels is compromised by factors including the obstructive presence of the lower ribs, long or inferiorly angulated transverse processes, the shallow position of the posterior visceral cavity in some patients and the kidneys and adrenal glands. Analysis of the MRI scan is advised to preoperatively check these features. When selecting the skin portal distance from the midline, the safest point is at the border of the thoracolumbar fascia at the upper border of the jig after displacement, to coincide with the lower margin of the rib. When venturing to use the ideal position more laterally, please proceed with caution, preserving a shallow approach initially and deepening after the border of the thoracolumbar facia has been traversed. The above technique has facilitated this approach in males and females of widely varying frames and also accommodates for variation in obesity and has avoided damage to perineural or visceral structures to date.

Experiences in 120 Cases with Percutaneous Non-endoscopic Laser Disc Decompression (PLDD) Using the Nd:YAG Laser System in the Cervical Spine – Retrospective Study of 40 Cases

K. Diehl · A. Ruffing · A. Wollny

Background

The Nd:YAG laser is well known for its ability to coagulate and vaporize tissue through flexible fibres. The application of the 1064-nm wavelength creates a homogeneous carbonized cavity in the disc space. At the same time, the surrounding tissue loses water and dries out, causing shrinkage of the disc.

Since the nucleus pulposus does not have any specific absorption in the wavelength of the Nd:YAG laser, energy application in noncontact mode causes strong scattering in the tissue, with possible coagulation within a range between 5 and 10 mm. Carbonization changes the optical properties of the tissue. Black carbonization completely absorbs the laser light into a small volume, causing a local temperature increase, which leads to vaporization of the surrounding tissue. This thermal effect is limited and there is macroscopically no irritation of the surrounding nerves. Our own experiments showed that the temperature doesn't increase by more than 8 °C when cadaveric spine is lased with energies of 600–800 J in the cervical spine and 1500–2000 J in the lumbar spine with the Nd:YAG laser at 1066 nm. Similar results have been reported by Siebert (1991).

Choy and Ascher (1992) used laser energy to treat the lumbar spine already in 1986. By 1990, Hellinger (1993) started treating cervical disc pathology with laser. Due to the gratifying results of the treatment of lumbar and cervical disc herniations with laser, we started using Nd:YAG laser in the cervical spine in 1993. The procedure has been described by Hellinger (1993).

Materials and Methods

Inclusion Criteria

Initially, clinical indication was restricted to monosegmental cervical radiculopathy without paresis. Later we included patients with multilevel pathology, whose clinical symptoms continued to deteriorate despite conservative treatment. This respresents a cohort integrity of 33 %.

Between August 1993 and July 1996, 120 patients were treated. All the patients were contacted for an examination in August 1996 for postoperative follow-up. We report here the results of 40 patients who took part in a postoperative examination in the hospital. The follow-up period ranged from 5 months to a maximum of 32 months. The average follow-up period was 21.6 months.

Preoperative Examinations

Before operation, each patient had a neurological examination in our department of neurology, including EMG examination and evoked potentials, to exclude onset myelopathy.

Imaging Procedures

An x-ray of the cervical spine was performed in four planes to show bone pathology. CT or MRI scans confirm the status of the discs and the spinal canal. If there is still uncertainty about the pathology, we perform myelography in flexion and extension positions, including CT myelography with 2-mm slices, especially in cases of lateral herniation of the disc.

Procedure

Thirty minutes before the beginning of the procedure, 2 Cephazolin 29 (Hexal) is administered intravenously. To reduce spinal oedema, we infuse 1 mg Methylprednisolone shortly before the start of the procedure. The procedure is performed under local anaesthesia and as necessary, additional intravenous anaesthesia (Remifentanil [Glaxo Wellcome] 0.03 µg/kg) or anaesthesia under spontaneous respiration is provided. The patient is made to lie on the back, with the head in a reclined position. A 2–4-kg skull traction is applied. Draping is done as for trauma surgery of the cervical spine.

The skin corresponding to the target disc space is marked after x-ray localization. The needle entry point is then infiltrated with local anaesthesia. We prefer the left side, independent of the side of the pathology. We use a cannula with a diameter of 1.6

mm. The anterior surface of the cervical spine is palpated, the trachea and oesophagus are displaced medially, and the common carotid artery and sternocleidomastoid muscle are displaced laterally. After a small skin incision has been made, the needle is inserted under x-ray (image intensifier) control in two planes with the needle directed towards the index disc level. After making contact with the vertebra or the disc, the deep tissues are infiltrated with local anaesthesia. The most uncomfortable time for the patient is during the deep palpation of the ventral cervical spine.

The AP x-ray view must show that the tip of the needle is in a medial position. Lateral x-ray control shows the needle at the disc under study. The needle is progressed in increments until the needle reaches the dorsal third of the disc diameter. After x-ray confirmation and photo documentation of the needle position, the laser fibre is inserted. The tip of the fibre is projected 2 mm beyond the tip of the needle. The energy is applied by a Dornier Nd:YAG laser system (Fibertom, 1064 nm) via a 0.6-mm glass fibre. The setting is 20 W and 0.3 s, which corresponds to approximately 7 J per pulse. No suction is used. After each 200 J of laser energy application there is a short break to check the neurology. After reaching 400 to 800 J, the procedure is stopped. Energy application is usually pain-free.

Occasionally, some patients experience nonspecific pain radiating to the neck and shoulder region. This pain ceases soon after laser energy application has been stopped. After the procedure, the patient wears a collar for 4 weeks. Isometric exercises are advised postoperatively.

Results

We report on the results of 74 segments treated with PLDD in 40 patients. In four cases we had C3/4 pathology, in 16 cases C4/5 pathology, in 32 cases C5/6 pathology, in 20 cases C6/7 pathology and in two cases C7/T1 pathology. Sixty percent of the patients had a double-level treatment and 12.5% had a triple-level treatment.

Infections

None of the patients had any infections postoperatively.

Complications

Two patients had postoperative swallowing complaints and one patient developed postoperative haematoma. One patient with level 3 PLDD had severe and persisting pain from facet-joint syndrome, which lasted several weeks.

Paresis

In 40% of patients paresis was noted preoperatively: this reduced to 5% of the cases after percutanous laser disc decompression. We didn't have worsening of paresis.

Sensory Impairment

Nearly 50% of the patients suffered sensory impairment before the operation. After the operation, the impairment had disappeared in six patients, and the remaining group reported improvement of their sensory impairment. In nearly half of the cases, improvement occurred immediately after the procedure. In approximately one-quarter of the cases, improvement occurred within 1 week. Between the third and fourth postoperative week, improvement occurred in one-fifth of the cases. After this time, we found no significant improvement in symptoms.

Postoperative Drug Consumption

Before the operation, 80% of the patients had used pain medication permanently. At the follow-up, 20% of patients used drugs occasionally.

Local Pain

Persistent cervical pain unresponsive to conservative treatment before the procedure was reported in 50% of the cases. At follow-up, only two patients had residual pain symptoms.

Radicular Pain

Radicular pain was found in more than 50% of the patients before the operation. At the final follow-up, 10% of the patients continued to have radicular symptoms.

Headaches

Headaches were reported in 40% of the cases before operation. Afterwards, it was found in less than 10% of the cases.

Cervical Lordosis

Preoperative lateral x-ray showed a decrease of the cervical lordosis in many cases. Return of the normal lordotic cervical curvature was observed in most of the patients who had a laser disc decompression. Deterioration of the cervical curvature was observed in none of the cases.

Height of the Disc Space

After the procedure, we found a decrease in disc height of 0.5 to 1 mm in the treated discs, especially in the dorsal region of the disc.

Laser Effect in the MRI

All cases showed signal enhancement of the adjacent vertebrae in the $T2$-weighted MR scan images performed almost immediately after the procedure. Gadolinium-enhanced MRI showed a strong uptake of gadolinium in the region. Initially this was interpreted as a bacterial infection. However, haematological parameters and CRP measurements, x-rays of the cervical spine and CT scans showed no evidence of infection. This reaction is interpreted as a transient benign reaction which resolves after 2 months.

Local Tissue Changes Following PLDD

In patients who had a cervical fusion after unsuccessful PLDD, no complications directly attributable to the foregoing PLDD procedure could be identified. Only the annulus was usually found to be very stiff. We assume this occurred as a result of shrinking and dehydration of tissues due to the application of laser energy.

References

[1] Choy DSJ, Altmann P (1995) Fall of intradiscal pressure with laser ablation. J Clin Las Med surg 13:149–152
[2] Choy DSJ, Ascher PW, Ranu HS, Saddekni S, Alkaitis D, Lieber W, Hughes J, Diwan S, Altman P (1992) Percutaneous laser disc decompression – a new therapeutic modality. Spine 7:949–956
[3] Choy DSJ, Case RB, Ascher P (1987) Percutaneous laser ablation of lumbar discs. A preliminary report of in-vitro and in-vivo experience in animal and/or human patients. In: 33rd Annual Meeting, Orthopeadic Research Scoiety 1:19
[4] Choy DSJ, Case RB, Fielding W, Hughes J, Liebler W, Ascher P (1987) Percutaneous laser nucleolysis of lumbar discs. New Eng J Med 317:771
[5] Choy DSJ, Michelsen, Getrajdman G, Diwans S (1992) Percutaneous laser disc decompression. An update. J Clin Laser Med Surg 6:177
[6] Choy DSJ (1995) Clinical experience and results with 389 PLDD procedures with ND:YAG laser, 1986 to 1995. J Clin Las Med Surg 13:209–214
[7] Ascher PW, Holzer P, Sutter B, Tritthard N (1991) Nucleus-pulposus-Denaturierung bei Bandscheibenprotrusionen. In: Siebert WE, Wirth CJ (eds) Laser in der Orthopadie. Thieme, Stuttgart, pp 169–172
[8] Ascher PW (1985) Status quo and new horizons of laser therapy in neurosurgery. Lasers Srug Med 5:499
[9] Hellinger J (1993) Simultane Lasernukleotomie bei zervikalen und lumbalen Bandscheibenvorfällen. Lasermed 9:121–122
[10] Siebert WE, Bisek K, Breitner S, Fritsch K, Wirth CJ (1988) Die Nucleus-pulposus-Vaporisation – Eine erneute Technik zur Behandlung des Bandscheibenvorfalles? Orthop Prax 12:732
[11] Siebert WE, Krohn D, Breitner S, Wirth CJ (1988) Laser in der Orthopädie – Gibt es sinnvolle Anwendungsmöglichkeiten? Orthop Praxis 11:667–669
[12] Siebert WE, Kinsik B, Wirth CJ, Seinmetz M, Mutschter R (1991) In vitro-Untersuchungen zur thermischen Belastung der Bandscheibe bei der Laserablation. In: Siebert WE, Wirth CJ (eds) Laser in der Orthopädie. Thieme, Stuttgart, pp 150–153
[13] Siebert WE (1989) Nucleus pulpsus vaporization experimental investigations on use of lasers on the intervertebral disc. In: Mayer HM, Brock M (eds) Percutaneous nucleotomy. Springer, Berlin Heidelberg New York
[14] Siebert WE (1995) Percutaneous laser disc decompression of cervical discs. J Clin Las Med Surg 13:205–209
[15] Siebert WE (1993) Percutaneous laser disc decompression: the European experience. Spine 7:103–133

Infrared Thermography and the Determination of the Ablation Volume in Cervical Laser Discectomy

S. Schmolke · L. Kirsch · F. Barth · F. Gossé

Introduction

Herniated cervical intervertebral discs and protrusions are frequently presented in neurosurgical and orthopedic patients.

The Rochester study on the epidemiology of cervical radiculopathy registered an incidence of radicular symptoms in 83 out of every 100,000 individuals. In around 22 % of cases, the cause was identified to be a herniated intervertebral disc [6, 10, 14, 23]. This suggests that almost 19 individuals in every 100,000 will suffer a herniated cervical intervertebral disc.

Over the last few years, there has been controversy over the type of surgical treatment for herniated cervical intervertebral discs and the extent of disc excision desired for a satisfactory clinical outcome. These days, minimally invasive therapy is the most frequently used method of treatment in many clinics. Compared to the "classic" surgical procedures that involve fusion of the affected spinal segment, the intradiscal decompressive procedure requires removal of only a relatively small section of the intervertebral disc material.

The procedure described by Cloward and Smith-Robinson and introduced in the middle of the 1950s has undergone great improvements and is cited as the standard surgical procedure for cervical disc herniation [1, 2, 3, 7, 10, 12, 16, 18, 21, 22, 27, 28].

Minimally invasive techniques, such as PLDD, can only be regarded as supplementary therapy due to their limited indication spectrum. Excision of herniated intervertebral discs, and sequestered discs in particular, may involve open as well as endoscopic surgery. After successful results have been reported for the treatment of herniated lumbar intervertebral discs in 1990, cervical PLDD has been performed more frequently [4, 5, 26]. Hellinger performed the first cervical PLDD in 1990. There have been reports of serious complications resulting from this procedure [26].

Until now, there has been no documented experimental basic research on temperature changes and reaction to ablation of intradiscal laser treatment in the region of the cervical spine. The aim of this study was to determine whether, within the presently used clinical parameters, laser treatment of the cervical disc can endanger the physical integrity of the neurovascular structures, and whether the technical parameters required further optimization. For this purpose, a thermal camera was used to determine the heat generated during laser treatment. The temperature measurements with the thermoscan would immediately indicate whether dangerous heating was likely to occur.

Materials and Methods

Mobile segments of the human cervical spine between C2-C7 were used in the study of the temperature assessment during laser treatment. The specimens were removed from the donors within 24 hours of death, packed in airtight containers, and frozen at –20 °C. Prior to testing, the specimens were thawed in a warm water bath and freed of remaining musculature. The second step involved removal of the vertebral arch. The prepared mobile segments were then tested in a specifically designed experimental setup (Fig. 1). A thermographic camera (Agema Thermovision 470 Pro, Rietberg, Germany) was used to detect the heat radiation. The camera demonstrated a thermal resolution (noise-equivalent temperature difference) of 0.02° at 30 °C ambient temperature. The emission constant c (the relation of specific radiation of a true body to an ideal "black body") was set at 0.95 for biological tissue (Fig. 2).

For the experiment, the thermograph camera was positioned behind the spine allowing the target region, that is, the dorsal intervertebral disc demarcation, to be in the focal zone of the camera. The ventral aspect of the intervertebral disc was punctured with a specially designed gold-covered laser cannula (Aesculap, Tuttlingen, Germany). The previously assessed and prepared laser fibers were then pushed through the cannula into the intervertebral disc space. The distance between the distal fiber end and the posterior longitudinal ligament could be determined from the length of the laser fiber mea-

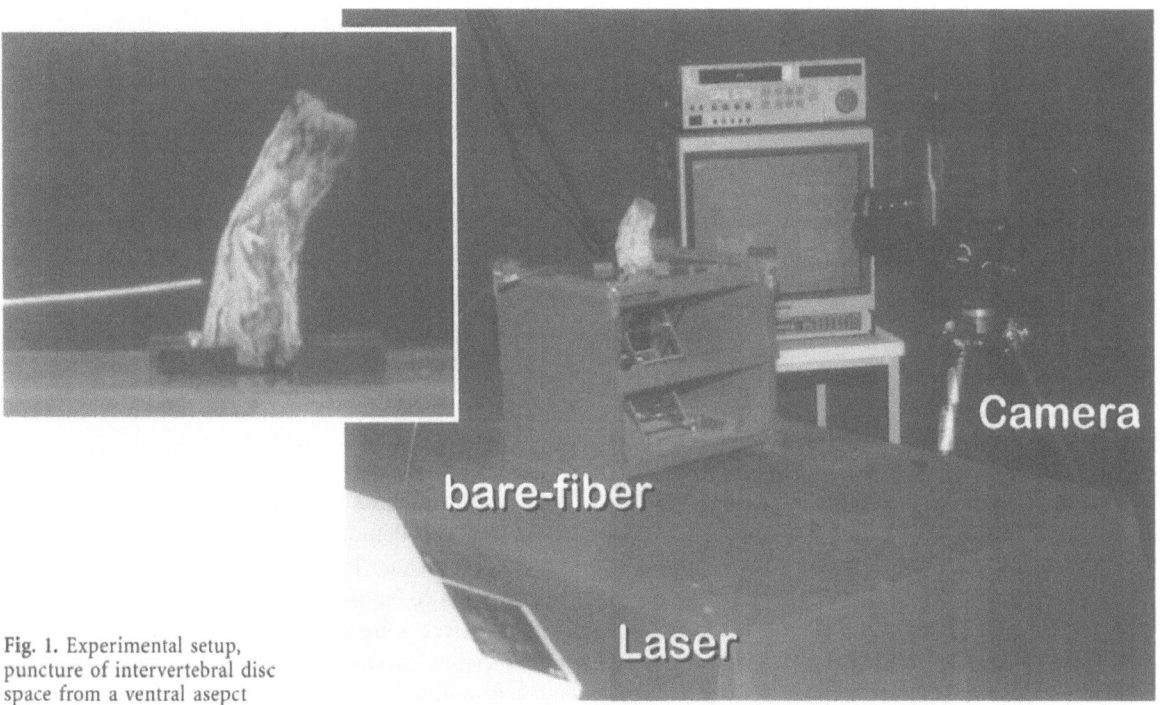

Fig. 1. Experimental setup, puncture of intervertebral disc space from a ventral asepct

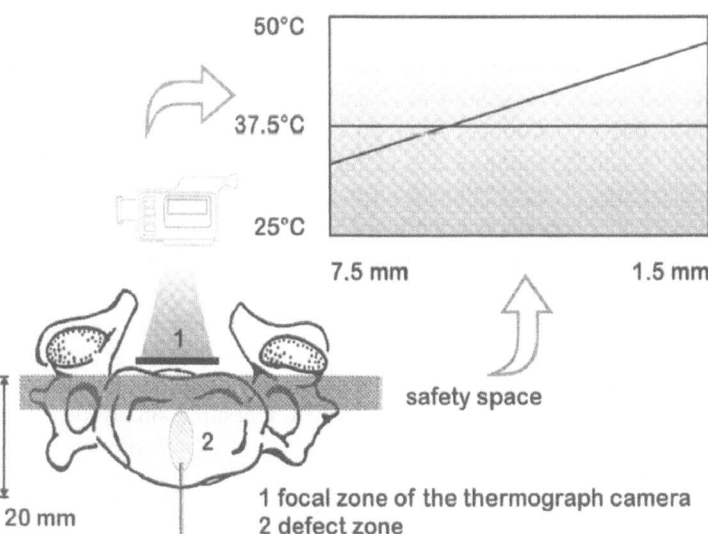

Fig. 2. Schematic experimental structure and maximal temperature values of thermography testing as a function of the width of the intervertebral space between the dorsal demarcation of the denaturation zone and posterior longitudinal ligament

sured in relation to specific points marked on the instruments in the experimental setup (Fig. 3).

The method of energy application and the applied energy was altered sequentially in an individual series of experiments to identify the most favorable combinations of parameters (Table 1). An Nd:YAG laser (MediLas 40 N, Firma Dornier Medizintechnik, Gemmaring, Germany) was used with a wavelength of 1064 nm. At the start of the energy application, the recording of the temperature was also initiated. This ensured monitoring and documentation of all changes on a continually running graph.

The results of the experiment were assessed at each stage. Firstly, the dimensions of the intervertebral discs were measured in the sagittal and the transverse plane. They were divided in the middle along the transverse plane, photographed to true scale, and digitally measured. The next step involved measurements in the sagittal plane (Fig. 3). The defect zone was also accurately documented and assessed in two planes. The digital measurements were carried out with the OPTIMAS 5.0 program (Optimas Corporation, Edmond, USA; Weskamp & Partner GmbH, Meerbusch, Germany). This made volumetric

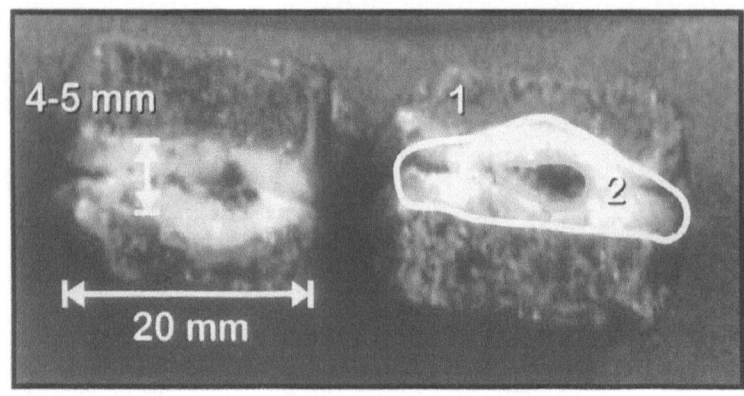

Fig. 3. Cut in sagittal area through cervical intervertebral disc 5/6

Table 1. Laser parameters

Parameter	
Laser output	5/10 W
Energy level conducted	400/600 J
Laser fiber diameter	200/400 µm
Width of intervertebral space between the dorsal demarcation of the denaturation zone and the posterior longitudinal ligament	1.5–4 cm

measurements possible. Assessment of the infrared thermograph pictures was given in a descriptive form, since numerous parameter variables would have been difficult to correlate and analyze statistically.

Results

Some new data were obtained, correlating laser energy application to the mass of disc ablated. The digitally measured areas of tissue which underwent macroscopic changes with laser radiation showed an average volume defect of 8.4 mm³ out of the total intervertebral disc volume of approximately 2000 mm³. This demonstrated that clinically acceptable energy levels cause less than 1 % of the intervertebral disc volume reduction [15].

The defect zone lay in a central position in the intervertebral space. Differentiation between the nucleus pulposus and the annulus fibrosus was not possible with the naked eye.

It was assumed that most of the nucleus pulposus was ablated by laser (Fig. 4). Earlier anatomical and planimetric investigations of the lumbar intervertebral disc between L1 to L5 demonstrated an average disc volume of 12 cm³, of which the nucleus pulposus accounted for 4 cm³. After laser application a defect volume of 5 % of the total intervertebral was determined: this corresponded to 15 % of the nucleus pulposus volume [24, 25, 29].

The applied energy level of 1500 J was 2–3 times higher than that applied to the cervical region. There is no relation between the rise in temperature and the volume of disc tissue ablated in the relatively large lumbar spinal column. In the cervical spine, the defect created measured on average 0.6 cm × 0.4 cm in the horizontal plane, with a surface area of 9 mm².

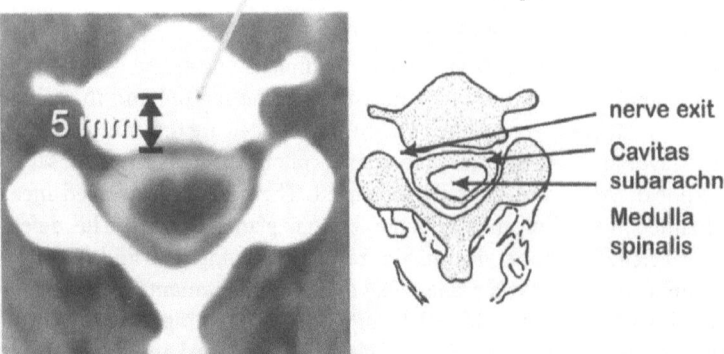

Fig. 4. Distance between laser fiber and myelin

Infrared Thermography

The influence of time on the temperature gradient could not be statistically correlated. Therefore, a descriptive account is presented with the aid of the IRVIN 2.07 program (Firma Agema Infrared Systems, Rietberg, Germany). Figures 5 and 6 show two typical temperature courses during laser application. In the experimental series shown in Fig. 5, the Nd:YAG laser was used with an output of 10 W. The energy applied amounted to 400 J when using a 200-μm fiber.

With 300 J, a true temperature of 45 °C was registered in the target region. This corresponds to a temperature increase of approximately 17 °C, with an initial tissue temperature of 28 °C. In other experimental series, shown in Fig. 6, a total of 600 J was applied to the intervertebral disc. The laser application was carried out with an output of 20 W. The temperature recorded here was 50 °C in the focal zone of the camera. Both produced a defect zone of 4 mm at the posterior longitudinal ligament.

Discussion

The results show that there is only a small loss of discal nucleus material with laser energy application. This suggests that a reduction in intradiscal pressure cannot be brought about by laser radiation [29]. This study also suggests that the symptomatic improvements observed in patients may have no bearing on the reduction in intradiscal pressure. Other factors appear to play a role in the described clinical success.

A number of studies have been carried out over the past few years to determine the biochemical changes occurring in damaged intervertebral discs [6, 7, 8, 11, 13]. It may be assumed that the initial beneficial results brought about by laser radiation in this region are a result of inactivation of inflammatory substances (e.g., phospholipase A^2), or results from the direct ablation of nociceptors. This could explain the lack of pain immediately following surgery. Anatomical–morphological studies by Mendel demonstrate that most of the pain-inducing nerve fibers are found in the posterolateral region of the intervertebral space [15, 17, 19]. They lie directly in the radiation field of the laser fiber. There are no reported studies on the dangers of laser treatment of cervical discs, especially the dangers to the important neurovascular structures such as the vertebral artery, nerve roots, and the dura.

Another important safety factor demonstrated with thermography is the distance of the tip of the laser fibers to the dorsal intervertebral disc–spinal canal interface (Fig. 4). During operations, the exact fiber position cannot be determined, even under the most favorable conditions involving image mag-

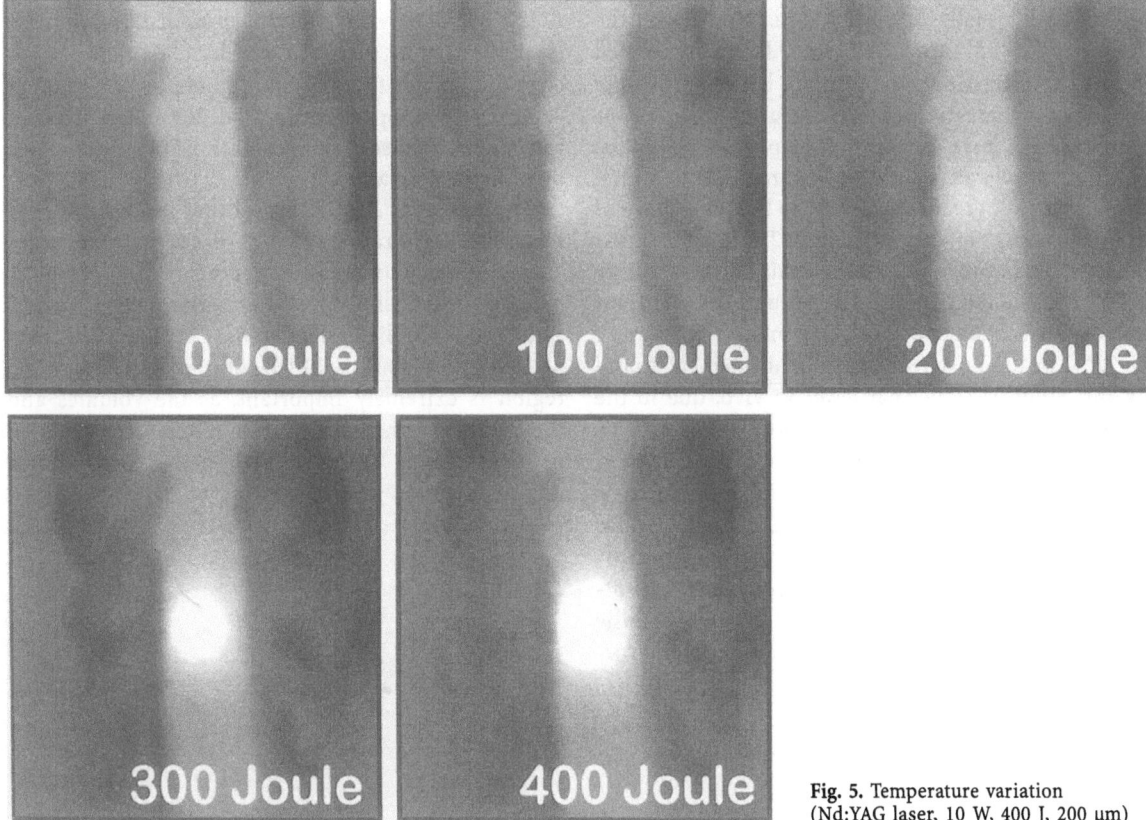

Fig. 5. Temperature variation
(Nd:YAG laser, 10 W, 400 J, 200 μm)

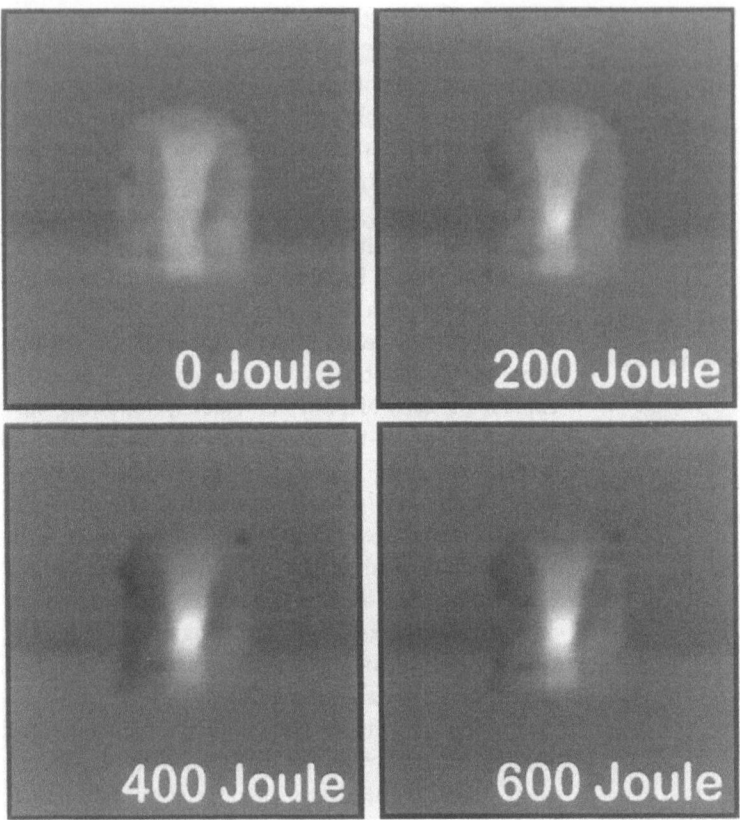

Fig. 6. Temperature variation (Nd:YAG laser, 20 W, 600 J, fiber diameter 400 μm)

nification and control. It has been reported that during perforation of the ventral annulus, no loss of resistance is usually felt. After initial resistance, the laser fiber is advanced by 5 mm. In the presented in vitro investigations, the distance between the dorsal line of demarcation of the denaturation zone after application of laser energy and the posterior longitudinal ligament was found to be approximately 5 mm. This space is of great significance in the prevention of thermal damage to the cord. Figure 2 shows the linear relationship between the width of this "thermal safety zone" and the temperature rise around the posterior longitudinal ligament. The maximum temperature of 50 °C in the posterior logitudinal ligament found by this study is somewhat lower in vivo, due to the blood flow in the epidural venous plexus. Any attempt to ablate a proportionately large area of disc tissue within the small cervical intervertebral disc space may possibly endanger neurovascular structure, due to the thermal effects of the laser. During controlled application of an energy of 600 J, a sufficient reserve space remained in the region of the posterior longitudinal ligament, even with unfavorable positoning of the laser fiber.

Conclusion

PLDD of the cervical intervertebral disc should only be performed by surgeons who have a sound knowledge of the laser technique, who have several years of experience in open surgery of herniated cervical intervertrbral discs, and who are well versed in the possible complications.

The results of PLDD suggest that it is an effective means of ameliorating cervical disc symptoms, probably by the ablation of nociceptors. PLDD is not as effective in reducing actual herniation in the cervical spine as it is in the lumbar spine. Correct positioning of the probe during PLDD of the cervical spinal region is extremely important, as the volumes and dimensions of the cervical disc render the posterior wall susceptible to potential injurious temperature increases.

References

[1] Bohlman HH, Emery SE, Goodfellow DB, Jones PK (1993) Robinson anterior cervical discectomy and arthrodesis for cervical radiculopathy. Long-term follow-up of 122 patients. J Bone Joint Surg Am 75:1298–1307

[2] Brigham CD, Tsahakis PJ (1995) Anterior cervical foraminotomy and fusion. Surgical technique and results. Spine 20:766–770

[3] Chesnut RM, Abitbol JJ, Garfin SR (1992) Surgical management of cervical radiculopathy. Orthop Clin North Am 22:461–473

[4] Choy DS, Botsford J, Black WA (1995) Patient selection: indications and contraindications. J Clin Laser Med Surg 13:157–160

[5] Choy DS (1995) Clinical experience and results with 389 PLDD procedures with the Nd:YAG laser, 1986 to 1995. J Clin Laser Med Surg 13:209–214

[6] Connell MD, Wiesel SW (1992) Natural history and pathogenesis of cervical disc disease. Orthop Clin North Am 22:369–380

[7] Connolly PJ, Esses SI, Kostuik JP (1996) Anterior cervical fusion: outcome analysis of patients fused with and without anterior cervical plates. J Spinal Disord 9:202–206

[8] Daftari TK, Levine J, Fischgrund JS, Herkowitz HN (1996). Is pathology examination of disc specimens necessary after routine anterior cervical discectomy and fusion? Spine 21:2156–2159

[9] Ebraheim NA, An HS, Xu R (1996) The quantitative anatomy of the cervical nerve root groove and the intervertebral foramen. Spine 21:1619–1623

[10] Fujiwara K, Yonenobu K, Ebara S, Yamashita K, Ono K (1989) The prognosis of surgery for cervical compression myelopathy. An analysis of factors involved. J Bone Joint Surg (Br) 71:393–398

[11] Hellinger J (1992) Die Laserosteotomie als Zugangsmöglichkeit zur lumbalen und zervikalen perkutanen Nukleotomie. Lasermedizin 8:105

[12] Hoogland T, Scheckenbach C (1995) Low-dose chemonucleolysis combined with percutaneous nucleotomy in herniated cervical discs. J Spinal Dis 8:228–232

[13] Kang JD, Georgescu HI, McIntyre-Larkin L, Stefanovic-Racic M, Evans CH (1995) Herniated cervical intervertebral discs spontaneously produce matrix metalloproteinases, nitric oxide, interleukin-6, and prostaglandin E2. Spine 20(22):2373–2378

[14] Kelsey JL, Githens PB, Walter SD, Southwick WO, Weil U, Holford TR, Ostfeld AM, Cologero JA, O'Connor T, White AA (1984) An epidemiological study of acute prolapsed cervical intervertebral disc. J Bone Joint Surg (Am) 66:907–914

[15] Lang J (1983) Funktionelle Anatomie der Halswirbelsäule und des benachbarten Nervensystems. In: Hohmann D, Kugelgen B, Liebig K, Schirmer M (eds) Neuroorthopädie 1, Halswirbelsäulenerkrankungen mit Beteiligung des Nervensystems. Springer, Berlin Heidelberg New York, pp 1–118

[16] Maurice-Williams RS, Dorward NL (1996) Extended anterior cervical discectomy without fusion: a simple and sufficient operation for most cases of cervical degenerative disease. Br J Neurosurg 10:261–266

[17] Mendel T, Wink CS, Zimny ML (1992) Neural elements in human cervical intervertebral discs. Spine 17:132–135

[18] Onik GM, Kambin P, Chang MK (1997) Controversy: minimally invasive disc surgery. Nucleotomy versus fragmentectomy. Spine 22:827–830

[19] Pait TG, Killefer JA, Arnautovic KI (1996) Surgical anatomy of the anterior cervical spine: the disc space, vertebral artery, and associated bony structures. Neurosurgery 39:769–776

[20] Panjabi MM, Duranceau J, Goel V, Oxland T, Takata K (1991) Cervical human vertebrae. Quantitative three-dimensional anatomy of the middle and lower regions. Spine 16:861–869

[21] Plotz GM, Benini A, Kramer M (1996) Micro-technological anterior discectomy without fusion in cervical disc displacement with radicular symptoms. Orthopäde 25:546–553

[22] Pointillart V, Cernier A, Vital JM, Senegas J (1995) Anterior discectomy without interbody fusion for cervical disc herniation. Eur Spine J 4:45–51

[23] Radhakrishnan K, Litchy WL, O'Fallon WM, Kurland LT (1994) Epidemiology of cervical radiculopathy. A population-based study from Rochester, Minnesota, 1976 through 1990. Brain 117:325–335

[24] Schlangmann BA, Schmolke S, Siebert WE (1996) Temperatur- und Ablationsmessungen bei der Laserbehandlung von Bandscheibengewebe. Orthopäde 25:3–9

[25] Schmolke S (1995) Experimentelle Untersuchungen zum Einsatz von Neodym:YAG Lasern bei der Perkutanen Laser Diskus Dekompression. Dissertation, Medizinische Hochschule, Hannover

[26] Siebert WE (1995) Percutaneous laser discectomy of cervical discs: preliminary clinical results. Clin Laser Med Surg 13:205–207

[27] Silvers HR, Lewis PJ, Suddaby LS, Asch HL, Clabeaux DE, Blumenson LE (1996) Day surgery for cervical microdiscectomy: is it safe and effective? J Spinal Disord 9:287–293

[28] Van den Bent MJ, Oosting J, Wouda EJ, van Acker EH, Ansink BJ, Braakman R (1996) Anterior cervical discectomy with or without fusion with acrylate. A randomized trial. Spine 21:834–839; discussion 840

[29] Zweifel K, Panoussopoulos A (1996) Laser und Bandscheibenchirurgie – Balgrist Erfahrungen. In: Berlien HP, Muller G (eds) Angewandte Lasermedizin, III-3.11.3. Ecomed, Landsberg

Percutaneous Cervical Discectomy with Forceps and Endoscopic Ho:YAG Laser

S.-H. LEE

Introduction

The spinal canal is usually entered when cervical discectomy, with or without fusion, is performed. This procedure has the potential risk of epidural bleeding, periradicular fibrosis, spinal cord ischemia or damage. These risks are in addition to the risk of general anethesia. The minimally invasive technique of percutaneous cervical discectomy under local anesthesia may avoid these complications.

After Tajima performed the first cervical percutaneous descectomy in 1981, three types of mechanical minimally invasive techniques have evolved to partially or wholly remove the soft cervical disc herniations. These are: manual percutaneous cervical discectomy (MPCD) developed by Gastambide [8] and Bornet [5], automated percutaneous cervical discectomy (APCD), of Theron [27], Algara [1] and Herman [10], and laser percutaneous cervical decompression (LPCD), by Siebert [22], Hellinger [9] and Bonati [4]. Although all three of these mechanical methods were reported to have good success rates and no side effects, allergic reactions, transverse myelitis, or subarachnoid hemorrhage, similar to those seen following chemonucleolysis treatment with chymopapain [13], there is some reported difficulty in removing enough of the posteriorly displaced herniated disc nucleus in patients with moderate and large disc herniations.

From October 1993 to December 1995, we performed a combination of MPCD and subsequent endoscopic Ho:YAG laser treatment (CPCD) in 143 patients with soft disc herniations contained by the posterior longitudinal ligament without much degenerative bone changes. The procedure focused on removal of the nucleus pulposus in the posterior quadrant of the disc immediately subjacent to the annular defect and on shrinkage of the protruded hernia mass itself.

Patients and Materials

Of the patients who presented with cervical disc herniation and who didn't improve with conservative therapy, 143 underwent the procedure. There were 80 male and 63 female patients, aged 20 to 79 years, with the majority aged 30 to 50 years (Table 1). The levels of the herniation were mostly between C5-6 and C6-7. The highest level was C3-4, in 3 cases (Table 2). We did not approach the C7–T1 level.

The average duration of symptoms was 2 years and 4 months. However, 59 patients were symptomatic for less than 1 year (Table 3). The majority had over 6 months of unsuccessful conservative management in the form of Oriental medicine, acupuncture, physical therapy, or chiropractic care.

Table 1. Compositon of patients by sex and age

Age	Male	Female
20–29	6	2
30–39	23	14
40–49	25	23
50–59	18	15
60–69	7	8
70–79	1	1
Total	80	63

Table 2. Level of herniation in the patients studied

Herniation level	No of patients
C4-5	18
C5-6	74
C6-7	29
C3-4 and C4-5	2
C3-4 and C6-7	1
C4-5 and C5-6	6
C5-6 and C6-7	10
C4-5, C5-6, and C6-7	3
Total	143

Table 3. Duration of symptoms in patients, prior to study

No of years	No of patients
< 1	59
1-2	16
2-3	24
3-4	21
4-5	9
5-6	4
6-7	1
7-8	3
8-9	1
9-10	3
> 10	2
Total	143

Average duration of symptoms: 2 years and 4 months.

Clinical Indications

Our principal clinical indication was sustained radiculopathy, unresponsive to conservative management. There were 131 patients with cervicobrachial neuralgia who had failed to respond to long terms of conservative treatment. The clinical symptoms and neurological signs of cervicobrachial neuralgia were correlated with positive CT and MRI findings.

We treated exclusive headache or neck pain as relative contraindications. However, four patients had cervicoencephalic syndrome, characterised by headache or dizziness with tiredness or poor concentration over 2 years. They presented with central cervical disc herniation at the C3–C4 or C4–C5 levels, which were evaluated by discography [2].

Most patients with myelopathy due to soft cervical disc herniations showed ruptured herniations through the posterior longitudinal ligaments. We regarded myelopathy with upper motor neuron signs, ataxic gait, or paraparesis as absolute contraindications. But if the risk of general anesthesia was too high and the patient feared paraplegia as a result of open cervical discectomy, we regarded this as a relative indication to perform the procedure. This was the case in eight patients.

Morphological Indications

The operation was indicated in patients with soft subligamentous disc herniations with mild bone spur formation or slight ossification of the posterior longitudinal ligament (Fig. 1). Although patients with large disc herniations were not contraindicated, patients with herniated disc masses occupying less than half of the spinal canal were considered good candidates for surgery. Two or three levels could be treated at the same time. Any form of disc herniation including central, paramedian, lateral and foraminal herniations was indicated (Fig. 2). Local disc protrusion and diffuse degenerative discs demonstrating epidural leakage of dye during discography were considered good indications.

The contraindications were migrated discal fragments, associated spinal stenosis, marked spondylosis, and ossification of posterior longitudinal ligaments.

Methods

The procedures were carried out under local anesthesia with the patients in the supine position. However, one patient desired surgery under general anesthesia. Local anesthesia with neuroleptics was recommended, to identify whether the patient's symptoms improved immediately and to protect the patient during surgery by identifiying paraparesis or weakness of the arms. If general anesthesia is used to control lancinating pain evoked in the supine position with neck extension or because of fear, it should be done without muscle relaxants, so as to recognise reflex movement of the arms if the laser energy approaches too close to the spinal cord or nerves.

To open the anterior intervertebral disc space, we kept the neck in mild extension. Hyperextension of the neck was avoided, as it could tighten the anterior neck structures, preventing manual displacement of these structures for safe access of the disc space. Some patients could not withstand the discomfort of neck or shoulder pain in prolonged hyperextension.

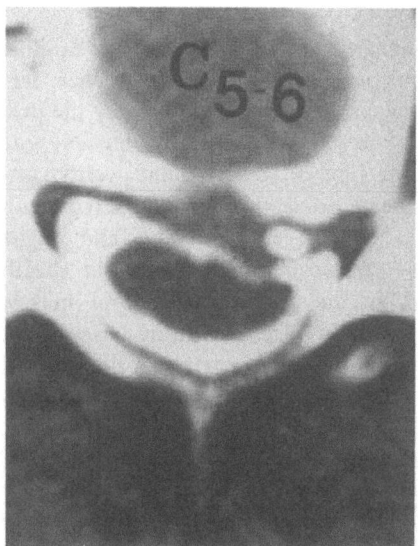

Fig. 1. The soft disc herniation with mild bone spur or slight ossification of the posterior longitudinal ligament was a strong indication

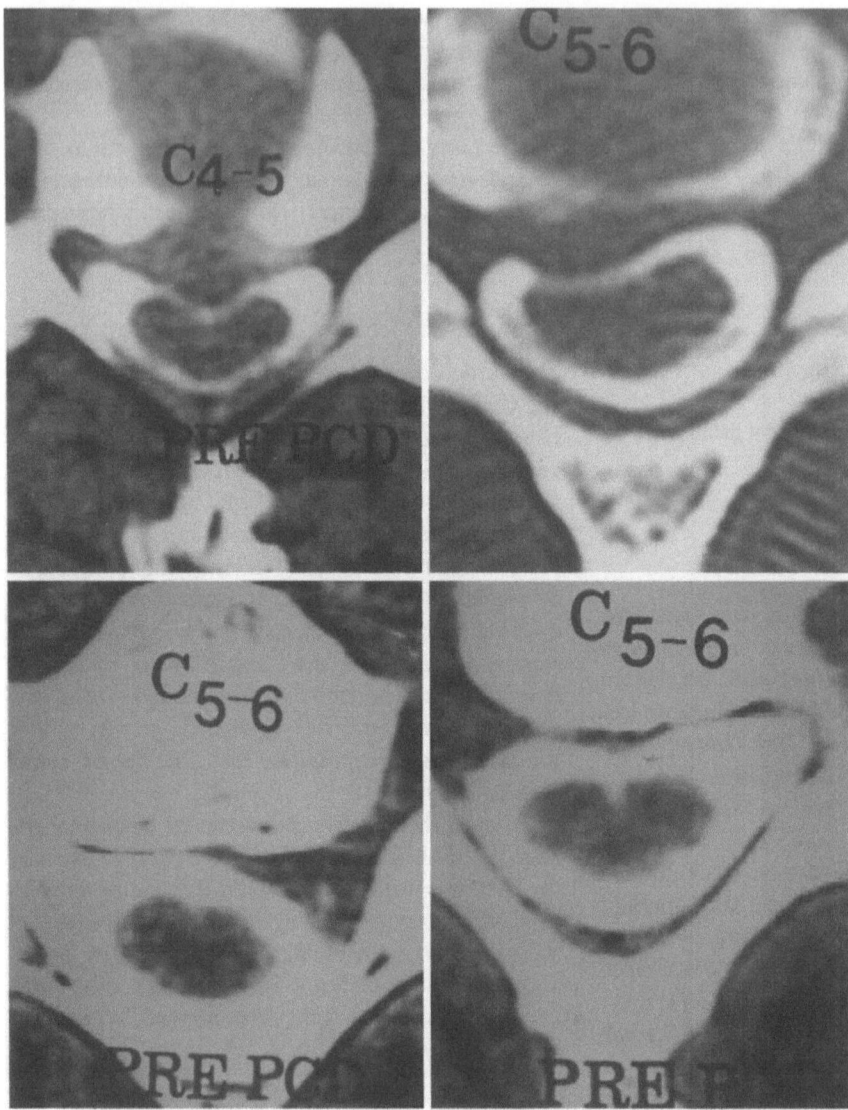

Fig. 2. Any of central, paramedian, lateral, and foraminal herniation was a strong indication

With our index fingers or we pushed the midline soft tissue structures thumb (thyroid, trachea, larynx, and esophagus), which are wrapped by the pretracheal layer of deep fascia, toward the opposite side of the lesion site (Fig. 3). We were not overtly concerned about the neuro-vascular structures (common carotid artery, internal jugular vein, and vagus nerve), which are enclosed by the carotid sheath and protected by the sternocleidomastoid muscle and are anatomically placed laterally away from the entry point on the ventral surface of the cervical disc. In the event of inadvertent puncture injury to the jugular vein, thyroid artery, or carotid artery, bleeding was easily controlled by digital pressure applied for about 5 min. But one must take care to move the carotid artery away from the puncture site, before inserting the cannula into the disc space.

Before 0.5-cm skin incision was made, soft disc herniations were confirmed by discography (Fig. 4). We inserted an 18-gauge needle into the disc space through the interval between the cervical midline structures and the vascular axis (Fig. 3). The entry point is 0.5 cm or more, lateral to the midline on the side of the pathology. This was done to reach the herniation directly. Approaching the disc from the contralateral side makes it difficult to place the laser near the herniated area due to the slope of the disc space (Fig. 4).

Initially, a thin K-wire is passed through an 18-gauge needle. After a 0.5-cm skin incision has been made, cannula is threaded over the K-wire, which is then replaced by a 25-mm dilator. A 4-mm working sleeve is then inserted under fluoroscopic guidance with gradual dilatation. The anterior annulus is cut with the trephine and the working cannula is pushed into the annulus to secure the sleeve. The internal

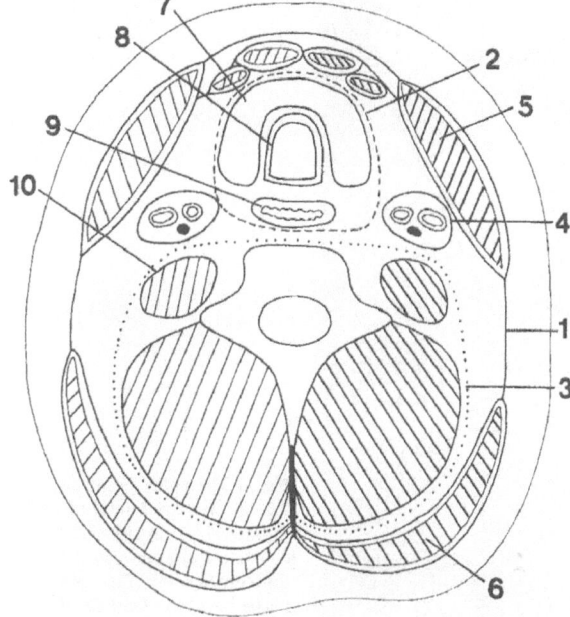

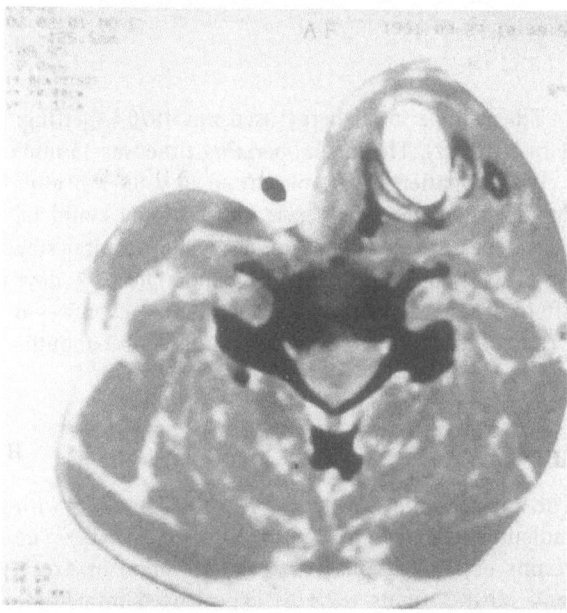

Fig. 3. Due to compartmentalization of the neck by deep fascia, the cleavage between the carotid sheath and the pretracheal layer over the pretracheal layer could be created easily by the index finger. Key to drawing: *1.* Superficial layer (investing layer); *2.* Pretracheal layer; *3.* Prevertebral layer; *4.* Carotid sheath, Internal jugular V., Common Carotid a., Vagus n.; *5.* Sternocleidomastoid m.; *6.* Trapezius m.; *7.* Thyroid gland; *8.* Trachea; *9.* Esophagus; *10.* Scalene m. (CT film produced by Daniel Gastambide; drawing from [30])

spire of the trephine allows automatic extraction of disc material [20].

The central and posterior part of the nucleus pulposus was removed with small thin forceps to decompress the disc space and to create adequate working space for the flexible endoscopic Ho:YAG laser fiber. We did not pass the forceps beyond the poster-ior vertebral body line, especially because one patient had increased paraparesis from further inward migration of the prolapsed disc into the spinal canal. The average amount of removed disc was 740 mg.

The laser fiber was inserted through the working sleeve (or the laser-working cannula), vaporizing the mucleus centrally and moving further posteriorly into the disc. We used an endoscopically controlled laser at a setting of 10 Hz and a performance of 1.2 J. The laser beam was directed as far posteriorly as possible, to ablate and shrink the herniated part of the discs directly (Fig. 5). We directed the end of the laser-working cannula with external diameter of 2.5 mm, paramedially, centrally, laterally, and far laterally, depending on the direction of the herniated disc. This was done through the manual working sleeve kept in line with the posterior vertebral body line. The direction of the laser-working can-nula could be controlled by anterioposterior fluoro-scopy. If we could not insert the laser-working can-nula close to the herniated disc, we widened the pos-terior discal space by flexing the neck mildly with a pillow under the head which allowed direct ablation of the herniated nucleus and shrinkage of the bulged annulus. The inside of the disc could be inspected visually for defects in the posterior edge of the end plate, the posterior area of the disc, the annulus, or the posterior longitudinal ligament. The proce-dure was carried out with continuous pumping irri-gation of the saline (1000 ml) mixed with cefazolin (1 or 2 g) (Fig. 6). It was only occasionally necessary to place the laser fiber tip a little beyond the poster-ior vertebral body line on the fluorscopic image (Fig. 5).

If a patient experienced reflex jerking of arms or legs, or complained of shoulder or arm pain during lasing, the laser tip was withdrawn, as it meant that the laser tip was too close to the spinal cord or nerve root.

Prior to the application of laser energy, we checked the depth of the laser fiber tip on the oblique or lateral fluoroscopy so as to confirm that the pos-terior longitudinal ligaments were not penetrated. The laser vaporizes or shrinks the discal herniation gradually without the possibility of compressing the spinal cord. This can occur with the use of manual instrumentation which may push the herniation further into the spinal canal.

If there was ossification of posterior ligaments or if bone spurs were identified, we tried to partially ablate the osteophytes with an endoscopic holmium laser, expecting delayed absorption of the spurs. Manual removal of osteophytes with forceps was impossible. However, ablation by Ho:YAG lasing leads to an acute and chronic reaction [24].

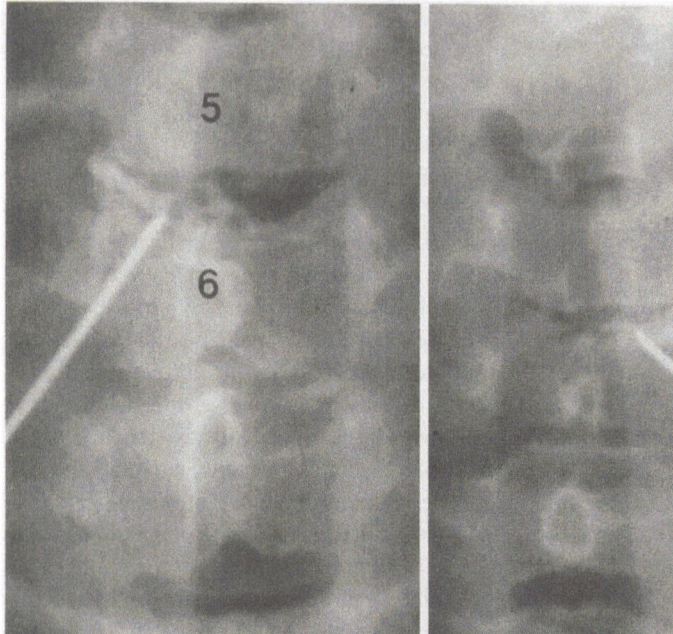

Fig. 4. The entry point is 0.5 cm or more lateral to the ipsilateral lesion side. With the contralateral approach it is difficult to touch the hernia mass, because of the slanted slope of the disc space

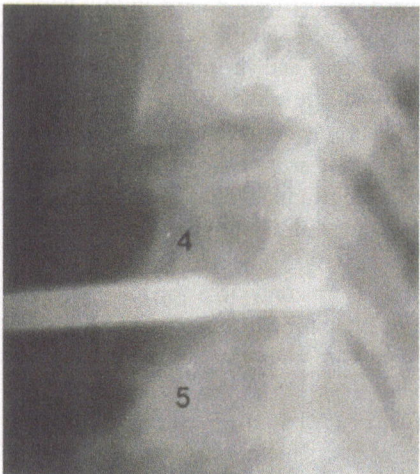

Fig. 5. The laser fiber is inserted through the working cannula as far posteriorly as possible, to directly vaporize and shrink the herniated part of the disc. Sometimes the laser fiber tip was slightly beyond the posterior body line

The average total energy used was 4870 J (setting: 0.8 J at 10 Hz). The mean operating time was 45 min.

All the patients were permitted to walk 3 h after surgery. Percutaneous cervical discectomy could be considered an outpatient surgery. The hospital stay was less than 24 h. Cervical collars for 3-7 days after surgery, and cervical strengthening exercises 6 weeks after the operation for a period of 3 months were recommended.

Results

The average follow-up time for the 131 patients with radiculopathy was 1 year (5 months – 2.7 years). The results of 119 patients (90.9 %) were good or excellent. Most patients (82.4 %) experienced immediate improvement of chronic radicular pain that they had prior to surgery or severe lancinating arm or

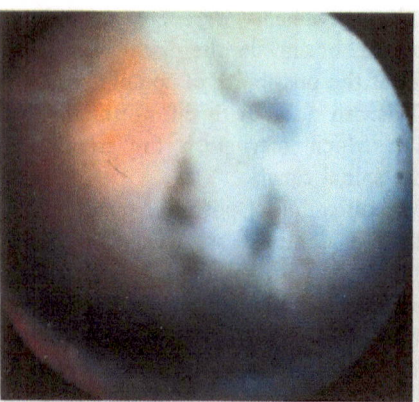

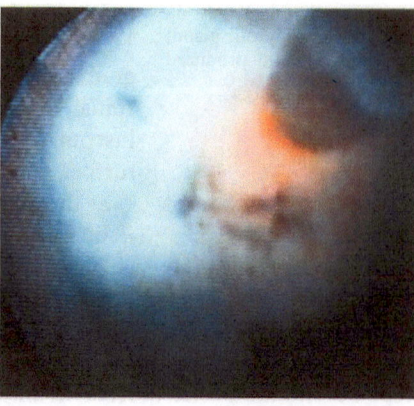

Fig. 6. The ablated defect of the posterior edge of the spine, annulus or herniated mass could be seen with endoscopic Ho:YAG laser

shoulder pain that they experienced during the operation. Most patients with radiculopathy had tearing of the outer layer of the annulus with the herniation contained by the posterior longitudinal ligament. No significant intraoperative or postoperative complications were noted in the radiculopathy group. However, some patients had some temporary discomfort in swallowing and one patient experienced transient hoarseness.

Only five of eight patients with myelopathy had good results. One patient with myelopathy had aggravation of paraparesis. He immediately underwent discectomy and anterior cervical spine fusion and recovered completely.

Of the four patients with cervicoencephalic syndrome (headache and dizziness), three had good or excellent results. There were no complications in this group.

The overall results of all 143 patients are as follows: 127 patients (88.8 %) had excellent or good results, the results of 12 (8.4 %) were fair, and 4

patients (2.8 %) had poor results, after a mean follow-up time of 1 year (Table 4).

The outcomes for patients with positive provocative cervical discography and patients with negative provocation were not different (Table 5). According to the type of discograph, we sub-stratified the results into those with protruded disc, extruded disc, and those who demonstrated epidural leakage, suggesting discal tear. There were no identifiable differences in outcome amongst the subgroups (Table 6).

We could obtain follow-up MRI or CT scans in only 33 patients 3 months after surgery (Table 7). In 18 patients, the disc herniation had either completely disappeared or had reduced significantly in size compared to preoperative scans (Figs. 7a, b, c). The patients whose scans were minimally different had a clinical success rate of 60 %. The success rate was 91 % in those with moderate changes and 100 % in those who had marked changes. These results suggest that the benefit obtained from percu-

Table 4. Overall results of the study

	Result[a]				Total patients
	Excellent[b]	Good[c]	Fair[d]	Poor[e]	
Myelopathy	–	5 (62.5)	2 (25.0)	1 (12.5)	8
Radiculopathy	14 (10.7)	105 (80.2)	10 (7.6)	2 (1.5)	131
Cervicoencephalic syndrome	2 (50.0)	1 (25.0)	–	1 (25.0)	4
Overall results	16 (11.2)	111 (77.6)	12 (8.4)	4 (2.8)	143

[a] Number of patients, percentage given in parentheses.
[b] Excellent: free of pain, no discomfort, no neurological signs.
[c] Good: free of pain, no neurological signs, but mild discomfort.
[d] Fair: partial pain relief of signs and symptoms.
[e] Poor: no pain relief and positive signs.

Table 5. Provocative discography and correlation with results

	Result				Total
	Excellent	Good	Fair	Poor	
Positive	11 (12.4)	68 (76.4)	8 (9.0)	2 (2.2)	89
Negative	3 (6.7)	38 (84.5)	4 (8.8)	–	45

See Table 5 for definitions of results.

Table 6. Results classified according to type of discograph

	Result			
	Excellent	Good	Fair	Poor
Protruded	6 (10.9)	44 (80.0)	5 (9.1)	–
Prolapsed	2 (2.9)	61 (89.7)	3 (4.5)	2 (2.9)
Epidural leakage	4 (26.4)	5 (45.5)	1 (9.1)	1 (9.1)
Total	12 (9.0)	110 (82.1)	9 (6.7)	3 (2.2)

Protruded: herniation between intradiscal space. Prolapsed: herniation extends beyond the intradiscal space.
See Table 5 for definitions of results.

Table 7. Postoperative change in CT or MRI and results

Postoperative change	Result			
	Excellent	Good	Fair	Poor
No change	–	–	–	1
Minimal change (< 2.5 %); success rate 60 %	–	3 (60)	1 (20)	1 (20)
Moderate (26-75 %); success rate 91 %	3 (27)	7 (64)	1 (9.0)	–
Marked change (75 % <); success rate 100 %	3 (60)	2 (40)	–	–
Total 22 cases	6 (27.3)	12 (54.5)	2 (9.1)	2 (9.1)

See Table 5 for definitions of results.

taneous cervical discectomy is not from reduction of intradiscal pressure but is from the decrease in the size of the herniation mass. There was no difference between the preoperative and postoperative MRI scans of the one patient who obtained no benefit. In three cases, postoperative MRI showed anterior herniation through anterior discal fenestration, which decreased intradiscal pressure and prevented recurrence of posterior herniation. In the postoperative MRI we sometimes observed a thermal effect on the end plate, produced by laser along with the density changes in the bone marrow, but these changes did not produce symptoms. The postoperative MRI and plain lateral films showed no narrowing of disc space or segmental instability (Fig. 8).

Discussion

Since Hirsch [11] reported the success (80 %) with simple anterior cervical discectomy without removal of posterior annulus and posterior longitudinal ligament without interbody fusion, many authors (Boldrey [3], Susen [25], Murphy [17], Martins [16], Dunsker [7], Wilson [28], Robertson [21], Pertuiset [19], Lunsford [15], Lee [14]) reported that only partial removal of a cervical disc with preservation of annulus, osteophyte and posterior longitudinal ligament by the anterior approach without interbody fusion can eliminate the patient's symptoms. From 1982 to 1992, Lee, one of the authors of this chapter, performed 49 simple partial anterior discectomies to treat soft cervical disc herniations at the same hospital. Only one out of 49 cases required re-operation with anterior interbody fusion.

The results of the experience with partial removal of cervical disc supported the concept that partial discectomy could provide a satisfactory outcome. It was felt that decompression could easily be achieved with automated percutaneous cervical discectomy. A percutaneous anterior approach to the disc with automated nuleotome was therefore attempted by the authors between May and October 1993 in 10 patients with severe radicular pain from herniated cervical

discs. Six patients (60 %) with mild to moderate disc herniation had excellent or good results, but four patients with large herniated discs did not improve. We then altered the method and combined manual discectomy with endoscopic Ho:YAG laser discectomy to treat the patients with moderate or large soft disc herniations.

Zweifel reported the results of experimental intervertebral laser disc surgery, and demonstrated that the Ho:YAG laser was the safest, with the most effective tissue ablation capability and with the least thermal damage produced through tissue penetration. The thermal penetration of the 2100-nm Ho:YAG laser is to a depth of less than 3 mm in human disc tissue in the absence of saline irrigation [29]. Microscopic examination of rabbit liver ablated by a pulsed holmium laser revealed zones of thermal damage extending 0.5-1.0 mm from the point of application [18]. But the relatively low penetration capability of the Ho:YAG laser allows safe clinical application in close proximity of neural structures, especially when continuous irrigation is used [29]. The endoscopic Ho:YAG laser worked precisely, obtaining a 0.3-0.5 mm cutting depth under continuous saline irrigation, allowing safe ablation of the tissue near or inside the herniated mass close to the posterior longitudinal ligament. This ensured that the spinal cord or nerve root was protected from any injury caused by laser energy (Fig. 9).

The authors estimate that the about 3 mm thick tissue consisting of posterior longitudinal ligament, epidural fat, dura mater, and subarachnoidal CSF maintained a safe margin protecting the spinal cord from the bubbling and thermal effects of the laser (Fig. 10).

To ablate the tissue near or inside the hernia mass we should try to see inside the disc, annulus, or posterior longitudinal ligament near the herniation. The pumping irrigation with a saline–antibiotic solution during operation has prevented discitis.

There are other percutaneous techniques available for treating herniated cervical discs. Buchheit reported excellent results in 100 cases, which

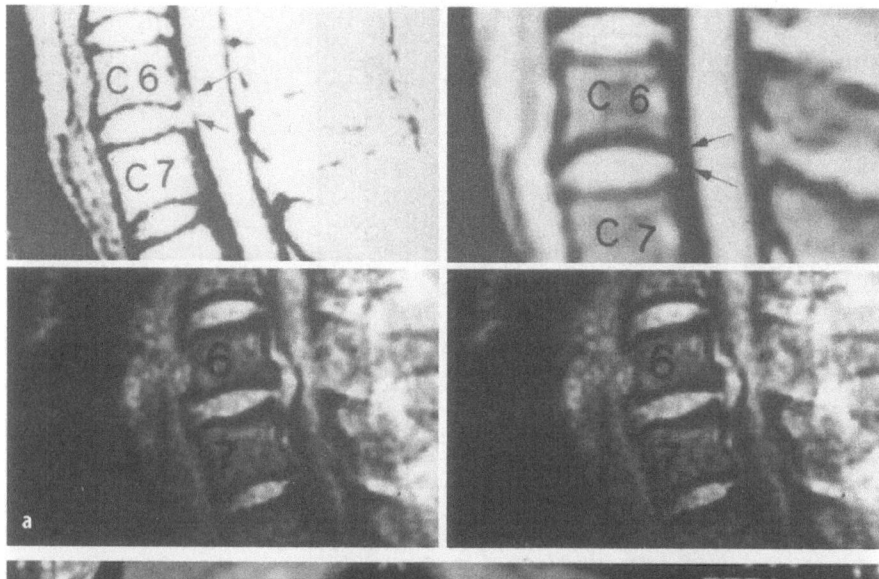

Fig. 7a. Posteriorly prolapsed discs were shrunk or vaporized by endoscopic Ho:YAG laser

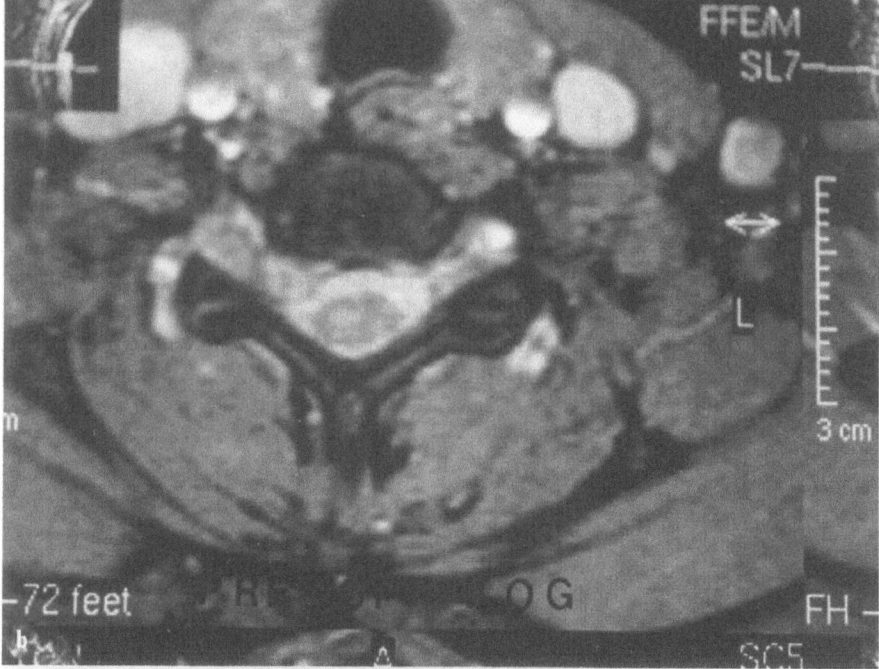

Fig. 7b. Right-sided cervical disc prolapse compressing exiting nerve (preoperative)

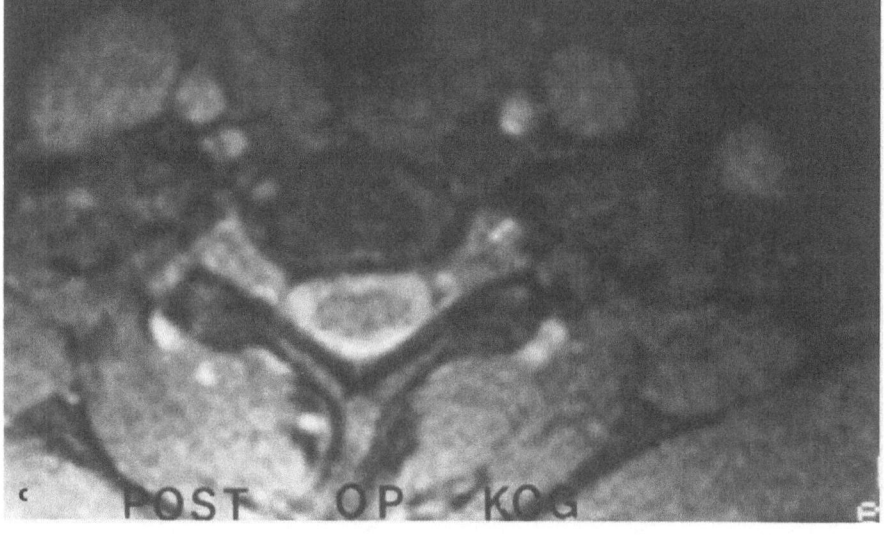

Fig. 7c. Postoperative MR scan showing adequate disc decompression

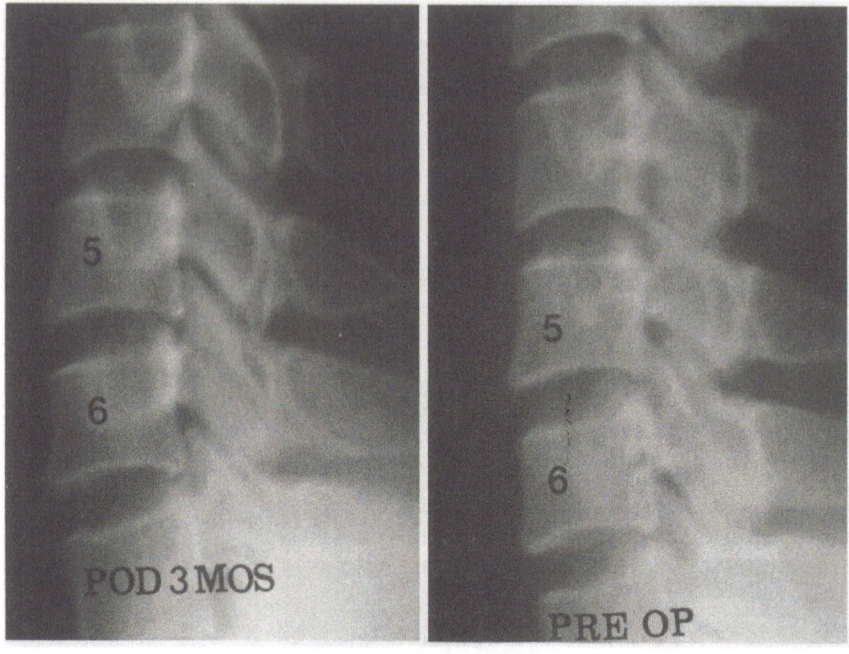

Fig. 8. The postoperative lateral view shows no change in disc height

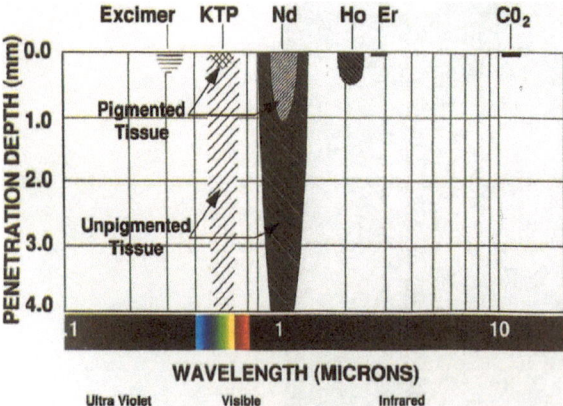

Fig. 9. The penetration depth of the Ho:YAG laser under saline irrigation is 0.3–0.5 mm

included large disc herniations of cervical discs when treated with chemonucleolysis with chymopapain [4]. But in Korea, one patient treated with chymopapain became quadriplegic, even though the discography showed no epidural leakage or intradural connection. Furthermore, the USA brochure for chymodactin contraindicates its use in cervical and thoracic discs, so we did not try chemical cervical discectomy with chymopapain.

Hoogland combined low-dose chemonucleolysis with percutaneous nucleotomy to wash out chymopapain immediately, and avoid the side effects of chymopapain. He suggested that the percutaneous approach to cervical disc herniation could become the treatment of choice in the future [12].

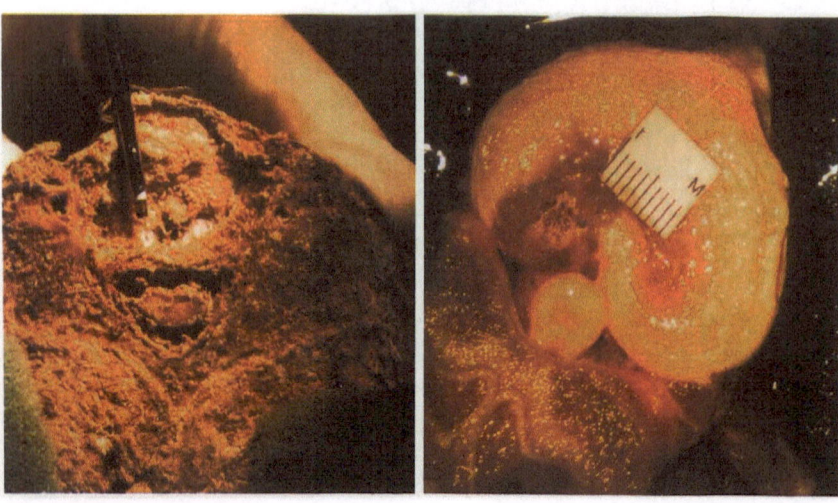

Fig. 10. The bulged annula and protruded hernia mass could be ablated precisely with endoscopic Ho:YAG laser under saline irrigation without spinal cord damage in the pig and in human cadaver

Satisfactory results were obtained for patients treated with MPCD by Tajima (78 % of 104 patients) [26] and Gastambide (80 % of 20 patients). Theron treated 80 % of 147 patients satisfactorily with APCD, and Bornert obtained 82 % satisfactory results among 212 patients treated with APCD and 128 patient treated with MPCD [5]. Bonati obtained satisfactory results in 51 out of 60 patients treated with LPCD [4]. Siebert treated 26 patients with LPCD [22], but cautioned against the use of laser in the cervical spine by the average conventional spine surgeon, unskilled in the use of laser in cervical spine, as the risk of complications from accidental damage could be disproportionately high.

Potential complications of MPCD, APCD, LPCD, and CPCD postulated by Gastambide are immediate vascular injury, pre-vertebral or epidural hematoma, laryngeal edema, esophageal perforation, lesion of recurrent nerve, superior laryngeal nerve, or large hypoglossal nerve, cervical cord compression or ischemia, secondary subacute discitis and epidural abscess. However, there are no serious complications noted so far in the literature, except for the one reported by Hellinger, who had reversible subtotal paraplegia in one case and intradiscal infections in 1.5 % of 154 cases treated with LPCD and Nd:YAG laser [9].

Conclusion

Although open anterior discectomy with fusion for cervical disc herniation has been reported to have a high success rate [2, 23], this standard approach has a higher potential morbidity. The advantages of combining percutaneous manual decompression with various forceps, with subsequent ablation of the posterior part of the disc with the endoscopic Ho:YAG laser are as follows:
- Possible direct extraction of the hernia itself after ablation and shrinkage
- Absence of epidural bleeding and prevention of periradicular fibrosis
- Segmental stability is maintained, with no reduction in disc height
- Discitis or epidural abscess is prevented with the use of antibiotic and saline irrigation in association with the antibacterial effect of the laser
- Reduced recurrence of disc herniation from anterior fenestration
- Reduced morbidity, short hospitalization and rapid return to routine activities

CPCD has the highest success rate of all the types of percutaneous procedures, and broadens the indication of the percutaneous approach. CPCD might become the treatment of choice in future, because

of the possibility of direct ablation of the herniated disc mass without the fear of paraplegia. Minimal invasive techniques have proven to be safe and effective for treatment of soft cervical disc herniations especially when percutaneous manual techniques are combined with endoscopic Ho:YAG laser discectomy.

References

[1] Algara M (1993) Automated percutaneous cervical discectomy. In: 4th annual meeting of the European Spine Society, 1993
[2] Blume HG (1995) Discography for the evaluation of cervicogenic headaches. In: 10th European congress of neurosurgery, Berlin 7–12 May 1995
[3] Boldrey EB (1964) Anterior cervical decompression without fusion. In: 25th annual meeting of the AANS, 12 November 1964, Florida
[4] Bonati AO (1991) Percutaneous cervical laser discectomy. In: International meeting of laser surgery, San Francisco, 26–29 Sept 1991
[5] Bornert D (1994) Cure chirurgicale de hernie cervicale par voie anterolaterale percutanee: analyse de six and d'experience. In: GIEDA Rachis, Paris, 15–17 Dec 1994
[6] Brodke DS, Zdeblck TA (1992) Modified Smith–Robinson procedure for anterior cervical discectomy and fusion. Spine 17S:427–430
[7] Dunsker SB (1977) Anterior cervical discectomy with & without fusion. Clin Neurosurg 24:516–521
[8] Gastambide D (1993) Percutaneous cervical discectomy nonautomatized, SICOT, ISMISS, Seoul, 27 Aug–3 Sept 1993
[9] Hellinger J (1994) Nonendoscopic percutaneous 1064 Nd:YAG laser decompression. In: 3rd symposium on laser-assisted endoscopic & arthrosopic intervention in orthopaedics. Zurich, 1–2 Dec 1994
[10] Herman S, Nizard RS, Witvoet J (1994) La discectomie percutanee au rachis cervical, Rachis cervical degeneratif et traumatique, Expansion scientifique francaise, pp 160–166
[11] Hirsch D (1966) Cervical disc rupture: diagnosis and therapy. Acta Orthop Scand 30:172–186
[12] Hoogland T, Scheckenbach D (1995) Low-dose chemonucleolysis combined with percutaneous nucleotomy in herniated cervical discs. J Spinal Disord 8(3):228–232
[13] Krause D, Drape JL, Jambon F, de Souza-Lima A, Tongio J, Maitrot D, Orenstein D, Giannetti A, Boyer P, Srour R et al. (1993) Nucleolyse cervicale: indication, technique, resultats. 190 patients. J Neuroradiol 20:42–59
[14] Lee SH (1982) Partial anterior cervical discectomy without interbody fusion for herniated cervical discs. J Pusan Med Assc. 18(4):21–24
[15] Lunsford LD, Bissonette DJ, Jannetta PJ (1980) Anterior surgery for cervical disease. J Neurosurg. 53:1–11
[16] Martins AN (1976) Anterior cervical discectomy with and without interbody bone graft. J Neurosurg 44:290–295
[17] Murphy AN, Gado M (1972) Anterior cervical discectomy without interbody bone graft. J Neurosurg 37:71–74
[18] Nishioka NS, Domankevitz Y, Flotte TJ, Anderson RR (1989) Ablation of rabbit liver, stomach, and colon with a pulsed holmium laser. Gastroenterology 96:831–837
[19] Pertuised B (1978) Recurrent instability of the cervical spine: advances, technical standards. In: Neurosurgery. Springer, Berlin Heidelberg New York
[20] Peyrou PL, Cazenave A, Guingand O, Krayenbuhl H, Brihaye J, Loew F, Logue V, Mingrino S, Pertuiset B, Symon L, Troupp II, Sagaigil M (eds) (1991) Discectomie percutanee par instrumentation courbe a extraction mecanique. Rev Med Orthop 26:27–32
[21] Robertson JT (1978) Anterior operations for herniated disc and for myelopathy. Clin Neurosurg 25:245–250

[22] Siebert WE (1993) Percutaneous laser discectomy. Spine (state of the art reviews) 7(1):129–130

[23] Snyder GM, Bernhardt M (1989) Anterior cervical fractional interspace decompression for treatment of cervical radiculopathy. Clin Orthop 246:92–99

[24] Stein E, Sedlacek T, Fabian RL, Nishioka NS (1990) Acute and chronic effects of bone ablation with a pulsed holmium laser. Lasers Surg Med 10:384–388

[25] Susen AF (1966) Simple anterior cervical discectomy without fusion. In: 27th annual meeting of the AANS. 17 Oct 1966

[26] Tajima T, Sakamoto H (1989) Discectomy cervicale percutane. Rev Med Orthop 17:7–10

[27] Theron J, Huet H (1994) Nucleotomie cervicale. In: GIEDA Rachis, Paris, 15–17 Dec 1994

[28] Wilson DH, Campbell DD (1977) Anterior discectomy without bone graft. J Neurosurg 47:551–555

[29] Zweifel K (1994) Laser tissue interactions: practical approach and real-time-MRI analysis of energy effects. In: 3rd symposium on laser-assisted endoscopic & arthroscopic intervention in orthopaedics, Zurich, 26–27 May 1994

[30] Chung IH (1996) Human anatomy.

Percutaneous Laser Disc Decompression (PLDD):
Twelve Years' Experience with 752 Procedures in 518 Patients

D. S. J. Choy

Introduction

Surgical treatment of intervertebral disc herniation by open discectomy, microdiscectomy, or automated nucleotome discectomy achieves its goals through reducing the volume of the nucleus pulposus. In 1984, this author first proposed pressure reduction by laser energy introduced through a needle, to vaporize a small volume of nucleus pulposus. Percutaneous laser disc decompression (PLDD) is based on the principle that a small reduction of volume in a closed hydraulic space such as intact disc results in a disproportionately large fall of pressure, an outcome first demonstrated through in vitro studies [4] (Fig. 1). The decrease in this pressure following laser application of 1000 J to the nucleus pulposus in 17 human lumbar discs [6] in a compression frame averaged 1344 ± 601 mmHg or 55.6% ($p = 0.0001$) (Fig. 2). A control determination, with the laser off, yielded a fall in intradiscal pressure of only 143 mmHg. It is hypothesized that a negative change in the pressure gradient between nucleus pulposus and the peridiscal tissue causes significant retraction of the herniation away

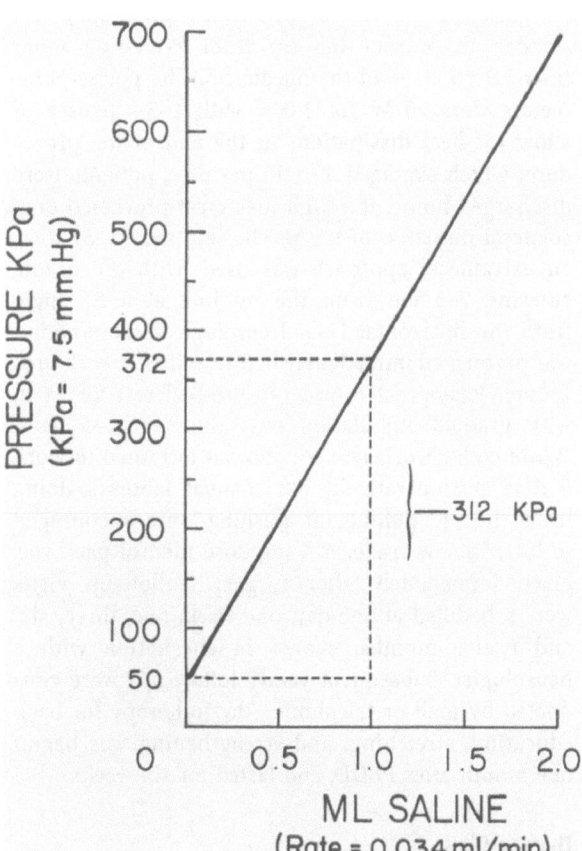

Fig. 1. Unloaded discs: change of intradiscal pressure as a function of volume of saline injected intradiscally. This is 312 kPa/ml and is linear. The initial pressure is 132.9 kPa

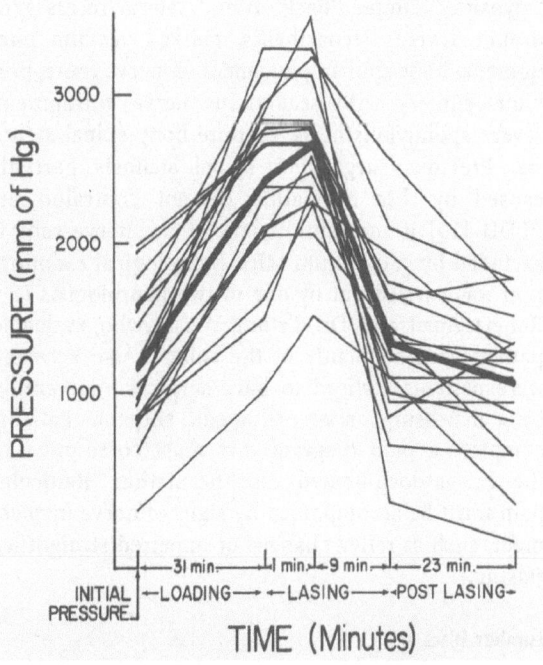

Fig. 2. The intradiscal pressure graph is divided into five parts: (1) the preload pressure (mean: 1175 mmHg), (2) the after-load pressure, stabilizing after 31 min (mean: 2419 mmHg), (3) the pressure change during the first minute of lasing, (4) the fall of pressure during the next 9 min of lasing (mean pressure at the end of lasing: 1346 mmHg), (5) the continued fall of pressure during the next 23 min after lasing with stabilization at the end; (mean pressure after stabilization: 1075 mmHg). The *heavy line* represents mean intradiscal pressures. Total fall of intradiscal pressure with 1000-J laser ablation: 1344 ± 601 mmHg, or 55.6% ($p = 0.0001$). The continued fall of intradiscal pressure after cessation of lasing may represent continued denaturation of disc

from the affected nerve root. This conclusion appears to be supported by clinical experience, in which most patients describe cessation of radicular pain immediately after and sometimes even during the procedure.

This is a report on 752 PLDD procedures in 518 patients, with a follow-up of as much as 12 years.

Materials and Methods

Patient Selection

Patients with current disc herniations and corresponding pain syndromes documented by magnetic resonance imaging (MRI) were treated. Failure of three months of conservative therapy was nesessary for inclusion, and a second concurring opinion was sought from a neurologist, neurosurgeon, or orthopedic surgeon. PLDD is based on the underlying principle that water is noncompressible. Thus, the disc herniation must be contained, or at least be contiguous with the parent disc. A free disc fragment is an absolute contraindication.

Excluded from PLDD are patients with cancer in the spine, fracture, infection, "litigation back disease," "myositis," simple "back strain," lateral recess syndrome, severe osteoarthritis, marked vacuum phenomena, bone spur impingement on nerve roots, previous surgery with scar tissue nerve entrapment, severe spondylolisthesis, or pure bony spinal stenosis. Previous surgery or spinal stenosis partially caused by disc herniation do not contraindicate PLDD [10] if scar entrapment of the nerve root is excluded by gadolinium MRI. Neurological examination was carried out by one of two neurologists (Dr. Robert April and Dr. Arthur Weiss) who evaluated patients independently of the author. Also accepted were patients advised to have surgical intervention by a neurosurgeon or orthopedic surgeon. Patients complete a pain diagram that must correspond to the image-documented disc herniation. Radicular pain must be accompanied by signs of nerve involvement, such as reflex changes or impaired straight leg raising.

Lumbar Discs

The lumbar group comprised 497 patients with 699 herniated discs. The last 350 of these patients received vancomycin (0.5 g in 500 mL saline infusion, intravenously) just prior to the procedure. The procedure, which has been described previously [9], consisted of a needle, guided by C-arm fluoroscopy, inserted percutaneously into a herniated disc under local anesthesia that did not extend past the skin and deep fascia. With the needle parallel to the disc, midway between the end plates, and the tip

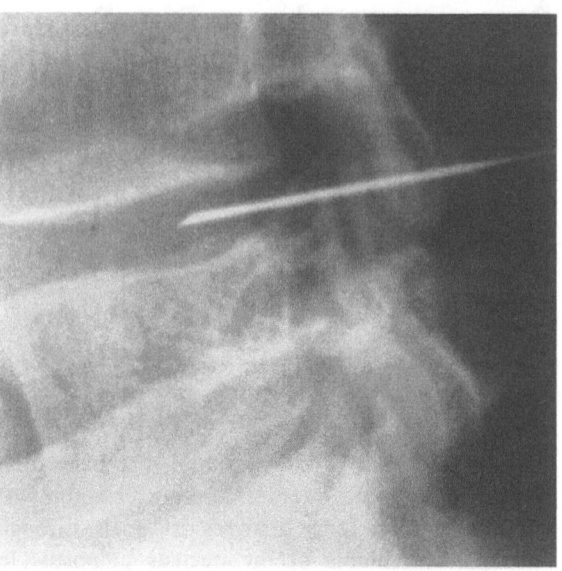

Fig. 3. Optimal position: the needle tip is just past the annulus with the needle midway between the end plates and parallel to the disc axis. The projected laser tract of 2 cm × 5 mm cannot damage the end plates or the opposite annulus

just past the annulus (Fig. 3), Nd:YAG (1.06 µm) laser, 1000 to 1200 J, was delivered through a 400-µm glass/glass fiber equipped with a proximal metal stopper to prevent the tip from extending more than 1.0 cm beyond the needle tip. The power parameters were 20 W for 1.0 s, with 4–5-s pauses to allow for heat dissipation. At the end of the procedure, which averaged 30 min per disc, patients were discharged home. If a high iliac crest prevented dorsolateral insertion of the needle into the L5–S1 disc, an extrathecal approach was used, with the needle entering 2–3 cm from the midline at a 5° angle from the horizontal [11]. Neurological examination was performed immediately before and after each procedure. Postoperative orders were bed rest for 24 h, with gradual ambulation over the next 2–3 days. White-collar workers were allowed to return to work 6 days postoperatively, but manual laborers doing heavy lifting, pulling, or pushing were encouraged to learn a new trade. A 4-mg dose medrol pack was given immediately after surgery. Follow-up visits were scheduled at one day, one week, one, three, six, and twelve months, shared in alternation with a neurologist. Subsequent yearly follow-ups were conducted by mail or telephone. Physiotherapy for back education, stretching, and strengthening was begun one month after PLDD, and lasted for six weeks.

Thoracic Discs

There were six patients with thoracic disc herniation, all of whom had pain in the dermatomes corre-

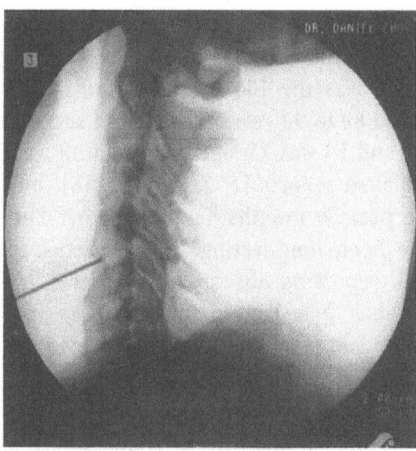

Fig. 4. Position of the needle for cervical disc laser decompression

sponding to the levels of herniation. Dorsolateral needle placement was performed as for lumbar discs, with care to avoid pneumothorax.

Cervical Discs

There were 27 patients with 47 cervical disc herniations. All had cervical pain with radiation down one arm, usually accompanied by digital tingling. Half of them had absent biceps or triceps reflexes. Needle insertion was anterior to the carotid sheath and lateral to the trachea and esophagus. Needle position was halfway between the superior and inferior end plates, and parallel to the disc axis with the tip just past the annulus (Fig. 4). A previously measured fiber (to extend no more than 1.0 mm from the needle tip) was inserted, and pulses of 20 W were delivered for 0.5 s until 300 J had been reached.

Results

A total of 752 procedures in 518 patients (Table 1) were performed from February 1986 to February 1998. The longest follow-up was 12 years, the mean was 84 months, and the shortest 3 months. All patients were evaluated with the MacNab criteria (Table 2). Of 317 male patients, 38 (12 %) were lost to follow-up at 6 months, and another 6 (1.8 %) at 12 months. Of 201 female patients, 36 (18 %) were lost at 6 months, and another 8 (4 %) at 12 months. Office evaluations were alternated between an independent neurologist and the author. Patients who did not return for examination were contacted by mail and/or telephone.

From February 1986 to March 1993, 236 procedures in 168 patients were performed at a teaching hospital. From April 1993 to February 1998, 516

PLDDs in 350 patients were performed at a private outpatient facility. Since more detailed data are available from the latter group, statistical analysis was carried out only for these patients. This group consisted of 120 (60 %) male and 140 (40 %) female patients. The age range was from 17 to 92 years, with a mean of 50.4 years. In females, the mean age was 52.8 ± 18.8, in males it was 48.8 ± 17.2. No significant difference in age was found between male and female patients (t (222) = 1.87, not significant (n. s.)). Likewise, there was no significant difference in outcome with respect to sex: χ^2 (3) = 3.705 (n. s.). There was no significant association between

Table 1. Summary–PLDD–Feb. 1986 to Feb. 1998

Number of procedures	752
Number of patients	518
Age range	17–92
Male	317
Female	201
C3–4	2
C4–5	9
C5–6	22
C6–7	14
T6–7	1
T9–10	1
T11–12	3
T12–L1	1
L1–2	9
L2–3	32
L3–4	65
L4–5	329
L5–S1	264
Longest follow-up	144 months
Mean follow-up	84 months
Overall success rate	75 %
Success rate past 36 months	89 %
Complication rate	< 1 %

Table 2. MacNab criteria of response to treatment

Good	Resumed preoperative function Occasional backache or leg pain No dependency-inducing medications Activity appropriate No objective signs of nerve root involvement
Fair	May be nonproductive if unchanged from preoperative status Intermittent episodes of mild lumbar pain and/or low back pain No dependency-inducing medications Acitivity appropriate No objective signs of nerve root involvement

Poor	Subjective:
	    No productivity
	    Continued pain behavior
	    Medication abuse
	    Inactive
	Compensation and/or litigation focus
	
	Objective: signs of continuing radiculopathy

sex and the level of disc: χ^2 (4) = 2.86 (n. s.). And there was no association between oucome and disc level: χ^2 (13) = 12.46 (n. s.). The preoperative duration of symptoms was more than 24 weeks in 305 (87 %) and less than 24 weeks in 45 patients (13 %). There was no association between outcome and duration of symptoms: χ^2 (3) = 2.59 (n. s.). The mean laser energy was 1358.27 ± 341.87 J, and analysis of variance revealed a significant difference in J between levels L4-5 and L3-4 at the 0.05 significance level. The mean severity of pain rated on a scale of one to ten, with the higher number signifying severe pain, was 7.27 ± 1.77; there was no difference in pain severity between sexes (t (221) = 0.75, n. s.). There was no significant difference in pain severity by level of involvement.

Two levels were decompressed during one procedure in 56 patients (16 female, 40 male) (16 %), three levels in 15 (2 female, 13 male) (4 %), four levels in 3 (1 female, 2 male) (0.8 %), and five levels in 1 (male) patient (0.29 %). The percentages of multiple discs according to patient age are shown in Table 3. The occurrence of multiple disc herniation was greater in the eighth and ninth decades in women (49–50 %), but did not seem to vary by decade in men. The number of patients peaked at the fourth and sixth decades in men, and in the fifth and sixth decades in women (Table 3). There were three repeat PLDDs in one male, three single repeat procedures in three males, and a single repeat PLDD in two females; all were due to re-injury.

Results by Sex and Age

Good to fair results, as distinguished from poor ones as defined by the MacNab criteria, laid out in Table 2, were analyzed by percentages and age/decades for male and female patients. The good to fair results were 76 % in males, and 82 % in females. Patients rated as good to fair were functioning as housewives or were gainfully employed at their previous occupations. White-collar workers were generally back at work on the fifth to sixth postoperative day. The poor results averaged 18 % in women in all decades,

with no particular trend. They averaged 24 % in the second through eighth decades in men.

Of special note was the 100 % failure rate in six male patients aged 80 to 92 years. The overall success rate (MacNab A and B) was 75 %, corresponding well with other published reports [1, 2, 3, 5, 12, 18], but the rate for the past 36 months has been 89 %. The remissions have been long-lasting, with patients at 10-12 years still reporting absence of sciatica. The recurrence rate has been approximately 5 %, and eventual open revision surgery was performed in 6 % of both men and women. This was not universally successful; 55 % of those who had open discectomy did not improve. It should be noted that free disc fragments were found in half of these (4 % of all patients), and may well have been the cause of PLDD failure. This problem will be discussed later. Five patients with disc protrusions with a 90 % turn inferior to the midlevel of the lower vertebra (Fig. 5) were treated in the past 6 months to "expand the envelope." Four of these obtained relief from pain. One did not respond. Three of the five also had foot drop, and of these, one improved by 50 % within 3 weeks, and two had 100 % improvement. In 80 % of all lumbar patients, complete relief of pain was seen immediately after PLDD, and sometimes during the surgery. When pain disappeared after PLDD, it was almost always absent at subsequent follow-up. By the first postoperative day, absent Achilles reflexes reappeared in 48 %, patellar reflexes in 58 %, and normal straight leg raising [13] in 79 %.

The six patients with thoracic disc herniations became free of symptoms, three immediately, one after two weeks, and two, four weeks after PLDD.

Table 3. Multiple discs

Age	Male (%)	Female (%)
20–30	0	0
30–40	24	9
40–50	28	13
50–60	25	11
60–70	26	10
70–80	33	49
80–92	28	50

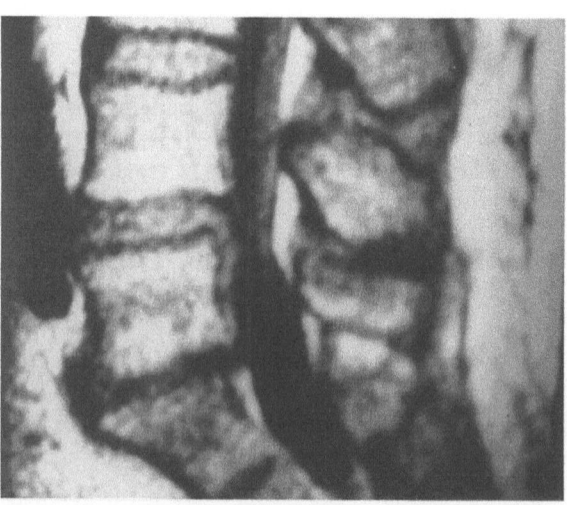

Fig. 5. A herniated L4–5 disc that has extended 90° toward the middle half of the L5 vertebral body. The patient had a foot drop that responded to PLDD after three weeks

No complications were seen in this group. Of the 27 patients with cervical disc herniations ($n = 47$), 20 had two discs involved and five of them had three involved discs. Eight such patients failed to obtain benefit (30 %). One had a repeat procedure, with benefit; two (7 %) required open surgery. Nineteen patients (70 %) became asymptomatic immediately after PLDD. There was one serious complication, which is discussed below.

Complications

Two patients with lumbar discs developed aseptic discitis 3–4 days after PLDD. Both responded to a brief hospitalization with bed rest and parenteral analgesics for 3–4 days. The sciatica was relieved. Two other patients with lumbar discs developed septic discitis, confirmed by MRI and needle puncture culture positive for *Staphylococcus aureus* three days after PLDD. Both responded to brief hospitalization with parenteral vancomycin continued on an outpatient basis for 6 weeks. The sciatica was relieved. One patient with cervical disc decompression developed a retroesophageal abscess, which was successfully drained surgically. This patient also required subsequent open discectomy and fusion.

Based on 518 patients, these five complications represent a rate of 1 %. Since vancomycin infusions were begun 5 years ago, no septic discitis in lumbar and thoracic cases has occurred. The single cervical complication was a retroesophageal abscess with no discitis. At no time was there damage to nerve roots or spinal cord.

Discussion

A radiograph from Dr. John Botsford (Fig. 6) shows a typical laser tract with gas formation in a lumbar disc treated with 800 J. This represents the mass of nucleus ablated by the laser.

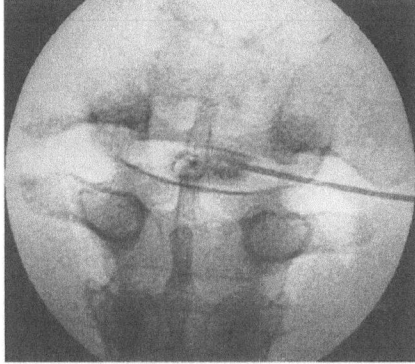

Fig. 6. A laser tract after 800 J; note the gas formation. The radiopaque dye is from a prior discogram. (Slide by courtesy of Dr. John Botsford)

At the Third Congress of the International Musculoskeletal Laser Society (IMLAS), November 7–10, 1996, at the University of Kassel, Germany, 20 neurosurgeons and orthopedic surgeons from the U.S., U.K., Germany, France, Switzerland, Austria, Slovenia, Spain, Argentina, Colombia, Korea, and Japan reported on 4560 patients with herniated lumbar and cervical discs treated with PLDD. The actual number of patients treated worldwide far exceeds this figure. The three lasers used were the KTP (532 nm), the Ho:YAG (2100 nm), and the Nd:YAG (1064 nm). Their combined success rate, by the MacNab criteria and the Oswestry score, was 75 % with a complication rate of 0.5–2.0 %. The shortest and longest follow-ups reported were 2 and 4 years, respectively. These results were comparable with those reported in this study.

Spinal stenosis in which bulging or protruding discs play a contributory role was found in 35 cases who responded to PLDD at rates comparable with open surgery [10]. Some surgeons [3] routinely perform preoperative discography. They report that injection of a small amount of dye, less than 0.5 ml, will reproduce the pain. Patients not experiencing this pain are not treated with PLDD and a 100 % success rate is claimed for procedures performed after this preliminary screening process. However, since the success rate in our series is 75–89 %, we prefer not to perform discography. Often the pressure of the needle point against the annulus will reproduce the sciatic pain. Futhermore, an extra procedure may cause increased morbidity.

As to the mechanism by which PLDD works, it may be postulated that the change in pressure gradient between the tissue adjacent to the herniation and the parent disc results in the movement, however minute, of the herniation away from the affected nerve root. This hypothesis is supported by an "experiment in nature," in which a stunt pilot with an L4-5 herniated disc experienced immediate severe sciatic pain in a pullout of 5-Gs from a dive (which greatly increased intradiscal pressure). He found immediate relief through performing an outside loop (minus 3 Gs, decreasing intradiscal pressure) [12].

In the first 100 of our cases where pain relief was complete, an MRI 6 weeks postoperatively demonstrated a decrease of disc herniation in only a third of the patients. Since the resolution of the best MRI is only 1.5–2.0 mm, any disc shrinkage of less than 1.5 mm will not be demonstrable. We believe that repeat MRIs after PLDD are indicated only when there is a complication. The usual cause for repeat PLDD was re-injury, that is, a new clinical presentation.

Cervical Discs

PLDD of cervical discs was first performed in Europe [19]. This series began in November 1994, and consisted of 47 discs in 27 patients, the commonest being C5-6 and C6-7 levels. Multiple discs were common: two of them in 20 patients and three of them in five. Despite its apparent simplicity, PLDD of cervical discs should not be performed except after strict tutorials, and then only under close supervision. The average height of these discs is only 4–5 mm; the needle diameter is 1.1 mm, so that the clearance on each side is only 1.4–1.9 mm, creating a considerable potential for poor results. PLDD of cervical discs should not be attempted with the Ho:YAG laser, because the smallest trochar in this system is 1.7 mm in diameter, imposing an even smaller clearance on each side.

In addition, the wavelength of the Ho:YAG laser (2100 nm) is too well absorbed by water, and necessitates cooling by saline irrigation; a separate channel must be provided, and this mandates a larger trochar. This is a five-step system, with a needle, a guide-wire, a trochar, dilators, and a trephine. The KTP laser has a wavelength of 532 nm; this approximates the color of the human intervertebral disc and is poorly absorbed. Moreover, the delivery system employs a side-firing fiber, improper placement of the needle has resulted in a number of burns through the end plates, with consequent necrosis of vertebral bodies. The poor results reported by Mathews [16] were probably due to his using the KTP. The Nd:YAG system is the simplest of all, with a single puncture of a 1.1-mm diameter needle through which is threaded a direct firing fiber that is completely controllable. Intradiscal pressure was measured with a Hewlett-Packard angioplasty pressure transducer in eight patients undergoing PLDD. A typical change from 300 to 154 mmHg is seen in Fig. 7.

What accounts for the failures in PLDD? One factor may be patient selection, and this in turn is dependent on the MRI received. There was a wide variation in the quality of the MRIs sent to us; some of these may have failed to detect extruded disc fragments. Another factor could have been vacuum phenomena undetected by MRI. It is known that the CT scan is better for such purposes. PLDD would be expected to work best in a disc with high water content and devoid of vacuum phenomena, in other words, a truly enclosed, homogenous hydraulic system. With aging, the water content of the lumbar disc is decreased. In the elderly, assessment of discs for degenerative changes and reduction of water content should be part of the pre-PLDD evaluation.

In half the patients undergoing subsequent open surgery, free disc fragments were found. It is known that even high-quality noncontrast MRI will fail to diagnose transligamentous ruptures in more than a third of all patients studied [14, 15, 20]. The failures in this series may have been caused by the inability to diagnose free fragments preoperatively.

PLDD offers a less invasive method of treating herniated intervertebral discs than automated discectomy with the nucleotome. Since the 18-guage needle is considerably thinner than the nucleotome trochar, and the procedure takes less time compared with chymopapain nucleolysis, PLDD does not have the side effects of anaphylaxis and leakage of chymopapain. Compared with open discectomy, PLDD has almost no morbidity and does not require general anesthesia or hospitalization. Questions of subsequent spinal instability do not arise with PLDD, since the amount of nucleus pulposus vaporised is very small. Failure of PLDD does not preclude subsequent surgery. Patients who are poor surgical risks through cardiopulmonary decompensation, renal, hepatic, and other major organ failures can be treated with PLDD, since only a local anesthetic is used.

Is PLDD still an experimental procedure? According to a recent paper in the New England Journal of Medicine [17], that is determined by market forces. Accordingly, Medicare, Blue Cross & Blue Shield, and several other major insurers have concluded that PLDD is not experimental, since they all reimburse for it. It is also FDA-approved.

With proper patient selection and meticulous attention to technique, PLDD with the Nd:YAG laser is both safe and effective. At least 5312 procedures have been performed worldwide. It is minimally invasive, is performed in an outpatient setting, requires no general anesthesia, results in no scarring or spinal instability, reduces rehabilitation time, is repeatable,

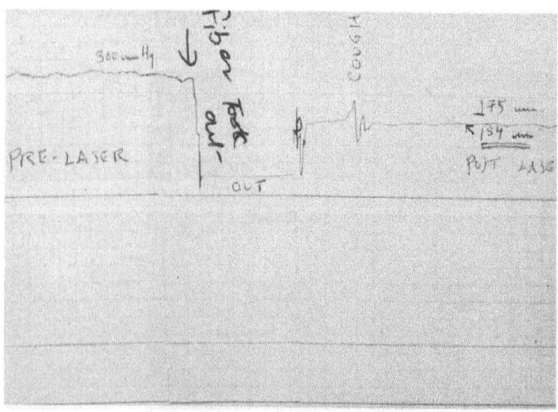

Fig. 7. In vivo measurement of intradiscal pressure before and after laser disc decompression. There is a fall in pressure from 300 to 154 mmHg. The manometrics are seen to be clear from the cough "spike"

and does not preclude open surgery, should that become necessary.

■ **Addendum.** The data have evolved since this article was originally submitted in 1998. The latest data from the author are given in Table 4.

■ **Acknowledgments.** The author is indebted to Milda Goldstein and Rhea Brown for proofreading, and to Drs. Robert April and Robert B Case for invaluable input in manuscript organization and editorial comment. Statistical analysis was performed by Emilia Bagiella, Columbia University School of Public Health. Kit Davidson edited the final manuscript.

Table 4. Summary of PLDD procedures, including the latest data from the author (up to March 31, 2000)

Number of procedures	1157
Number of patients	707
Age range	17–92
Male	442
Female	265
C3–4	6
C4–5	11
C5–6	32
C6–7	22
T5–6	2
T6–7	2
T7–8	1
T8–9	1
T9–10	1
T10–11	1
T11–12	4
T12–L1	2
L1–2	14
L2–3	49
L3–4	120
L4–5	475
L5–S1	414
Longest follow-up	171 months
Mean follow-up	102 months
Success rate past 75 months	89%
Complication rate	0.12%

References

[1] Ascher PW (1986) Application of the laser in neurosurgery. Lasers Surg Med 291–297
[2] Black WA Jr (1995) A neurosurgical perspective on PLDD. J Clin Laser Med Surg 13(3):167–171
[3] Botsford JA (1994) CT discography: prognostic value in patient selection for percutaneous laser disc decompression (PLDD). In: 94th annual meeting of the Am Roentgen Ray Society (ARRS), New Orleans, 24–29 April 1994; Abstract 265
[4] Case RBC, Choy DSJ, Altman P (1985) Intervertebral disc pressure as a function of fluid volume infused. J Clin Laser Med Surg 13:143–147
[5] Caspar GD, Hartman VL, Mullins LL (1996) Results of a clinical trial of the Holmium:YAG laser in disc decompression utilizing a side-firing fiber: a two-year follow-up. Lasers Surg Med 19:90–96
[6] Choy DSJ, Altman P (1993) Fall of intradiscal pressure with laser ablation. Spine 7(1):23–29
[7] Choy DSJ, Altman PA, Case RB, Trokel SL (1991) Laser radiation at various wavelengths for decompression of intervertebral disc. Clin Ortho Rel Res 267:245–250
[8] Choy DSJ, Case RB, Fielding W, Hughes J, Liebler W, Ascher P (1987) Percutaneous laser nucleolysis of lumbar discs. N Engl J Med 317:771–772
[9] Choy DSJ, Ascher PW, Saddekni S, Alkaitis D, Lieber W, Hughes J, Diwan S, Altman P (1992) Percutaneous laser lumbar disc decompression – a new therapeutic modality. Spine 17(8): 949–956
[10] Choy DSJ, Ngeow J (1998) Percutaneous laser disc decompression in spinal stenosis. J Clin Laser Med Surg 16(2):123–125
[11] Choy DSJ (1995) The problem of the L5-S1 disc solved by needle entry with an extrathecal apporach. J Clin Laser Med Surg 12(6):321–324
[12] Choy DSJ (1997) Positive and negative gravitational forces and herniated-disc sciatic pain. N Engl J Med 337:1396–1397
[13] Choy DSJ (1996) Immediate reversal of neurologic deficits after percutaneous laser decompression. J Clin Laser Med Surg 14(1):13–15
[14] Greenspan A (1993) CT discography vs MRI in intervertebral disk herniation. Appl Radio 34–40
[15] Joubert JM, Laredo JD, Ziza JM et al. (1992) Gadolinium-enhanced MR imaging in the preoperative evaluation of lumbar disc herniations. In: 78th scientific assembly and meeting of the RSNA, Chicago, 29 Nov–4 Dec 1992, Abstract 304
[16] Mathews HH, Kyles MK, Fiore SM, Long BH (1994) Laser disc decompression with KTP 532 wavelength: a two-year follow-up. In: Amer Acad of Ortho Surg, New Orleans, February 1994, Abstract 292
[17] Newcomber LN (1997) Defining experimental therapy: a third party payer's dilemma. Sounding board. N Engl J Med 323:1702–1704
[18] Sherk H, Black J, Rhodes A, Lane G, Prodoehl JU (1993) Laser discectomy. Clin Sports Med 12:569–577
[19] Siebert W (1995) Percutaneous laser discectomy of cervical discs: preliminary clinical results. J Clin Laser Med Surg 13(3):205–207
[20] Thornbury JR, Fryback DG, Turski PA Javid MJ, McDonald JV, Beinlich BR, Gentry LR, Sackett JF, Dasbach EJ, Martin PA (1993) Disc-caused nerve compression in patients with acute low back pain. Diagnosis with MR, CT myelography and plain CT. Radiology 186:731–738

Lumbar Disc Operation:
Results of Percutaneous Laser Disc Decompression (PLDD)

U. Pfeil · W. Siebert

Introduction

Minimally invasive procedures for lumbar disc herniation reduce postnucleotomy syndrome (PNS) [2, 3, 11, 16, 18, 20]. One risk factor for PNS is extensive disc excision [1, 10, 12, 17, 18]. The removal of facets and disc excision create instability. Examinations from Weber and Saal showed no difference between patients treated surgically and nonsurgically: 60 % were free of pain after 10 years [15, 19]. The results from Hakelius demonstrated that surgical intervention improved the short-term outcome for patients with sciatica, but after seven years the study showed little difference between conservative and surgical groups. The patients who did not receive surgery had more episodes of low back pain and sciatica and more sick leave from work [6].

To improve the surgical results, the indications and contraindications for lumbar disc surgery must be strictly and carefully observed. Prior conservative therapy should last for 6 weeks to 3 months or more, except where the patient is experiencing progressive neurologic deficit or cauda equina syndrome [1, 7].

A CT or MRI scan can distort and misrepresent the size of nuclear material and thereby the size of a disc herniation may be overestimated. The misinterpretation of the true volume of the disc material arises because the disc material incites an inflammatory reaction in the epidural space. On the MRI scan we have to distinguish the efffects of a combination of disc material, inflammatory tissue, epidural hematoma and oedema in deducing the disc protrusion volume [5, 6, 7, 9, 10, 13 14].

The inflammatory potential of the disc can be reduced by an epidural corticoid injection. Conservative therapy (injections, physical therapy, etc.) may successfully reduce the pain symptoms in many patients with a lumbar disc herniation [2, 4, 13]. If this nonoperative intervention is not effective, then surgery should be considered.

Percutaneous Laser Disc Decompression

Percutaneous laser disc decompression (PLDD) has some advantages for the patient:
- The surgical procedure can be done under local anesthesia.
- The patient is awake and monitored neurologically during the whole procedure.
- The dorsolateral access does not leave any epidural scars.

We did not observe any complications in all 165 patients treated with this method in our clinic.

Indications:

- Patients with lumbar sciatica that is resistant to conservative treatment
- Computer tomography or MRI examination that shows a disc protrusion without extrusion or sequestration in the spinal canal or lateral recess

Contraindications:

- Sequestrated herniation, cauda equina symptoms
- Spinal canal stenosis
- Prior index level surgery
- Spondylolisthesis
- Early pension, psychosociological factors

Surgical Procedure for PLDD

The patient is placed prone in a kyphotic lumbar spine position on a radiolucent X-ray surgery table. The patient is awake and under local anesthesia 8–10 cm laterally from the spinous processus. After the correct disc level is identified, the skin is infiltrated with 0.5 % to 1.0 % local anesthesia, and a depot of 10 ml 0.75 % carbostesin is injected through a small incision. The side is punctured with an 18 g needle under radiologic control, generally on the side with sciatica. A water-soluble contrast medium is injected into the intervertebral space, and often provokes memory pain. If an abnormal disc is observed during the discography, the inner guide needle is removed and the guiding cannula is inserted.

The laser fiber is pushed through the cannula until 2 to 4 mm protrudes beyond the cannula tip. We use the following energy parameters: holmium:YAG laser (2.1 μm), 3.6–4.8 W, pulse rate 6–10 Hz, with impulses repeated at 3–5 times per second intervals. The procedure is carried out with continuous intradiscal flushing with isotonic saline solution and constant verbal communication with the patient. The procedure should cause no pain to the patient.

Postoperative Treatment

After application of a sterile bandage, patients should remain in bed in the supine position for several hours postoperatively. We then prescribe supervised physical therapy, including back training. Patients are encouraged to sit in a correct position for periods of 10–15 minutes, initially.

Material and Methods

From 1. 7. 1994 to 1.10. 1997 we treated 168 patients with lumbar disc protrusion and prolapses with PLDD. In a follow-up examination, which included questions on persistent or recurring back and/or leg pain similar to preoperative symptoms, 131 patients took part. The patients graded their pain on a visual analogue scale ranging from 0 to 10 (0: no pain, 10: unbearable pain). They also graded the postoperative increase of daily activities on a scale from 10 to 100 %. Furthermore, we asked the patients if they would have agreed to undergo further PLDD if surgery was again necessary.

Results

Out of 168 patients (82 female and 86 male), 131 patients (78.0 %) were included in this clinical trial. The mean age was 43 years; the mean time for the postoperative follow-up examination was 24 months. The disc level L4–L5 was most frequently affected (66 cases), the disc level L5–S1 was involved in 51 cases, and both levels were affected in 42 cases; there were four cases with level L3–L4 and L4–L5, three cases with level L3–L4, one case with levels L3–S1 and also one case with level L2–L3. Following PLDD in our clinic, 27 patients out of a total of 168 had received microdiscectomy at an average period of 7.5 months. During the follow-up examination, a further 18 patients reported reoperation at the same disc level in another hospital. In this study, our success rate for PLDD surgery was 60 % of the patients; 66.7 % ($n = 86$) had moderate pain (grade 1–5) on a visual analogue scale from 1–10. The self-rated increase of postoperative daily activities ranged from 40 to 100 %. Ninety-four patients (72.9 %) would agree to PLDD again.

Conclusion

Minimal invasive procedures such as percutaneous laser disc decompression have advantages over other open surgical techniques. In our examination, the success rate of PLDD-treated patients was only 60 %. This rather poor result shows that a precise indication for this surgical procedure is necessary. The use of other minimally invasive procedures such as endoscopic discectomy should increase, because these have shown better results in our hands.

References

[1] Andersson G, Weinstein J (1996) Disc herniation editorial. Spine 21/24:1–9
[2] Bookwalter JW, Busch MD, Nicely D (1994) Ambulatory surgery is safe and effective in radicular disc disease. Spine 19:526–530
[3] Bush K, Cowan N, Katz DE Crishen P (1992) The natural history of sciatica associated with disc pathology. A prospective study with clinical and independent radiologic follow-up. Spine 17:1205–1212
[4] Dilke TF, Burry HC, Graham R (1973) Extradural conticosteroid injection in management of lumbar nerve root compression. Br Med J 867:635–637
[5] Gundry CR, Heithoff KP (1993) Epidural hematoma of the lumbar spine: 18 surgically confirmed cases. Radiology 187:427–431
[6] Hakelius A (1970) Prognosis in sciatica: a clinical follow-up of surgical and non-surgical treatment. Acta Othop Scand 129 (Suppl):1–76
[7] Herzog R (1996) The radiologic assessment for a lumbar disc herniation. Spine 2:19–38
[8] Jensen MC, Brant-Zawadzki MN, Obuchowski N, Modic MT Malkasian D, Ross JS (1994) Magnetic resonance imaging of the lumbar spine in people without back pain. N Engl J Med 331:69–73
[9] Kimori H, Shinomiya K, Nakai O, Yamaura I, Takeda S, Furnya K (1996) The natural history of herniated nucleus pulposus with radiculopathy. Spine 21:225–229
[10] McCaron RF, Winjed MW, Hudgins PG, Laros GS (1987) The inflammatory effect of nucleus pulposus: a possible element in the pathogenesis of low back pain. Spine 12:760–764
[11] Nachemson AL (1985) Advances in low-back pain. Clin Orthop 200:266–278
[12] Newman MH (1995) Outpatient conventional laminotomy and disc excision. Spine 20:353–355
[13] Olmarker K, Blomquist J, Strömberg J, Nannmark U, Thomsen P, Rydevik B (1995) Inflammatogenic properties of nucleus pulposus. Spine 20:665–669
[14] Saal JS (1995) The role of inflammation. Spine 20/16:1821–1827
[15] Saal JA, Saal JS (1989) Nonoperative treatment of herniated lumbar intervertebral disc with radiculopathy. Spine 14/4:431–437
[16] Saal JA, Saal JS, Herzog RJ (1990) The natural history of lumbar intervertebral disc extrusions treated nonoperatively. Spine 15:683–686
[17] Shekelle PG, Adams AH, Chassin MR,. Hurwitz EL, Brook RH (1992) Spinal manipulation for low-back pain. Br Med J 1117:590-598
[18] Siebert WE, Berendsen BE, Toligaard J (1996) Die perkutane Laserdiskus-Dekompression (PLDD). Orthopäde 25:41–48
[19] Weber H (1983) Lumbar disc herniation: a controlled, prospective study with ten years of observation. Spine 8:141–140
[20] Weber H (1994) The natural history of disc herniations and the influence of intervention. Spine 19/19:2234–2238

Lumbar Percutaneous KTP 532-nm Laser Disc Decompression and Disc Ablation in the Management of Discogenic Pain

M. Knight · A. Goswami

Introduction

Laser disc decompression (LDD) can be performed with the KTP 532-nm or Ho:YAG wavelengths but with different tissue effects and thus differing applications. Potassium titanyl phosphate (KTP) laser disc decompression (KTP LDD) is an intradiscal decompressive technique that diminishes intradiscal pressure by 50%, thus reducing the compression upon the adjacent nerve roots [1–4]. The therapeutic effect of KTP percutaneous laser disc decompression is based on the reduction of intradiscal pressure by vaporisation of degenerate disc tissue [3]. Nachemson's [5] studies of intradiscal pressure measurements demonstrated significant pressure elevation with weight lifting and in specific postures. Choy and Ascher [2] reported that the intradiscal application of 1000–1850 J of Nd:YAG laser energy consistently reduced intradiscal pressure by more than 50% in vivo.

Several basic science and histological studies suggest that apart from mechanical factors, non-compressive local inflammation is also a major cause of back and nerve-root pain. Alteration in pH, liberation of various kinins, nitric oxide, neuropeptides, phospholipase A_2 (PLA_2), CGRP (calcitonin gene related protein), neuropeptides, TGF-β (transforming growth factor β) and several metalloproteinases have been implicated in the causation of chronic back pain [6] Freemont et al. [7] have demonstrated that neovascularisation and neoneuralisation within the disc may be implicated in the causation of discogenic pain. These findings are supported by unpublished data from this centre, where histological data were correlated with operative details obtained from operating on patients in the conscious state with endoscopic laser foraminoplasty. This might explain why it was very often difficult to correlate a disc bulge or prolapse to the patients' radicular symptoms. The published evidence from basic science studies on the mechanisms of back pain [6] made it obvious that the mere presence of a disc bulge or herniations could not explain discogenic pain. Studies on disc pathology indicate that KTP LDD attenuates intradiscal inflammation and in addition has a thermoplastic annealing effect on the damaged disc wall [8].

To understand the pain mechanism in patients with back pain and radicular symptoms, more discrete methods of isolating the pain source was needed. This was made possible with the introduction of spinal probing and discography. Further information could be obtained by endoscopic examination of spinal tissue with the patients in the conscious state giving feed-back on painful sites during surgery. This made correlation of the discographic findings with the pathological disc easier, reducing the chance of false positive results. Collected data and experience with endoscopic surgery allowed us to rely on probing and discographic findings and hence we extended the indication for laser disc decompression to discs which reproduced pain associated with painful tears during discography, irrespective of disc bulge or prolapse.

Published articles on percutaneous laser disc decompression suggest excellent to good results in 70–87% of patients [2, 9–12]. Such gratifying results were obtained when patient selection was confined to those who had contained disc herniations and with short-term studies.

In this study we present our experience with the side-firing potassium titanyl phosphate (KTP) laser on 579 consecutive cases treated between 1992 and 1997. To observe the long-term outcome of laser disc decompression we followed these patients up for a minimum period of three years. These procedures were performed for treating painful disc protrusions, annular tears and painful disc pathology.

Materials and Methods

All patients with chronic back pain unresponsive to conservative management were included in this study. All patients filled in a questionnaire on their disability; this also included psychometric profile data, a pain mannikin and desired targets to be achieved at the end of the management protocol, together with a visual analogue pain scale and Oswestry Disability Score. The patients were assessed clinically with x-rays, including dynamic views in flexion and extension. Any olisthesis or retrolisthesis was observed in these dynamic views. All patients then underwent a kinetic muscle balancing programme of physiotherapy for a minimum period of 3 months. On failure of conservative management, patients were reviewed with MR scans and reassessed clinically. Spinal probing and discography was performed as the first step towards identification of the source of pain.

Inclusion criteria:
- Disc bulge (broad-based)
- Contained disc prolapse
- MRI or clinically suspected radial tears of the discs
- Painful discs as proven by spinal probing and discography
- Patients presenting with stenotic symptoms not proven on MRI scans

Exclusion criteria:
- Spinal stenosis (including lateral and foraminal) as determined by MR or CT scans
- Disc sequestration
- Cauda equina syndromes and any neurological emergencies
- Associated tumours
- Acute trauma

Operative Technique

This procedure was performed in the prone position on a specially designed table. Patients were mildly sedated with the neurolept analgesic fentanyl, titrated by the anaesthetist to permit adequate assessment of pain reproduction during provocative discography. A single dose of 1.5 g of intravenous cefuroxime was routinely used as prophylaxis against infections. A designated nurse would record distribution and reproduction of pain while the surgeon probed different structures of the spine and during discography.

The posterolateral approach was used to gain access to the intervertebral disc. A special jig was used to facilitate locating the entry site (Chapter 14). The skin, subcutaneous tissue and paravertebral muscles were anaesthetised with 10 ml of 0.25 % lignocaine. Under C-arm image-intensifier control, a blunt, 2-mm probe was guided towards the posterolateral corner of the intervertebral disc. Pain produced on probing the facet joint and disc annulus was noted. The probe was positioned in line with the posterior disc margins on the lateral projection and in the mid-pedicular line on the postero-anterior projection. A 22-gauge needle was

then introduced into the disc. Discography was performed to evaluate disc containment, configuration of the degeneration within the disc, disc-wall protrusion and the acceptance volume. Any pain reproduction was noted during discography at the presumed index level and adjacent degenerate segments.

Once a symptomatic, degenerate, prolapsed and contained segment was identified, it was injected with 0.5 ml of indigo carmine, used as an external chromophore to augment absorption of 532-nm laser waves [13]. With the discography needle as a guide, the guiding tube for the laser fiber was advanced on to the disc wall. A trephine was passed down the cannula and the disc wall was opened. The laser fiber and suction sheath was inserted into the disc. Its position was confirmed in the anteroposterior and lateral plane with the image intensifier. Laser energy was then delivered through a 400-μm optical fiber encased in a probe that incorporated suction and deflected the laser beam laterally by 90° (Spinestat Laserscope, CA). A standard energy dose of 1250 J of 20 W laser energy was delivered in pulses of 0.2 s every 0.5 s. If local heat was perceived by the patient, lasing was briefly discontinued and resumed once discomfort was alleviated. The laser beam was directed towards the site of disc protrusion and away from the vertebral body end plates. Typical procedure time for a two-level discography and KTP percutaneous laser disc decompression was 30–45 min.

Post-Operative Regimen and Follow-up

Patients were discharged from hospital on the same day or the day following the procedure. All patients underwent a programme of graduated kinetic muscle-balancing physiotherapy 24 to 48 hours after surgery and continued for six sessions over 3 months. Patients in sedentary work were allowed to return to work 5–21 days following surgery. Those involved in physically demanding occupations were cautiously allowed into work in 6–12 weeks, depending on the response to the procedure.

Follow-up
Patients were followed-up at 6 weeks, 3 months, and 6 months after operation and thereafter on a yearly basis. Questionnaires were filled in at each visit.

Data Collection
Outcome analysis was based on the Oswestry disability index (ODI), the visual analogue pain scale (VAPI), patient target achievement score (PTAS) and patient satisfaction scores (Table 1). Review was done during clinical assessment and by postal questionnaires where necessary.

Table 1. Indices and scores

$$\text{Disability: } \Delta DI = \frac{\text{Preoperative DI} - \text{Postoperative DI}}{\text{Preoperative DI}} \times 100$$

$$\text{Pain: VAP Index} = \frac{\text{Preoperative score} - \text{Postoperative Score}}{10} \times 100$$

$$\text{Targets: PTAS} = \frac{\text{Points}}{25} \times 100$$

DI, disability index

Results

A total of 576 consecutively operated patients were followed for a minimum period of 3 years. The number of levels operated on were 687. While the outcome data for all the patients were available in the first year of the follow-up, the cohort integrity was compromised at the second and subsequent years. We wanted to know the long-term outcome of laser disc decompression, and used all clinical data and follow-up details which were available in 388 patients at the time of this report. The cohort integrity of this study is therefore 67%. The average follow-up time was 5.33 years (range 3–9 years). The average age of the patients at the time of operation was 43 years (range 18–80 years).

The average duration of symptoms prior to intervention was 4.7 years (range 8 months to 22 years). The symptoms were of insidious origin in 63% of the patients, and 22% of the symptoms appeared following trauma.

The symptoms of back, buttock or leg pain varied from a minimum of 8 months to a maximum of 18 years. Of the patients 18% had previous open surgical interventions including discectomy and fusion procedures. Different coping courses on pain and physiotherapy were undergone by 7% of the patients. MR scans showed that 62% of the patients had multiple level disc degeneration.

Oswestry Disability Score

The Oswestry disability score results are summarised in Table 2.

Back pain: At the end of the first year after laser disc decompression, 60% of the patients demonstrated good to excellent results while the response for another 21% was satisfactory. However, follow-up of patients in the third year showed that the good to excellent outcomes were limited to 52% of the patients, while 24% demonstrated a satisfactory response.

Buttock pain: The initial response was good to excellent in 57% of the cases, with another 18%

demonstrating satisfactory improvement. These results declined to 48% and 23%, respectively.

Leg pain: The results were excellent to good in 60% of the cases while another 19% showed initial improvement, but in the third year these values deteriorated to 51% and 22%, respectively.

Visual Analogue Pain Scores

On the visual analogue pain scale, 12% of the patients were pain-free at the end of 3 years. A more than 50% reduction in the pain scale was found in 51%, while 8% had deterioration of pain symptoms.

Patient Target Achievement Score (PTA)

More than 50% of the preoperative rehabilitative objectives, selected as goals prior to surgery, was achieved by 56% of the patients. Another 12% were satisfied with the targets achieved.

Patient Satisfaction Scoring

At the end of follow-up, 61% of the patients were satisfied with the overall outcome of the procedure.

Complications

Four patients developed aseptic discitis with increased pain and muscular spasms. Blood investigation and culture and subsequent biopsy failed to identify any infective pathology. No neurological complications occurred in patients in this series. Further disc prolapse occurred at the same level in 2% of the patients.

Further intervention in the form of endoscopic laser foraminoplasty for foraminal and lateral recess decompression was required by 17% of patients. These patients demonstrated an initial improvement lasting between 6 months and 5 years. Endoscopic laser foraminoplasty in these patients resulted in the improvement in symptoms in 12% of the patients.

Table 2. Response to PLDD on the Oswestry disability index

		Back (348)	Buttock (292)	Leg (310)
1st year	Good/excellent	210	165	184
	Satisfactory	72	52	58
	Poor	55	67	59
	Worse	11	8	9
2nd year	Good/excellent	192	145	173
	Satisfactory	82	65	63
	Poor	60	71	65
	Worse	14	11	9
3rd year	Good/excellent	181	140	158
	Satisfactory	86	68	67
	Poor	71	73	75
	Worse	10	11	10

Discussion

It is well recognised that the primary purpose of disc decompression is to relieve nerve-root irritation or compression due to herniated disc material in patients with disc prolapse. Minimal invasive techniques for the treatment of back, buttock and leg pain are attractive because of the advantages such as reduced complication rates, early functional recovery, their outpatient nature and because they do not jeopardise future surgical procedures. The benefits of minimal intervention are only relevant if outcome results are comparable to those of conventional methods.

The review of the Cochrane Database [21] suggests that surgical discectomy produced better clinical outcomes than chemonucleolysis with chymopapain, and chemonucleolysis produced better clinical outcomes than placebo. There is also some evidence that the surgical outcome of microdiscectomy is almost that of open discectomy. Three trials of percutaneous discectomy provided moderate evidence that it produces poorer clinical outcomes than standard discectomy or chymopapain.

The outcome is directly related to patient selection with all surgical methods for treatment of sciatica from lumbar disc prolapse. However, the ideal candidate with predominantly sciatic pain of anatomic dermotomal distribution, without significant spondylosis or facet osteroarthritis and with ample bony canal is relatively rare to find in most back pain referral centres [14, 15]. Matters are further complicated by associated factors such as depression from chronic pain and ongoing cases for compensation following injuries sustained during work or road traffic accidents. The majority of the referrals will have one or more factors associated with a less than optimal outcome. This study sought to evaluate the efficiency of KTP percutaneous laser disc decompression on a diverse group, typical of referrals to specialist units.

As is the case for most percutaneous discectomy techniques, the indications for KTP percutaneous laser disc decompression were restricted to contained disc protrusions. In this unit, this is defined as annular containment without the breach of the posterior longitudinal ligament. This inclusion criteria included cases with annular leaks. It has been argued that only a minority of patients with a contained disc prolapse will present with symptomatology sufficient to warrant surgical intervention [16]. Our patient population suggests that this is not the case. Our patients with contained disc prolapse had had prolonged symptomatology resistant to adequate and sustained conservative treatment. In addition, most had suffered from recurrent sciatic episodes for several years with the resultant disruption in social and work-related activities.

The long-term follow-up of patients who underwent laser disc decompression and laser disc ablation suggests that following an initial gratifying result there is some deterioration of the clinical condition with time. However, the principal deterioration occurs in the first and second years. Further follow-up of the patients in the fifth and the sixth years showed only minimal subsequent deterioration and the results are sustained with 50 % good to excellent outcomes. We believe there are several factors that may be directly involved in the relatively worse than expected outcomes in patients with laser disc decompression:

1. Our patients consituted a spectrum including some ideal and some less than ideal candidates for surgery. The criteria for the selection of the patients for LDD were unlike those in other published papers. The selection criteria were not confined to the contained disc bulges/prolapses but were extended to painful discs that demonstrated tears or provoked pain during probing and discography.

2. Strict criteria were used to assess patients; one of these is the Oswestry disability index. We regarded an index value of more than 50 to be good to excellent and a value of more than 20 on the ODI represented a satisfactory response to the surgery.

3. Of the patients in the study, 23 % had previous open surgical interventions such as open disc decompression and fusions. Painful discs identified by discography, with or without leakage of dye, were treated with laser disc ablation. The results in these patients were less gratifying than in the rest of the group. This, we believe, is secondary to inflammatory processes in the disc, which we failed to address adequately with the laser disc ablation in all patients.

4. Progressive clinical deterioration was secondary to further reduction in the disc height. This led to the development of lateral recess or foraminal stenosis. These patients (17 %) were treated subsequently with endoscopic laser foraminoplasty with success.

Early lateral recess stenosis may limit the effectiveness of KTP 532-nm-wavelength percutaneous laser disc decompression. Most of the patients in this group had initial relief of their leg pain, which later recurred as an activity-related ache rather than with irritative characteristics.

Retrospective analysis of the failures indicate that KTP 532-nm-wavelength laser disc decompression is not suitable for hourglass disc protrusions, disc segments subjected to prior surgery, weight-bearing disc heights of less than 4 mm, flexion–extension listhesis of 3 mm or more or in case of lateral recess stenosis. Endoscopic laser foraminoplasty was used in these patients with success. The application of these guidelines in more recent cases confirmed the appropriateness of these indications. The lasting outcome is better than with conservative and conventional techniques, and bodes well for the long term.

Our experience with no neurologic, septic or vascular complications supports the generally accepted concept that percutaneous techniques have lower complication rates than open discectomy [17–20]. KTP percutaneous laser disc decompression allows treatment with no risk or araphylaxis and is technically relatively simple. The side-firing probe tip permits controlled delivery of laser energy, thus contributing to its safety. In our hands it has proven to be an effective day-case method of surgical intervention for the alleviation of back pain, buttock pain and leg pain, as an alternative to conventional open discectomy.

Conclusions

KTP LDD has proven to be an effective "day-case" minimal means of treating contained lumbar disc prolapse causing sciatica in patients with wide-based disc protrusions and annular tears and leaks, limited olisthesis and preserved disc height on bending x-rays of 4 mm or more. The restoration of activity levels, sustained in the long term, for appropriately indicated patients is encouraging. It offers excellent and good results in 52 % of patients followed up for more than three years. The method permits outpatient treatment of lumbar disc prolapse with minimal local morbidity, minimal disruption of patients' work and social activities and does not preclude or jeopardise future surgery if required. KTP percutaneous laser disc decompression is a safe minimal intervention technique. The incidence of complications is less than that reported for open discectomy.

References

[1] Choy DSJ, Altman P (1995) Fall of intradiscal pressure with laser ablation. J Clin Las Med Surg 13:149–152
[2] Choy DSJ, Ascher PW, Ranu HS, Saddekin S, Alkaitis D, Liebler W, Hughes J, Diwan S, Altman P (1992) Percutaneous laser disc decompression – a new therapeutic modality. Spine 7:949–956
[3] Choy DSJ, Case RB, Fielding W, Hughes J, Lieber W, Ascher P (1987) Percutaneous laser nucleolysis of lumbar discs. New Engl J Med 317:771
[4] Choy DSJ, Michelsen J, Getrajdman G, Diwans S (1992) Percutaneous laser disc decompression. An update. J Clin Laser Med Surg 6:177
[5] Nachemson A (1965) The effects of forward leaning on lumbar intradiscal pressure. Acta Orthop Scan 35:314–328
[6] Cavannaugh JF (1999) Innervation of the lumbosacral spine. In: Willis WHK, Barnard TN Jr (eds) Managing low back pain. Churchill Livingstone, Pittsburgh, Pennsylvania
[7] Freemont AJ, Peacock TF, Coupville P, Hoyland JA, O'Brien J, Jayson MIV (1997) Nerve ingrowth into diseased intervertebral disc in chronic back pain. Lancet 350:178–181
[8] Hayashi K, Thabit G 3rd, Vailas AC, Bogdanske JJ, Cooley AJ, Markel MD (1996) The effect of nonablative laser energy on joint capsular properties. An in vitro histologic and biochemical study using a rabbit model. Am J Sports Med 24(5):640–646
[9] Hihikata S (1989) Percutaneous nucleotomy. A new concept technique and 12 years' experience. Clin Orthop 238:9–23
[10] Kambin P, Schaffer K (1989) Percutaneous lumbar discectomy. Review of 100 patients and current practice. Clin Orthop 238:24–34
[11] Ohnmeiss DD, Guyer RD, Hochschuler SH (1994) Laser disc decompression. The importance of proper patient selection. Spine 19:2054–2058
[12] Schreiber A, Suezawa Y, Leu H (1989) Does percutaneous nucleotomy with discoscopy replace conventional discectomy? Clin Orthop 238:35–42
[13] Jacques SL (1993) Laser-tissue interactions. Surg Clin N Am 72:531–558
[14] Abramovitz J, Neff S (1991) Lumbar disc surgery: results of the prospective lumbar discectomy study of the joint section on disorders of the spine and peripheral nerves of the American Association of Neurological Surgeons and the Congress of Neurological Surgeons. Neurosurgery 29: 301–308
[15] Maroon JC, Onik G, Vidovich DV (1993) Percutaneous discectomy for lumbar disc herniation. Neurosurg Clin N Am 4:125–134
[16] Herkowitz H (1993) Automated percutaneous lumbar discectomy versus chemonucleolysis in the treatment of sciatica. Adv Orthop Surg 17:38–40 (commentary)
[17] Caspar W, Campbell B, Barbier D, Kretschmmer R, Goffried Y (1991) The Caspar microsurgical discectomy and comparison with a conventional standard lumbar disc proceudre. Neurosurgery 28:78–87
[18] Davis GW, Onik G, Helms C (1991) Automated percutaneous discectomy. Spine 16:359–363
[19] Maroon JC, Onik G, Vidovich DV (1993) Percutaneous discectomy for lumbar disc herniation. Neurosurg Clin N Am 4:125–134
[20] Tregonning GD, Transfeldt EE, McCulloch JA, MacNab I, Nachemson A (1991) Chymopapain versus conventional surgery for lumbar disc herniation: 10-year results of treatment. J Bone Joint Surg 73B:481–486
[21] Gibson JNA, Grant IC, Waddell G (1999) The Cochrane Review of Surgery for lumbar disc prolapse and degenerative lumbar spondylosis. Spine 24(17):1820–1832

Laser Foraminoscopic Surgery

G. D. Casper

Introduction

Laser foraminoscopic surgery of the spine has developed as a consequence of the search for minimally invasive techniques to address certain pathologic entities such as herniated nucleus pulposus in the lumbar spine. The overall goal of minimally invasive approaches to spinal pathology is to at least simulate the results of open laminectomy or microdiscectomy, while providing the added value of decreased morbidity and complications.

The work of Hihikata [1], Kambin [2] and others [3–5] has clearly shown that a safe approach to the intradiscal area can be accomplished. This work was expanded upon by Mathews [6, 7] with his description of a transforaminal approach with a working channel endoscope for addressing pathology within the foraminal space. The safe use of laser energy for intradiscal decompression by Choy et al. [5], Sherk [8], and Lane et al. [9] has also been expanded from the original Nd:YAG laser to the use of other forms of thermal energy, such as the KTP and the Ho:YAG wavelengths.

The ability to "aim" the laser energy has also afforded certain potential advantages to the use of thermal energy in the intradiscal space [10]. Laser foraminal endoscopic surgery has evolved as an alternative approach for the removal of disc material that is accessible within the foraminal space by endoscopy and directable laser energy. It is hoped that the long-term results from this procedure will, indeed, simulate open laminectomy or microdiscectomy in terms of results and will also be comparable to percutaneous endoscopic or nonvisualized procedures in terms of relative morbidity when compared to open laminectomy or microdiscectomy [3].

Indications

The indications for laser foraminoscopic surgery are contained or noncontained disc herniations within the lumbar region (i.e., from L1 to S1) that are endoscopically accessible via a foraminal approach. These would include the following:

1. Far-lateral disc herniations
2. Contained or noncontained foraminal disc extrusions or herniations
3. Certain paramedian disc herniations that are endoscopically accessible

Clinically, the patient would present with signs and symptoms compatible with lumbar radiculopathy persisting over a period of six weeks despite intense, adequate conservative management (e. g., physiotherapy, chiropractic therapy, nonsteroidal anti-inflammatory medication, epidural steroids, selective nerve blocks, etc.).

Confirmation of the aforementioned disc pathology would need to be obtained by MRI (preferred), CT, myelogram with or without CT, or discogram with or without CT. Once the clinical and radiographic diagnosis of disc herniation is confirmed, the procedure itself can be accomplished.

Surgical Procedure

The procedure is performed under a local anesthetic, with managed anesthesia care, in a fully equipped operating suite including appropriate video equipment, radiolucent frame, and imaging capabilities for both AP and lateral views throughout the procedure. Although the prone position is most frequently utilized, some physicians prefer the lateral position. The hips are always slightly flexed to decrease lumbar lordosis and to open the foraminal space. The appropriate level is identified radiographically, and local anesthetic solution is placed in the skin parallel to the involved disc space approximately 12 cm lateral to the midline.

A generous skin weal is made, and the local anesthetic is carried down through the lumbosacral fascia at roughly a 60° angle. A small skin incision is made utilizing a no. 11 blade. A 0.62-mm guide wire is inserted to a position just anterior to the facet, and advanced to the annulus fibrosis. During placement of the guidewire, the wire itself will strike the lateral portion of the facet during insertion. The surgeon simply backs off, slightly raising the hand and guiding the wire just beneath the facet. Once the fiber is in its ideal position it will project fluoroscopically as being at the interpedicular line on the AP projection, and at the posterior vertebral body line on the lateral projection.

At this point, the guide wire can be inserted further into the disc space for anchorage. The dilator mechanism is placed over the guide wire and directed into the foraminal area. If a large extrusion occupies the foraminal space, it may not be possible to completely seat the dilator cannula against the annulus fibrosis. Thus, the docking of the dilator may strike free disc material first. Under these circumstances, the tip of the dilator will be projected away from the ideal fluoroscopic position.

Once the foraminal space has been approached with the dilator, a cannula for the endoscope is placed over the dilator. The dilator is withdrawn and an endoscope is introduced. The working channel endoscope is then connected with irrigation of normal saline solution at 40–60 cm^3 per minute, and a passive outflow is established. This allows the foraminal space to remain slightly distended with good visualization as the procedure progresses.

At this point, endoscopic visualization and placement will allow navigation throughout the foraminal space. Also, this allows visualization of disc material, and frequently the traversing and exiting nerve roots.

The laser fiber can then be inserted via the working channel within the endoscope, and the offending disc material can be removed. The author's preference is to use a 90° side-firing Ho:YAG laser fiber so that 360° rotation is available and aiming of the fiber is precise.

Disc removal is continued until the traversing and/or exiting nerve roots are well-visualized and found to be no longer compressed by displaced nuclear or annular material. Frequently this occurs concurrent with the patient's resolution of presenting symptoms. The laser fiber and endoscope are withdrawn and the skin is closed with a suture.

Postoperatively, the patients are discharged with analgesics, a steroid pack and nonsteroidal anti-inflammatory medication. Further care is modified to the patient's need, much as one would manage a standard microdiscectomy or lumbar laminectomy.

Early Results

Foraminal laser endoscopic disc ablation (FLEDA) has resulted in success rates comparable to microdiscectomy [3, 6, 11], ranging from 75 to 80 % surgical success.

In one series, Casper et al. [3] provided preliminary findings of 20 patients having received FLEDA for treatment of sequestered herniated nucleus pulposus, foraminal disc extrusions or far-lateral disc hernia-

tions. Patients were evaluated by an independent interviewer immediately postoperatively, at three months, six months and annually thereafter. Ratings were based upon the modified Macnab criteria [12]. Postoperative follow-up at six months yielded a surgical success rate of 75 %, including ten excellent and five good Macnab ratings. Surgical failures include two patients with fair ratings and three patients requiring open laminectomy. No intraoperative complications were encountered within this group of patients.

It is important to note that a steep learning curve for this procedure does exist. This is evident from the fact that the first ten patients from this study had a surgical success rate of 60 % and that the second group of ten patients had a 90 % success rate. This is comparable to outcome breakdowns of similar studies [11, 13].

Endoscopic Laser Foraminotomy (ELF)

Laser energy is also being utilized for bone removal in selected cases of foraminal stenosis. Although at the present time true lateral and central stenosis cannot yet be addressed endoscopically, foraminal stenosis lends itself to the aforementioned endoscopic approach. The approach for ELF is exactly as described previously, with the exception that docking of the endoscope would be lateral to the facet. With that in mind, one can visualize the anterior surface of the facet or dome of the foramen. The laser fiber can then be inserted under direct visualization, and laser energy can be utilized in a side-firing mode to remove bone and to open the foraminal space. Decompression can be inferred when a 4.6-mm endoscope can be slowly advanced and comfortably fitted into the foraminal space without the patient complaining about radicular discomfort. The efficacy of this procedure continues to be evaluated.

Early Results

Preliminary findings of 21 patients having received endoscopic laser foraminotomy (ELF) for foraminal stenosis yielded a 76 % surgical success rate at an average of two years post-ELF. Surgical failures include three patients requiring open lumbar decompression and two patients receiving additional pain management. The preliminary findings suggest that ELF provides satisfactory surgical outcomes in a carefully selected patient population. Clearly, the diagnosis of this entity can be difficult, and this author's preference has been to utilize discography with CT, as well as selective nerve-root blocks to determine the precise level of foraminal stenosis. To date, we have limited our experience to patients who have only single-level disease.

Conclusion

In conclusion, laser foraminoscopic surgery for lumbar disc disease and stenosis appears to represent a viable alternative to other open surgical procedures. It is advisable that in vitro training be accomplished prior to performing in vivo application of this technology.

References

[1] Hihikata S, Yamagishi N, Nakayama T et al. (1975) Percutaneous discectomy: a new treatment method for lumbar disc herniation. J Toden Hospital 5:5

[2] Kambin P, Gellman H (1983) Percutaneous lateral discectomy of the lumbar spine: preliminary report. Clin Orthop 174:127

[3] Casper GD, Hartman VL, Mullins LL (1996) Foraminal laser endoscopic disc ablation for the treatment of lumbar disc disease: preliminary findings. In: Procdings of the 1st European advanced spinal surgery forum. Manchester 1996, Abstract no. 28

[4] Casper GD, Hartman VL, Mullins LL (1996) Results of a clinical trial of the Holmium:YAG laser in disc decompression utilizing a side-firing fiber: a two-year follow-up. Lasers Surg Med 19:90–96

[5] Choy DJS, Case R, Fielding W et al. (1987) Percutaneous laser nucleolysis of lumbar discs (Letter). N Engl J Med 12:86–91

[6] Mathews HH, Firoe M, Molligan H, Long B (1996) Foraminoscopic approach to lumbar disc sequestrum: a surgical technique. In: Proceedings of the 9th annual meeting of the North American Spine Society. Minneapolis 1996, Abstract no. 65

[7] Methews HH (1996) Transforaminal endoscopic microdiscectomy. Neurosurg Clin N Am 7:59–63

[8] Sherk HH (1993) The use of lasers in orthopaedic procedures. J Bone Joint Surg 75:768–776

[9] Lane GT, Prodoehl JA, Black SJ, Lee SJ, Rhodes A, Sherk HH (1993) An experimental comparison of CO_2, argon, Nd:YAG and Ho:YAG laser ablation of intervertebral discs. State of the art review. Spine 7:1–10

[10] Uppal C, Smith R, Hawver J (1995) In vivo comparison of two infrared laser wavelengths and two delivery systems used for lumbar disc decompression. Contemp Orthop 30:123–126

[11] Siebert WE (1996) Endoscopic foraminoscopic surgery with laser supplementation. In: Proceedings of the 1st European advanced spinal surgery forum. Manchester 1996, Abstract no. 26

[12] Tregonning GD, Transfeldt EE, McCulloch JA, Macnab I, Nachemson A (1991) Chymopapain versus conventional surgery for lumbar disc herniation: 10-year results of treatment. J Bone Joint Surg Br 73:481–486

[13] Knight M, Jakab GV (1996) Endoscopic laser foraminoplasty and intradiscal discectomy: an alternative to decompression and fusion. In: Proceedings of the 1st European advanced spinal surgery forum. Manchester 1996, Abstract no. 27

Endoscopic Foraminoplasty:
An Independent Prospective Evaluation

M. T. N. KNIGHT · A. GOSWAMI · J. T. PATKO · N. BUXTON

Introduction

Conventional spinal surgery is confined to patients with physical compression of nerves within the spinal canal and foramen or is only used for the treatment of back pain by means of tissue immobilisation by fusion.

Recent appreciation of neural mechanisms of pain, pain mediators in and around the spinal canal and pain modulation in the peripheral and central nervous system has cautioned us against excessive dependence on purely mechanical concepts of back pain [31, 32, 33, 34, 35, 36]. Endoscopic aware-state studies and anatomical studies of the foramen have pointed out the various factors that cause compressive entrapment or irritation of the nerve root [41, 42, 43, 61] and presence of other painful foraminal tissues in a degenerate spine.

The sensitivity, reliability and the predictive value of diagnostic tools such as magnetic resonance scans, computer assisted tomograms, myelograms, discography, alone or in combination, cannot reliably establish the source and cause of back pain [37, 38, 39, 40]. Current concepts in the management of degenerative disease of the spine are hampered by indirect diagnosis and by operating on the unresponsive patient.

Open surgical procedures for the management of spinal pain give unpredictable results and may cause additional morbidity. Widely varying claims of success are attributed to these techniques [4, 5]. The Cochrane Collaboration [62] statement that "there is no evidence that any form of surgery is helpful in the management of lumbar spondylosis" has fueled the quest to reduce tissue trauma and morbidity by minimal decompressive disc procedures such as fenestrectomy and midline microdiscectomy with encouraging results [6, 7, 8, 9].

Endoscopic techniques allow for direct visual inspection of discs and zones in and around the spine with the patient in the aware state, and can be combined with intradiscal decompression [10, 11, 12]. These techniques have, however, not addressed pathology in the foramen, extraforaminal zone, epidural space and posterior disc wall.

Laser as a tool for tissue ablation is being used in several surgical disciplines with encouraging results [13, 14, 15, 16, 17, 18, 19]. Not only has it been effective in "precision surgery" [18], but it has also been shown to reduce morbidity associated with conventional surgery [20]. In 1984 laser disc decompression was introduced by Choy and others [21, 22, 23] and recently it has been combined with endoscopy to effect intradiscal clearance [23, 24, 25]. Its wider application as a "surgical tool" in spinal surgery remained underestimated until it was used to ablate bone and scar tissue [26]. That it is safe to use in human spinal tissue has been confirmed in animal studies and histological studies in human tissues [63].

In this prospective study we present the results of the management of back pain by the "viviprudence" system [64] of "aware-state" and endoscopic diagnosis of the causes of pain, followed by causal-pain-source ablation in the epidural, foraminal and extraforaminal zones, combined with lateral recess and intradiscal decompression by endoscopic laser foraminoplasty. The results of this study have been independently reviewed by a neurosurgical unit from a separate health service region in the United Kingdom.

Materials and Methods

Study Construct and Data Acquisition

The study was designed prospectively and consisted of 250 consecutive patients treated between March 1994 and June 1997; the results were independently evaluated. Details of history and symptoms were recorded in preoperative and postoperative questionnaires involving a pain manikin, a visual analogue pain scale (VAP) and an Oswestry disability score. Patients were evaluated at six and 12 weeks and at six months following surgery and reviewed at yearly intervals unless clinical symptoms required closer supervision. The data were entered by bar coding and computerised for subsequent comparison during follow-up. Full clinical, neurological and postural analysis was performed together with plain AP and neutral weight-bearing x-rays and a dynamic series of digitised "instability" radiographs in flexion and extension during both sitting and standing.

Patient Selection

Muscle balance physiotherapy for a period of three months was prescribed to patients. If the pain intensity remained high, and the response to physiotherapy remained inadequate, patients were re-evaluated with an MR scan. Gadolinium enhancement was added where prior spinal surgery had been involved or perineural scarring was suspected.

Inclusion and Exclusion Criteria

The clinical indication was the persistence of back pain, buttock pain and leg pain or a combination of these at a disabling level for over three months, failure to respond to advanced muscle-balancing physiotherapy or other conservative methods (see also Table 1).

Table 1. Inclusion and exclusion criteria for endoscopic laser foraminoplasty

Inclusion criteria:
  Compressive radiculopathy with sensorimotor impairment
- Disc extrusion or sequestration with predominantly back pain or leg pain
- Degeneration and settlement and predominantly back pain, buttock pain or leg pain
- Non-compressive irritative radiculopathy
- Non-radicular pain persisting despite facet joint injection
- Lateral recess stenosis with dynamic compressive radiculopathy
- Lateral recess stenosis with dynamic non-compressive radiculopathy
- The above with prior conventional surgery at the index level
- The above with perineural scarring at the index level
- Spondylolytic spondylolisthesis
- Failed back syndrome

Exclusion criteria:
- Cauda equina syndrome
- Painless motor deficit
- Tumours

Definitions

If the MR scan clearly identified loss of foraminal space and loss of perineural fat and a foraminal dimension of less than 5 mm, then patients were deemed to have lateral recess stenosis.

Surgical Protocol

Patients were consented for a staged procedure consisting of:

- Spinal probing and discography at suspected levels approached on the side of maximal symptoms
- Endoscopic laser foraminoplasty consisting of exploration of extraforaminal, foraminal and epidural zones with flexible endoscopic intradiscal discectomy, neurolysis, undercutting of facets and osteophytectomy as required
- However, the final decision for the second stage (endoscopic laser foraminoplasty) was made only after spinal probing and discography had reproduced pain of type, intensity and distribution corresponding to that which the patient normally experienced
- Where symptom reproduction was imperfect, a differential discogram was performed with the instillation of 2 ml methylprednisolone acelate (Depomedrone, Upjohn) at the presumend level. If post-intervention observation revealed a reduction of symptoms for five to ten days, then the symptoms affected could be expected to be modified by endoscopic laser foraminoplasty at the said level

Spinal probing differs from discography in that it relies upon specific probing of the anterior margin of the facet joint, perineural structures and the disc wall at several points. The essential and distinctive steps in "viviprudence" are therefore spinal probing and differential discography [64]. Discography defines the distribution of degeneration within the disc and the acceptance volume and the presence of annular leaks. If discography on a contained disc produces radicular pain then this further endorses that that disc is the index level for the pain. Similarly, if a leak reproduces the patient's pain then this identifies the targeted disc as a contributor to the evoked pain.

Operative Technique

Neurolept (aware-state) analgesia was performed with 0.03 mg/kg midazalam (Hypnovel Roche) bolus at the onset of the operation, 2–5 µg/kg fentanyl and 30–70 µg/kg droperidol. Patient feedback is essential in these cases, where the presence of perineural scarring is often unexpectedly dense and masks the neural structures. A bolus dose of 1.5 g cefuroxime was given at the onset of the operation. The skin and subcutis was infiltrated with the local anaesthetic anhydrous lignocaine hydrochloride (Xylocaine, Astra) 0.25 % (0.75–1.5 mg/kg) with 1:200 000 adrenaline.

Lasing Technique

The probe was replaced with a guide wire, and under biplanar x-ray control, a 5.0 mm dilator tube was railroaded to the exit-root foramen. During the entire procedure an image intensifier was used at intervals to ensure the correct position of the endoscope and the laser probe. The trocar was removed and a Richard Wolf endoscope with an eccentrically placed 2.5-mm working channel and two irrigation channels was inserted. A side-firing 2.1-mm diameter laser probe with internal irrigation was inserted through the endoscope. The extraforaminal zone and margin of the foramen were cleared. The ascending and descending facet-joint surfaces were excavated and undercut to allow admission of the endoscope beyond the isthmus of the foramen into the epidural space. Vertebral body and facet-joint osteophytes, ligamentum flavum and superior foraminal ligament, perineural and epidural scarring were ablated and the facet joint undercut until the annulus and epidural space were displayed.

The exiting and transiting nerve roots were mobilised and decompressed medially and laterally until the functional axilla of the root at the apex of the safe working zone was displayed. The nerve was cleared of perineural fibrosis. The bone margin of the superior notch and the superior foraminal ligament were addressed. Osteophytes along the ascending facet joint and in the superior notch, dorsum of the vertebral margin and the vertebral shoulder (shoulder osteophytes) were ablated under endoscopic vision. In the presence of a disc protrusion in the epidural or foraminal zone, disc degeneration, annular collection or leaks, the disc was entered and cleared by laser ablation and manual punches.

Follow-up

Patients were discharged the day following surgery. The muscle-balance physiotherapy regime was recommenced on the first day following surgery and amplified with neural mobilisation drills. Patients were encouraged to carry out these self-help drills twice a day until review.

A daily pain diary was maintained by patients to identify the intensity and location of residual pain. Patients were followed up at 6 and 12 weeks, 6 months, and annually thereafter, unless clinical indications required closer supervision. Patients no longer requiring support were contacted by postal questionnaire combined and reinforced by telephone appraisal and confirmation.

Statistical Analysis

The analysis of the data was done with the SPSS (Statistical Package for Social Sciences, SPSS Inc.). Parametric analysis of the data was effected because the distribution of the preoperative scores for back, buttock and leg pain and preoperative Oswestry scores demonstrated a normal distribution pattern. A two-tailed paired t-test was carried out individually for back, buttock and leg pain for functional outcomes.

Independent Evaluation

A total of 58 (24 %) patients were randomly selected to assess the accuracy with which the clinical and questionnaire results had been recorded. The patients were interviewed by telephone. The questionnaires were then checked against the computerised data for each patient to assess the accuracy of the prior established data record. Of those selected, 48 (20 %) patients could be directly contacted by telephone; those who could not be contacted by telephone had their computer record checked against the original follow-up questionnaire. Of all the data recorded, the only inaccuracy detected was the transcription of a VAP score from the questionnaire to computer (marked 4, i.e., moderate in the questionnaire but marked 6 in the computer, i.e., distressing but bearable for some time). This was rectified and the relevant results recalculated.

Analysis

Oswestry Disability Scores and Oswestry Disability Index (ODI)

Oswestry disability scores were substratified for back, buttock and leg pain. The outcome was measured by observing the percentage change in the Oswestry disability score [46]. An index of 100 % was deemed excellent, result greater than 20 % deemed improved whilst less than 20 % was deemed poor, and negative values were deemed a worse result. The change in the Oswestry disability score (ΔDI) was calculated as follows:

$$\Delta DI = \frac{\text{preoperative DI} - \text{postoperative DI}}{\text{preoperative DI}} \times 100$$

Percentage Change in Visual Analogue Pain Scores (VAP Index)

Preoperative and follow-up visual analogue pain levels were measured by a visual analogue pain scale with the following guidelines to patients: pain level 10: excruciating pain, unbearable for any time, 9: horrible pain bearable for only a short time, 6: distressing pain bearable for some time, 3: mild pain, 0: no pain. An index of 100 % was deemed an excellent result, more than 50 % deemed good, greater than 20 % deemed improved whilst below 20 % was deemed poor, and negative values were deemed a worse result.

Results

The demographics of the patients under study are given in Table 2. All patients had back, buttock or leg pain with or without sciatica syndrome. Of the patients, 137 had predominantly left-sided leg pain and 133 right-sided leg pain. All underwent a hospital stay of less than 24 hours.

Table 2. Patient demographics

- Number of patients 250 (consecutive)
- Cohort integrity at follow-up: 97%; Patients lost to follow-up: 6; Died: 2
- Period of study: March 1994 – June 1999
- Males: 121; Females 129
- Age: 21–86 years; Mean: 48 years; SD: 13.21
- Period of follow-up: 24–48 months; Mean: 30 months, SD: 5.87
- Duration of symptoms: Mean 6.1 years (range 5–21 years, SD: 2.4)
- Prior open surgery (N, 75): one prior op.: 62; two prior op.: 7, three prior op.: 6
- Patients with failed laser disc decompression surgery: 3
- Levels Operated: L2-4 = 16; L4–5 = 110; L5–S1 = 155 (Total: 281)
- Work accidents: 36
- Litigation and compensation cases: 18
- Patients on MST: 19
- Patients with prior coping courses: 90
- Patients with multiple opinions: 142

The overall results of this study are summarised in Table 3.

Of the patients, 142 had obtained opinions from one or more spinal or orthopaedic surgeons or neurosurgeons prior to referral to the unit and had been deemed unsuitable for surgery. These patients included 75 patients with prior failed open conventional lumbar spinal surgery.

Of the patients, 90 had been through residential coping courses which included pain-clinic visits, facet-joint injections, epidural injections, extensive physiotherapy with or without the use of MST, acupuncture treatment, and transcutaneous electrical nerve stimulation. A pre-emptive trauma history was obtained from 67 patients [work: 36, home: 14, games: 2; RTA (road traffic accidents): 15] Of these incidents, 36 were work-related while 15 arose from road traffic accidents.

If all the patients in this study were taken as a group, the Oswestry disability index on a global scale demonstrated that 61% had excellent or good results for their back pain (17% excellent results and 44% good results), 65% for their buttock pain, and 65% for their leg pain. However, clinically discernible improvement was observed in 76% patients (ODI ≥ 20). For patients who had no previous operations, the corresponding figures for the excellent or good category were 67%, 72% and 71%, while clinical improvement in patients (ODI ≥ 20) occurred in 82%, 80% and 81% for back, buttock and leg pain, respectively. At the two-year follow-up review, 7% of the patients evidenced continuing degeneration and were worse on their Oswestry disability index (N, 17) and pain scores (N, 15).

Visual analogy pain scores demonstrated that 16% were pain-free, 40% had a visual analogue pain index

of or above 50% while 6% were worse at the two-year review.

Of the patients 79% achieved more than 50% of their preoperative rehabilitation objectives, selected prior to surgery, within the patient target achievement score. Seventy-five percent of the patients were satisfied with their management and the results obtained.

■ **Prior Open Operations.** There were 75 patients who had between one and three conventional open operations on the spine. Perineural fibrosis with or without epidural fibrosis was identified in all these patients. This was confirmed both with MR scanning in those cases without instrumented fusion and by the operative endoscopic findings. Endoscopic laser foraminoplasty resulted in an excellent or good Oswestry disability index of 50% for back pain, 46% for buttock pain and 51% for leg pain. The results were the same regardless of whether the patients had one or more prior open operations.

■ **Coronary and Vascular Disease.** Eight patients had severe coronary and peripheral or cerebral vascular disease. Six out of these eight patients were considered inoperable by means of open surgery because of significant anaesthetic risk. Of these patients 62% had an excellent or good outcome.

■ **Preoperative Foot Drop.** There were ten patients who had foot drop, grade 1–2, prior to surgery. All these patients had had the foot drop for more than 2.5 years. All except one demonstrated improvement in the dorsiflexion power at the ankle at the end of two years (grade 4 or weak 5) although none reached normal power.

■ **Revision Surgery.** Five percent of patients (N, 13) required revision surgery. Four patients underwent a revision endoscopic laser foraminoplasty at the index level, while another four required endoscopic

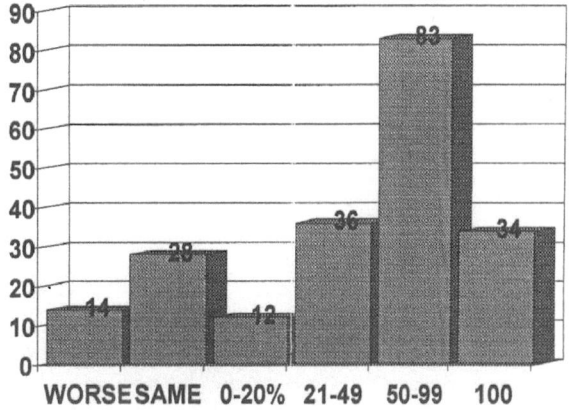

Fig. 1. Percentage alteration in pain (VAP score)

Table 3. Overall results of this study

Group (Total N, 250)	N (*Data available on)	ΔDI ≥ 50	ΔDI 20-49	ΔDI < 20	Comments
Overall group	242*				
Back pain	232	61%	13%	26%	42E, 98G, 35S. 19P, 22U, 15W
Buttock pain	209	66%	11%	23%	78E, 58G, 22S, 19P, 18U, 13W
Leg pain	231	65%	10%	25%	72E, 79G, 24S, 19P, 20U, 17W
					5 patients showed reversal of leg/back/buttock change (2%)
Patients with no previous operations	167*				
Back pain	160	67%	15%	18%	36E, 68G, 24S, 11P, 15U, 6W
Buttock pain	148	72%	8%	20%	64E, 43G, 10S, 8P, 17U, 6W
Leg pain	165	71%	10%	19%	59E, 56G, 16S, 11P, 15U, 8W
Patients with prior open operations	75*				Statistics of period between ops: Avg: 53 months; SD: 53.86; Median: 66 months; Min: 6 months; Maximum: 239 months
Back pain	73	50%	14%	36%	7E, 29G, 11S, 11P, 6U, 9W
Buttock pain	64	46%	19%	35%	15E, 14G, 12S, 12P, 3U, 8W
Leg pain	69	51%	12%	37%	12E, 23G, 8S, 9P, 7U, 10W
Patients with one prior operation	62*				
Back pain	61	49%	15%	36%	7E, 22G, 9S, 9P, 6U, 7W
Buttock pain	53	46%	20%	34%	13E, 19G, 6S, 7P, 6U, 8W
Leg pain	57	51%	10%	39%	10E, 19G, 6S, 7P, 6U, 8W
Previous coping courses	84*/90				
Back pain	80	56%	10%	34%	15/84 (18%) E, 30G, 9S, 8P, 10U, 8W
Buttock pain	70	60%	7%	33%	29/70 (41%) E, 13G, 5S, 10P, 8U, 5W
Leg pain	80	60%	10%	30%	26/80 (33%) E, 22G, 8S, 7P, 10U, 7W
Multiple opinions	138*/142				
Back pain	131	57%	17%	26%	19E, 56G, 22S, 9P, 14U, 11W
Buttock pain	119	65%	11%	24%	45E, 32G, 14S, 9P, 11U, 8W
Leg pain	132	64%	11%	25%	38E, 47G, 15S, 8P, 14U, 10W
Rheumatoid (3) and seronegative spondyarthritis (4)	6*/7				
Back pain		2	1	3	1E, 1G, 1S, 1P, 1U, 1W
Buttock pain		2	2	2	1E, 1G, 2S, iU, 1W
Leg pain		3	1	2	2E, 1G, 1S, 1U, 1W
					One patient had marked improvement with leg (100%) pain but poor results with back (12%) and satisfactory results with leg (21%) pain
Spondylolytic spondylolisthesis	23 (Cr1: 16, Cr2: 7)				
Back pain		17	1	5	3E, 14G, 1S, 3P, 2W
Buttock pain		18	1	4	6E, 12G, 1S, 3P, 1W
Leg pain		17	2	3	8E, 9G, 2S, 2P, 1W (22/23 had leg pain)
Coronary and vascular disease: considered inoperable for anaesthetic risk.	8	62%	20%	18%	3E, 2G, 2SA, 1US
Preoperative foot drop	10				9 Gr 4-5; 1 Unchanged (6/6 with painful foot drop improved)
MST usage	19				2 still on MST
Back pain	19	53%	11%	36%	4E, 6G, 2S, 3P, 3U, 1W
Buttock pain	17	47%	11%	41%	7E, 1G, 2S, 5P, 1U, 1W
Leg pain	18	56%	-	44%	6E, 4G, 2P, 5U, 1W
Multiple sclerosis	4	-	75%	25%	80% on satisfaction scoring (> 70% relief in pain)
Litigations and compensations	18	51%	13%	36%	Consists of patients who have had previous operations, MST users and patients with multiple opinions

N = no of patients; DI = Oswestry disability index
E = excellent (100), G = good (50-99), S = satisfactory (20-49), P = poor (1-19), U = unchanged (0), W = worse (< 0)

laser foraminoplasty at adjacent level with success. Five underwent exploration and fusion at other centres.

■ **Complications.** One patient suffered neurological deficit following surgery. Despite the use of light aware-state analgesia and sedation, we failed to establish good communication with this woman who was not conversant with the English language. She suffered severe dysaesthesia postoperatively with ipsilateral (grade 2) foot drop. Nerve-conduction studies suggested diminished nerve-conduction velocity at the foramen. However, two years later her power had recovered considerably (grade 4), but she still experiences some dysaesthesia in the L5 dermatome.

One patient had aseptic discitis. He had symptoms of severe painful discitis, but was afebrile and had normal blood values. Because of persistent back pain and spasm, he was treated empirically with antibiotics. He recovered progressively over a three-month period. A biopsy was not acceptable to the patient.

Discussion

The function of the foramen is a delicate balance between the size of the foraminal boundaries and the status of their contents. This balance is easily compromised by pathological changes in the tissues, irritation or sensitisation of tethered tissues, aided by abnormal motion at the index segment. Aware-state patient feedback combined with posterolateral endoscopy has revealed this site to be a potent cause of back pain, buttock pain and sciatica.

MRI Scans and Their Shortcomings

Endoscopy revealed that static magnetic resonance (MR) imaging fails to demonstrate the tethering and impaction of the superior facet joint, the tethering to infolded ligamentum flavum, facet joint capsule and the superior foraminal ligament on the nerve. Endoscopy demonstrated that dorsal and shoulder osteophytes not only encroach upon the foramen but tether to the nerves, and that dorsal osteophytes may impinge upon the posterior longitudinal ligament. MR imaging fails to demonstrate the degree of inflammation and irritation within these structures, the disc pad and in the disc. The presence of disc protrusions may be directly misleading when compared to the size and site of the true irritative pathology as could subsequently be located by aware-state endoscopy. The MR scans fail to demonstrate that nerves may become directly adherent to the disc wall and may become displaced from their normal path and be distorted. Endoscopy also

revealed that the MR scan underestimates the degree of local scarring and the vascular hyperaemia and thrombosis occurring within.

Visual Analogue Pain Index

On the visual analogue pain scale, 56 % patients had more than a 50 % improvement, while 6 % of patients had deterioration of pain symptoms following surgery.

Revision Surgery

For 97 % of patients, treatment without the need for open surgery was possible. This technique may be envisaged as a means of filtering the number of patients needing open surgery as well as a means of effectively offering a treatment algorithm where treatment is currently denied.

Multiple Sclerosis

Multiple sclerosis patients are susceptible to complications following general anaesthesia. These include altered sensations in the legs. Many patients are therefore managed non-operatively. The patients in this study had marked improvement in pain levels following endoscopic laser foraminoplasty and some functional improvement, despite the underlying irreversible status of their pathology. The marked improvement in pain levels benefited the quality of life of these patients and the authors feel that aware-state viviprudence and minimally invasive surgery can benefit these patients immensely.

Dynamic and Adynamic Lateral Recess Stenosis

The management of lateral stenosis conventionally leads to conservative management, decompression or fusion. The extent of bone excision needed to bring about adequate decompression is not defined [49, 50, 51, 52, 53]. The excision of bone at the time of decompression may cause an increase in motion of the spinal segment, but, depending upon extent, may or may not amount to "instability" [54]. Weight-bearing x-rays performed standing and sitting both in flexion and extension serve to demonstrate dynamic and adynamic degenerative spondylolisthesis and retrolisthesis. Endoscopic visualisation of the foramen has enabled us to identify impaction of soft tissues and indenting facet-joint osteophytes, dorsal or shoulder osteophytes or overriding hyperflexing or hyperextending hypertrophic facet joints upon the nerves.

Impact of Multiple Operations

Seventy-five of the patients in this study had had conventional surgical interventions without any improvement in their preoperative condition. Careful application of the diagnostic tools of spinal probing and differential discography and deliberate attempts to identify the exact source of pain endoscopically have allowed us to assist these patients. Identification and resection of scar tissue, removal of tethering of the nerve to the shoulder, superior-notch and dorsal osteophytes, mobilisation of the nerve from adherent disc wall, posterior longitudinal ligament and superior foraminal ligament, resection of the ascending facet joint and rectification of the distorted pathway of the nerve contributed variously to the amelioration of symptoms. The inflamed tissues produced unexpected atypical distributions of pain. Endoscopic laser foraminoplasty achieved discrete and precise ablation and consequential resolution of the pain.

Postoperative Flares

Postoperative flares occurred in 28 % of patients and were significant in 12 %. The flare represented a recurrence of symptoms usually between 5–21 days following surgery. The onset of such symptoms coincides with the inflammatory process and may represent "revascularisation" and remodelling of the laser-ablated tissues along with accumulation of breakdown products in the small operative space caused by the intervention. Timely caudal epidural steroid infiltration with manipulation under anaesthesia has helped to relieve these symptoms, maintain neural mobility and restore patients to their appropriate physiotherapy regime with satisfactory outcome.

Neurological Recovery

Visualisation of the foramen under endoscopic vision demonstrated combinations of severe foraminal and epidural scarring, osteophytic encroachment and/or extraforaminal bone hypertrophic paravertebral bone graft compressing the exiting nerve at the index level. Conventional midline exploration would have had limited access to these pathological entities; this has led to the prevalent belief that re-exploration for the relief of long-standing compressive neuropathy is unrewarding.

Scarring

Scarring was far more prevalent and dense than preoperative MR scanning would suggest. Mature scarring arising from operations carried out over three years prior was certainly significantly underestimated. Postoperative scarring found in patients with significant early postoperative symptoms with prior operations demonstrated haemosiderin pigmentation, suggesting postoperative occult bleeding as an aetiology of postoperative morbidity.

Scarring was almost always associated with vascular bands. The exiting or traversing nerve was often hyperaemic and particularly tender at discrete points along its course. The discrete inflamed length would be tethered to inflamed perineural scarring the adjacent impacting ascending facet joint, superior foraminal osteophytes, the superior foraminal ligament, the foraminal ligament, the facet joint capsule and be adherent to the disc wall or shoulder or dorsal osteophytes. Conversely, scarring could be found at areas of quiescent nerve but under these circumstances, inflammation was absent.

In addition, swelling and engorgement of veins and thrombosis therein was noted endoscopically in the perineural region. These features have been suggested to cause lateral recess stenotic symptoms by compromising the space in the spinal exit foramen or compromising neural drainage [56, 57, 58].

It is likely that chemical irritants may cause oedema of the nerve and irritation of adjacent tissues and scar [59]. Dynamic stenosis arising either from lateral recess encroachment or from disc settlement combined with abnormal movements such as olisthesis or facet joint overriding could lead to further irritation and compression of the nerve, causing a vicious cycle of compression, irritation, oedema and further compression. Endoscopic visualisation of the oedematous inflamed sheath has been done in this study and in particular in those patients with dynamic anterior olisthesis or retrolisthesis and settlement, flexion or extension overstrain confirmed by dynamic digitised radiographs.

Sequestration

Ten out of 14 patients who had sequestration of disc material had excellent to good results with foraminoplasty. Four patients had a poor outcome, with persistent back pain and were operated elsewhere for residual sequestrectomy and fusion. ELF can be used for sequestrectomy and results reflect experience with the technique.

Untreatable Patients

Of these patients, 42 were considered untreatable by surgeons elsewhere because they had either been operated before with conventional surgery or no "treatable" pathology was identifiable on the MR scan. An additional group of patients had been offered surgery on a deferred basis, pending the outcome of pain-management therapy. This indicates that here is a well-found reticence to offer conventional surgery, except to the most classical of presenting pathology. This results in a large number of patients being consigned to coping courses and psychological counselling. The outcome of such conservative management in these patients had not been encouraging.

Ninety patients had participated in coping courses or pain-management programmes for extended periods of time until frustration at the enduring symptoms and degraded lifestyle led them to cease attendance. Two-thirds of these patients benefited from the foraminoplasty, with more than 60 % being in the "excellent" category. Viviprudence and keyhole day-case surgery therefore offers a promising opportunity to ameliorate their symptoms, with sustained results and, additionally, benefit to the exchequer.

Morphine Sulphate (MST) Users

Nineteen patients in this series were on constant MST therapy. Regular MST utilisation is a caveat to surgical intervention for many spinal surgeons, yet, with endoscopic laser foraminoplasty, this group of patients fared well, with only two requiring medication two years later. These findings call into question the appropriateness of the prescription of long-term high doses of MST, and raises the possibility that these patients need further due diligence with vivipridence to find the source of their pain and an appropriate ablative treatment thereof.

Learning-Curve Effect

It should be stressed that this report represents our preliminary surgical experience with this technique, a technique which has been evolving during the treatment of this cohort. The first 98 patients were treated with a fiber-optic endoscope and the remainder with a solid round rod-lens endoscope developed with Richard Wolf Endoscopes and company. Our report encompasses all the patients treated with this technique, without preferential exclusion of the early group. With experience, the completeness of undercutting and pain-source ablation increased and laser energy usage diminished from 120 kJ to the current average usage of 60 kJ per intervention.

Shortcomings of Endoscopic Laser Foraminoplasty

Endoscopic laser foraminoplasty is ideally applied to the treatment of unilateral unisegmental pathology. However, in many cases of bilateral pain, both symptomatic sides improve with endoscopic foraminoplasty performed unilaterally, and we presume that this is due to the removal of breakdown products from the index level, thus amelioration of irritation on the contralateral side. Endoscopic laser foraminoplasty can only address one level at a time, and this may be a disadvantage. Adjacent-level pathology may be supplemented with a minimal laser disc decompression with benefit. This was not effected in this reported series. However, it is interesting that in so many cases of multiple-level pathology, only 3 % required adjacent-level intervention. This suggests that current open bilateral multilevel intervention may be overcomprehensive.

Endoscopic laser foraminoplasty is a technically demanding procedure, which usually requires 90–120 min to effect once the learning curve has been surmounted.

Conclusion

Endoscopic laser foraminoplasty offers a minimalist procedure, which may have increasingly wider application in the future as an alternative to conventional discectomy, decompression and "soft" and "solid" fusion, and, in addition, may be used increasingly to treat patients currently denied surgery and destined to pain-clinic and coping courses until frustration causes these patients to cease further participation.

The prinipal cause for the "failure" of conventional spinal surgery is attributed to "operating on the wrong level" [60]. Viviprudence and endoscopy indicates that the cause of failure is in reality not only failure to identify the level but failure to define the pain site therein.

References

[1] Nettelbladt E (1985) Antalet reumatikerinvalder I Sverige under en 30-arsperiod. OPMEAR 30:54–56
[2] Report of the Commission on the Evaluation of Pain (1987) Soc Security Bull 50(1):13–44
[3] Fairbank JCT (1986) The incidence of back pain in Britain. In: Hukins DWL, Mulholland RC (eds) Back pain. Methods for clinical investigation and assessment. Manchester Universtiy Press, Manchester
[4] Nachemson A (1985) Recent advances in the treatment of low back pain. Int Orth 9:1–10
[5] Mooney V (1988) The failed back: an orthopaedic view. Int Disabil Stud 10:32–36
[6] Caspar W, Campbell B, Barbier D, Kretschmmer R, Gotfried Y (1991) The Caspar microsurgical discectomy and comparison with a conventional standard lumbar disc procedure. Neurosurgery 28:78–87
[7] Mayer HM (1994) Spine update. Percutaneous lumbar disc surgery. Spine 19:2719–2723
[8] Onik G, Mooney V, Maroon JC, Wiltse L, Helms C, Schweigel J, Watkins R, Kahanovitz N, Day A, Morris J et al. (1990) Automated percutaneous discectomy: a prospective multi-institutional study. Neurosurgery 26:228–232
[9] Hihikata S (1989) Percutaneous nucleotomy: a new concept technique and 12 years' experience. Clin Orthop 238:9–23
[10] Kambin P (1996) Diagnostic and therapeutic spinal arthroscopy. Neurosurg Clin N Am 7:65–76
[11] Kambin P (1993) Arthroscopic microdiscectomy of the lumbar spine. Clin Sports Med 12(1):143–150
[12] Kambin P, Casey K, O'Brien E, Zhou L (1996) Transforaminal arthroscopic foraminal decompression of lateral recess stenosis. J Neurosurg 84(3):462–467

[13] Gerber BE, Siebert WE, Morscher E (1996) Chirurgische Laseranwendung am Berwegungsapparat (Surgical use of laser on the locomotor apparatus). Orthopäde 25:1–2 (editorial)

[14] Gerber BE, al Khodairy AT, Morscher E, Hefti E (1996) Offene Laserchirurgie am Berwegungsapparat (Open laser surgery on the locomotor apparatus). Orthopäde 25:56–63

[15] Sherk HH (1993) The use of lasers in orthopaedic procedures. J Bone Joint Surg 75-A:768–776

[16] Mathews HH (1996) Transforaminal endoscopic microdiscectomy. Neurosurg Clin N Am 7:59–63

[17] Quigley MR, Maroon JC (1994) Laser discectomy: a review. Spine 19:53–56

[18] Quigley MR (1996) Percutaneous laser discectomy. Neurosurg Clin N Am 7:37–42

[19] Scholz M, Deli M, Wildforster U, Wentz K, Becknagel A, Preuschaft H, Harders A (1996) MRI-guided endoscopy in the brain: feasibility study. Minim Invasive Neurosurg 39:33–37

[20] Simpson JM (1996) Indications for laser surgery in the treatment of degenerative disc disease of the lumbar spine. J South Orthop Assoc 5:174–180

[21] Choy DS, Michelsen J, Getrajdman G, Diwan S (1992) Percutaneous laser disc decompression: an update-spring 1992. J Clin Laser Med Surg 10:177–184

[22] Casper GD, Hartman VL, Mullins LL (1996) Results of a clinical trial of the holmium:YAG laser in disc decompression utilizing a side-firing fiber: a two-year follow-up. Lasers Surg Med 19:90–96

[23] Casper GD, Mullins LL, Hartman VL (1996) Laser assisted disc decompression: an alternative treatment modality in Medicare population. J Oklahoma State Med Assoc 89(1):11–15

[24] Knight MTN (1996) Laser assisted percutaneous and endoscopic lumbar discectomy. In: Ramani PS (ed) Textbook of spinal surgery. Dept. of Neuro and Spinal Surg Mumbai, India, pp 449–454

[25] Knight MTN, Pantoja S (1996) KTP/532 Percutaneous laser disc decompression for lumbar disc prolapse. Clin Neurosci 49:330–336

[26] Knight MTN, Vajda A, Jakab GV, Awan S (1998) Endoscopic laser foraminoplasty on the lumbar spine-early experience. Minimally Invasive Neurosurg 41(1):5–9

[27] Roberts S, Eisenstein SM, Menage J, Evans EH, Ashton IK (1995) Mechanoreceptors in the intervertebral discs. Morphology, distribution and neuropeptides. Spine 20(24):2645–2651

[28] Anand P, Gibson SJ, Yiangou Y, Christophides ND, Polak JM, Bloom SR et al (1984) PHI-like immunoreactive colocates with the VIP-containing system in human lumbosacral spinal cord. Neurosci Lett 46:191–196

[29] Henry JL (1976) Effects of substance P on functionally identified units in cat spinal cord. Brain Res 114:439–451

[30] Kushlick SD, Ulstrom CL, Michael CJ (1991) The tissue origin of low back pain: a report of pain response to tissue stimulation during operations on lumbar spine using local anaesthesia. Orth Clin North Am 22(2):181–187

[31] Almay BGL, Johansson F, Von Knorring L, Le Greves P, Terenius L (1988) Substance P in CSF of patients with chronic pain syndromes. Pain 33:3–9

[32] Andersson SA, Carlsson CA, Eriksson M (1984) Akupunktur: fran to till vetenskap. Malmo, Liber, Forlog

[33] Terenius L (1981) Endorphins and pain. Frontiers Hormone Res 8:162–167

[34] Von Knorring, Almay BGL, Johansson F et al (1978) Pain perceptions and endorphin levels in cerebrospinal fluid. Pain 5:359–365

[35] Parke WW, Watnabe R (1985) The intrinsic vasculature of the lumbosacral nerve roots. Spine 10:508–515

[36] Rydevik B, Brown MD, Lundborg G (1984) Pathoanatomy and pathophysiology of nerve root compression. Spine 9:7–15

[37] Quebec Task Force on Spinal Disorders (1987) Scientific approach to the assessment and management of activity-related spinal disorders: a monograph for clinicians. Spine 12(suppl):S1–S59

[38] Angtuaco EJC, Holder JC, Boop WC, Biner EF (1984) Computed tomographic discography in the evaluation of extreme lateral disc herniation. Neurosurgery 14:350–351

[39] Weber H (1978) Lumbar disc herniation: a prospective study of prognostic factors including a controlled trial. Part I. J Oslo City Hosp 28:33–40

[40] Weber H (1978) Lumbar disc herniation: a prospective study of prognostic factors including a controlled trial. Part II. J Oslo City Hosp 28:89–95

[41] Varga PP (1995) Lumbalis spinalis stenosis. Springer, Berlin Heidelberg New York

[42] Regan JJ, McAfee PC, Mack MJ (1995) Atlas of endoscopic spine surgery. Quality Medical, St. Louis

[43] Kambin P, Casey K, O'Brien E, Zhou L (1996) Transforaminal arthroscopic decompression of lateral recess stenosis. J Neurosurg 84:462–467

[44] Shapiro R (1986) Lumbar discography: an outdated procedure (letter). J Neurosurg 64:686

[45] Evans JG (1964) Neurogenic intermittent claudication. Br Med J 2:985–987

[46] Little DG, MacDonald D (1994) The use of percentage change of Oswestry disability index score as an outcome measure in lumbar spinal surgery: Spine 19:2139–2143

[47] Deyo RA, Battie M, Beurskens AJ, Bombardier S, Croft P, Koes B, Malmivaara A, Roland M, Von Korff M, Waddell A (1998) Outcome measures for low back pain research: a proposal for standardised use: Spine 23(18):2003–2013

[48] Kirkaldy-Willis WH (1984) The relationship of the structural pathology to the nerve root. Spine 9:49–52

[49] Goel VK, Goyal S, Clark C, Nishiyama K, Nye T (1985) Kinematics of the whole lumbar spine: effects of discectomy. Spine 10:543–554

[50] Tibrewal SB, Pearcy MK, Portek I, Spivey J (1984) A prospective study of lumbar spinal movements before and after discectomy. In: Proceedings of the international society for the study of lumbar spine, Montreal, 3–4 June 1984

[51] Lehmann TR, Wilson MA, Corwninshield RD (1981) Load response characteristics of lumbar spine following surgical destabilisation. In: 28th Annual ORS:240, New Orleans, 19–21 Jan 1981

[52] Lee CK (1983) Lumbar spinal instability: (olisthesis) after extensive spinal decompression. Spine 8:429–433

[53] Johnsson K, Willner S (1986) Post operative instability after decompression of lumbar spinal stenosis. Spine 11:107–110

[54] Posner I, While AA III, Edwards WT, Hayes WC (1982) A biomechanical analysis of the clinical stability of the lumbar and the lumbosacral spine. Spine 7:374–389

[55] Goswami AKD (1994) Laminotomy versus laminectomy: is there a difference in stability? – A biomechanical study on cadaveric spines. MCh(Orth), thesis, University of Liverpool

[56] Parke WW, Watnabe R (1985) The intrinsic vasculature of the lumbosacral spine nerve roots. Spine 10:508–515

[57] Parke WW, Gammell K, Rothman RH (1981) Arterial vascularisation of the lumbosacral spinal nerve roots. J Bone Joint Surg 63A:53–62

[58] Evans G (1964) Neurogenic intermittent claudication. Br Med J 2:985–987

[59] Hoyland JA, Freemont JA, Jayson MIV (1989) Intervertebral foramen venous obstruction – a cause of perineural fibrosis. Spine 14:558

[60] McCulloch J (1987) Complications of lumbar microdiscectomy. Acta Orth Belg 53(2):272–275

[61] Rauschning W (1999) Surgical and imaging anatomy of the lumbar spine. In: Proceedings of the 9th international conference of lumbar fusion and stabilisation, Cheshire, 31 May – 4 June 1999

[62] Gibson JNA, Grant IC, Waddell G (1999) The Cochrane Review of surgery for lumbar disc prolapse and degenerative lumbar spondylosis. Spine 24(17):1820–1832

[63] Hafez M, Zhou S, Coombs RRH, McCarthy ID (2000) Assessment of temperature changes in surrounding structures during endoscopic laser foraminoplasty. In: Proceedings of Orthopaedic Research Society annual meeting, paper no 133, Orlando, 12–15 March 2000

[64] Knight MTN, Goswami AKD, Patko J (1999) Endoscopic laser foraminoplasty and aware state surgery: a treatment concept and outcome analysis. Arthoscopie 12:62–73

Endoscopic Percutaneous Lumbar Disc Decompression with the Ho:YAG Laser (Ho:YAG EPLDD)

Y. Nishijima · H. Ishizika

Introduction

Compared to open nucleotomy, percutaneous lumbar disc decompression (PLDD) has several advantages for treating lumbar herniated nucleus pulposus (HNP). PLDD can be performed under local anesthesia and as an outpatient procedure. This allows earlier return to normal daily activity. From the surgical point of view, it requires no muscular and ligamentous tissue dissection and does not lead to intraoperative nerve injuries or perineural fibrosis. Since first introduced by Hijikata [2] percutaneous discectomy has undergone several modifications. Onik [7] developed automated nucleotomy, and Schreiber [9] performed the procedure under a discoscope, in an attempt to improve the technique. However, its disadvantages have also been reported and include limited indication, relatively low response rate (70 % at the most), long x-ray exposure time, the difficulty in lumbosacral puncturing, and contamination. Because of these disadvantages, PLDD is not yet fully accepted as a routine clinical procedure.

We have performed endoscopic PLDD with the Ho:YAG laser (Ho:YAG EPLDD) since June 1994. Compared to mechanical procedures, laser ablation decompresses the intradiscal pressure less invasively, and the delivery system's small diameter enable us to reach the L5-S level; endoscopic images guarantee safe practice and decreased x-ray exposure time. In this report we discuss Ho:YAG EPLDD and the findings after a one-year follow-up, to emphasize the efficacy of Ho:YAG EPLDD in properly selected patients with HNP.

Materials and Methods

Technique

The patient was placed in a lateral pisition with the affected side up. The point of entry was 10–12 cm lateral to the dorsal midline, and a point 7–8 cm lateral, on the iliac crest line was chosen for the lumbosacral approach. After local anesthesia, the 21-gauge, 22-cm-long needle was inserted into the disc under

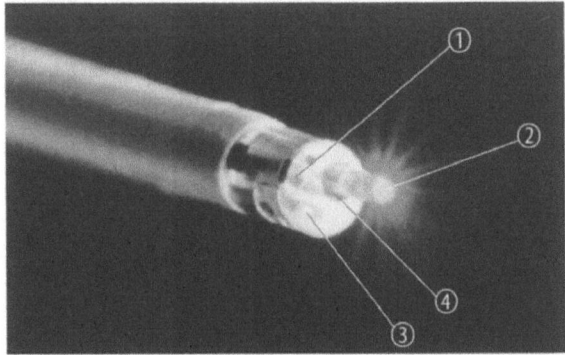

Fig. 1. LASE endoscope (Clarus) and delivery system (outer diameter: 1.7 mm) of Ho:YAG laser used in EPLDD. *1.* Video monitor image fiber. *2.* Laser fiber. *3.* Illumination fiber. *4.* Irrigation tube

fluoroscopic observation, and we confirmed annular resistance on the line connecting the posterior vertebral edges, to avoid irritating the nerve roots. A 3-mm skin incision was made to introduce the flexible trocar along the needle, and a straight cannula of 1.7 mm diameter was next inserted along the trocar onto the surface of the annulus, which was further deepened into the nucleus pulposus. A LASE endoscope (Clarus, USA) (Fig. 1), inserted through the straight cannula, was connected with Versa Pulse or Versa Pulse Select (Coherent, USA), an illuminator, and a video monitor through the optical fiber. The tip of the laser fiber was irrigated with saline at a flow rate of 30 ml/min, and was controlled by endoscopic monitoring throughout surgery. The final setup is shown in Fig. 2. Once a clear endoscopic image of the disc was obtained, we initiated nuclear ablation (Fig. 3) with the laser set at 1.0 J and 10 Hz; if the patient experienced no pain during initial ablation, the setting was changed to 1.2–1.5 J and 12–15 Hz. The ablation of the nucleus pulposus is essentially painless; thus, if the patient complained of any pain, the endoscopic image was carefully checked. During nucleus ablation, the patient experienced a decreased degree of pain, numbness, and motor weakness in their legs. The ablation of the end plate or the annular ligaments, on the other hand, is usually associated with some pain.

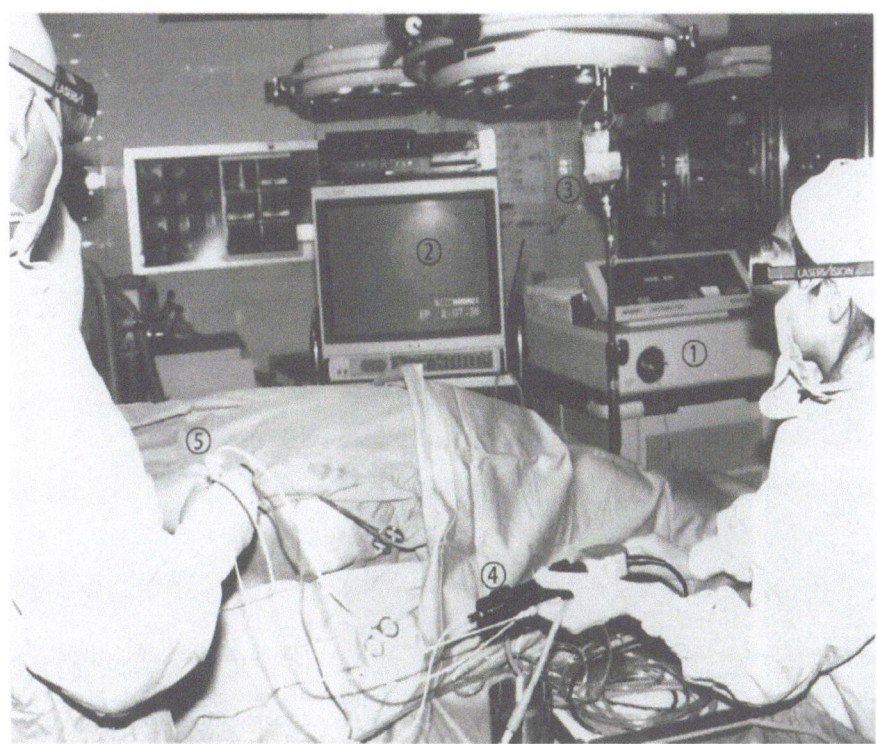

Fig. 2. The final setup of Ho:YAG EPLDD. *1.* VersaPulse (Coherent). *2.* Video monitor. *3.* Irrigation root. *4.* Video camera. *5.* LASE endoscope (Clarus)

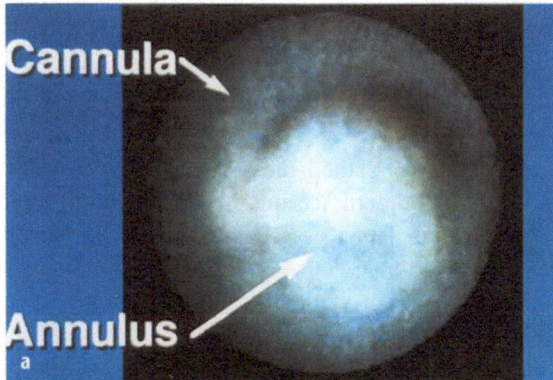

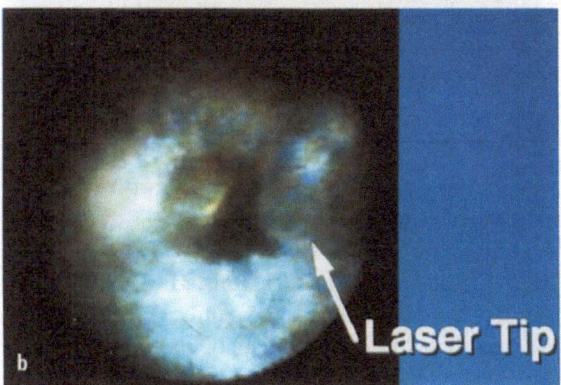

Fig. 3a, b. An endoscopic view during Ho:YAG EPLDD. **a** The surface of the annulus. **b** The laser tip, indicated by the *white arrow,* ablated the nucleus pulposus and created a cavity

The intradiscal pressure was monitored by observing the endoscopic image of the cavity created by ablation. Although the cavity immediately closed during the initial stage of ablation as a result of high intradiscal pressure, once the pressure decreased sufficiently, the cavity no longer collapsed, suggesting decompression of the disc had been achieved (Fig. 4). We used the following criteria for deciding when laser disc decompression was complete: (1) diminished patient symptoms with regard to leg pain, numbness, and motor weakness, (2) an endoscopic image revealing no collapsing of the cavity created by ablation, and (3) a total energy of around 20 kJ has been reached. The incision was finally covered with skin tape. We do not provide any special postoperative care, and we allow our patients to go home on the day of the surgery or the day thereafter; they may resume desk work on the next day, but heavier work may be resumed only three weeks later.

Inclusion Criteria

The criteria for patient selection were as follows:
1. The contained HNP (McCulloch [5]) (Fig. 5) demonstrated by MRI was responsible for the symptoms.
2. The patients had been under conservative treatment for at least three consecutive months.

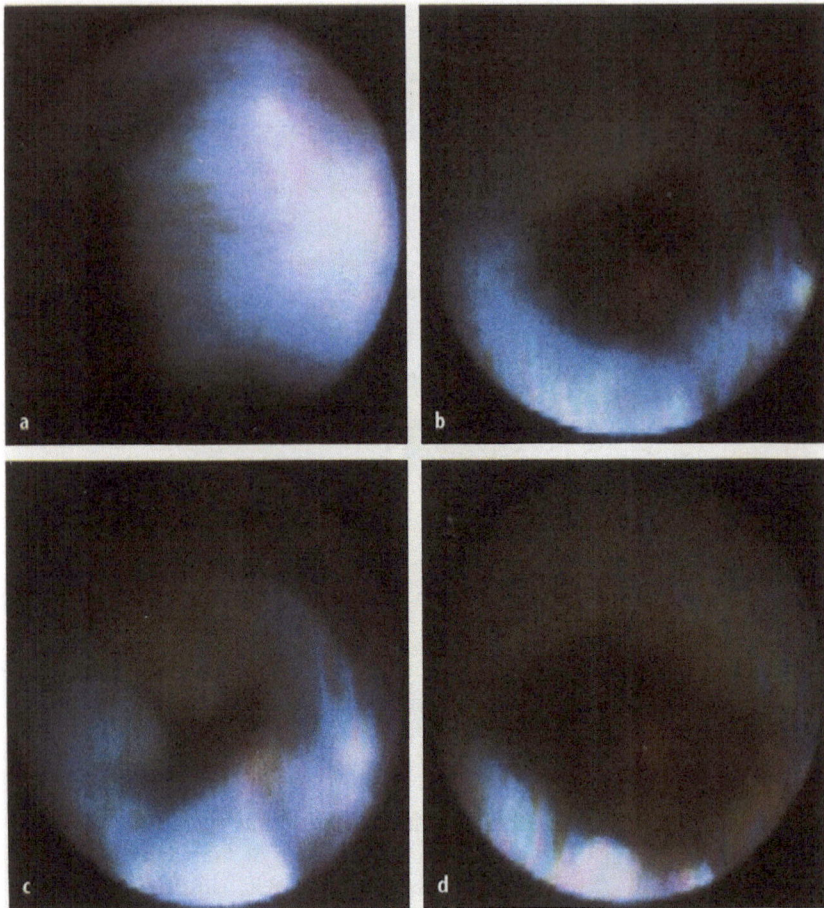

Fig. 4a–d. Sequential changes of the nuclear view associated with decrease of intradiscal pressure achieved with laser ablation. a The nucleus pulposus is pushed into the cannula due to high intradiscal pressure. b Laser ablation is started and a cavity is created. c The cavity immediately closes under high pressure. d After sufficient ablation, the cavity remains open

3. The Japanese Orthopedic Association score (JOA score), a standard scoring system for lower back problems in Japan, was less than 20. The details of this scoring system are shown in Table 1.

Exclusion Criteria

Patients with noncontained discs, spinal stenosis, intraspinal canal ossification, history of previous disc surgery, tumours, infectious diseases, or compensation problems were excluded.

Demographics

Since L5–S disc punctures failed in two of the 438 patients who met our selection criteria and underwent Ho:YAG EPLDD from June 1994 to December 1995, a total of 436 patients, consisting of 345 males and 91 females, entered the study. Table 2 shows the age distribution of the patients. Figure 6 lists the treated disc levels; we performed double-level treatments in 40 patients with the same setting. We measured both the x-ray exposure time and total energy of the Ho:YAG laser applied.

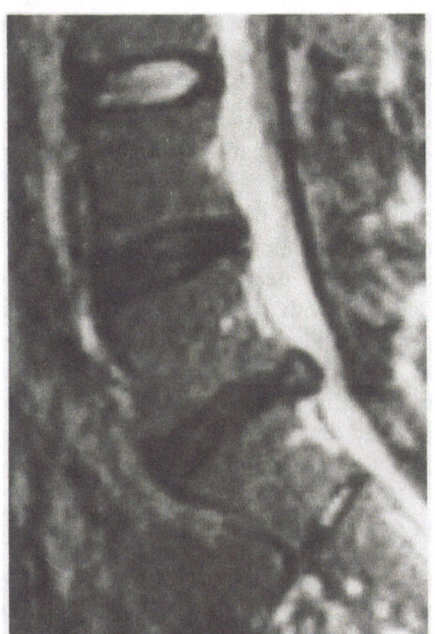

Fig. 5. A typical MRI image of the contained HNP (T2-weighted). The image of the protruded HNP in L5-S1 is contained within the low signal band image (*black line*)

Table 1. Japanese Orthopedic Association score for low back pain (JOA score)

I. Subjective (9)
A. Low back pain
  a. none   3
  b. sometimes   2
  c. always   1
  d. always severe   0
B. Numbness or pain in lower legs
  a. none   3
  b. sometimes   2
  c. always   1
  d. always severe   0
C. Gait disturbance
  a. none   3
  b. no, but some pain or numbness   2
  c. cannot walk more than 300 m   1
  d. cannot walk more than 100 m   0

II. Objective (6)
A. SLR
  a. more than 90°   2
  b. 30–70°   1
  c. less than 70°   0
B. Sensory
  a. normal   2
  b. mildly disturbed   1
  c. severely disturbed   0
C. Motor
  a. normal   2
  b. mildly disturbed   1
  c. severely disturbed   0

III. ADL (14)
a. rotating and turning
  easy   2
  difficult   1
  very difficult   0
b. standing up
  easy   2
  difficult   1
  very difficult   0
c. washing one's face
  easy   2
  difficult   1
  very difficult   0
d. standing for a long time
  easy   2
  difficult   1
  very difficult   0
e. sitting for a long time
  easy   2
  difficult   1
  very difficult   0
f. lifting up a weight of more than 20 kg
  easy   2
  difficult   1
  very difficult   0
g. walking
  easy   2
  difficult   1
  very difficult   0

Recovery rate = (postoperative JOA score – preoperative JOA score) × 100/(29 – preoperative JOA score)

Table 2. Age distribution of patients

Age	Number of cases
14–19	37
20–29	81
30–39	101
40–49	141
50–59	58
60–72	18

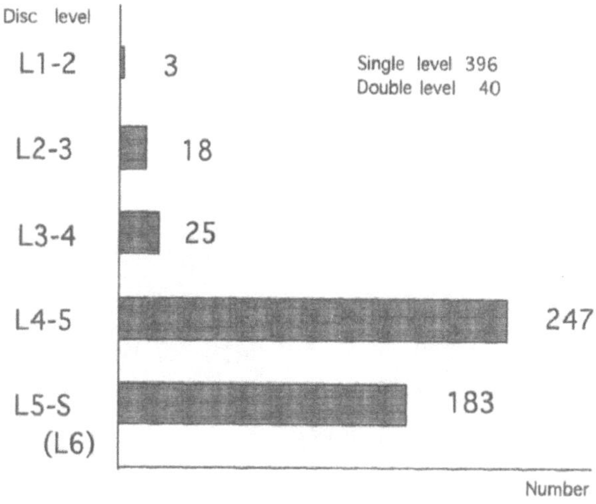

Disc level

L1-2	3
L2-3	18
L3-4	25
L4-5	247
L5-S (L6)	183

Single level 396
Double level 40

Number

Fig. 6. Distribution of 476 discs in 436 patients

Data Analysis

The clinical results were evaluated on the basis of the JOA score at one day, six months, and 12 months after the operation. The recovery rate was calculated with the formula shown in Table 1; we defined recovery rates above 25% as successful outcomes. Statistical analysis was performed by comparing pre- and postoperative JOA scores.

Results

None of the patients encountered neurological complications, postoperative discitis, or an increased amount of leg or low back pain. The incised skin healed without any complications.

The total x-ray exposure time was 2.2 + 1.5 min on average. Although the average x-ray exposure time of 2.1 + 1.4 min in L1–2 to L4–5 procedures was shorter than the 2.5 + 1.7 min used for L5–S procedures, there was no significant difference between the two values. The total energy for disc ablation ranged from 5.4 to 28.5 kJ, with an average of 15.5 kJ. Pre- and postoperative MRIs are illustrated in Fig. 7 for comparison. The postoperatively protruding HNP had decreased in mass and the dura was no longer being compressed.

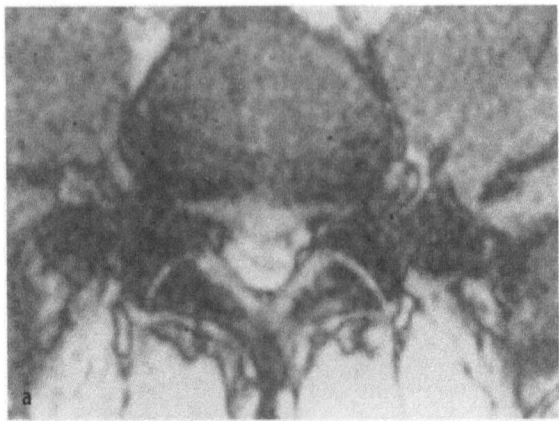
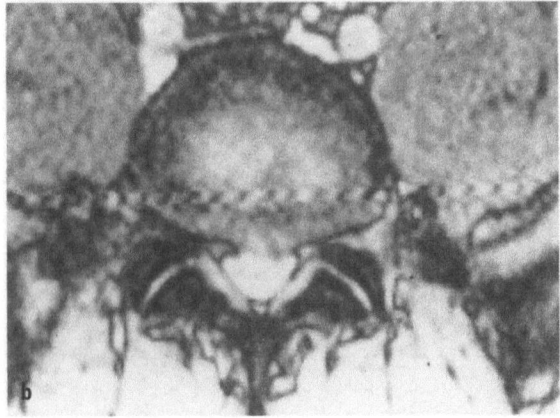

Fig. 7a, b. Disappearance of the HNP following Ho:YAG EPLDD due to contained HNP on the left-hand side of the spine in the L5–S1 level (a). The sciatica immediately recovered, and MRI at one month later showed no protrusion of the disc (b)

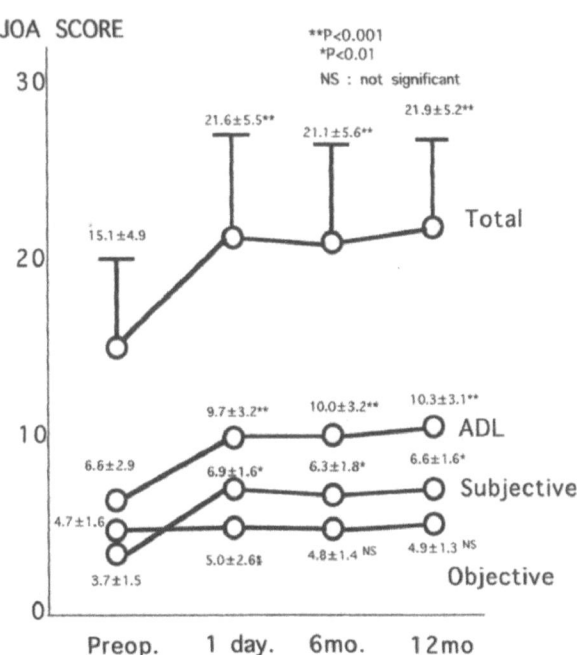

Fig. 8. Clinical results of Ho:YAG EPLDD, evaluated by JOA score

All 436 patients (100%) answered the questionnaires one day after surgery; the questionnaires were completed by 211 patients (69.2%) after 6 months and 106 patients (58.6%) after 12 months. The preoperative and postoperative JOA scores are shown in Fig. 8. At all postoperative periods, there was a statistically significant improvement in subjective, ADL, and total scores. One day after the operation, there was a statistically significant improvement in the objective scores; however, the scores at 6 and 12 months were not significantly higher than the preoperative findings. The success rate was determined to be 80.0%, 72.5% and 80.2% at one day, 6 months, and 12 months, respectively. As for patient satisfaction, 77.7% were satisfied with the outcome at one day after surgery, 73.1% at 6 months, and 74.6% at 12 months.

A second trial was performed in 13 patients whose initial Ho:YAG EPLDD failed. In five of these cases, a new disc level was ablated and improvement was obtained. In these cases, the new level had already been suspected as a site of an HNP on the previous MRI. A second ablation at the same level was performed in the remaining eight patients, of whom four experienced a diminished amount of pain; the other four all nedded surgical interventions: microscopic nucleotomy for subligamentous sequestered discs was performed in three of them and posterior lumbar interbody fusion (PLIF) for rotatory spinal instability was performed in one patient.

On the patients whose Ho:YAG EPLDD interventions failed, we performed then microscopic nucleotomies for subligamentally sequestered disc fragments and two PLIF operations for accompanied rotatory instability.

Discussion

In laser PLDD with Ho:YAG [8, 10, 11], Nd:YAG [24], or KTP [6], the laser energy is applied to ablate the nucleus pulposus, thus decreasing the intradiscal pressure and relieving pain [1, 4, 6, 8, 10, 11]. Of the lasers used today, Ho:YAG results in less thermal damage, with the temperature of the surrounding tissue rising only by 5 °C and with lowest tissue penetration depth of 0.5 mm [12]. Macroscopic and microscopic views of a disc ablated by Ho:YAG are shown in Fig. 9, revealing no thermal effects or mechanical tears in the ablated tissue. We believe that Ho:YAG laser is safe enough to be applied in EPLDD. Regardless of the introduction of laser for PLDD when treating patients with HNP, the criteria for candidate selection established for mechanical PLDD [2, 3, 7, 8] should also be used. Except for the addition of the JOA score, a scoring system widely accepted in Japan and other Asian countries for evaluating

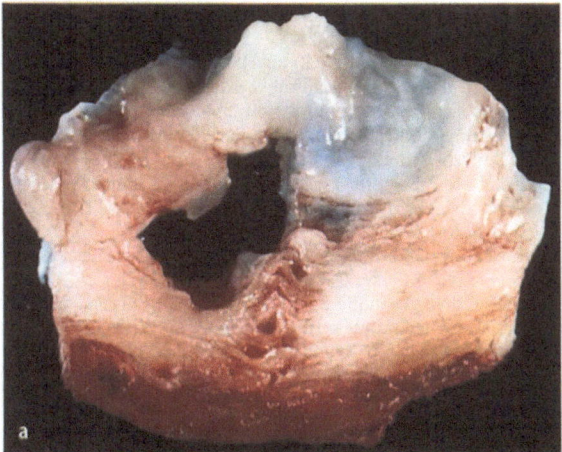
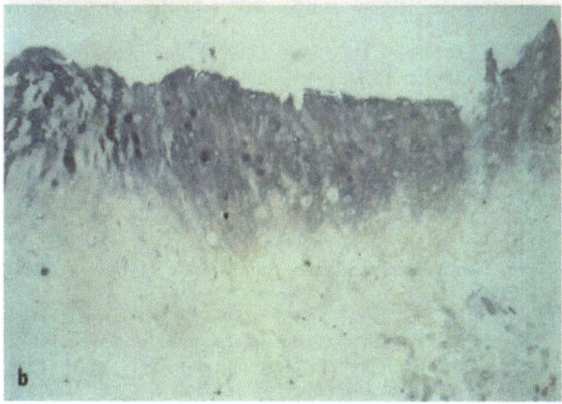

Fig. 9a, b. Macroscopic and microscopic findings of a disc ablated by Ho:YAG laser. Neither the macroscopic (a) nor the microscopic (b) photo shows thermal effects around the edge of the ablated disc

lower back problems, our criteria is identical to the previous criteria. Patients who score less than 20 points usually require some operative intervention.

The most important criterion, however, was that the contained HNP had to be confirmed [5]; this depended on the black line on either the sagittal or the transaxial MRI image. The black line shown as a low-signal intensity band behind the disc represents the posterior ligament complex including the posterior annular ligament and the posterior longitudinal ligament, and the posterior part of the HNP contained within the black line was defined as contained (Fig. 3).

Ho:YAG EPLDD solved several of the problems associated with conventional mechanical PLDD. First, the new procedure significantly reduced the rate of contamination. We have not yet encountered any discitis.

Secondly, lumbosacral puncturing was easier in Ho:YAG EPLDD; the procedure failed in only two of the 185 cases we tried for lumbosacral puncturing. Hijikata [2] stated that lumbosacral puncturing was impossible in one-third of L5-S candidates. Onik

[7] recommended employing a curved cannula for L5-S puncturing. We have no experience in using the curved cannula, but the straight cannula proved to be adequate for accessing the lumbosacral disc. The lower iliac wing in Asian people may also make it easier to access the L5-S disc.

Thirdly, the x-ray exposure time was significantly shortened with the use of an endoscope, which clearly showed the location of the optical fiber tip. Without the endoscope, an image intensifier was constantly needed to check the intradiscal position of the instruments. Although there is no literature on the x-ray exposure time, we believe the exposure time with the endoscope is much shorter than that without it.

Fourthly, we were able to confirm completion of disc decompression by using the endoscopic image. Mechanical PLDD is known to require extensive removal of the nuclear material in order to relieve the pain; excess excision, however, may result in narrowing the disc space, resulting in postoperative low back pain. The endoscope allows confirmation of the change in pressure by observing the cavity in the nucleus created by laser ablation. While the cavity closes immediately under high intradiscal pressure, as the pressure is decreased, the cavity closes more slowly, and, finally, remains open when complete decompression is achieved.

Finally, provided that the surgeon keeps the following points in mind, Ho:YAG EPLDD is absolutely painless: (1) Never irritate the exiting nerve root passing over the disc surface. (2) Never ablate the surface of the annulus or the end plate. (3) Never advance the laser tip into the cavity when the intradiscal pressure is high, because this will further increase the intradiscal pressure, due to water pressure produced by the irrigation pump: this will lead to severe sciatica. Our recommendation is to ablate only the wall of the cavity.

Our clinical results are comparable to those of Choy who reported [1] a 78% success rate with Nd:YAG-PLDD and those of Ohmesis [6] who reported a 70.7% success rate with KTP. On the other hand, the success rate of mechanical PLDD was found to be approximately 70% (72% by Hijikata [2] and 72.5% by Schreiber [9]), although Kambin [3] obtained a higher success rate of 87%. We believe that Ho:YAG EPLDD done in properly selected patients may result in a success rate of around 80%, which is higher than that of mechanical PLDD, but lower than that of open nucleotomy, with which a 90% success rate is obtained [13].

The JOA score recorded one day after surgery showed a statistically significant improvement, which remained unchanged at both 6 months and 12 months later, suggesting that immediate postoperative improvement is maintained for at least one year after surgery. Since the root pain is relieved with Ho:YAG EPLDD because of the decrease in the intradiscal pressure, this result is quite understandable. Of the subjective, objective, and ADL scoring categories, the objective category score did not show statisically significant improvement; although in some patients muscle weakness or sensory disturbance had recovered, the average value indicated no improvement. On the other hand, the ADL and subjective scores had statistically significantly improved. In general, the patients treated with Ho:YAG EPLDD had no difficulty in their daily life, but experienced slight low back pain or numbness, muscle weakness, and pain in the legs for some postoperative period.

Conclusion

We have performed endoscopic percutaneous lumbar disc decompression using the Ho:YAG laser (Ho:YAG EPLDD) since June 1994 in 436 patients. This method decompresses the intradiscal pressure in a less invasive manner than mechanical procedures do and allows safe practice and confirmation of decreased intradiscal pressure through endoscopic monitoring. Ho:YAG EPLDD is virtually painless and did not lead to any neurological or infectious complications, and disc puncture failed in only two of the 185 lumbosacral procedures. The success rate was 80.0 %, 72.5 %, and 80.2 % at one day, 6 months, and 12 months, respectively. We believe that Ho:YAG EPLDD is a safe and promising method for the treatment of contained HNP.

References

[1] Choy DSJ, Ascher PW, Ranu HS, Saddekin S, Alkaitis D, Liebler W, Hughes J, Diwan S, Altman P (1992) Percutaneous laser disc decompression. Spine 17:949–956
[2] Hijikata S (1989) Percutaneous nucleotomy. A new concept technique and 12 years' experience. Clin Orthop 238:9–23
[3] Kambine P, Schaffer J (1989) Percutaneous lumbar discectomy. Review of 100 patients and current practice. Clin Orthop 238:24–34
[4] Kosaka R, Onomura T, Yonezawa T (1994) Laser disc ablation. Rinsho Seikei Geka 29:431–440
[5] McCulloch JA, Inoue S, Moriya H (1990) Surgical indications and techniques. In: Weinstein JN, Wiesel SW (eds) The lumbar spine. Saunders, Philadelphia, pp 303–421
[6] Ohnmeiss DD, Guyer RD, Hochschuler SH (1994) Laser disc decompression. The importance of proper patient selection. Spine 19:2054–2058
[7] Onik G, Helms CA, Ginsberg L et al (1975) Percutaneous lumbar discectomy using a new aspiration probe. AJNR 290–293
[8] Rodes A, Black J, Lane GJ et al (1993) Clinical use of the 2.1 micron holmium:YAG laser and percutaneous discectomy. Spine (State of the Art Rev) 7:17–22
[9] Schreiber A, Suezawa Y, Leu H (1989) Does percutaneous nucleotomy with discoscopy replace conventional discectomy? Clin Orthop 238:35–42
[10] Sherk HH (1992) Current concepts review. The use of lasers in orthopaedic procedures. J Bone Joint Surg 75A:768–776
[11] Siebert W (1993) Percutaneous laser disc decompression: the European experience. Spine (State of the Art Rev) 7:103–133
[12] Trost D, Zacker A, Smith MFW (1992) Surgical laser properties and their tissue interaction. In: Smith MFW, McElveen JT Jr (eds) Neurological surgery of the ear. Mosby Yearbook, St. Louis, pp 131–162
[13] Spangfort EV (1972) The lumbar disc herniation - a computer-aided analysis of 2,504 operations. Acta Orthop Scand 142 (suppl):1–95

Percutaneous Transforaminal Laser-Assisted Surgery in the Epidural Space for Noncontained Herniated Discs

R. STUCKER

Introduction

Disadvantages of conventional lumbar disc surgery are epidural scarring and instability. Many of the so called "failed backs" are results of either one or the other of these complications. Extensive scarring is often accompanied by some residual complaints after disc surgery. Recently, Ross et al. [1], in a double-blind multicentre study, were able to show that patients with extensive scarring complain two to three times more often of low back pain after disc surgery than patients with minor epidural scarring do.

Instability is more likely caused by the evacuation of the disc space during conventional surgery, with subsequent narrowing of the disc space. It has been shown by several investigators that preserving the disc space and the nucleus pulposus during surgery results in less postoperative narrowing of the disc space and less postoperative back pain. To minimise morbidity after disc surgery, minimal invasive techniques were developed in the past. Disadvantages of chemonucleolysis, percutaneous automated or non-automated nucleotomy, laser nucleotomy and uniportal or biportal intradiscal endoscopic surgery are that these procedures are indicated for contained herniated discs only.

This is a report on a series of 85 patients who were treated for noncontained herniated discs by a new endoscopic technique, which uses mechanical instruments and laser vaporisation in the epidural space to remove sequestered disc material.

Study

Indications and Contraindications

Good indications for transforaminal endoscopic eidural laser-assisted surgery are
- young patient
- pathology at disc level
- no previous disc surgery
- disc space narrowing < 50 %
- no lateral recess stenosis

The only contraindications are sequestered disc material not located at disc level and cauda equina syndrome. A narrow intervertebral foramen, old age and disc space narrowing more than 50 % are relative contraindications, but can be managed with experience. The disc space L5/S1 is more difficult to approach than the other lumbar levels, especially if the iliac crest is high above the L4/L5 interspace and if L5 has a big transverse process.

Patients

From November 1993 until September 1996, 85 patients were treated for noncontained herniated lumbar discs. The first 20 patients were retrospectively analysed. The mean follow-up time was 16 months. An analysis of the last 65 patients is currently being performed. The first 20 patients make up our "learning curve" and consist of 12 men and 8 women. The average age was 41.5 years, and range from 21–72 years. All patients were treated conservatively for at least six weeks. Two patients had disc herniation at the L3/L4 level, ten patients at L4/L5, seven patients at L5/S1, and one patient at L5/L6. Two patients had an extraforaminal herniation, two patients an intraforaminal herniation, eight patients a mediolateral and seven a medial noncontained disc herniation.

In each case, laser energy was used for tissue ablation or to obtain haemostasis. The applied laser energy ranged from 1.5 to 9.5 kJ, with a mean of 3.8 kJ. A Ho:YAG (2100 nm) laser was used because of its ability to vaporise disc tissue and because of low tissue penetration of heat, only 1 mm compared to 2–6 mm for a Nd:YAG laser. A laser fiber which can deliver energy at a 90° angle is recommended.

Patients were examined clinically and completed a questionnaire. On a visual analogue scale from one to ten, patients had to assess their back pain and leg pain preoperatively, one day postoperatively and finally at follow-up. A value of zero represented no pain, a value of ten excruciating pain. They also rated their sensory loss on a scale of one to four, where one was normal and four represented numbness.

Operative Techniques

Operations of the first 50 patients were performed under local anaesthesia, and for the last 35 patients under general anaesthesia.

Patients were positioned prone on a radiolucent table; they were supported by a soft pillow, to correct some of the lumbar lordosis, a blunt K-wire was introduced percutaneously about 12–14 cm from the midline and was aimed towards the disc space under image-intensifier control. It was guided through the foramen and pierced the posterior longitudinal ligament at the line connecting both medial borders of the adjacent pedicles. Through a small skin incision, a cannulated dilator was used and was advanced through the foramen. Then a cannula with a 6.4-mm outer diameter was placed over the dilator. It was only advanced to a line connecting both centres of the adjacent pedicles, so that dilator and cannula were shaped like a bullet.

A 4.6-mm endoscope with a 2-mm working channel was introduced through the cannula on top of the K-wire after removal of the dilator. The endoscope was connected to an irrigation system. We recommend cold Ringer solution with the addition of epinephrin (1.5 mg for 3 l fluid). The irrigation fluid should be stored in a refrigerator for at least 2 hours prior to surgery. A suction tube is also connected to the scope; however, permanent suction is not necessary. We recommend that suction is controlled by, and adjusted according to the preference of, the surgeon. If these recommendations are adhered to, no bleeding will be encountered during surgery.

The next steps depend on the existing pathology. In case of a disc fragment under the posterior longitudinal ligament, a small hole is made through this ligament and decompression can safely be performed under that ligament even to the midline. In case of a free fragment, surgery has to be performed posterior to the posterior longitudinal ligament and under the traversing nerve root. In the case of a foraminal or extraforaminal herniation, the same approach is used. In the safe working zone axilla and exiting nerve root are inspected by levering the endoscope cranially. With a nerve hook, the tension on the exiting nerve root can be checked readily. Decompression can be performed with manual instruments such as forceps, punches, hooks or with a laser fiber. After decompression, both the traversing and exiting nerve roots should be without tension. At the end of the procedure, the author of this chapter prefers to use a laser fibre to seal the posterior longitudinal ligament, using the tissue-shrinking effect of laser energy.

Results

The results of our first 20 patients ("learning curve") are given in Figs. 1–2. On a visual analogue 0–10 scale (0 = no pain, 10 = excruciating pain) leg pain decreased from 6.2 preoperatively to 2.5 one day after surgery to 1.8 at follow-up. Back pain changed from 4.9 preoperatively to 1.5 and 2.6 respectively.

On a 1–4 scale (1 = normal, 4 = numbness), patients rated their sensory deficits with 2.2 preoperatively, and 3.4 at follow-up. According to the criteria of McNab, 65 % of patients had a good and very good result, 15 % a satisfactory and 20 % a bad outcome. Revision surgery was performed in 25 % of the "learning curve" patients, whereas only two patients of the last 65 cases needed surgery for true recurrent herniation; this was again managed by endoscopic surgery. During open revision of the four patients of our learning curve, no significant scarring was encountered. In each case, decompression was found to be incomplete, that is, due to limited experience of the surgeon and not due to a true reherniation. All four patients were rated to have a poor result.

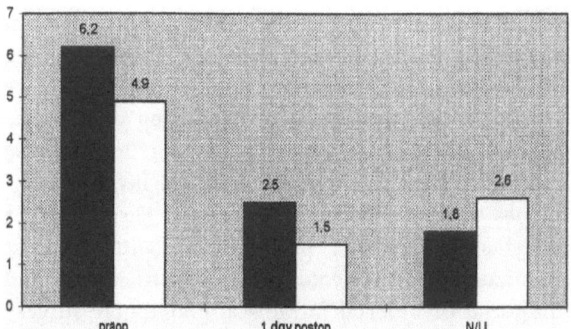

Fig. 1. Back pain and leg pain in the first 16 patients before operation, 1 day after, and during follow-up. Patients rated their pain on a visual analogue scale from 0 to 10 where 0 = no pain and 10 = excruciating pain

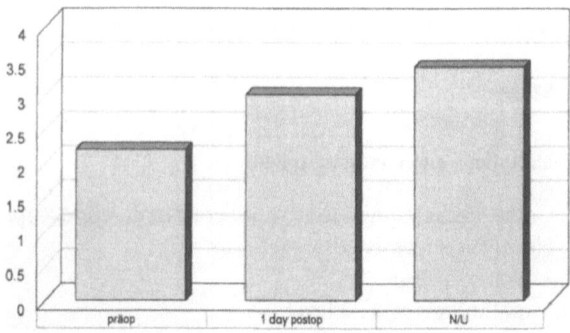

Fig. 2. Sensory deficits of 16 patients before operation, 1 day after, and during follow-up. Patients rated their sensory deficit on a scale of 1 = no sensory loss to 4 = complete sensory loss

Discussion

The so-called "failed backs" after conventional lumbar disc surgery are most likely either due to instability following severe disc-space narrowing or due to epidural scarring. Both complications significantly account for the postoperative back pain developing in up to 30 % of cases after lumbar discectomy. To avoid disc-space narrowing, it has been suggested that only the herniated fragment should be removed and that the nucleus pulposus should be retained. Furthermore, it has been shown that preserving the nucleus pulposus during conventional surgery does not increase the reherniation rate, but lowers the incidence of postoperative back pain significantly.

The procedure presented here may avoid both complications mentioned. Our limited experience with postoperative MRI did not demonstrate significant epidural scarring after endoscopic surgery. On performing four open revisions during our learning curve and two endoscopic revisions for the true reherniations later on, we encountered no difficulties, during surgery, as a result of epidural scarring.

Our follow-up period is not long enough for us to comment on disc-space narrowing after endoscopic surgery, but we can speculate that there is no difference compared to the natural behaviours of noncontained herniated discs.

The incidence of revision surgery for our last 65 patients is different compared to that during our "learning curve." Only two true reherniations were observed during the former period, suggesting that the recurrence rate is not different to that of currently employed open procedures.

A very useful tool during endoscopic surgery in the epidural space is laser energy from a Ho:YAG laser delivered by a laser fiber through the working channel of an endoscope. Vaporisation of disc tissue is easily accomplished and bleeding from epidural vessels is safely controlled. We also used laser energy to decompress the lateral recess and remove bony appositions and osteophytes of facet joints successfully in two patients.

So far, we have not encountered any adverse effects of laser surgery. No other complications such as haematoma, infection or others were observed. Nevertheless, endoscopic manipulation in the epidural space is demanding surgery, requiring a long learning period. It should be performed by experienced spine surgeons only.

In conclusion, epidural scarring and disc-space narrowing produced by conventional open procedures may be avoided by endoscopic transforaminal surgery in the epidural space and thus may improve the prognosis of noncontained herniated discs significantly. As a minimally invasive procedure, it causes little morbidity to the patient and the average hospital stay is reduced. Our first experiences with operations on 85 patients are very encouraging, but a longer follow-up time is required to assess the indications for the different types of disc lesions. We are already able to treat about 80 % of our patients with non-contained herniated discs in this manner and we firmly believe that endoscopic surgery in the epidural space will replace open surgery for most indications.

References

[1] Ross JS, Robertson JT, Fredrickson RC, Petrie JL, Obuchowski N, Modic MT, de Tribolet N (1996) Association between peridural scar and recurrent radicular pain after lumbar discectomy: Magnetic resonance imaging. ADCON-L European Study Group. Neurosurgery 38(4):855–861; Discussion 861–863

Percutaneous Foraminal Endoscopic Lumbar Discectomy – Evolution from a Laparoscopic Technique

T. G. OBENCHAIN · D. W. CLOYD

Introduction

Minimally invasive techniques for the removal of herniated discs are in a continual state of evolution. Transperitoneal anterior lumbar discectomy was first carried out in 1991 [1]. The authors subsequently had experience with twenty-nine cases, all performed in an outpatient setting, with an approximately 80 % success rate. The procedure, however, is moderately difficult and is sufficiently technologically demanding to discourage widespread acceptance by spine surgeons. The authors therefore developed a retroperitoneal balloon technique [2] which not only could be achieved under local anesthesia, but was technically less demanding that the transperitoneal method. By either route, however, entry into the anterior portion of the disc space was achieved with an 8-mm trephine-utilizing fluoroscopic guidance for disc removal. In the latter cases, an endoscope with a straight working channel was utilized for visualization. In six of the ten latter cases, postoperative x-rays revealed some narrowing of the operated disc space. Two of the six patients had significant low back pain, leading the senior author (Cloyd) to develop an even less invasive form of discectomy. This method involves entry through the foramen, thereby avoiding any removal of normal disc en route to the herniated portion of the disc. The penultimate step in development involved balloon dissection of the retroperitoneal space combined with a posterolateral (discographic) entry into the disc space. With further experience retroperitoneal dissection has been found to be unnecessary. The subject of this report is the latest iteration of a stereotactic entry into the foramen for removal of the disc herniation.

Indications

Percutaneous foraminal endoscopic discectomy can be recommended for patients with virtually any type of lumbar disc herniation, who have been unresponsive to conservative treatment. Imaging studies should reveal a herniation consistent with the patient's clinical picture. The herniation is amenable to this form of treatment regardless of whether it is contained within the posterior longitudinal ligament (PLL) or is an extruded or sequestered fragment. Foraminal endoscopic discectomy is well suited to treatment of discs heriated centrally, posterolaterally, in the foramen or in the far lateral position. The only contraindication is a deep-seated L5–S1 disc space with a high-riding iliac crest.

Technique

Percutaneous foraminal discectomy is carried out under local anesthesia, with the patient's symptomatic side upward. A standard posterolateral, fluoroscopically guided needle entry into the disc space is achieved. This needle serves as a guide pin. Over the guide pin, an 8-mm nerve-deflecting needle with a conduit is inserted, with the conduit directed caudally (Fig. 1). When the tip of the needle is in the disc space, it is rotated 90° so that the conduit is facing laterally thereby serving as a conduit from the retroperitoneal space to the foraminal space. Next, a stereotaxic arm is secured onto the needle. A second entry site is made in the skin at the end of that stereotaxic arm. A T-handled trocar is inserted approximately 3 cm to penetrate the muscular layers. To avoid visceral penetration, the sharp tip is replaced by a blunt-tipped trocar which traverses the rest of the retroperitoneal space until its tip engages the lateral aspect of the conduit. A rigid rod lens endoscope with a straight working port and distal suction/irrigation capability is inserted down the shaft. Once the ligamentous lateral wall of the foramen is encountered, the stem of the universal joint is secured to the operating table by means of a laparoscopic holder (Fig. 2). At this point, the nerve-deflecting conduit is no longer needed and is therefore removed (Fig. 3). While the lateral aspect of the foramen is visualized, the universal joint can be adjusted for an optimal position relative to the foramen.

A corkscrew grasping trephine is now inserted through the working port to traverse and excise a

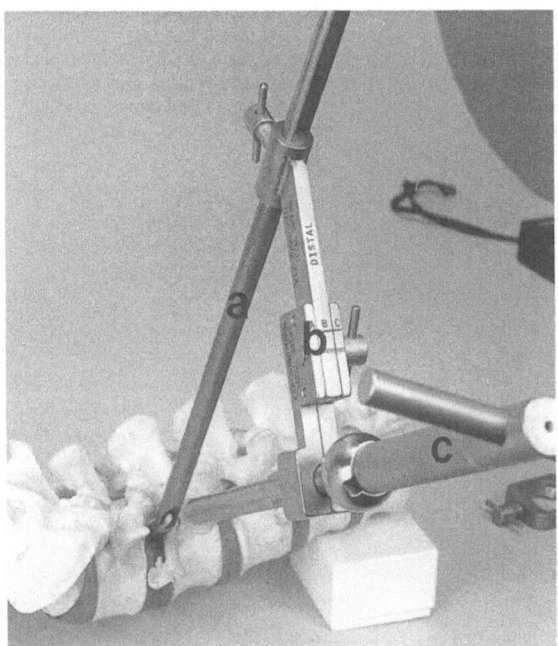

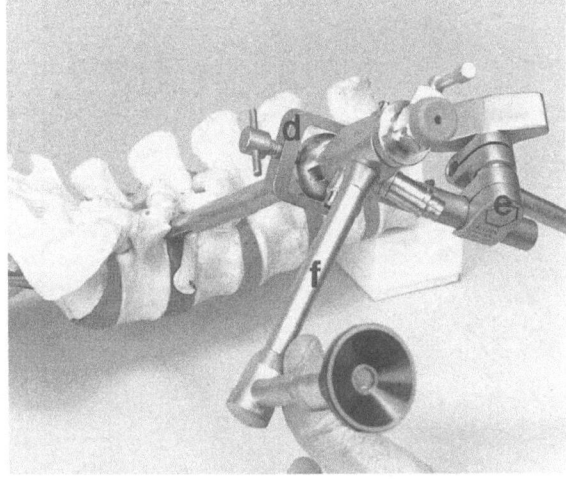

Fig. 3. Items *a*, *b*, and *c* have now been removed. The surgeon now has a straight port into the lateral foramen. Change of position can now be achieved by adjustments at the universal joint. A parallel eye-beam endoscope with a straight working port is in position *f*

Fig. 1. The large needle (*a*) has a "heel" which tends to deflect the emergent nerve. The large hole or conduit is directed laterally. A sterotaxic arm (*b*) is then attached. Through the opening, a cannula with T-handled trocar (*c*) is inserted until its tip encounters the lateral end of the conduit

sions or sequestra, the surgeon can remove the disc without entering the disc space proper. For a contained herniation, the disc space is entered to initiate disc removal. The inferior portion of the superior articular facet can also be removed if there is significant foraminal stenosis.

Upon completion of the operation, the entry ports are closed with single inverted subcutaneous sutures and steri-strips are applied. The patient is discharged from the recovery room to home two to three hours after surgery.

Clinical Experience

Clinical experience thus far includes a total of eight patients, as summarized in Table 1. Three patients underwent open laminectomy at the same sitting, that is, when the foraminal approach could not be technically achieved. One failure was due to inability to enter the foramen. A second was due to endoscopic visual loss when a lens dislodged. A third case was converted to laminectomy because of bleeding which was mild, but significant enough to obscure endoscopic visualization. The other five cases were all successfully treated percutaneously. They include herniations at L1–2, L4–5 and L5–A1. Four of the five patients have had excellent results and one patient with aposterolateral herniation had a fair result by the criteria of MacNab. Mean follow-up for that group of five patients is six months. Apart from the patients requiring open laminectomy, all were treated in an outpatient setting and were discharged home from the recovery room two to three hours after surgery. None has required reoperation.

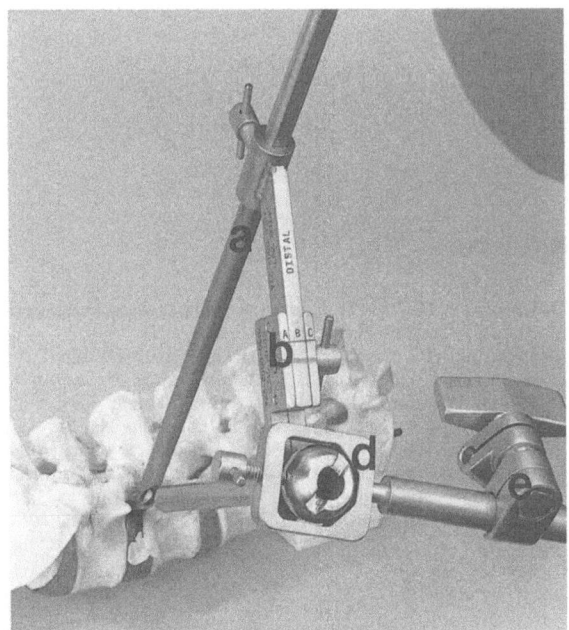

Fig. 2. A universal joint (*d*) is attached onto the cannula. This apparatus is now stabilized with a holder (*e*) affixed to the operating table

core of ligament from the foramen. A variety of bone shavers, coagulating forceps, Kerrison ronguers, interspace ronguers and curettes can be inserted to remove bone, ligament and/or disc tissue (Fig. 4). Tissue is removed until the nerve root at that level is decompressed. For far-lateral herniations, extru-

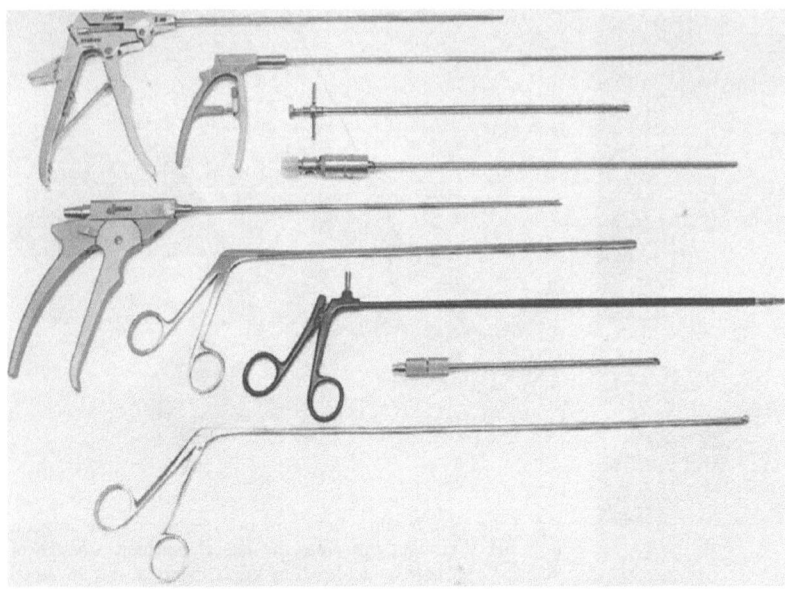

Fig. 4. All instruments can be passed through the straight working port of the endoscope. This includes trephines, Kerrison and interspace ronguers, suction ronguers, coagulating forceps and automated shavers

Table 1. Clinical cases

Patient	Level	Herniattion	Follow-up results	Month	Failure/open
RP	L4–5	Foraminal	Excellent	10	
PR	L4–5	Foraminal	Fair	8	Opened, poor visibility
MC	L4–5	Post/Lat.	Fair	8	
CM	L3–4	Post/Lat.	Excellent	5	Opened, scope failure
JK	L1–2	Far Lat.	Excellent	5	
GP	L4–5	Extrusion	Excellent	4	
RH	L5–S1	Post/Lat.	Excellent	3	
WT	L4–5	Foraminal	Excellent	2	Opened, bleeding

Conclusions

Clinical experience is thus far too limited to make any sweeping conclusions regarding the clinical effectiveness of foraminal endoscopic discectomy. But the technique is feasible. However, today, where the decision for surgery must be based on evidence of its effectiveness, further studies may be necessary and the outcome measured and compared to more widely used procedures such as microdiscectomy. The advantages of the foraminal endoscopic discectomy are that (a) it is performed in an awake patient, (b) it is less invasive, (c) it is performed consistently on an out-patient basis, and (d) its entry does not require removal of significant amounts of ligament, bone, muscle, or disc tissue. The likelihood of significant epidural scarring is minimal. Foraminal endoscopic discectomy can be achieved in the awake patient under local anesthesia in an out-patient setting with minimal use of oral narcotics postoperatively.

References

[1] Obenchain TG (1991) Laparoscopic lumbar discectomy; case report. J Laparoendosc Surg 1:145–159
[2] Obenchain TG, Cloyd DW (1995) Laparoscopic lumbar retroperitoneal and transperitoneal discectomy. In: Regan J, McAfee PC, Mack MJ (eds) Atlas of endoscopic spine surgery. Quality Medical Publishers, St. Louis, pp 243–245
[3] Obenchain TG, Cloyd DW (1996) Laparoscopic lumbar discectomy; description of transperitoneal and retroperitoneal techniques. Neurosurg Clinics North Am 7:77–85
[4] MacNab I (1971) Negative disc exploration. JBJ S(A) 52:891–903

Complications of Percutaneous Laser Disc Decompression (PLDD)

H. Grasshoff · K. Mahlfeld · R. Kayser

In 1984, Choy and Ascher developed the method of percutaneous disc decompression by laser energy. One cause of development was the decrease of the complication rate of other percutaneous methods in disc surgery, such as chemonucleolysis. A number of experiences with PLDD at different laser wavelengths and delivery systems have been described since then [1, 2, 3, 4, 6, 7, 8, 9, 11, 12, 13, 14, 16, 18]. The success rates, in terms of pain relief and return of normal function for PLDD, are reported to be between 64–80 % [1, 2, 3, 8, 18]. Complications after PLDD are rare, but include nerve-root irritations and dural injuries, and damage to retroperitoneal structures is possible. Post-operative bleeding and delayed infections may occur as well. Hellinger (1994) reported a complication rate of 0.6 % in 1437 cases of PLDD with the ND:YAG laser. Choy (1991) described discitis in one case out of 560 patients treated with PLDD. Ascher (1991) and Sibert et al. (1996) described one case of discitis each, out of 210 and 180 cases of PLDD, respectively. Simons et al. (1994) presented 50 cases of PLDD with one case of lasting back pain and damage of the vertebral zone in MRI. Thermal changes in the vertebral body after PLDD were observed by Witte et al. (1995). In the published literature [3, 9, 10, 14, 18], few complications have been reported for PLDD (e. g., Choy 1991; Mayer et al. 1989; Liebler 1995; Ruffing et al. 1994; Siebert et al. 1996).

Between 1992 and 1995 we treated 347 patients with PLDD for contained and bulging symptomatic discs (136 females and 211 males, average age 42.6 years). The L3–4, L4–5 and L5–S1 discs were affected in 13, 178 and 156 cases, respectively. The Nd:YAG laser at 1320 nm was used to ablate the disc. Water was used for cooling along with local anaesthesia as described by Rudolph (1994). Discography was performed to exclude disc perforation and to use the patient's response to assess what contribution the disc makes to the condition. A double-lumen 3.0-mm spinal needle was positioned in the centre of the disc by the standard posterolateral approach. An average laser energy of 2718 J and 2385 J was delivered at the L4-5 and L5–S1 interspace, respectively.

Complications occurred in nine of 347 cases (2.6 %). All nine patients (8 male and 1 female, average age 37.5 years) showed signs of discitis or discitis-like disease. The levels involved were L4–5 in five cases and L5–S1 in four cases. The applied energy was found to be higher in patients presenting with symptoms of discitis when compared to the unaffected ones. In the affected patients the laser energy averaged: 3012 J at the L4–5 disc and 3500 J at the L5–S1 disc. The clinical and laboratory findings are shown in the Table 1.

The discitis was identified with diagnostic tools such x-ray, MRI scans, bone scans and leukocyte bone scans, and needle bone aspiration or open biopsy have been performed in six cases. In all cases the initial x-rays exhibited no change. The bone scan was positive for discitis in all cases. In the leukocyte bone scan, however, a higher activity was observed in the cases of real discitis. In all other cases, thermal damage of the vertebral bone was presumed.

We observed a number of MRI changes in patients with complications after PLDD. In the T-1-weighted images a decreased signal intensity in the disc and in the end plate of the vertebral bone was observed. The contrast enhancement was positive in all cases.

Table 1. Clinical and laboratory findings on complications after PLDD

Clinical findings	Laboratory findings
– lasting pain after 10 (1...21) days, $n = 9$	– elevated sedimentation rate, $n = 9$
– local tenderness, $n = 9$	– elevated white blood cell count, $n = 9$
– inability to flex the spine, $n = 9$	– elevated level of CRP, $n = 9$
– temperature above 38.5 °C, $n = 1$	

Table 2. Differentation between thermal bone damage and acute spondylitis after PLDD

Thermal end plate reaction	Acute spondylitis
– lasting back pain	– lasting back pain
– slight elevation of white blood cell count, sedimentation rate and CRP	– large elevation of white blood cell count, sedimentation rate and CRP
– MRI changes	– MRI changes
– positive bone scan	– positive bone scan
– negative leukocyte scan	– positive leukocyte scan
– no bacterial detection and no inflammation	– bacterial detection possible
– histological signs of acute inflammation	– histological signs of an acute pyogenic inflammation

Needle bone aspiration found no signs of discitis and no organisms grew when the aspirate of patients with aseptic discitis (23 %) was cultured. In the one patient (0.3 %) with septic discitis, open biopsy was positive for *Staphylococcur aureus*. The histological features of acute osteomyelitis were found.

All patients with discitis-like lesions were treated with bed rest for 10 days, spine immobilization with plaster cast for 4–8 weeks, along with parenteral and oral antibiotics. Abscess drainage was needed for acute spondylitis.

A number of differences between patients with aseptic discitis with thermal end-plate reaction and acute spondylitis afer PLDD were observed (Table 2).

In our study we found a discitis complication rate of 2.6 % and severe complications due to acute infective discitis were found in 0.3 % of the cases. In eight cases, thermal end-plate reactions in the vertebral bone were observed. Possible causes of these thermal bone damages are non-central needle position, disc space height of less than 12 mm in the x-rays and an excessively high laser energy. However, we consider the needle position to be the most important factor if unwanted bone heating during OLDD is to be avoided.

In respect to the above, the rare but potential hazards, such as nerve root or vascular injuries, as well as infectious complications must be considered. However, we suggest PLDD as a procedure with fewer complications than the standard and percutaneous disc surgical techniques.

References

[1] Ascher DW, Holzer P, Sutter B, Tritthart H (1991) Nucleuspulsus Denaturierung bei Bandscheibenprotrusionen. Siebert WE, Wirth UCJ (eds) Laser in der Orthopädie. Thieme, Stuttgart, pp 169-172
[2] Bonati AO (1991) Arthroscopic lumbar laser disectomy. In: 1st international symposium lasers in orthopaedic surgery, 26-29 Sept 1991, San Francisco, pp 4-5
[3] Choy DSJ, Ascher PW, Saddekui S, Alkaitis D, Liebler W, Hoghes J, Diwan S, Altman P (1992) Percutaneous laser disc decompression. Spine 12:949-956
[4] Choy DSJ, Michelsen J, Getrajdman G, Diwan S (1992) Percutaneous laser disc decompression. An update-spring 1992. J Clin Laser Med Surg 177-184

[5] Choy DSJ (1991) Percutaneous laser disc decompression (PLDD). In: 1st international symposium lasers in othropaedic surgery, 26-29 Sept 1991, San Francisco, p 24
[6] Grifka J (1994) Intradiscal laser therapy: indications, technique. In: 3rd Symposium on laser-assisted endoscopic intervention in orthopaedics, 26-27 May 1994, Zurich, p 6
[7] Hellinger J, Nonendoscopic percutaneous 1064-Nd:YAG laser decompression: mechanism, technique and experience. In: 3rd Symposium on laser-assisted endoscopic intervention ind orthopaedics, 26-27 May 1994, Zurich, p 6
[8] Leu HJ, Stalder H, Elsig JP, Perrenoud A, Schreiber A (1994) Percutaneous endoscopic lumbar disc surgery: a minimally invasive alternative. In: Wittenberg RH, Steffen R (eds) Chemonucleolysis and related intradiscal therapies. Thieme, Stuttgart, pp 110-124
[9] Liebler WA (1995) Percutaneous laser disc nucleotomy. Clin Orthop 310:58-66
[10] Mayer HM, Brock M, Stein E, Muller G (1989) Percutaneous endoscopic laser discectomy-experimental results. In: Mayer HM, Brock M (eds) Percutaneous lumbar discectomy. Springer, Berlin Heidelberg New York, pp 187-196
[11] Ohumeiss DD, Guyer RD, Hochschuler SH (1994) Laser disc decompression. The importance of proper patient selection. Spine 19:2054-2059
[12] Quigley MR, Shih T, Alrifai A, Maroon JC, Lsiecki ML (1992) Percutaneous laser discectomy with the Ho:YAG laser. Lasers Surg Med 12:621-624
[13] Rudolf J, Studtmann V (1994) Der Lasereinsatz in der perkutanen Therapie lumbar Bandscheibenschäden. In: Berlien HP, Muller G (eds) Angewandte Lasermedizin. Ecomed Landsberg, Munich, vol 1, pp 1-12
[14] Ruffing A, Diehl K, Wolf A, Hager H, Weber I (1994) Percutaneous Nd:YAG and Ho:YAG laser-decompression in cervical and lumbar disc herniations. In: 3rd Symposium on laser-assisted endoscopic intervention in orthopaedics, 26-27 May 1994, Zurich, pp 7-8
[15] Schlangmann BA, Schmolke S, Siebert WE (1996) Temperatur- und Ablationsmessungen bei der Laserbehandlung von Bandscheibengewebe. Orthopäde 254:3-9
[16] Sherk HH, Black JD, Prodoehl JA, Cummings RS (1993) Laser discectomy. Orthopedics 16:573-576
[17] Siebert WE, Ksinsik B, Wirth CJ, Stienmetz M, Muschter R (1991) In-vitro-Untersuchungen zur thermischen Belastung der Bandscheibe bei der Laserablation. In: Siebert WE, Wirth CJ (eds) Laser in der Orthopädie. Thieme, Stuttgart, pp 150-153
[18] Siebert WE, Berendsen BT, Tollgard J (1996) Die perkutane Laserdiskusdekompression (PLDD). Orthopäde 25:42-48
[19] Simons P, Lensker E, Wild KV (1994) Percutaneous nucleus pulposus denaturation in treatment of lumbar disc protrusions-a prospective study of 50 neurosurgical patients. Eur Spine J 3:219-221
[20] Witte H, Recknagel S, Grifka J, Lesch C, Rao JG (1995) Mechanische und thermische Begleitentwicklungen der Laseranwendung bei der Spinaloskopie - eine in vitro-Studie. Med Orth Techn 115:88-90

Bone Necrosis Adjacent to the Disc After Percutaneous Laser Disc Decompression – An Analysis of Magnetic Resonance Imaging

R. Kosaka · M. Abe · T. Yonezawa · Y. Ichimura · T. Onomura

Introduction

After the first clinical report [2] of percutaneous removal of a herniated lumbar disc by a laser system, a considerable number of clinical and experimental studies on the use of laser were conducted. With the increasing application of laser in recent years, several authors have reported laser-induced osteonecrosis in the knee after arthroscopic laser surgery [3, 8]. However, there are few scientific literature references discussing the incidence of bone necrosis in patients treated with percutaneous laser disc decompression (PLDD). In the present study, we examine pre- and postoperative magnetic resonance imaging (MRI) in patients receiving PLDD, to identify the risk factors causing bone-marrow lesions adjacent to the disc.

Materials and Methods

Forty-two patients with herniated lumbar discs underwent PLDD between February 1992 and September 1997. Following PLDD, the preoperative and postoperative MR scans of the 42 discs were evaluated and compared. Age at the time of PLDD ranged from 14 to 62 years, with the average being 27.2 years. The distribution of the disc levels treated with PLDD was L4-5 in 23 patients, L5-6 in three patients and L5–S1 in 16 patients. Twenty-five patients were male and 17 were female. Laser equipment employed in this study were the Nd:YAG laser of 1064-nm wavelength in 39 patients, and endoscopically assisted laser ablation with the Ho:YAG laser of 2100 nm in three patients. The clinical background of the patients treated with either laser system was similar (Table 1). The total amount of applied energy was 1450 J on average in Nd:YAG, and 19400 J in Ho:YAG, with the use of lavage fluid for endoscopy. The clinical parameters for the laser irradiation are given in Table 2.

MRI scanning was done in all 42 patients with a 1.5-T superconductive magnet, with similar imaging sequences (Table 3). Images were obtained between one and 88 days (mean, 17 days) prior to PLDD,

Table 1. Details of patients according to laser system used

	Nd:YAG	Ho:YAG	p
Number of pts.	39	3	
Age at PLDD	26.7 ± 11.3	33.0 ± 13.2	0.281
Male:female	24:15	1:2	0.556
Disc level (L5–S1)	14 (35.9 %)	2 (66.7 %)	0.547

Table 2. Parameters of laser radiation

Nd:YAG laser, 1064 nm (under air irrigation)	
power	10–15 W (0.3-s pulse/1.7-s interval)
energy	970–2000 (avg. 1450) J/disc
fiber diameter	200 μm
Ho:YAG laser, 2100 nm (under saline irrigation)	
power	1.0–1.4 J
rate	10 Hz
energy	15.2–41.6 (avg. 19.4) kJ/disc
fiber diameter	400 μm

Table 3. MRI imaging details

Magnet	1.5-T superconductive magnet (General Electric, Signa Unit)
Coil for imaging	surface coil for spine imaging
Imaging sequence	spin echo technique T1-weighted images of sagittal and axial images pulse repetition time (TR) = 500 ms; echo time (TE) = 20 ms T2-weighted images of sagittal images TR = 2000; TE = 80 ms
Matrix elements	256 × 192
Slice thickness	6 mm

and postoperatively between one and 43 days (mean 19 days). Preoperative and postoperative signal changes in the T1- and T2-weighted sagittal images of the vertebral body marrow adjacent to the end plate were evaluated and compared. The pattern of the signal in the marrow was evaluated according to Modic's classification [7] (Table 4). The findings of MRI were compared to several clinical parameters of the patients such as age, gender, disc level, quan-

Disc Height Ratio, DHR

$$\text{DHR L3-4} = \frac{a+b}{A} \times 100$$

$$\text{DHR L4-5} = \frac{c+d}{B} \times 100$$

Disc Height Index (DHI)
$$= \text{DHR L4-5} / \text{DHR L3-4}$$

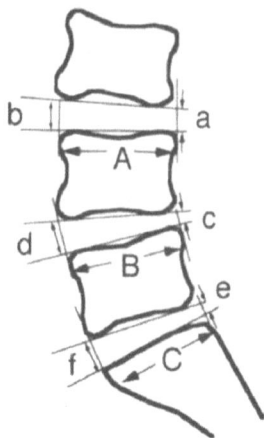

Fig. 1. Disc height ratio (DHR) and disc height index (DHI) on plain lateral x-ray

Table 4. Classification according to Modic

Type 1	Decreased signal intensity on T1-weighted images; Increased signal intensity on T2-weighted images
Type 2	Increased signal intensity on T1-weighted images; Same or slightly increased signal intensity on T2-weighted images
Type 3	Decreased signal intensity on both T1- and T2-weighted images

tum of irradiated energy (in patients treated with Nd:YAG), and the therapeutic outcome after PLDD. Preoperative disc height ratio (DHR) and the disc height index (DHI) were based on measurements obtained from plain lateral x-ray, as shown in Fig. 1, and were compared with the MRI findings. From these data, the incidence of postoperative marrow change in MRI was statistically analyzed by the chi-squared test or Fisher's exact test.

Results

On preoperative MRI, four patients showed preexisting signal changes in the marrow. According to the Modic classification system, two patients showed type 1 change, and two patients showed type 2 change. Postoperatively, three out of the four showed deterioration of signal change in the same Modic typing, while in one there was a change from Modic type 2 to type 1. In addition, two patients presented with type 1 changes, postoperatively. Overall, six patients (14.3%) demonstrated signal changes in the marrow adjacent to the irradiated disc. Modic type 1 change was identified in five of the six patients (Figs. 2–4).

No evidence of infection was detectable in blood tests in patients demonstrating the signal changes. Clinical backgrounds in six patients with signal change and 36 patients without signal change are summarized in Table 5. All six of the patients showing postoperative signal changes in the marrow were females and were relatively older. In five of the

six patients (83.3%), the changes involved the L5–S1 disc level. There was no correlation between the occurrence of marrow change and the total amount of applied energy in patients treated with Nd:YAG ($p = 0.547$). Preexisting narrowing in disc height was notably significant in the six patients with postoperative signal change in bone marrow ($p = 0.001$) when compared to the rest of the group.

Signal change in the marrow was not directly linked to the final clinical outcome in each patient ($p = 0.076$). However, it related to some transient increase in low-back pain immediately after PLDD (four of six patients, $p = 0.021$). The disc level of L5–S1 ($p = 0.044$), age older than 30 years ($p = 0.021$), preoperative narrowing in disc height on plain x-ray (DHI < 0.75; $p = 0.001$) and the preexisting signal change in the marrow close to the end plate on MRI ($p = 0.0001$) were found to be risk factors for postoperative marrow lesion.

In subsequent MRI after an average of 6.8 months following PLDD (range 3–11 months), the signal changes in three of the six patients had returned to normal. Two patients with Modic's type 1 changes changed to type 2 or 3. At the final follow-up, signal change in the marrow was identified in three of 42 patients (7.1%) (Table 6).

Table 5. Background of patients according to whether signal changed or not

	Signal change (+)	Signal change (–)	p
Number of pts.	6	36	
Male:female	0:6	25:11	0.002
Age at PLDD	37.0 ± 12.1	25.6 ± 10.6	0.029
Disc level (L5–S1)	5 (83.3%)	11 (30.6%)	0.023
Applied energy[a]	1550 ± 385	1440 ± 440	0.547
Preop. DHI[b]	0.76 ± 0.10	1.01 ± 0.16	0.001

[a] For patients treated with Nd:YAG laser.
[b] DHI: disc height index.

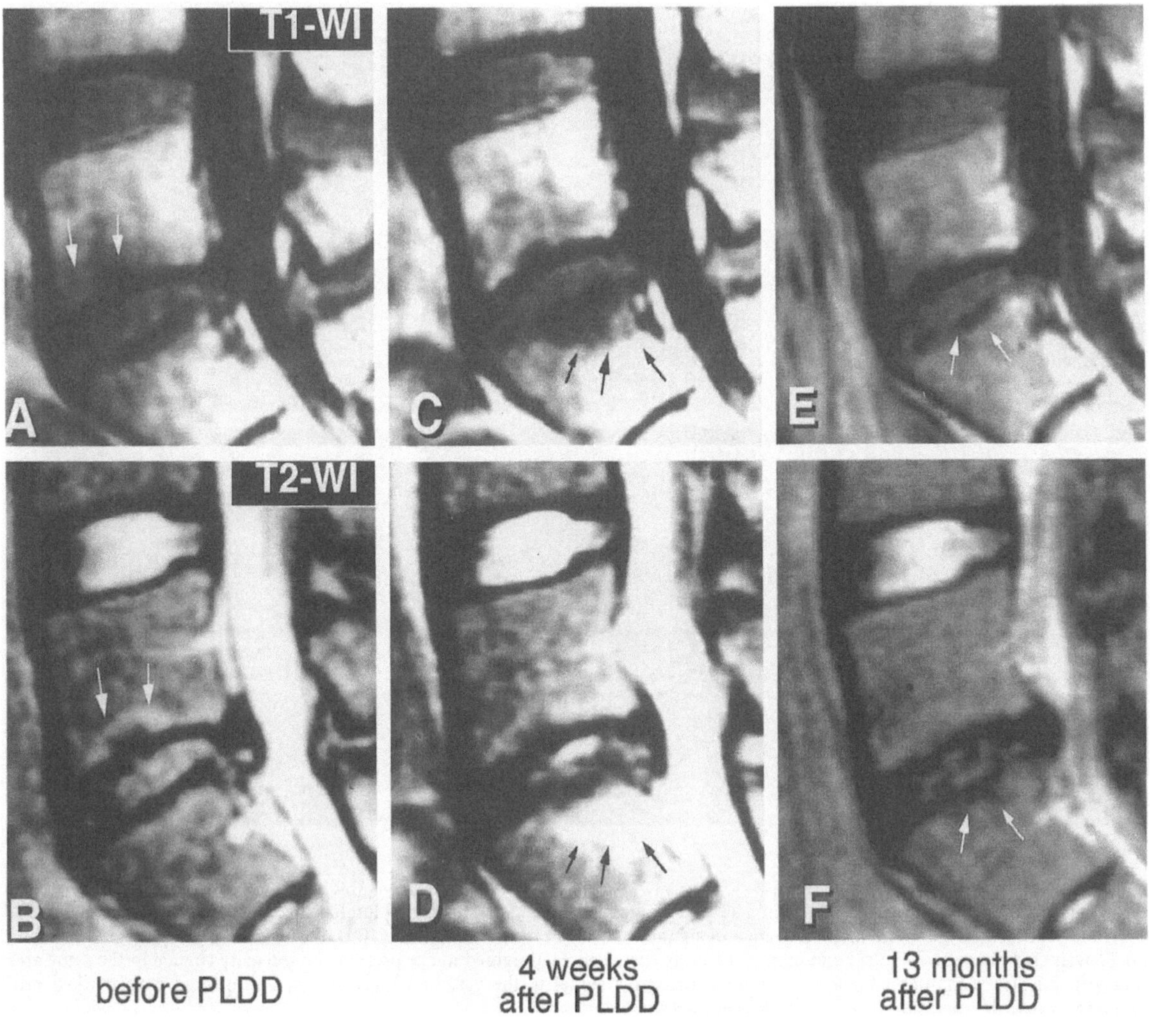

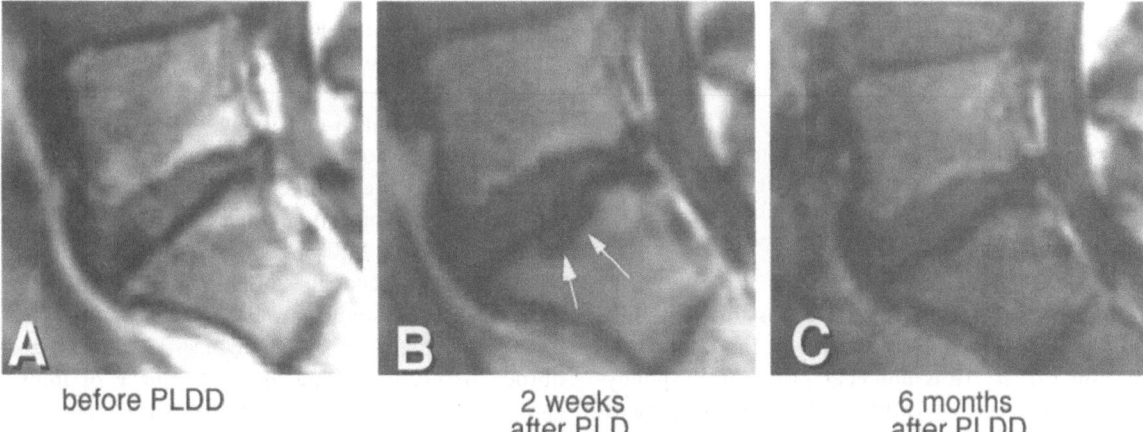

Fig. 2A–F. MR images after Nd:YAG PLDD in a 34-year-old female with L5–S1 herniated lumbar disc. **A,B.** Preoperative *T1*- and *T2*-weighted sagittal scan shows protruded disc herniation at L5–S1. Note the preexisting type-1 change at the lower end plate of L5 body (*arrows*). **C,D.** Modic type 1 change of S1 body (*arrows*). This patient complained of increased low-back pain immediately after PLDD. **E,F.** Thirteen months after PLDD. Abnormal marrow signal in the vertebral body disappeared, with a slight irregularity in the upper end plate of S1 (*arrows*). Note marked degradation of L5–S1 disc signal in *T2*-weighted image

Fig. 3A–C. MR images after Ho:YAG PLDD in a 48-year-old female with L5–S1 herniated lumbar disc. **A.** Preoperative *T1*-weighted sagittal scan shows protruded disc herniation at L5–S1. Preexisting high signal intensity at the lower end plate of L5 and the upper end plate of S1 is identified. **B.** *T1*-weighted scan obtained 2 weeks after PLDD presents an additional low-intensity area at the upper end plate of S1 body (*arrows*). **C.** Six months after PLDD. Abnormal marrow signal in the vertebral body almost disappeared

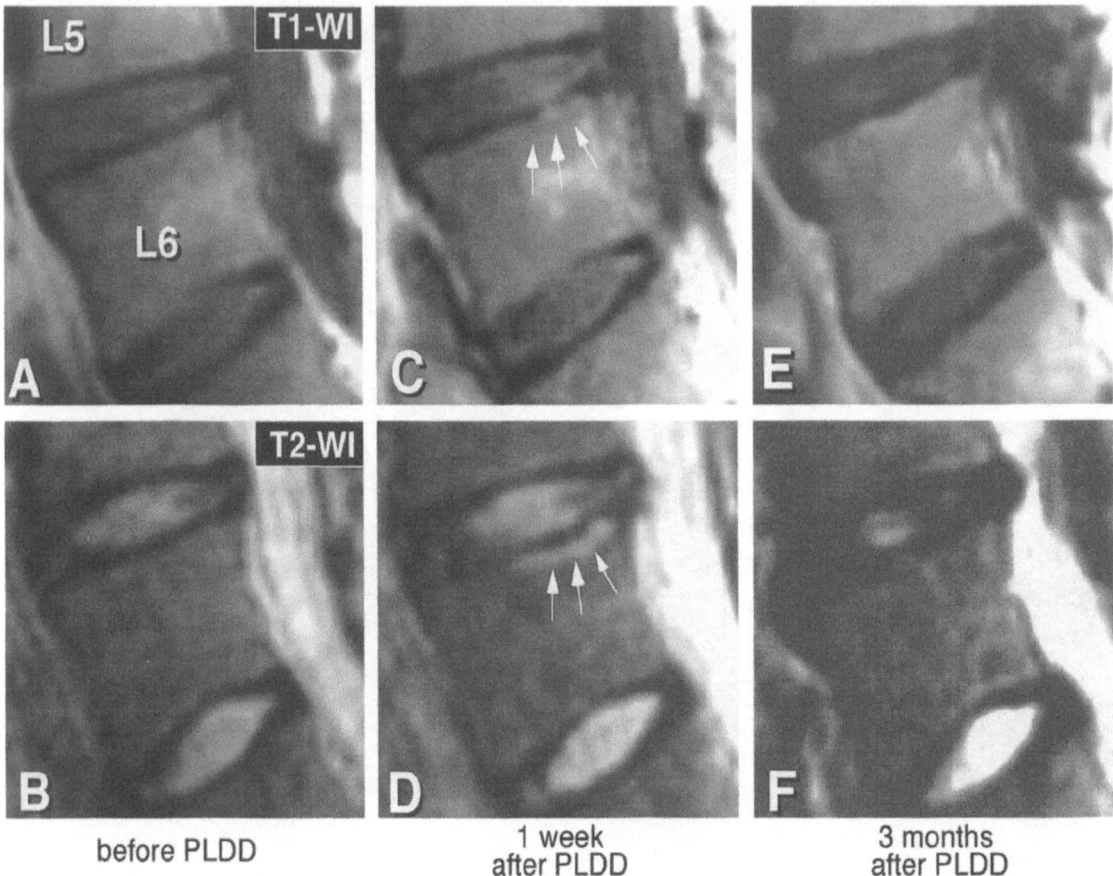

Fig. 4A–F. MR images after Ho:YAG PLDD in a 23-year-old female with L5–L6 herniated lumbar disc. **A,B.** Preoperative T1- and T2-weighted sagittal scan shows no marked change in signal intensity of the vertebral body. **C,D.** Postoperatively, high signal intensity on T2-weighted image at the upper end plate of L6 body (*arrows*); T1-weighted image presents no intensity change in the same area (*arrows*). **E,F.** Three months after PLDD. Abnormal marrow signal in the vertebral body almost disappeared with marked progression of disc degeneration in L5–6 on T2-weighted image

Table 6. Signal intensity pattern of patients whose signals of the marrow changed over time

Modic's classification	Before PLDD	After PLDD	Follow-up[a]
Type 1	2	5	0
Type 2	2	1	2
Type 3	0	0	1
Total no. of patients	4	6	3

[a] Follow-up: 3–11 months (average 6.8 months)

Discussion

Laser-induced osteonecrosis is a possible complication in arthroscopic laser surgery of the knee [3, 8]. In spine surgery, Grasshoff et al. [4] reported spondylitis-like changes on MRI in nine of 347 patients (2.6 %) treated with Nd:YAG of 1320-nm wavelength. They postulated that this occurs due to thermal damage of the vertebral body. Casper et al. reported end-plate damage, identifiable on MRI after PLDD

with Ho:YAG of 2100-nm wavelength, in 13 of 223 patients (5.8 %). Despite the large number of patients in these reports, there was scant information available on the prevention of marrow damage in PLDD. We conducted this study to find out the incidence of bone necrosis after PLDD, to identify the risk factors causing marrow lesions, and to prevent possible complications.

Change in signal intensity in the vertebral body marrow adjacent to the end plates is a common finding in MRI of degenerative disc disease. Modic et al. reported three major types of signal change in the bone marrow on MRI in degenerative disc disease [8]. Modic type 1 change is often observed in patients treated with chemonucleolysis [5] and is considered to be histologically associated with vascularized fibrous tissue, indicating an acute phase of injury and repair of the vertebral end plates [7]. Type 2 or 3 changes, on the other hand, are believed to suggest a chronic state. According to Modic, type 2 changes reflect the histological red marrow replacement by yellow (fat) marrow, and type 3 changes correspond to the relative absence of marrow, and its replacement with dense woven bone in areas of advanced sclerosis [7]. In the present study (Table 6), six of the 42 patients (14.3 %) demonstrated postoperative signal changes in the marrow. Modic type 1 change, which most likely indicated thermal damage of the tissue, was identified in five of the six patients. On the follow-up MRI's meanwhile, signal changes in three of the six patients returned to normal. These observations indicate that bone lesions identified on the MRI are mild and reversible thermal changes.

Risk factors identified in the present study appeared to be related to each other from the clinical point of view. The disc of L5–S1 is usually accompanied by disc-height narrowing, and this narrowing is often observed in the elderly patients with a degenerate disc. At L5–S1, it is usually difficult to introduce the needle-tip at the center of the disc, especially in female patients with a higher iliac crest. High-dose laser irradiated close to the end plate cause damage to the marrow, causing signal changes on the MRI scans. Marrow signal changes adjacent to the end plate are often observed on MRI scans in patients with severely degenerate discs, with longer preoperative periods of morbidity.

In the present sudy, preexisting degeneration around the disc could have played an important role in the occurrence of signal change in the marrow. Preoperative marrow changes in MRI scans may reflect the vulnerability of the disc to preceding degeneration of the end plate (Fig. 5).

In this study, we examined MRI scans of patients 2.5 weeks after treatment with PLDD. We had previously reported that the length of time after PLDD might influence the morphological changes around the disc, possibly due to the structural changes following disc decompression [6] (Fig. 6, see p. 350). In this study, postoperative MRI scans were obtained very early after PLDD, to detect the immediate effects of laser on the spine.

In this study, signal change in the marrow immediately after PLDD was more frequently observed in patients treated with Ho:YAG laser (two of three patients) than in those treated with the Nd:YAG laser (four of 39 patients), despite the similarity in patient backgrounds for the two groups. We consider this to be mainly because we are still at the beginning of the learning curve in the use of the new technique involving the Ho:YAG laser, and the mean energy values applied were relatively high even after the energy loss in the fluid medium is taken into account.

In conclusion, laser energy caused signal changes in the marrow adjacent to the irradiated disc after PLDD especially in relatively older patients, and patients with symptomatic degenerate L5–S1 discs, with decreased disc height, and/or with preexisting signal changes close to the end plate. Signal changes in the marrow were observed on the MRI scan immediately after PLDD in six of 42 patients (14.3 %). However, some of the marrow lesions on the MRI scans changed to normal between three to 11 months. To prevent marrow damage by PLDD, it is crucial to follow the correct technique of needle-tip introduction and placement, to use an appropriate laser energy setting [the same or lower than that used by the authors (Table 2)], and to exclude patients with preexisting MRI signal changes in the bone marrow when selecting patients for PLDD.

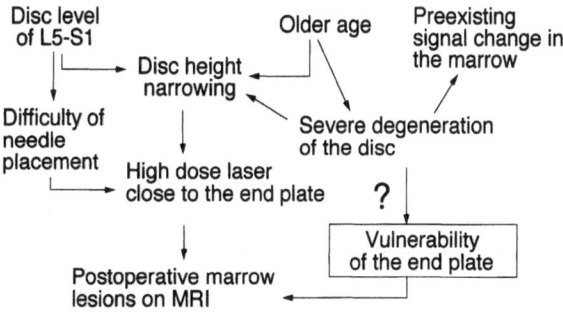

Fig. 5. Risk factors for bone marrow lesions after PLDD

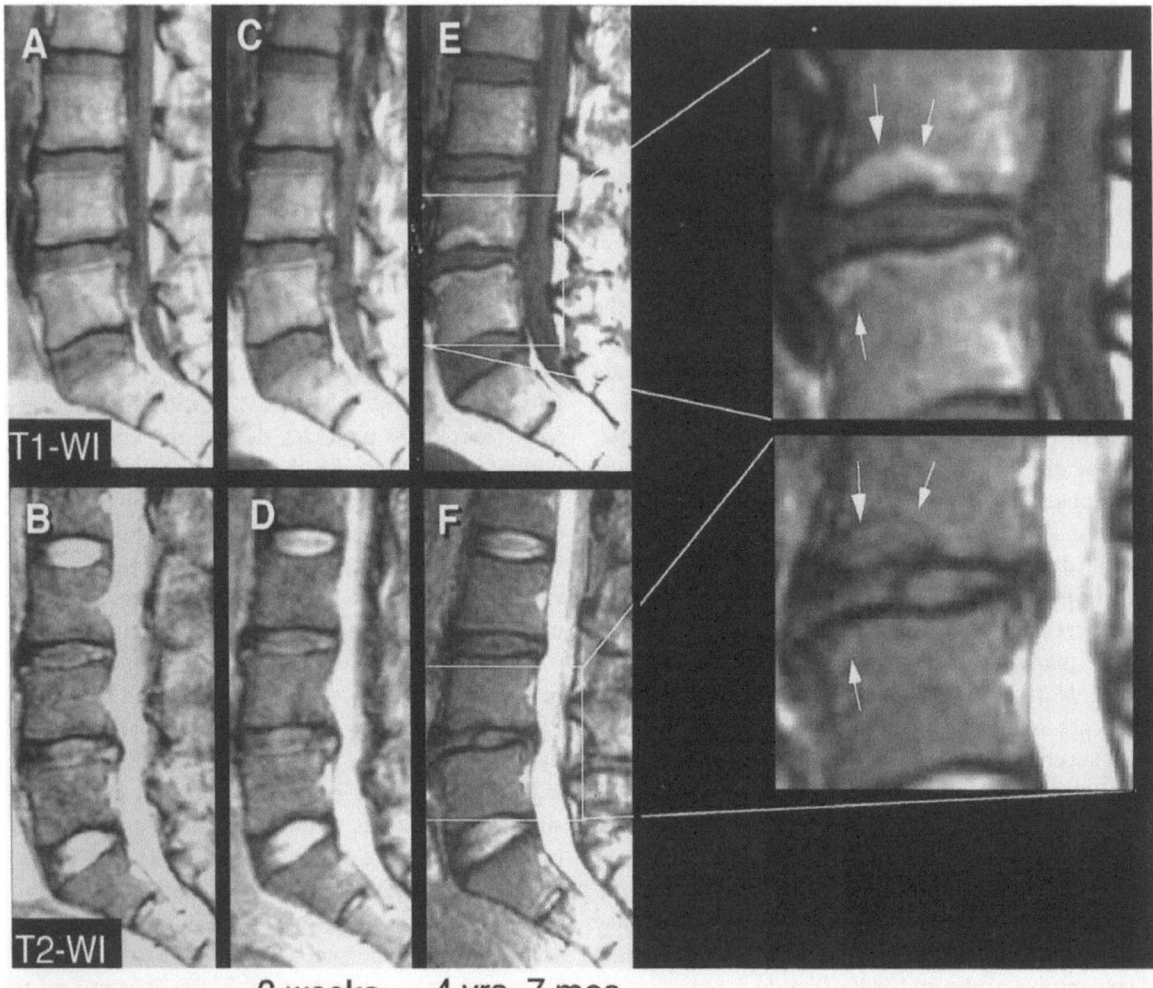

before PLDD   3 weeks
after PLDD   4 yrs. 7 mos.
after PLDD

Fig. 6A–F. MR images after Nd:YAG PLDD in a 28-year-old female with L4–L5 herniated lumbar disc. **A,B.** Preoperative T1- and T2-weighted sagittal scan shows protruded disc herniation at L4–L5. Marked change in signal intensity at the vertebral body is not observed. **C,D.** There are no changes in signal intensity in the marrow on T1 and T2 scans taken 3 weeks after PLDD. **E,F.** Four years and 7 months after PLDD. High signal intensity on T1 image and same intensity on T2, corresponding to type 2 of Modic's classification (*arrows*), accompanied with marked disc height narrowing and reduction in signal intensity inside L4–L5 disc

References

[1] Casper GD, Hartman VL, Mullins LL (1995) Percutaneous laser disc decompression with the Ho:YAG laser. J Clin Laser Med Surg 13(3):195–203
[2] Choy DSJ, Case RB, Fielding W, Hughes J, Liebler W, Ascher P (1987) Percutaneous laser nucleolysis of lumbar discs. N Engl J Med 317:771–772
[3] Garino JP, Lotke PA, Sapega AA, Reilly PJ, Esterhai JL (1995) Case report: osteonecrosis of the knee following laser-assisted arthroscopic surgery: a report of six cases. Arthroscopy 11(4):467–474
[4] Grasshoff H, Kayser R, Mahlfeld K (1996) Complication of percutaneous laser disc decompression. In: 3rd IMLAS conference, 7–10 Nov 1996, Kassel
[5] Kato F, Mimatsu K, Kawakami N, Iwata H, Miura T (1992) Serial changes observed by magnetic resonance imaging in the intervertebral disc after chemonucleolysis. A consideration of the mechanism of chemonucleolysis. Spine 17:934–939
[6] Kosaka R, Yonezawa T, Onomura T, Ichimura Y, Abe M (1996) Magnetic resonance imaging findings for more than 1 year after Nd:YAG-PLDD. In: 3rd IMLAS conference, 7–10 Nov 1996, Kassel
[7] Modic MT, Masaryk TJ, Ross JS, Carter JR (1988) Imaging of degenerative disc disease. Radiol 168:177–186
[8] Rozbruch SR, Wickiewicz TL, DiCarlo EF, Potter HG (1996) Case report: osteonecrosis of the knee following arthroscopic laser meniscectomy. Arthroscopy 12(2):245–250

Potential Operative Complications of Percutaneous Laser Discectomy

J. A. Botsford

Introduction

Percutaneous laser discectomy (PLD) is a safe and effective alternative treatment of the symptomatic contained lumbar disc herniation. Its success depends on appropriate patient selection and careful attention to operative technique. Several articles dealing with the radiology of patient selection have been published [1–3]. Others have discussed the basic surgical prinicples of the percutaneous approach to the lumbar intervertebral disc [4–7]. When rigid preoperative selection criteria are applied and careful operative technique is used, treatment failure is usually related to potentially avoidable operative complications. The number-one axiom in PLD is "laser not in disc, disc not lased."

Many of the theoretical complications of laser discectomy are the same as those described for discography. They include sterile or infectious discitis, retroperitoneal or epidural hemorrhage, and direct trauma to the nerve root or dural sac. Other complications are unique to this technique and include thermal trauma to adjacent bone and/or soft tissues, needle or trephine injury to the annulus and/or dural sac, and laser fiber or catheter vaporization, fracture or dissociation. While routine radiography, myelography and computed tomography (CT) are useful in some of these conditions, magnetic resonance imaging (MRI) is the modality of choice in evaluating patients thought to have experienced an operative complication. Nearly all of the aforementioned PLD-related complications have been seen by the author over the last several years. They will be individually presented in this review and their imaging will be discussed. This paper reviews the complications in a group of 250 consecutive patients treated with PLD.

The Postoperative Lumbar Spine – The Normal Case

In order to appreciate the "abnormal" post-PLD imaging examination, one must recognize findings that should be considered "normal." While routine radiography, myelography and CT have been used in the past, contrast-enhanced MR imaging is the preferred method of imaging the postoperative lumbar spine [8]. It is clearly superior to all other imaging modalities in patients with recurrent radicular symptoms or failed back syndrome [9, 10]. The MRI appearance of recurrent disc herniation and epidural scar has been thoroughly reviewed elsewhere [11–12]. Little attention has been paid to the postoperative appearance of the lumbar herniated nucleus pulposis (HNP) successfully treated by surgery. Theoretically, the herniating disc signal material seen on cross-sectional imaging (CT or MRI) should be reduced in volume by open discectomy. However, recent investigations of now asymptomatic open surgical patients demonstrated the presence of a persistent anterior epidural mass on MRI at the site of the original HNP despite the complete relief of leg pain [13, 14]. This intermediate signal intensity tissue was present in all patients imaged and was contiguous with the disc space, mimicking a recurrent disc. The persistence of a residual mass despite relief of symptoms may support the work of others who believe it is disc pressure not mass effect that induces clinical symptoms [15, 16]. In the majority of patients, this nondiscal residual epidural tissue resolved over a six-month period as part of an orderly regression of other imaging abnormalities.

A comprehensive discussion of the MR appearance of the patient successfully treated by PLD has been published elsewhere [7]. This report and the findings seen in additional asymptomatic PLD-treated patients recently imaged at the Deaconess Hospital have recently been reviewed. Based on this information, the expected postoperative appearance of the treated central nucleus, the contained herniated fragment, and the peridiscal bone and soft tissues can now be described.

The Treated Nucleus

To observe the MR changes in spine following the application of laser energy, MR imaging of the cadaveric lumbar spine was performed at the Deaconess

Hospital both before and after laser-energy application using Nd:YAG and Ho:YAG wavelengths. Both produced a distinctive MR defect in the cadaveric nucleus after delivery of 1000 J, which corresponds to the laser track upon histologic examination of the treated disc. There was little change in the size of the defect when the delivered energy was increased beyond 1800 J.

However, no similar MR defect has yet been identified in the central nucleus of the PLD-treated patient even when imaged within one hour of the therapy. No successfully treated PLD patient has demonstrated a significant focal or generalized change in the $T1$ signal within the nucleus. No abnormal $T1$ nuclear enhancement has been noted after Gd-DTPA administration, although some have shown a thin line of enhancement along the peripheral aspect of the disc just adjacent to the bony endplates, similar to that reported in the open discectomy patient [14]. A minority of patients have shown a uniform decrease in $T2/T2*$ signal throughout the entire disc within two weeks of PLD, possibly related to an overall decrease in intradiscal water content.

The Herniated Fragment

No characteristic or consistent changes could be identified in the $T1$ or $T2/T2*$ signal within the herniated fragment in any of the PLD-treated patients even where there was complete resolution of symptoms. However, unlike in surgical patients undergoing open procedures, a definite decrease in the epidural mass of the herniating fragment has been identified in the MR image of the many successfully treated PLD patients. The majority showed at least a 50 % reduction in the volume of posteriorly projecting disc material, while a few showed complete resolution. Only a small minority have shown no definite MRI change in the size of the fragment or the degree of dural-sac compression following PLD, despite symptomatic improvement.

Peridiscal Bone and Soft Tissues

Although little change occurs within the disc itself, MR bone marrow signal alterations have been identified adjacent to the vertebral endplates in the majority of patients. Bands of slightly decreased $T1$ and increased $T2/T2*$ signals can be seen in the vertebral bodies above and below the treated interspace for up to three months after intradiscal therapy. This is similar to the findings in open discectomy patients. There appears to be no consistent relationship between the width of this stripe and the type of laser wavelength or system employed or the amount of energy delivered to the disc. There may be mild $T1$ enhancement of this stripe with Gd-DTPA administration. Unlike the diffuse enhancement of the bone, disc and epidural structures in patients with discitis, this enhancement is completely confined to the subendplate vertebral marrow. Successfully treated asymptomatic patients may show the same marrow-signal changes as those whose radiculopathy persists or even those who develop symptomatic thermal injury, to be discussed later.

No consistent pattern of MR signal alteration within the soft tissues of the successfully treated PLD patient has yet been identified. None of the patients have shown any epidural soft tissue signal changes unless they presented with symptoms of a sterile or infectious postoperative discitis or a new/recurrent disc herniation. Paravertebral or posterior soft-tissue signal alterations were observed when there was suspected direct thermal trauma or hemorrhage.

The Postoperative Lumber Spine – The Complications

Assuming careful patient selection, treatment failure in percutaneous laser discectomy may be related to an operative complication. These complications are avoidable by strict adherence to proper operative techniques. Axiom number two in PLD is "laser not in disc, laser causes big trouble." The complications reviewed herein are based on the cumulative experienced gained in performing over 250 PLD procedures at the Deaconess Hospital since 1992.

For ease of discussion, the theoretical complications of PLD are arbitrarily divided into a generic and a specific group. "Generic" complications can occur whenever a disc space is entered. These are the same as those described for lumbar discography [17, 18]. They include sterile or infective discitis, retroperitoneal or epidural hemorrhage, and direct needle trauma to the nerve root or dural sac. "Specific" complications unique to PLD include thermal trauma to adjacent bone and soft tissues, thermal and/or trephine injury to the annulus or dural sac, and laser fiber or catheter vaporization, fracture or dissociation. Many of these procedural complications result in similar clinical symptoms and require radiologic imaging for the correct diagnosis to be established. While both routine radiography, myelography and CT are useful in some of these conditions, MR is the primary tool in evaluating patients thought to have experienced PLD-procedure complications. All of the PLD generic and specific complications listed above have been experienced and imaged at the Deaconess Hospital.

Discitis: Sterile or Infective

Discitis in the PLD patient may be sterile or infectious. Sterile discitis is probably related to an inflammatory response to the thermal trauma that normally accompanies laser vaporization. Pyogenic discitis is a bacterial infection most likely related to operative contamination. The patient with postoperative discitis classically presents with new back pain and fever. However, the pain pattern may be confusing and the fever low-grade or absent. The erythrocyte sedimentation rate (ESR) is usually normal with thermal injury and generally elevated with true infection. Fluoroscopic- or CT-guided thin-needle disc aspiration for bacterial culture is mandatory to separate aseptic from pyogenic discitis.

So far there have been five cases of presumed discitis in over 250 PLD-treated patients at the Deaconess hospital (2.0%). Four of these cases were culture-negative (sterile) and occurred in patients to whom relatively high levels of energy were delivered (1800 J), supporting a heat-related reaction. One case was culture-positive (< 0.5%), presumably from direct operative contamination.

MRI is the procedure of choice to diagnose postoperative sterile or infectious discitis. The MR findings in discitis are characteristic of this process and have been described thoroughly elsewhere [19]. They are similar in both the sterile and pyogenic forms of inflammation. However, the sterile-discitis patients all had less severe findings and all changes completely resolved by three months after the procedure. The single infectious discitis patient had destructive alterations which persist to this day.

Hemorrhage: Retroperitoneal/Paraspinal and Epidural

Hemorrhage into the retroperitoneal or paraspinal musculature is usually the result of aggressive puncture with larger-caliber laser systems. It is more frequent in patients with diminished muscle tone or mass and in patients with preexistent bleeding disorders. The typical patient presents with deep or superficial muscle pain and decreasing hematocrit. A palpable paraspinal hematoma mass may be present. The process is usually self-limiting. Epidural bleeding is rare, but unpredictable. If uncontrolled, it can produce a neurologic deficit from cauda equina syndrome.

Although frequently cited as a complication in the discography literature [17], no documented case of abnormal bleeding has occurred in my practice in literally thousands of disc-entry procedures for discography and PLD. However, other laser physicians using larger-caliber systems have seen four cases from this study group (< 2.0%). Careful attention to technique, constant monitoring of needle position and the use of smaller-caliber needles appear to be effective in preventing hemorrhagic complications.

Both MR and CT are equally reliable examinations for the diagnosis of retroperitonal or paraspinal hemorrhage. While MR may be more sensitive for the diagnosis of epidural bleeding [20], as a general rule, hematoma is usually better appreciated on CT and is my personal preferece for imaging when acute bleeding is suspected. The CT findings are diagnostic and consist of a high-density mass expanding and distorting normal anatomy in the involved area.

Needle Trauma of Nerve Root and Dural Sac

Direct nerve-root trauma usually results in new radicular symptoms including paresthesia. It is most likely to occur in the oversedated patient whose response to root irritation is diminished. Although usually self-limiting, injury can theoretically be permanent. Two cases have been seen (< 1.0%), both in patients who were heavily sedated during the PLD procedure.

Dural-sac laceration results in a cerebrospinal fluid leak and a "spinal headache." It occurs if the puncture needle, trephine or laser system is directed too posteriorly. It too may be self-limiting, but a dural fat patch may be necessary to close a persistent leak. A blood patch may be used to stop bleeding. A single case of dural injury occurred (< 0.5%) from a too vertical approach, which traversed the edge of the dural sac.

Imaging plays a lesser role when direct nerve-root trauma is suspected. Water-soluble CT myeolgraphy can be used to demonstrate a CSF leak from an inadvertent dural-sac puncture. Both types of injury can be avoided by using a cautious, constantly monitored approach to the interspace and adjusting needle position when new radicular and/or dermatomal pain is elicited.

Thermal Trauma of Vertebral Body and Paraspinal/Epidural Soft Tissues

Direct thermal trauma to an adjacent vertebral endplate and the underlying bone marrow has been identified in eight patients (< 4.0%) and has been the most common complication specific to PLD. With two exceptions, it has been confined to patients in whom a side-firing laser system was used. The pain pattern experienced in patients with vertebral thermal injury is characteristic. Intense central-low back pain unrelieved by antiinflammatory agents is typical of this. Only high-dose steroids have shown to produce a significant improvement in the clinical symptoms, presumably caused by iatrogenic thermal bone injury.

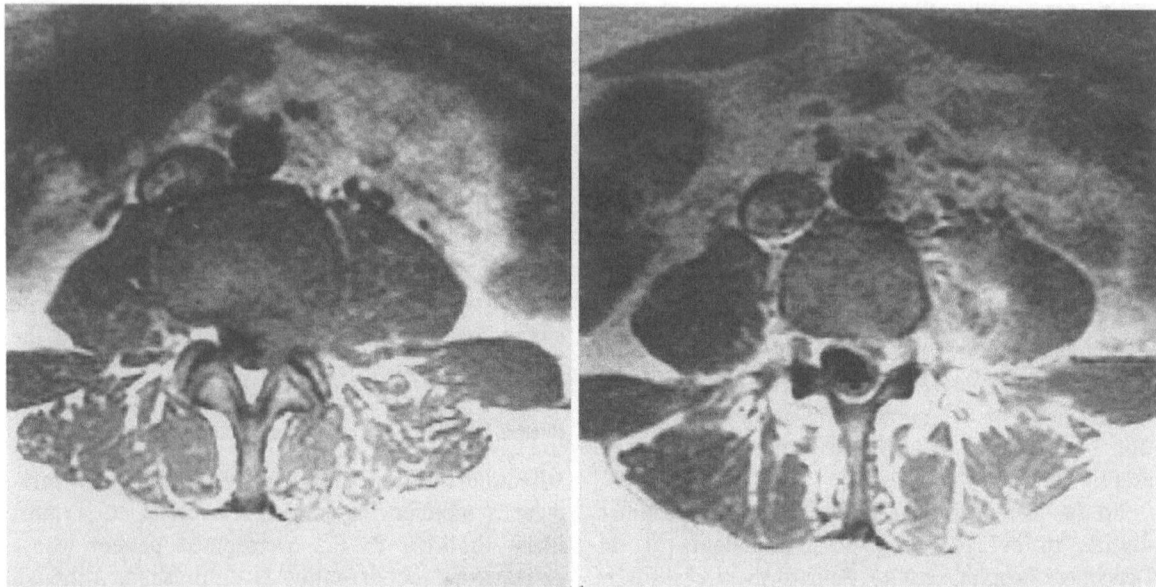

Fig. 1. Noncontrast (*left*) and contrast-enhanced (*right*) MRI demonstrates marked enhancement of injured epidural and paraspinal soft tissues along entry tract after laser thermal trauma

Thermal injury to the soft tissues or paraspinal muscles has been seen in four patients (< 2.0%) and again has been more frequent in those treated with a multistep system. It is the result of direct exposure to laser in the affected area. It occurred from unrecognized malpositioning of the laser system and after sheath dislodgment away from the annulus during laser-catheter removal and reinsertion. These iatrogenic soft-tissue laser injuries could be theoretically avoided if imaging guidelines previously referred to were strictly followed. One additional patient experienced heat-related soft tissue damage from inadvertent needle heating, an injury unpreventable by imaging but unlikely if the patient response is monitored during surgery.

Direct vertebral thermal injury presents a characteristic MR appearance. There is a well defined, usually arcuate area of decreased $T1$ and increased $T2$ signal within the subendplate marrow adjacent to the point of injury. The abnormality occurs directly beneath a sharply circumscribed defect in the overlying bony cortex. The margins of the semilunar signal alteration undergo intense $T1$ enhancement upon intravenous Gd-DTPA administration. Retrospective review of the intraoperative spot films on these patients has consistently shown inappropriate angulation of the laser cannula toward the injured endplates. The importance of disc entry directly parallel to the interspace to avoid this preventable complication cannot be emphasized enough.

Direct soft-tissue injury also shows a relatively characteristic MR appearance. There is a loss of normal $T1$ soft tissue/fat planes and increased $T2/T2^*$

signal in the damaged region, probably secondary to reactive edema. $T1$ contrast enhancement is dramatic and parallels the laser entry tract (Fig. 1). This enhancement is seen for at least six weeks in the injured tissues and may theoretically persist even longer [8].

Trephine/Cannula Laceration of Annulus Fibrosis and Dural Sac

Annular or dural-sac laceration occurs as the result of large-bore injury to these usually durable soft-tissue structures. Annular laceration results in leakage of soft nuclear material along the puncture, irritating the adjacent tissues including the exiting root. The injured patients usually present with new pain in a radicular distribution corresponding to the level and side of entry. The symptoms usually resolve but can be severe. It has been documented in two patients (< 1.0%). Dural-sac laceration results in a CSF leak, sometimes lasting longer than with needle injury, with protracted clinical symptoms. It may require surgical intervention to arrest the leak.

Although MR can suggest the diagnosis, annular tear can best be diagnosed by CT discography (Fig. 2). Post-PLD dural-sac laceration and CSF leak can best be identified with CT myelography.

Laser Fiber/Catheter – Vaporization and Fracture/Dissociation

Nd:YAG laser fiber vaporization with foreshortening results in abnormal needle heating. Recently this has been clinically and visually recognized, but this

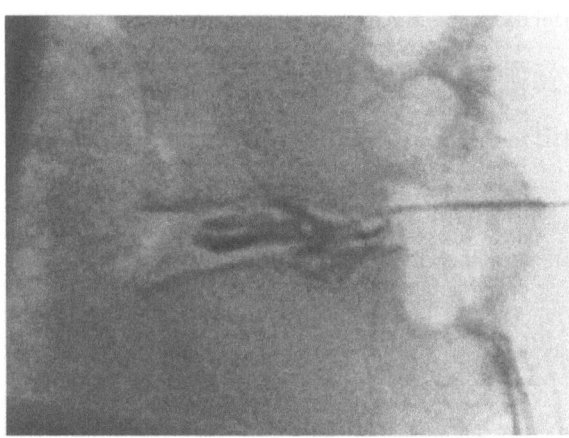

Fig. 2. Lateral spot film from discogram demonstrating contrast filling a large posterolateral defect in the annulus following PLD

cannot be "seen" or recognized fluoroscopically. It results in a direct heat injury to the tissues surrounding the guiding needle. The patient characteristically presents with intense, immediate local pain after the application of a laser-energy pulse. Removal and visual inspection of the laser fiber will reveal tip charring and fiber foreshortening. Intermittent direct inspection of fiber length after each application of 200 J should be employed to prevent the soft-tissue thermal injury that could result with a "hot" needle or guiding sheath.

Seventeen cases of Nd:YAG fiber foreshortening have been documented (< 8.0 %), but only four resulted in clinical symptoms. This complication may be of little concern in the future, as the manufacturer has recently switched to a fiber with a significantly higher melting point (Personal communication, M Johnson, Percudisc).

Laser catheter tip dissociation from "meltdown" has also been identified in two patients (< 1.0 %) with a multistep system. This occurs most likely from inadequate fluid cooling from inflow or outflow obstruction. The presence of a fractured or dissociated catheter tip may well be clinically asymptomatic, but this may have profound medico-legal implications. Although a laser tip left in the disc space is an FDA-approved biocompatible device (personal communication, Coherent Laser Systems), its long-term effect on the nucleus is unknown. Routine

radiography or fluoroscopic spot films are adequate to demonstrate the radiopaque portion of the separated catheter fragment, implying that the majority of the catheter tip is radiolucent.

Other Complications

Although not a "normal" postoperative finding, several successfully treated PLD patients in the above group experienced recurrent symptoms more than three but less than six months after their initial improvement. Two developed a transligamentous disc extrusion, both with new contralateral symptoms at the treated level, which improved following open laminotomy and discectomy. Two more developed a new symptomatic contained herniation on CT discography at a different untreated level and improved following PLD. Finally, two additional patients developed a recurrent symptomatic contained herniation at the same level and improved following repeat PLD.

Conclusion

The complication rate for PLD at the Deaconess Hospital is based on 250 cases and is summarized and presented in Table 1. The most common complication, laser-fiber foreshortening, has been essentially eliminated by recognizing the problem and improving the equipment. Secondly, the second and third most common complications, thermal vertebral and soft-tissue injury, have been reduced by more meticulous attention to operative detail and reduced total energy delivery. Finally, hemorrhagic events have been reduced by utilizing a slower, more delicate approach to disc entry and cannula introduction.

Diagnostic radiology plays a major but previously underemphasized role in the diagnosis and treatment of the PLD patient. A clear understanding of fundamental radiologic principles combined with state of the art intraoperative imaging will result in rapid accurate positioning of the laser of choice within the central nucleus, improving the chances for symptomatic improvement by PLD. When treatment is ineffective or new clinical symptoms develop, diagnostic imaging can accurately diagnose the postoperative complication usually responsible for failure.

Table 1. Complication rate for PLD at the Deaconess Hospital, based on 250 cases

Discitis:	Thermal Trauma:	Hemorrhage:
Sterile < 2.0 %	Vertebral body < 4.0 %	Intramuscular < 2.0 %
Infective < 0.5 %	Soft tissues < 2.0 %	Epidural 0.0 %
Trephine/cannula laceration:	Needle trauma:	Laser fiber/catheter:
Annulus < 1.0 %	Nerve root < 1.0 %	Vaporization < 8.0 %
Dural sac < 0.5 %	Dural sac < 0.5 %	Dissociation < 1.0 %

References

[1] Botsford JA (1993) Radiological considerations: percutaneous laser disc decompression. J Clin Laser Med Surg 11(5):229–231

[2] Botsford JA (1994) Radiological consideration: patient selection for percutaneous laser disc decompression. J Clin Laser Med Surg 12(5):255–259

[3] Botsford JA (1994) CT discography: prognostic value in patient selection for percutaneous laser disc decompression (PLDD). In: 94th annual meeting of the American Roentgen Ray Society (ARRS), New Orleans, LA, April 2 and 29, 1994; Abstract no 265

[4] Choy DSJ, Ascher PW, Saddekni S, Alkaltis D, Liebler M, Hughes J, Diwan S, Altman P (1992) Percutaneous laser disc decompression. Spine 17:949–956

[5] Hijikata S, Yamagishi M, Nakayama T, Oomori K (1975) Percutaneous discectomy: a new treatment for lumbar disc herniation. J Toden Hosp 5:5–13

[6] Choy DSJ (1994) The problem of the L5–S1 disc solved by needle entry with an extrathecal approach. J Clin Laser Med Surg 12(6):321–324

[7] Botsford JA (1995) The role of radiology in percutaneous laser disc decompression. Clin Laser Med Surg 13(3):173–186

[8] Hueftle MG, Modic MT, Ross JS, Masaryk TJ, Carter JR, Wilbur G, Bohlman H (1988) Lumbar spine: postoperative MR imaging with Gd-DTPA. Radiology 167:817–824

[9] Ross JS, Delamarter R, Hueftle MG, Masaryk TJ, Alkawa M, Carter JR, VanDyke C, Modic MT (1989) Gadolinium-DTPA enhanced MR imaging of the postoperative lumbar spine: time course and mechanism of enhancement. AJNR 10:37–46

[10] Georgy BA, Hesselink JR (1992) Gadolinium-enhanced fat suppression MR imaging of the postoperative back. In: 78th scientific assembly and meeting of the Radiological Society of North Amerikca (RSNA), Chicago, Illinois, November 29 to December 4, 1992; Abstract no 303

[11] Soropoulos S, Chafetz NI, Lang P, Winkler M, Morris JM, Weinstein PR, Genant HK (1989) Differentiation between postoperative scar and recurrent disc herniation: prospective comparison of MR, CT, and contrast enhanced VCT. AJNR 10:639–643

[12] Bundschuh CV, Modic MT, Ross JS, Masaryk TJ, Bohiman H (1988) Epidural fibrosis and recurrent disc herniation in the lumbar spine: MR imaging assessment. AJNR 9:169–178

[13] Boden SD, Davis DO, Dina TS, Parker CP, O'Malley S, Sunner JL, Wiesel SW (1992) Contrast enhanced MR imaging performed after successful lumbar disc surgery: prospective study. Radiology 182:59–64

[14] Dina TS, Boden SD, David DO (1995) Lumbar spine after surgery for herniated disc: imaging findings in the early postoperative period. AJR 164:665–671

[15] Brock M, Gorge H, Curio G (1984) Intradiscal pressure volume response: A methodological contribution to chemonucleolysis. J Neurosurg 60:1029–1032

[16] Choy DSJ, Altman P (1993) Fall of intradiscal pressure with laser ablation. Spine: State of the art reviews 7(1):23–29

[17] Bernard TN (1990) Lumbar discography followed by computed tomography. Spine 15:690–707

[18] Collis JS Jr, Gardner WJ (1962) Lumbar discography: an analysis of one thousand cases: J Neurosurg 19:452–461

[19] Boden SD, David DO, Dina TS, Sunner JL, Wiesel SW (1992) Postoperative discitis: distinguishing early MR imaging findings from normal postoperative disc-space changes. Radiology 184:767–771

[20] Gundry CR, Heithoff KB (1993) Epidural hematoma of the lumbar spine: 18 surgically confirmed cases. Radiology 187:427–431

Subject Index